Iron
and
Human Disease

Edited by

Randall B. Lauffer

NMR Center
Massachusetts General Hospital
and
Harvard Medical School
Boston, Massachusetts

CRC Press
Boca Raton   Ann Arbor   London   Tokyo

Library of Congress Cataloging-in-Publication Data

Iron and human diseases / editor, Randall B. Lauffer.
    p.   cm.
    Includes bibliographical references and index.
    ISBN 0-8493-6779-4
    1. Iron--Metabolism--Disorders.   2. Iron in the body.   3. Iron-
-Pathophysiology.   4. Iron--Toxicology.   I. Lauffer, Randall Byron,
1957-   .
    [DNLM: 1. Disease--etiology.   2. Iron--metabolism.   QV 183 I701]
RC632.I7I74   1992
616.3'99--dc20
DNLM/DLC
for Library of Congress   92-7846
                                                 CIP

© 1992 by CRC Press, Inc.

International Standard Book Number 0-8493-6779-4

Library of Congress Card Number 92-7846

Printed in the United States of America 1 2 3 4 5 6 7 8 9 0

Printed on acid-free paper

Contents

PART IV: ROLES FOR IRON IN CARDIOVASCULAR DISEASE

PART V: ROLES FOR IRON IN OTHER COMMON DISEASES

PART VI: IMPLICATIONS FOR PREVENTION AND THERAPY

The Editor

Randall B. Lauffer, Ph.D., is Assistant Professor of Radiology at Massachusetts General Hospital and Harvard Medical School in Boston.

He graduated in 1979 from Wake Forest University with a B.S. degree in chemistry (magna cum laude) and obtained his Ph.D. degree in inorganic chemistry from Cornell University in 1983.

Dr. Lauffer was a National Institutes of Health Postdoctoral Fellow from 1984 to 1986 and an NIH New Investigator from 1986 to 1990 in the Department of Radiology at Massachusetts General Hospital, where he served as Director of the NMR Contrast Media Laboratory. He was appointed Assistant Professor at Harvard Medical School in 1987 and is also a member of the American Chemical Society and the Society for Magnetic Resonance in Medicine.

Dr. Lauffer has authored more than 40 publications and given 30 invited presentations in the areas of NMR studies of iron-containing oxidase enzymes and model complexes, the design and testing of paramagnetic NMR imaging contrast agents, and the role of iron in human health and nutrition. He is the author of *Iron Balance* (St. Martin's Press, 1991), an account of the dangers of high iron levels written for the lay reader.

Dr. Lauffer is also the founder, Chairman, and Chief Executive Officer of Metasyn, Inc. (Cambridge, Mass.), a pharmaceutical development company focused on the development of NMR imaging contrast agents and therapeutic strategies based on bioinorganic chemistry.

Contributors

D. BEN-SHACHAR, Department of Pharmacology, Technion-Bruce Rappaport Faculty of Medicine, Haifa, Israel

DAVID R. BLAKE, Inflammation Group, London Hospital Medical College, London, England

JEREMY H. BROCK, Department of Immunology, Western Infirmary, Glasgow, Scotland

ULF BRUNK, Department of Pathology II, University Hospital, University of Linköping, Linköping, Sweden

ARTHUR I. CEDERBAUM, Department of Biochemistry, Mt. Sinai School of Medicine, New York, New York

JAMES R. CONNOR, Department of Neuroscience and Anatomy, M. S. Hershey Medical Center, Penn State University, Hershey, Pennsylvania

ROBERT R. CRICHTON, Unité de Biochimie, Université Catholique de Louvain, Louvain-la-Neuve, Belgium

PHILIP E. HALLAWAY, Biomedical Frontiers, Inc., Minneapolis, Minnesota

JUNE W. HALLIDAY, University of Queensland and Queensland Institute of Medical Research, Herston, Brisbane, Australia

BARRY HALLIWELL, Pulmonary Medicine, UC Davis Medical Center, Sacramento, California

BO E. HEDLUND, Biomedical Frontiers, Inc., Minneapolis, Minnesota

CHARLES B. JONES, Department of Pathology II, University of Linköping, Linköping, Sweden

RANDALL B. LAUFFER, NMR Center, Massachusetts General Hospital and Harvard Medical School, Boston, Massachusetts

BARBARA A. LEGGETT, Department of Gastroenterology, Royal Brisbane Hospital, Herston, Brisbane, Queensland, Australia

MASSOUD R. MARZABADI, Department of Pathology II, University of Linköping, Linköping, Sweden

JOE M. McCORD, Webb-Waring Lung Institute, University of Colorado, Denver, Colorado

CHRISTOPHER MORRIS, Bone and Joint Research Unit, London Hospital Medical College, London, England

SAMPATH PARTHASARATHY, Department of Medicine, University of California, San Diego; La Jolla, California

LAWRIE W. POWELL, University of Queensland and Queensland Institute of Medical Research, Herston, Brisbane, Australia

JOHN E. REPINE, Department of Medicine, Webb-Waring Lung Institute, Denver, Colorado

JACK T. ROGERS, Department of Hematology, Brigham & Women's Hospital, Boston, Massachusetts

RICHARD STEVENS, Life Sciences Center, Pacific Northwest Laboratory, Richland, Washington

JEROME L. SULLIVAN, Laboratory Service, VA Medical Center, Charleston, South Carolina

LANCE S. TERADA, Department of Medicine, Webb-Waring Lung Institute, Denver, Colorado

Charles W. TRENAM, Bone and Joint Research Unit, London Hospital Medical College, London, England

ROBERTA J. WARD, Clinical Biochemistry, King's College Medical School, London, England

EUGENE D. WEINBERG, Department of Biology, Indiana University, Bloomington, Indiana

IRENE R. WILLINGHAM, Department of Neurosurgery, University of Colorado Health Sciences Center, Denver, Colorado

PAUL G. WINYARD, Inflammation Research Group, London Hospital Medical College, London, England

MOUSSA B. H. YOUDIM, Department of Pharmacology, Technion-Bruce Rappaport Faculty of Medicine, Haifa, Israel

JAY L. ZWEIER, Department of Medicine, Johns Hopkins School of Medicine, Francis Scott Key Medical Center, Baltimore, Maryland

Preface

The accumulation of evidence implicating iron in the pathophysiology of several common diseases prompted the need for this book. An assortment of literature and ideas on the subject has existed for some time without a common home, a home with a hard cover. The ideas are scattered throughout the biomedical world — from molecular biology and biochemistry to cell biology to medicine — requiring someone with an equally scattered set of interests to pull them together into a useful whole. One hopes that this book will encourage a re-examination of the role of iron in human health and nutrition.

This is also a good time to review some of the exciting new aspects of iron biochemistry, its regulation *in vivo*, and its pivotal role in oxidative stress. Many new findings evoke the naturalist's awe in their beauty and efficiency; others make us wonder whether there are not some serious oversights inherent in the system. On the one hand, we see that nature provided the cell with efficient translational mechanisms for the regulation of ferritin and transferrin receptor synthesis in response to changes in iron availability. Similar mechanisms are at work in restricting iron availability during the acute phase response. On the other hand, we see the considerable mischief caused by mixing iron and oxygen in inopportune ways, and we have to wonder whether nature has simply done the best it can in controlling some tough and often uncooperative starting materials. It is also time to ask whether the high iron stores in Western people are normal and healthy and whether the lack of a regulated iron excretion mechanism poses a threat to well-fed or, perhaps, over-fed, populations.

Iron and Human Disease, like most scientific books today, represents the collective effort of many scientists and physicians from many different disciplines. The book is essentially a meeting ground for their excellent contributions and provocative ideas. My greatest thanks go out to them for allowing me the privilege of acting as their secretary and coach.

I also thank Phil Aisen, Jeremy Brock, June Halliday, and Gene Weinberg for their early suggestions on the book, including its authors and title.

RANDALL B. LAUFFER

Foreword

The present book edited by Randall Lauffer is timely because nutritional problems in industrial countries today arise from overnutrition rather than from undernutrition. This is true not only for energy, saturated fat, and omega-3 fatty acids, but also for iron. The severe degrees of iron deficiency described by Jan Waldenström in 1946 are now almost unknown. The incidence of iron deficiency (normal hemoglobin, increased iron binding capacity and depleted iron stores) has decreased greatly. It was 25% in women in the fertile age groups in 1966, and only 5% in 1975 in Sweden. At that time, 16 to 25% of women in the same age groups had signs of latent iron deficiency.[1]

Since then, expanding health care facilities in industrialized countries, including pregnancy and well-baby clinics, industrial medicine, and regular checkups, have facilitated early diagnosis of anemia and iron deficiency. Early diagnosis is thus simple and common, and treatment with iron supplements easy.

This suggests that the benefits of preventive measures have decreased with time and that there is a need for the present book dealing with the cost of preventive measures in terms of damage to biomolecules and lysosomes, reduced defense against microbial and neoplastic invasion, and oxidative damage to lipids and synovial membranes. However, there are also other problems resulting from overnutrition with iron:

1. The overprescribing of iron tablets in Sweden, where only 43% of those with prescriptions had confirmable deficiency,[2] may lead to premature manifestations of porphyria cutanea tarda or hemochromatosis. The carrier rate of the autosomal recessive gene for hemochromatosis has been described in 10 to 16% of Danes.[3]
2. Prescribing iron tablets to elderly patients with iron deficiency without identifying its cause can mask anemia caused by bleeding gastrointestinal tumors and delay their diagnosis.
3. The prevalence of tablets containing unphysiologically large amounts of ionizable iron contributes to the incidence (20,000 cases/year in the U.S.[3]) of sometimes lethal iron poisoning in children.

Preventive measures directed at entire populations in industrialized countries thus need to be reconsidered. Perhaps we should switch toward targeted prevention in relatively few children, women in the fertile age groups, and blood donors. It is also possible that relatively unphysiological, sometimes toxic, several-hundred-milligram doses of ionizable iron could be replaced by heme-iron, which cannot be absorbed in excessive amounts and which does not give rise to free radicals in the intestinal lumen. At present it is a waste product in the form of cattle hemoglobin.[4]

In developing countries, iron deficiency anemia is still a major problem. Globally, 600 million people suffer from hemoglobinopathies, g-6PD deficiency, and iron deficiency anemias.

Dr. Lauffer and CRC Press are to be congratulated for a necessary and timely book which discusses and debates the most important parts of recent information concerning iron as a risk factor for various common diseases. Other sources[5] have even suggested that iron could have been a risk factor during the epidemics of bubonic plague in Europe in the 15th and 16th centuries, where strong, young, rich, iron-replete men were more frequent victims than poor and anemic women and children.

PETER REIZENSTEIN
Division of Hematology
Karolinska Hospital
Stockholm, Sweden

References

1. **Reizenstein, P., Ehn, L., Forsberg, K., Kuppevelt, A. V., and Liéden, G.,** Prevention of iron deficiency with ferrous iron and haemaglobin iron in subjects with controlled blood loss in iron metabolism and its disorders, *Exc. Medica,* Kief, H., Ed., Amsterdam, 1975.
2. **Reizenstein, P., Ljunggren, G., Smedby, B., Agenäs, I., and Penchansky, M.,** Overprescribing iron tablets to elderly people in Sweden, *Br. Med. J.,* 2, 962, 1979.
3. **Weinberg, E. D.,** Cellular iron metabolism in health and disease, *Drug Metab. Rev.,* 22(5), 531, 1990.
4. **Reizenstein, P.,** Hemoglobin fortification of food and prevention of iron deficiency with heme iron, *Acta Med. Scand. Suppl.,* 629, 1980.
5. **Palmblad, J.,** Lecture, Sept. 15, 1991.

Iron
and
Human Disease

Introduction

Iron, Aging, and Human Disease: Historical Background and New Hypotheses

RANDALL B. LAUFFER

*NMR Center, Massachusettes General Hospital
and Harvard Medical School,
Boston, Massachusetts*

I. INTRODUCTION

The possibility that iron, the most highly utilized transition metal in biology, could be a risk factor for human disease is a concept foreign to most biomedical researchers and physicians. The widespread problem of iron deficiency anemia in developing countries and in defined segments of more advanced societies elevated iron's status as an empowering nutrient. Throughout most of this century, the developing picture of iron's importance and versatility, particularly in regard to iron's central role in oxygen transport and electron transfer, implanted only positive images in the minds of most researchers. This was perhaps amplified by popular notions of iron as a strength-promoting nutrient, a cure-all for fatigue.[1]

The mounting evidence presented in this book suggests that iron indeed plays a role in some of the most deadly and widespread diseases in developed countries. Whether or not reduction of iron levels in the body will be an effective means to reduce the prevalence or severity of these conditions remains for future research. What is clear, however, is that defined roles for iron have been discovered, and future research should focus more on iron's darker side rather than on deficiency conditions which are suffered by a dwindling percentage of the developed world.

This chapter places the new information about iron in proper historical context. Also discussed are ways in which iron-catalyzed oxidative reactions may fit into current theories of aging. Finally, I offer some views on hypothesis formation and evaluation in this highly multidisciplinary area. It is hoped that these topics will serve as a fitting introduction to the more detailed accounts provided in this book.

II. EVOLUTION OF THE CONCEPT OF IRON AS A POSSIBLE RISK FACTOR IN HUMAN DISEASE

A number of excellent accounts of the history of iron in medicine[2] or important findings in the biochemistry and physiology of iron have been presented.[3-5] This section will highlight key findings from several lines of research which form the basis for continued scrutiny of the role of iron in common diseases. The most important discoveries can be grouped in three categories: (a) average iron stores in "Western" peoples are generally high due to high intake and limited excretion, (b) iron is a limiting nutrient for cell growth, and high iron levels may predispose a subject to infection and cancer, and (c) iron is a key catalyst for oxidative damage stemming from partially reduced oxygen metabolites.

A. HIGH IRON STORES ARE COMMON IN WESTERN SOCIETIES

> "It is suggested, therefore, that iron is excreted in very small amounts both by the bowel and kidney . . . . It is doubtful whether the intestine has any power of regulating iron excretion."
>
> McCance and Widdowson, 1937[6]

McCance and Widdowson were first to point to what could be viewed as a defect in the regulation of iron balance in the human body.[6] In contrast to the efficient regulation of other inorganic elements like sodium and potassium, there appeared to these authors to be no evidence in the literature for an efficient excretion pathway to get rid of excess iron. They proposed that the significant iron stores in the body — again, in contrast to the lack of sodium or potassium stores — must be in equilibrium with plasma iron, and that iron balance is somehow achieved by the regulation of the absorption of iron by the intestines in response to the level of plasma iron. The enhancement of iron absorption with decreasing iron stores was later shown experimentally in dogs by Hahn and co-workers[7] in 1939 and in humans by Ross and Chapin[8] in 1941.

How good is this "one-way" regulatory mechanism? Beginning in the 1940s, debate centered on whether there existed a "mucosal block" that would completely inhibit iron absorption when sufficient iron stores were present.[9,10] Despite being rather thoroughly discredited (or, at least, drastically modified) by subsequent research, this concept guided the thinking of more than one generation of investigators. While some regulation of iron absorption does occur in the intestines, it does not afford an absolute block and applies only to relatively small amounts of iron; it can easily be overloaded.

These studies focused on non-heme iron from inorganic salts or plant sources. With the discovery in 1951 by Moore and Dubach,[11] confirmed by many subsequent reports, that heme iron from meat is absorbed to a greater extent that non-heme iron, another pathway to the accumulation of high iron stores became evident. Bothwell, Charlton, and co-workers[12] showed in 1983 that, while the percentage of non-heme iron absorbed clearly decreases with increasing oral doses, the percentage of heme iron absorbed remains the same (approximately 20% in their studies) over a tenfold dose range. As discussed recently by Cook,[13] the lack of a saturation effect with large amounts of heme iron could definitely contribute to high iron stores in people who consume large amounts of meat.

Meat intake is one of the most important reasons for the higher iron stores in Western societies. One of the largest cross-cultural studies, performed by Charlton et al.[14] showed that hepatic iron stores in Western countries were greater than that of Japan and developing countries. As discussed further by Leggett and Halliday in Chapter 3, the iron stores (as estimated by serum ferritin readings) of office workers in Australia were recently noted to be among the highest recorded for apparently "normal" populations.[15] High meat intake was one of the factors discussed.

With the less-than-perfect "mucosal block", one might expect iron levels to increase with age. Three studies using serum ferritin to estimate iron stores are consistent with this notion. Age appeared to be significantly related to serum ferritin levels in an Italian study by Casale et al.[16] and the Australian study mentioned above.[15] A more detailed picture of age- and sex-differences in iron accumulation is evident in the study of Cook et al.[17] (see Chapter 19, Figure 1). Iron stores appear to rise rapidly in young men and continue to rise at a lower rate in later years. Menstruation and pregnancy keep the stores of premenopausal women relatively low; however, after menopause, their rate of iron accumulation appears to exceed that of men. Whether serum ferritin levels accurately reflect iron stores in older subjects is a matter of debate. Thus it is difficult to conclude at the present time that iron stores continue to increase in old age. Nonetheless, iron accumulation seems to be a fact of life in Western populations over most if not all of their lifespan.

B. IRON AS A LIMITING NUTRIENT FOR BACTERIA AND TUMOR CELLS

"In the contest between the establishment of a bacterial or mycotic disease and the successful suppression of the disease by animal hosts, iron is the cation whose concentration . . . at present appears to be the most important."

Weinberg, 1966[18]

" . . . a battle of chelating agents . . . "

Glynn, 1972[19]

The second group of crucial discoveries relates to the role of iron in enhancing infection or neoplasia. These topics are discussed in detail by Weinberg in Chapter 6 and Stevens in Chapter 13.

Iron has been found necessary for life for all but lactic acid bacteria. Discoveries related to the need for iron by bacteria date back to 1912 with the finding by Twort and Ingram[20] of a special "growth factor" for a mycobacterial strain. As was shown many years later, the growth factor turned out to be a hydroxamate siderophore, an organic iron-chelating agent used by bacteria to acquire iron. In the 1950s a number of labs isolated new siderophores.[21]

The discovery in the 1940s by Shade and Caroline[22,23] that the bacteriostatic properties of conalbumin and transferrin are due to strong iron binding underlined the importance of minimizing iron availability *in vivo*.

The existence of a more active and dynamic iron withholding defense became evident through the work of many investigators. In 1932 Locke and co-workers[24] described a profound drop in serum iron concentrations experienced in patients with infection, cancer or inflammatory disease. In 1962 Kampschmidt and Upchurch[25] found that serum iron concentrations decreased after injecting plasma containing what is now known as interleukin-1, a cytokine induced by the introduction of bacterial endotoxin. The mechanism of the iron withholding effect was investigated by Freireich et al.,[26] who found that the rate of iron release into plasma from catabolized red blood cells was reduced in animals with experimentally induced inflammation. In 1977 Konijn and Hershko[27] hypothesized that the hypoferremia was due to enhanced apoferritin synthesis. Indeed, recent studies, discussed by Rogers in Chapter 2, show that interleukin-1 enhances the translation of apoferritin mRNA. This discovery provides an important new link between iron metabolism and the important acute phase response.

Though it was recognized early on that the hypoferremia of inflammation was not dangerous to the patient,[28] the term widely used — "anemia of chronic disease" — still implied a pathological rather than a physiological response, possibly delaying the appreciation of iron's vital role in these conditions. Over the years, Weinberg has summarized the evidence for the clinical importance of the iron-withholding defense in infection.[29,30]

Weinberg also suggested that hypoferremia may also be a useful defense against neoplasia.[29,31] In addition to serving as a limiting nutrient for tumor cell growth (especially for the iron enzyme, ribonucleotide reductase, which is required for the synthesis of DNA), iron could serve as a catalyst for DNA damage stemming from oxygen free radicals.

Following studies by Blumberg and co-workers[32,33] revealing increased serum iron levels in chronic hepatitis B carriers, Stevens et al.[34] found that serum ferritin levels were positively associated with overall mortality rates of Solomon Islanders. The causes of death were not available in this study. However, additional studies by Stevens et al.[35,36] and Selby and Friedman[37] have indicated that high iron levels are associated with increased risk of death from cancer.

C. IRON AS A CATALYST FOR OXYGEN FREE RADICAL-INDUCED TISSUE DAMAGE

" . . . it seems probable that the iron acts in a manner usually termed 'catalytic,' a very small quantity of iron being sufficient to determine the oxidation . . . of an almost unlimited amount of tartaric acid."

Fenton, 1894[38]

"It is a sobering thought that the hydroxyl radical, earlier thought of only in connection with the effects of ionizing radiation, may in fact be produced in respiring biological systems.''

Fridovich, 1975[39]

Partially reduced oxygen byproducts from respiration present a formidable challenge to the maintenance of biological structure and function. It is surprising that powerful chemical oxidants, usually thought of only in the context of organic reaction chemistry or radiation chemistry, are encountered in everyday life. The formation of the most common forms of these reactive species — equivalent to internally generated ''radiation'' — require transition metal catalysts, especially iron.

In 1894 Fenton showed the power of trace amounts of ferrous ion, Fe(II), in catalyzing the oxidation of tartrate by hydrogen peroxide.[38] The so-called ''Fenton's reagent'' — hydrogen peroxide plus a ferrous salt — proved to be a versatile oxidant of a wide variety of organic substrates.[40]

With the discovery of superoxide dismutase by McCord and Fridovich in 1969,[41] it became apparent that nature had a high degree of respect and fear for reduced oxygen species. The possible role of metal ion catalysis was suggested in 1970 by Beauchamp and Fridovich in studies on the production of ethylene from methional in a xanthine/xanthine oxidase system.[42] They showed that, in addition to superoxide and hydrogen peroxide, an even more powerful oxidant is involved in the reaction. This latter oxidant could even react with ethanol or benzoate! The authors proposed that the oxidant is the hydroxyl radical, OH·, generated by the well-known Haber-Weiss reaction proposed in 1934:[43]

$$O_2^{\cdot-} + H_2O_2 \xrightarrow{\text{iron salts}} O_2 + OH^- + OH^{\cdot} \tag{1}$$

However, another interpretation is that the active oxidant in these systems is the ferryl ion, Fe(IV)=O^{2+}, first proposed in 1932 by Bray and Gorin.[44] This species could be formed from ferrous ion and hydrogen peroxide:

$$Fe(II) + H_2O_2 \rightarrow Fe(IV)=O^{2+} + H_2O \tag{2}$$

Further aspects of the current debate over the actual reactive species are discussed by Halliwell in Chapter 7 and McCord in the Epilogue.

The pathophysiological significance of oxygen free radicals — and, likewise, transition metal catalysts — has grown tremendously since these seminal discoveries. The number of human conditions thought to have some free radical component extends to every organ system and includes important and often life-threatening process such as inflammation, neoplasia, neurodegenerative disease, and ischemia/reperfusion injury.[45] The most important of these are discussed in Parts IV and V of this book.

The role of oxygen free radicals in cardiovascular disease deserves special mention, as it occupies an entire section of this book (Part IV). Few other areas of relevance to the free radical hypothesis have received more attention. This is undoubtedly due to the immense medical implications, and therefore "fundability," of this research. The free radical hypothesis should, of course, not be discarded if it ends up contributing little to the prevention and treatment of cardiovascular disease; its relevance to other forms of pathophysiology may remain strong.

In the case of coronary artery disease (CAD), two possible roles have emerged for reduced oxygen species and their transition metal collaborators: one role at the "beginning" of the disease — atherogenesis — and one at the "end" — ischemic injury to myocytes. In regard to the former, it had been known since the 1950s that atherosclerotic plaque contained ample quantities of peroxidized lipids, implicating perhaps some derangement of lipoprotein handling.[46] It had also been shown that low density lipoprotein (LDL) is particularly susceptible to oxidation, and copper(II) had been shown to stimulate this degradation.[47] Steinberg et al. have now developed a promising mechanism for atherogenesis:[48]

1. Oxidation of LDL lipids, most likely in the artery wall, is the committed step.
2. Through a chain reaction or via oxidation byproducts, this leads to covalent modification of apoprotein residues.
3. This in turn permits avid uptake by macrophages in the artery wall via a special scavenging receptor.
4. The lipid-loaded macrophage becomes a foam cell, the foundation of atherosclerotic plaque.

Parthasarathy, in Chapter 9, discusses the possible role of iron or iron-containing lipoxygenases in the initial oxidation step.

The actual damage to the heart muscle in CAD is most likely due to reperfusion injury. By the time superoxide and its dismutase were widely known, it had been discovered that myocyte injury occurs not during ischemia but during reflow; oxygen was shown to be responsible for the damage.[49] Oxygen free radicals were first shown to be involved in this process by Guarnieri et al. in 1980.[50] A paper by Myers et al.[51] in 1985 was the first of several to show that desferrioxamine, the iron-chelating drug, protected the heart from reperfusion injury, presumably by inhibiting the formation of hydroxyl or ferryl radicals. Further evidence for the role of iron in reperfusion injury came from a study by van der Kraaij et al.[52] which showed that reperfusion injury was more severe in iron-loaded rat hearts. This topic is further discussed by Zweier in Chapter 10 and McCord in the Epilogue.

Oxygen radicals have been shown to be involved in reperfusion injury to the intestine, liver, pancreas, skin, skeletal muscle, and kidney.[53] Similar data appear to be accumulating for the brain. In preliminary studies by Babbs,[54] brain cell damage was presumably reduced by the administration of desferrioxamine, which increased survival rates of animals subjected to total circulatory arrest. Furthermore, Repine and co-workers[55] found that gerbils fed low-iron diets, which led to lower brain iron levels, were protected from reperfusion injury of the brain. Repine and co-workers discuss this data in more detail in Chapter 12.

The accumulated data on possible roles for iron in cardiovascular conditions, especially in reperfusion injury, have greatly strengthened the prescient 1981 hypothesis of Sullivan that the sex difference in heart disease risk can be ascribed to the greater level of iron stores in men.[56] Sullivan noted that the temporal pattern of heart disease risk, with men acquiring high risk some 10 years earlier than women, matched that of iron accumulation. He also proposed that the rarity of heart disease in developing countries could be due in part to lower overall iron levels and outright iron deficiency.

Some data supporting these ideas are available. I recently found that published hepatic iron levels in male and female subjects from 11 countries are better correlated with CAD mortality rates than are cholesterol levels; the best index found was the *liver iron-serum cholesterol* product, which has a correlation coefficient to CAD rates of 0.74 ($p < 0.005$) (see Figure 1).[57] This is only a preliminary study based on an inadequate data base; a more complete international study using serum ferritin in a larger number of subjects is needed.

In one of the most exciting developments in this field, the CAD risk from high iron stores has been confirmed in a large study from Kuopio, Finland which has recently been presented in preliminary form.[58] Serum ferritin values in over 1900 men were found to be directly correlated ($p < 0.01$) to the incidence of acute myocardial infarction. Confirmation in other study populations is eagerly awaited.

In a review article[58a] and in Chapter 11, Sullivan summarizes the provocative links between iron and CAD. Because of the importance of the subject and the availability of voluminous but still not adequate data, the CAD area has become an important testing ground for hypotheses in the epidemiology of iron and human disease. Sullivan draws attention to the ease in which the iron links can be erroneously dismissed. Some additional thoughts on this problem are presented below in Section IV.

III. IRON, OXIDATIVE STRESS, AND AGING

The growing number of conditions in which iron and oxidative stress are thought to be important includes the aging process itself. Since aging is a cause, or at least a risk factor, for disease,[59] the discovery of any preventive measures, such as reducing iron levels, is of profound importance to advanced societies where decreased morbidity, rather than just increased lifespan, is

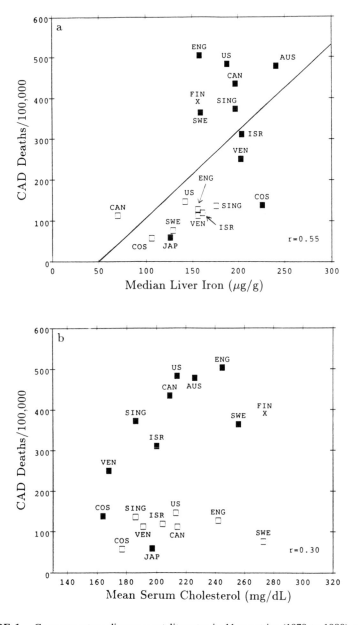

FIGURE 1. Coronary artery disease mortality rates in 11 countries (1978 to 1980) vs. corresponding estimates of liver iron (a), serum cholesterol (b), and the liver iron-serum cholesterol product (c). Values shown are for men (filled squares), women (open squares), and a single entry for Finland that is an average of both men and women (X). The lines shown in (a) and (c) are fits to all of the data with the correlation coefficient r given as shown. The countries included are: U.S., Canada, England, Australia, Sweden, Finland, Israel, Singapore, Costa Rica, Venezuela, and Japan. (From Lauffer, R. B., *Med. Hypoth.*, 35, 96, 1991. With permission.)

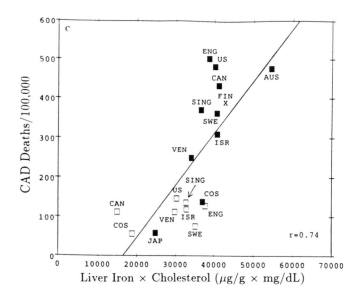

FIGURE 1c.

likely to become a major public health goal. While little direct evidence of a role for iron in aging has been presented, the involvement of oxygen free radicals is often discussed, and this justifies inquiries into iron. Unfortunately, research into the biochemical mechanisms of aging to date has not adequately proved any of the competing theories. Nonetheless, one can still see a possible role for oxidative stress.

A. GENETIC, DAMAGE-BASED, AND UNIFIED THEORIES OF AGING

A rather stark polarity has existed in the area of aging theories. Genetic or programmed aging theories seem to attract wider attention than damaged-based theories, but it is difficult to discern whether this is due to overall merits or the fashionable nature of molecular biology and the greater number of investigators who focus in this general area.

The genetic theories of aging point to the consistent characteristics and patterns of aging — e.g., the existence of species-specific lifespans and the consistency of aging rates — as evidence that aging is under developmental and thus genetic control. Evidence in favor of this theory includes the well-known observation that human fibroblasts stop dividing after a well-defined number of population doublings.[60] It is thought that, as for other fundamental events in the cell, DNA-binding proteins involved in cellular senescence eventually will be isolated.[61,62] Further evidence for genetic control is the discovery of nemotode mutants, involving so-called *age-1* mutations, with increased lifespan.[63]

A number of deficiencies of the genetic theory of aging have been discussed. For example, it is difficult to see why nature would have favored programmed cell and organism death for some obscure advantage, e.g., to allow greater resources (food, etc.) for younger, reproductively active individuals in a given species. Most animals in the wild are killed before they reach old age, and this would obviate the need for a defined mechanism to "weed out" resource-demanding older members.[64] Another observation is that, in the context of genetic theories, cellular senescence represents a *gain* in a genetic function with age, i.e., involving specific DNA-binding proteins.[65] The idea that a cell, experiencing a general decline in function, could exhibit a new function is at least a little difficult to accept. In addition, the aging-related inhibition of DNA synthesis observed in cell culture could be a result of an accumulation of defects which masquerade as a specific activation of a genetic program. And finally, while genetic theories nicely describe the *relative* consistency of aging rates in a given species, they may not allow adequately for the significant heterogeneity which still must exist.

Most readers of this book are probably more familiar with the free radical theory of aging,[59,66] the most popular damage-based theory, where reactive radicals, most notably those derived from molecular oxygen, inflict damage at a rate beyond the capacity of antioxidant defense and repair processes. The accumulated damage leads to altered cell function and eventually cell death. The most persuasive evidence in favor of the oxygen free radical theory is the correlation between basal metabolic rate and species' lifespans.[67] Presumably, a greater rate of metabolism and, therefore, respiration leads to increased "leakage" of reduced oxygen species and a higher degree of cellular damage. The likely source for these free radicals is the mitchondria, especially considering the prevalence of mitochondrial DNA mutations which could have extensive and severe effects on the net oxidative stress experienced in the cell.[68,69]

The oxygen free radical theory, on its own, has considerable deficiencies. The most important of these is the difficulty of ascribing the characteristic pattern and *relative* consistency of aging to a completely stochastic model of random damage to biomolecules. Many investigators are concerned that the increased lipid peroxidation and age pigment accumulation, while useful markers of aging, may not be reflecting the true, original cause of the decline in cell function. In terms of endogenous antioxidant defenses, such as superoxide dismutase, catalase, glutathione, and vitamins C and E, there is now little evidence that increased concentrations of these substances increase life span, and the same holds for exogenous antioxidants. In fact, there appears to be a preset balance between anti- and prooxidants in the cell which, though shifting toward a more oxidizing state in aging, nevertheless cannot be greatly altered by added substances.[70] (However, there is some evidence, presented in Section III.B below, that iron may lie outside this homeostatic system.)

A partial resolution of these two opposing theories seems to be creeping into current debate.[65,70,71] Oxidative stress is seen as being directly linked to cell death programs, the acquired lack of control over cell differentiation (which could lead to cancer as well as aging), or other changes in gene regulation. This unified approach encompasses the positive attributes of each theory — such as the reasonably consistent nature of aging in the genetic theory and the correlation between lifespan and metabolic rate which is supportive of the free radical theory — while it avoids the deficiencies.

There is increasing evidence that free radicals could influence gene regulation in a general way. Blake and co-workers discuss in Chapter 16 the possibility that reactive oxygen species could be used by cells as second messengers, much as nitric oxide is employed in the endothelium and in the brain. In an environment where free radicals are continuously generated, cells may have evolved not only ways to detoxify these radicals but also utilize them at reasonable concentrations as effective regulators of the expression of genes unrelated to detoxification. It is easy to see that this would be a dangerous game for the cell to play over extended periods of time: every successfully delivered message would be accompanied by some probability of collateral damage which, in turn, could inappropriately affect gene regulation.

B. IRON AND OXIDATIVE BALANCE

In Chapter 7 Halliwell discusses in detail the role of iron in oxidative tissue damage. The following brief account compliments his chapter, especially with respect to aging mechanisms.

There is some evidence that iron is involved in the aging process or at least in the chemistry that occurs along with aging. For example, age pigments contain rather large amounts of iron, and it is thought that transition metal catalysis is required for pigment formation.[64] Enhanced iron levels in animals in animals and humans have been reported to increase age pigment formation, while desferrioxamine inhibits its accumulation.[72,73] (This is discussed further by Brunk and co-workers in Chapter 8). In addition, elevated iron levels have been found in the cerebrospinal fluid of victims of neuronal ceroid lipofuscinosis, an inherited disorder characterized in part by pigment accumulation throughout the body.[64] These patients also exhibit enhanced iron absorption from the intestines.

Iron has been implicated in the oxidative modification of proteins via two distinct mechanisms. The first is oxidative glycosylation where glycated adducts on proteins, formed by the nonenzymatic addition of glucose to amine groups, are irreversibly oxidized with catalytic iron to, for example, N^ϵ-(carboxymethyl)lysine residues or other products including protein cross-links.[74,75] Thus, advanced glycosylation end products, which form the basis for still another aging theory and for the proposed mechanism for diabetic complications,[76] may require iron for their formation. A second role for iron in protein modification is in the direct oxidation of amino acid residues to carbonyl derivatives and other products. Carbonyl adducts increase with age in animals and human cell lines, and cells from patients with premature aging syndromes (progeria or Werner's syndrome) exhibit increased carbonyl content.[77]

Whether the above chemical observations have direct relevance to aging is not known. There is little information relating animal lifespans to iron levels. However, some provocative information has been obtained in studies of flies. Iron accumulation in fruit flies increased with increasing temperature, while life spans decreased with increasing temperature.[78] Administration of iron in the drinking water of houseflies shortened their life spans by one half and increased the accumulation of age pigment.[79] Other forms of oxidative stress, such as superoxide generation, catalase inactivation, or glutathione oxidation, did not increase the concentration of age pigment. From these data it appears that, as opposed to other oxidatively active substances which are in balance with one another,[70] iron is unique in that it accumulates with age and appears to shorten lifespan under different circumstances.[80]

Some crude parallels exist between these data and some observations on humans. Iron appears to accumulate with aging, as described in Section II.A. Men in advanced societies possess greater iron levels than women and shorter lifespans; in developing countries, where iron levels of the two sexes are comparable (and lower than in advanced countries), life expectancies are similar.[4,81] And finally, iron overload clearly offsets the oxidative balance in the body as evidenced by reduced concentrations of ascorbate and alpha-tocopherol.[4] The effect of moderately elevated iron levels on these substances is apparently unknown.

It should be pointed out that the hypothesis that iron contributes to aging does not *require* that iron must accumulate with age. A constant level of iron and oxidative stress over time would be sufficient to lead to the gradual accumulation of modified biomolecules, age pigments, and organ damage.

IV. HYPOTHESIS EVALUATION

Seeking epidemiologic links between iron and human diseases and affirming them in clinical trials will be undoubtedly a complex task. The multicausal nature of most diseases and the possible correlation between iron indices and other diet-related risk factors such as fat and cholesterol will frustrate attempts to assign a relative value to iron as an additional risk factor. One has only to look at the confusion that still permeates the well-studied cholesterol-heart disease relationship for a glimpse of the difficulty in store. In addition, looking for the role of a catalyst such as iron may likely be more difficult than examining substances like cholesterol which are more direct participants and are found in diseased tissue in relatively large quantities.

The following ideas may be helpful in guiding the development and testing of new hypotheses in this area. This discussion is meant to complement those in the rest of this book, especially that of Sullivan in Chapter 11 which is focused on ischemic heart disease.

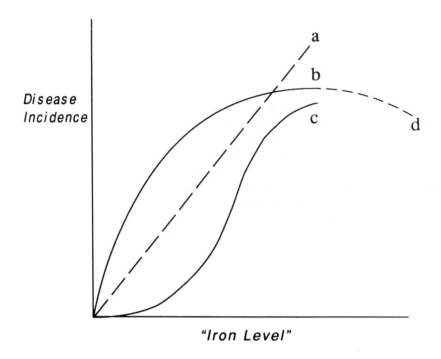

FIGURE 2. Hypothetical plots of disease incidence vs. some measurement of "iron level". The dependence could be linear (a), "saturable" (b), S-shaped (c), or parabolic (d).

The relationship between disease incidence and iron levels may not be straightforward. This concept is critical in the design of epidemiologic and clinical studies. As shown in Figure 2 (a to c), hypothetical plots of disease incidence vs. iron levels could take on several forms. If the dependence is linear, then it may be straightforward to detect a relationship as long as the populations considered vary significantly in their iron levels. However, if disease incidence reaches a plateau over a common range of iron levels in the population (Figure 2b), for example, the range exhibited by men and postmenopausal women, then a study focused on only these groups may yield no dependence. With reference to the apparent protection from ischemic heart disease exhibited by premenopausal women, Sullivan emphasizes in Chapter 11 that it may be iron *depletion* that is protective; once a moderate level of iron is reached, further increases may be of little effect. In this context, it appears that the S-shaped curve in Figure 2c should be considered because it allows for disease incidence to be low over some range of iron levels which might be typical of premenopausal women.

The obvious practical guideline stemming from these considerations is that a population selected for study would have to contain subjects with widely varying iron levels, including some with very low levels. If a study were to focus on men, for example, strict vegetarians, frequent blood donors, or others who exhibit lower iron levels would have to be included. In addition, studies focused solely on the effect of iron depletion through blood donation should also be performed.[82]

The apparent lack of increased risk for a given disease in iron overload victims does not necessarily argue against a role for iron in that disease. While it is most likely that the extremely high iron levels of hemochromatosis and transfused thallassemia patients should put them at high risk for iron-related diseases, it is also possible that iron overload and the organ damage thereof *favorably* alters the risk profile for a given disease.

For example, an objection to the proposed link between iron and coronary artery disease is that, according to simple clinical observations, hemochromatosis victims, while suffering the direct cardiotoxicity of iron, do not appear to suffer unduly from conventional ischemic heart disease. However, no studies of the incidence of either heart attacks or the severity of atherosclerosis in these patients have actually been reported. Moreover, one can envision how one disease — iron overload — could alter risk factors for a second disease in a *positive* manner. In the case of atherosclerosis in hemochromatosis victims, it is possible that the liver disease these patients experience could alter their lipid profile significantly. For example, it has been suggested that chronic liver disease may lead to decreased lecithin cholesterol acyl transferase (LCAT) activity in hepatocytes which, in turn, could lead to decreased atherogenic potential of LDL particles due to a lower degree of cholesterol esterification.[83] Thus, a graph of disease incidence vs. iron levels could actually be parabolic, as shown in Figure 2d, reflecting the multiparametric nature of the disease.

For those diseases in which iron depletion is ineffective, a role for iron may still exist. In the brain, for example, there is some evidence that iron levels are not very responsive to changes in overall iron status, perhaps due to the blood-brain barrier.[84] For any brain disease that might involve iron, such as Parkinson's or Alzheimer's disease, disease incidence may not relate to the general body iron levels and may not respond to conventional treatments that would reduce iron levels. Nonetheless, the role of iron in the pathophysiology should be fully investigated since more aggressive treatments, such as chelating drugs that cross the blood-brain barrier, could be designed.

Studies pointing to iron-related risk factors, such as male sex, red meat intake, etc., should be scrutinized for more direct evidence for a contribution from iron. Epidemiological studies of heart disease, cancer, and other conditions continue to be interpreted in terms of conventional theories. Thus, a dependence on male sex is interpreted as reflecting a hormonal contribution, and a dependence on meat intake is usually interpreted as stemming from fat intake. However, these and other risk factors, including the lack of both exercise and whole grain consumption (see Chapter 19), may be indirectly reflecting a role for iron as a dominant risk factor. The data bases collected to date are potentially fruitful testing grounds for the evaluation of iron as an independent risk factor.

New studies directly examining iron levels and disease incidence should be performed. There exists no more universal and multifaceted potential risk factor than iron. Its proposed role in cancer, heart disease, and other major killers in Western countries is provocative and, even if it is shown to be relevant only to a subset of these conditions, there will be extensive public health implications.

Future broad-based epidemiologic studies utilizing biochemical data should include complete screens of iron levels in the body, at the very least serum ferritin and transferrin saturation. In addition, if future research shows that these and other conventional measures of iron levels appear to inadequately reflect the concentrations of catalytically active forms of iron, i.e., the "chelatable iron pool" (see Chapter 1), new tests which can be given to large numbers of subjects should be developed.

V. CONCLUSIONS

There seems to be a growing realization that iron, like cholesterol, is a true double-edged nutrient. While nature has put this most abundant of the heavy metals to astoundingly good use in biological systems, the scientific findings of the past decade, as summarized in this book, have cast a long shadow over this nutrient of strength and vigor. Despite this, physicians, nutritionists, and the public continue to view iron in far too rosy a light. Outdated science, cultural notions, and even commercial advertising may have had a role in delaying our appreciation of the prevalence of iron overload and the risks from even moderately elevated iron levels. One hopes that the new climate afforded by recent findings will allow full and open discourse (and of course ample funding) to fully expose iron's darker side and set a proper balance for this nutrient in human health.

ACKNOWLEDGMENTS

The author thanks E. D. Weinberg, R. S. Sohal, and J. L. Sullivan for helpful discussions on this chapter.

REFERENCES

1. **Lauffer, R. B.,** *Iron Balance,* St. Martin's Press, New York, 1991, chap. 1 and 3 to 5.
2. **Fairbanks, V. F., Fahey, J. L., and Beutler, E.,** *Clinical Disorders of Iron Metabolism,* Grune & Stratton, New York, 1971, chap. 1.
3. **Jacobs, A. and Worwood, M., Eds.,** *Iron in Biochemistry and Medicine,* Academic Press, New York, 1974.

4. **Bothwell, T. H., Charlton, R. W., Cook, J. D., and Finch, C. A.,** *Iron Metabolism in Man,* Blackwell, Oxford, 1979.
5. **Jacobs, A. and Worwood, M.,** Eds., *Iron in Biochemistry and Medicine,* Vol. 2, Academic Press, New York, 1980.
6. **McCance, R. A. and Widdowson, E. M.,** Absorption and excretion of iron, *Lancet,* 2, 680, 1937.
7. **Hahn, P. F., Bale, W. F., Lawrence, E. O., and Whipple, G. H.,** Radioactive iron and its metabolism in anemia: its absorption, transportation, and utilization, *J. Exp. Med.,* 69, 739, 1939.
8. **Ross, J. F. and Chapin, M. A.,** The selective absorption of radioactive iron by normal and iron-deficient human subjects, *J. Clin. Invest.,* 20, 437, 1941.
9. **Hahn, P. F., Bale, W. F., Ross, J. F., Balfour, W. M., and Whipple, G. H.,** Radioactive iron absorption in gastro-intestinal tract: influence of anemia, anoxia, and antecedent feeding distribution in growing dogs, *J. Exp. Med.,* 78, 169, 1943.
10. **Granick, S.,** Ferritin: its properties and significance for iron metabolism, *Chem. Rev.,* 38, 379, 1946.
11. **Moore, C. V. and Dubach, R.,** Observations on the absorption of iron from foods tagged with radioiron, *Trans. Assoc. Am. Physicians,* 64, 245, 1951.
12. **Bezwoda, W. R., Bothwell, T. H., Charlton, R. W., Torrance, J. D., Macphail, A. P., Derman, D. P., and Mayet, F.,** The relative dietary importance of haem and non-haem iron, *S. Afr. Med. J.,* 64, 552, 1983.
13. **Cook, J. D.,** Adaptation in iron metabolism, *Am. J. Clin. Nutr.,* 51, 301, 1990.
14. **Charlton, R. W., Hawkins, D. M., Mavor, W. O., and Bothwell, T. H.,** Hepatic storage iron concentrations in different population groups, *Am. J. Clin. Nutr.,* 23, 358, 1970.
15. **Leggett, B. A., Brown, N. N., Bryant, S. J., Duplock, L., Powell, L. W., and Halliday, J. E.,** Factors affecting the concentrations of ferritin in serum in a healthy Australian population, *Clin. Chem.,* 36, 1350, 1990.
16. **Casale, G., Bonora, C., Migliavacca, A., Zurita, I., and deNicola, P.,** Serum ferritin and ageing, *Age Ageing,* 10, 119, 1981.
17. **Cook, J. D., Finch, C. A., and Smith, N. J.,** Evaluation of the iron status of a population, *Blood,* 48, 449, 1976.
18. **Weinberg, E. D.,** Roles of metallic ions in host-parasite interactions, *Bacteriol. Rev.,* 30, 136, 1966.
19. **Glynn, A. A.,** Bacterial factors inhibiting host defense mechanisms, *Symp. Soc. Gen. Microbiol.,* 22, 75, 1972.
20. **Twort, F. W. and Ingram, G. L. Y.,** A method for isolating and cultivating the *Mycobacterium enteriditis* chromicae pseudotuberculosis bovis, Johne, and some experiments on the preparation of a diagnostic vaccine for pseudotuberculosis enteritis of bovines, *Proc. R. Soc. London Ser. B,* 84, 517, 1912.
21. **Nielands, J. B.,** Some aspects of microbial iron metabolism, *Microbiol. Rev.,* 21, 101, 1957.
22. **Shade, A. L. and Caroline, L.,** Raw hen egg white and the role of iron in growth inhibition of *Shigella dysenteriae, Staphylococcus aureus, Escherichia coli,* and *Saccharomyces cerevisiae, Science,* 100, 14, 1944.
23. **Shade, A. L. and Caroline, L.,** An iron-binding component in human blood plasma, *Science,* 104, 340, 1946.
24. **Locke, A., Main, E. R., and Rosbach, D. O.,** The copper and non-hemoglobinous iron contents of the blood serum in disease, *J. Clin. Invest.,* 11, 527, 1932.
25. **Kampschmidt, R. F. and Upchurch, H. F.,** Effects of bacterial endotoxin on plasma iron, *Proc. Soc. Exp. Biol. Med.,* 110, 191, 1962.
26. **Freireich, E. J., Miller, A., Emerson, C. P., et al.,** The effect of inflammation on the utilization of erythrocyte and transferrin bound radioiron for red cell production, *Blood,* 12, 972, 1957.

27. **Konijn, A. M. and Hershko, C.**, Ferritin synthesis in inflammation. I. Pathogenesis of impaired iron release, *Br. J. Haematol.*, 37, 7, 1977.
28. **Cartwright, G. E. and Lee, G. R.**, The anaemia of chronic disorders, *Br. J. Haematol.*, 21, 147, 1971.
29. **Weinberg, E. D.**, Iron and susceptibility to infectious disease, *Science*, 184, 952, 1974.
30. **Weinberg, E. D.**, Iron withholding: a defense against infection and neoplasia, *Physiol. Rev.*, 64, 65, 1984.
31. **Weinberg, E. D.**, Iron and neoplasia, *Biol. Trace Elem. Res.*, 3, 55, 1981.
32. **Sutnick, A. I., Blumberg, B. S., and Lustbader, E. D.**, Elevated serum iron levels and persistent Australia antigen (HBsAg), *Ann. Intern. Med.*, 81, 855, 1974.
33. **Blumberg, B. S., Lustbader, E. D., and Whitford, P. L.**, Changes in serum iron levels due to infection with hepatitis B virus, *Proc. Natl. Acad. Sci. U.S.A.*, 78, 3222, 1981.
34. **Stevens, R. G., Kuvibidila, S., Kapps, M., Friedlaender, J., and Blumberg, B. S.**, Iron-binding proteins, hepatitis B virus, and mortality in the Solomon Islands, *Am. J. Epidemiol.*, 118, 550, 1983.
35. **Stevens, R. G., Beasley, R. P., and Blumberg, B. S.**, Iron-binding proteins and risk of cancer in Taiwan, *JNCI*, 76, 605, 1986.
36. **Stevens, R. G., Jones, D. Y., Micozzi, M. S., and Taylor, P. R.**, Body iron stores and the risk of cancer, *N. Engl. J. Med.*, 319, 1047, 1988.
37. **Selby, J. V. and Friedman, G. D.**, Epidemiologic evidence of an association between body iron stores and risk of cancer, *Int. J. Cancer*, 41, 677, 1988.
38. **Fenton, H. J. H.**, Oxidation of tartaric acid in the presence of iron, *J. Chem. Soc.*, 65, 899, 1894.
39. **Fridovich, I.**, Superoxide dismutases, *Annu. Rev. Biochem.*, 44, 147, 1975.
40. **Walling, C.**, Fenton's reagent revisited, *Acc. Chem. Res.*, 8, 125, 1975.
41. **McCord, J. M. and Fridovich, I.**, Superoxide dismutase: an enzymic function for erythrocuprein (hemocuprein), *J. Biol. Chem.*, 244, 6049, 1969.
42. **Beauchamp, C. and Fridovich, I.**, A mechanism for the production of ethylene from methional; the generation of the hydroxyl radical by xanthine oxidase, *J. Biol. Chem.*, 245, 4641, 1970.
43. **Haber, F. and Weiss, J.**, The catalytic decomposition of hydrogen peroxide by iron salts, *Proc. R. Soc. London Ser. A*, 147, 332, 1934.
44. **Bray, W. C. and Gorin, M. H.**, Ferryl ion, a compound of tetravalent iron, *J. Am. Chem. Soc.*, 54, 2124, 1932.
45. **Cross, C. E., Halliwell, B., Borish, E. T., Pryor, W. A., Ames, B. N., Saul, R. L., McCord, J. M., and Harman, D.**, Oxygen radicals and human disease, *Ann. Intern. Med.*, 107, 526, 1987.
46. **Glavind, J. and Hartman, S.**, The occurrence of peroxidized lipids in atheromatous human aortas, *Experientia*, 7, 464, 1951.
47. **Ray, B. R., Davisson, E. O., and Crespi, H. L.**, Experiments on the degradation of lipoproteins from serum, *J. Phys. Chem.*, 58, 841, 1954.
48. **Steinberg, D., Parthasarathy, S., Carew, T. E., Khoo, J. C., and Witztum, J. L.**, Beyond cholesterol: modifications of low-density lipoprotein that increases its atherogenicity, *N. Engl. J. Med.*, 320, 915, 1989.
49. **Hearse, D. J., Humphrey, S. M., and Bullock, G. R.**, The oxygen paradox and the calcium paradox: two facets of the same problem?, *J. Mol. Cell. Cardiol.*, 10, 641, 1978.
50. **Guarnieri, C., Flamigni, F., and Caldarera, C. M.**, Role of oxygen in the cellular damage induced by re-oxygenation of hypoxic heart, *J. Mol. Cell. Cardiol.*, 12, 797, 1980.
51. **Myers, C. L., Weiss, S. J., Kirsh, M. M., and Shlafer, M.**, Involvement of hydrogen peroxide and hydroxyl radical in the "oxygen paradox": reduction of creatine kinase release by catalase, allopurinol or deferoxamine, but not by superoxide dismutase, *J. Mol. Cell. Cardiol.*, 17, 675, 1985.

52. **Van der Kraaij, A. M. M., Mostert, L. J., van Eijk, H. G., and Koster, J. F.**, Iron-load increases the susceptibility of rat hearts to oxygen reperfusion damage: protection by the antioxidant (+)-cyanidanol-3 and deferoxamine, *Circulation*, 78, 442, 1988.

53. **McCord, J. M.**, Oxygen-derived radicals: a link between reperfusion injury and inflammation, *Fed. Proc.*, 46, 2402, 1987.

54. **Babbs, C. F.**, Role of iron ions in the genesis of reperfusion injury following successful cardiopulmonary resuscitation: preliminary data and a biochemical hypothesis, *Ann. Emerg. Med.*, 14, 777, 1985.

55. **Patt, A., Horesch, I. R., Berger, E. M., Harken, A. H., and Repine, J. E.**, Iron depletion or chelation reduces ischemia/reperfusion-induced edema in gerbil brains, *J. Pediatr. Surg.*, 25, 224, 1990.

56. **Sullivan, J. L.**, Iron and the sex difference in heart disease risk, *Lancet*, 1, 1293, 1981.

57. **Lauffer, R. B.**, Iron stores and the international variation in mortality from coronary artery disease, *Med. Hypoth.*, 35, 96, 1991.

58. **Salonen, J. T., Salonen, R., Nyyssönen, K., and Korpela, H.**, Iron sufficiency is associated with hypertension and excess risk of myocardial infarction: the Kuopio I schaemic Heart Disease Risk Factor Study (KIHD), *Circulation*, 85, 864, 1992.

58a. **Sullivan, J. L.**, The iron paradigm of ischemic heart disease, *Am. Heart J.*, 117, 1177, 1989.

59. **Harman, D.**, The aging process: Major risk factor for disease and death, *Proc. Natl. Acad. Sci. U.S.A.*, 88, 5360, 1991.

60. **Hayflick, L. and Moorhead, P. S.**, The serial cultivation of human diploid cell strains, *Exp. Cell Res.*, 25, 585, 1961.

61. **Smith, J. R.**, DNA synthesis inhibitors in cellular senescence, *J. Gerontol. Biol. Sci.*, 45, B32, 1990.

62. **Goldstein, S.**, Replicative senescence: the human fibroblast comes of age, *Science*, 249, 1129, 1990.

63. **Johnson, T. E.**, Increased life-span of *age-1* mutants in *Caenorhabditis elegans* and lower Gompertz rate of aging, *Science*, 249, 908, 1990.

64. **Halliwell, B. and Gutteridge, J. M. C.**, *Free Radicals in Biology and Medicine*, 2nd ed., Clarendon Press, Oxford, 1989, chap. 8.

65. **Holliday, R.**, The limited proliferation of cultured human diploid cells: regulation or senescence?, *J. Gerontol. Biol. Sci.*, 45, B36, 1990.

66. **Harman, D.**, Aging: a theory based on free radical and radiation chemistry, *J. Gerontol.*, 11, 289, 1956.

67. **Cutler, R. G.**, Antioxidants, aging, and longevity, in *Free Radicals in Biology*, Vol. 6, Pryor, W. A., Ed., Academic Press, New York, 1984, 371.

68. **Linnane, A. W., Marzuki, S., Ozawa, T., and Tanaka, M.**, Mitochondrial DNA mutations as an important contributor to ageing and degenerative diseases, *Lancet*, 642, 1989.

69. **Bandy, B. and Davison, A. J.**, Mitochondrial mutations may increase oxidative stress: implications for carcinogenesis and aging, *Free Rad. Biol. Med.*, 8, 523, 1990.

70. **Sohal, R. S. and Allen, R. G.**, Oxidative stress as a causal factor in differentiation and aging: a unifying hypothesis, *Exp. Gerontol.*, 25, 499, 1990.

71. **Cutler, R. G.**, Antioxidants and aging, *Am. J. Clin. Nutr.*, 53, 373S, 1991.

72. **Katz, M. L. and Robison, W. G.**, Nutritional influences on autoxidation, lipofuscin accumulation, and aging, in *Free Radicals, Aging, and Degenerative Disease*, Johnson, J. E., Walford, R., Harman, D., and Miquel, J., Eds., Alan R. Liss, New York, 1986, 221.

73. **Marzabadi, M. R., Sohal, R. S., and Brunk, U. T.**, Effect of ferric iron and desferrioxamine on lipofuscin accumulation in cultured rat heart myocytes, *Mech. Ageing Devel.*, 46, 145, 1988.

74. **Baynes, J. W.**, Role of oxidative stress in development of complications in diabetes, *Diabetes*, 40, 405, 1991.

75. **Wolf, S. P., Jiang, Z. Y., and Hunt, J. V.,** Protein glycation and oxidative stress in diabetes mellitus and aging, *Free Rad. Biol. Med.,* 10, 339, 1991.
76. **Brownlee, M., Cerami, A., and Vlassara, H.,** Advanced glycosylation end products in tissue and the biochemical basis of diabetic complications, *N. Engl. J. Med.,* 318, 1315, 1988.
77. **Stadtman, E. R. and Oliver, C. N.,** Metal-catalyzed oxidation of proteins, *J. Biol. Chem.,* 266, 2005, 1991.
78. **Massie, H. R., Aiello, V. R., and Williams, T. R.,** Iron accumulation during development and ageing of *Drosophila, Mech. Ageing Devel.,* 29, 215, 1985.
79. **Sohal, R. S., Allen, R. G., Farmer, K. J., and Newton, R. K.,** Iron induces oxidative stress in the housefly, *Musca Domestica, Mech. Ageing Devel.,* 32, 33, 1985.
80. **Sohal, R. S.,** personal communication, 1991.
81. **Waldron, I.,** Sex differences in human mortality: the role of genetic factors, *Soc. Sci. Med.,* 17, 321, 1983.
82. **Sullivan, J. L.,** Blood donation may be good for the donor: iron, heart disease, and donor recruitment, *Vox Sang.,* 61, 161, 1991.
83. **Miller, J. P.,** Dyslipoproteinaemia of liver disease, *Bailliere's Clin. Endocrinol. Metabol.,* 4, 807, 1990.
84. **Yehuda, S. and Youdim, M. B. H.,** Brain iron deficiency: biochemistry and behaviour, in *Brain Iron (Topics in Neurochemistry and Neuropharmacology, Vol. 2),* Taylor & Francis, London, 1988, 89.

Part I
Chemistry and Molecular Biology of Iron
and Iron-Binding Proteins

1. Structure and Molecular Biology of Iron Binding Proteins and the Regulation of 'Free' Iron Pools

ROBERT R. CRICHTON and ROBERTA J. WARD

*Unité de Biochimie, Université Catholique de Louvain,
Louvain-la-Neuve, Belgium; and Department of Clinical Biochemistry,
King's College Medical School, London, U.K.*

I. INTRODUCTION

A. THE ESSENTIAL NATURE OF IRON

Although the essential nature of iron for normal cellular function is beyond doubt, our understanding of its metabolism within the cell in most regards is conspicuous by its absence. Only in the last two decades has its uptake and regulation via transferrin receptors (Tf receptors) been relatively well understood, while the identification of iron-responsive element binding proteins (IREBP) has occurred only in the last two to three years. The paucity of our understanding is illustrated by the fact that we do not know the mechanism of iron absorption across the gastrointestinal tract, which is of great importance in understanding the origins of both iron deficiency and iron overload.

B. IRON METABOLISM IN MAN

Humans, in common with other multicellular organisms, must obtain the iron they require for growth, maintenance, and cellular division from dietary sources. The situation of man with regard to iron at the global level is summarized in Figure 1. We absorb 1 to 2 mg of our dietary iron by a yet unidentified protein carrier and excrete roughly the same amount under normal conditions. This means that iron metabolism in man is essentially conservative. In this respect man distinguishes himself from all other mammals, in that a small shortfall in iron absorption over excretion can result in iron deficiency, while a small excedent in absorption over excretion can result in iron overload. That these are major causes for concern is reflected in recent statistics. On the basis of WHO (World Health Organization) criteria some 1.3 billion people, an estimated 30% of the world population, are anemic, of whom 500 to 600 million people suffer from iron deficiency. Among mammals man is the only species to manifest a parenchymal iron overload of sufficient importance to cause tissue damage. The homozygous state for hereditary (idiopathic) hemochromatosis may affect as many as 0.5% of the U.S. population, an incidence more than twice that of iron deficiency anemia among adult men, and may attain levels of up to 10% in some Northern European populations. Secondary iron overload associated with refractory or transfusion-dependent anemias, such as thalassemia major, is also widespread. It is estimated that over 100,000 individuals are born each year with thalassemic syndromes and are at risk from iron loading (reviewed in References 1 and 2).

C. THE CHEMISTRY OF IRON

Iron is involved in a great many biological functions. By varying the ligands to which it is coordinated, iron has access to a wide range of redox potentials and can participate in a wide range of electron transfer reactions, spanning the standard redox potential range from $+300$ to -500 mV. It is also involved in oxygen transport, activation, and detoxification, in nitrogen fixation, and in many of the reactions of photosynthesis.

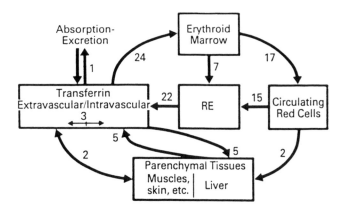

FIGURE 1. The amounts of iron (mg/day) exchanging between different body compartments in a 70-kg subjects. These data are largely based on ferrokinetic analyses. (From Bothwell, T. H., Charlton, R. W., Cook, J. D., and Finch, C. A., *Iron Metabolism in Man*, Blackwell Scientific, Edinburgh, 1979. With permission.)

In aqueous solution the two principal oxidation states of iron, ferrous Fe(II) and ferric Fe(III), exist respectively as the hydrated ions $Fe(H_2O)_6^{2+}$ and $Fe(H_2O)_6^{3+}$. In the absence of oxygen or other oxidants, ferrous salts give solutions of ferrous aqua ion $Fe(H_2O)_6^{2+}$. In contrast, between pH 5 and 9, ferric salts lose protons (hydrolyze) and polymerize precipitating hydrated ferric oxides. In biological media, as in natural waters, therefore, hydrated ferrous ions are real species, whereas except at low pH, hydrated ferric ions are rare. See Reference 3 for a more detailed account of the solution chemistry of iron in biological media.

D. THE NEED FOR IRON-BINDING PROTEINS (IBPs)

In light of the solubility problems of iron in biological mileu (with its inexorable tendency to hydrolyze and polymerize), it is not surprising that nature has evolved a number of iron-binding proteins (IBPs). These serve, on the one hand, to bind iron in a stable, soluble, and, where appropriate, cell-assimilable form, in the various iron transport proteins, or transferrins; within cells, in addition to iron present in a variety of hemoproteins, iron-sulfur proteins and non-heme, non-iron-sulfur iron containing enzymes, iron is stored in the iron storage proteins known respectively as ferritins and hemosiderins. Small amounts of iron not bound to IBP will be present in the cytosol of the cell to act as a reservoir to supply this essential element for incorporation into cytosolic enzymes and proteins. The nature of this pool (LMW Fe-pool) is unknown (see Section IV), but probably consists of both Fe^{2+} and Fe^{3+}. The presence of both ferric and ferrous forms of iron in the cytosol, possibly as ternary Fe(II)-O-Fe(III) complexes,[4] is an important pre-requisite for the initiation of lipid peroxidation. However, provided that the concentrations of such iron species in the cytosol are small and there are adequate antioxidants and cytoprotective enzymes available to scavenge any free radical species produced, propagation of these potentially damaging reactive oxygen species, especially hydroxyl radicals, will not be enhanced.

The hydroxyl radical can be produced from superoxide and peroxide, via the reactions described in Equations 1 and 2:

$$Fe(III) + O_2^{\cdot -} \rightarrow Fe(II) + O_2 \tag{1}$$

$$Fe(II) + H_2O_2 \rightarrow Fe(III) + OH^- + OH^{\cdot} \tag{2}$$

Superoxide and peroxide are, respectively, the products of reduction of dioxygen concomitant with oxidation of hydrated ferrous iron, and the dismutation of superoxide to yield hydrogen peroxide and molecular oxygen (Equations 3 and 4):

$$Fe(II)aq + O_2 \rightarrow Fe(III)aq + O_2^{\cdot -} \tag{3}$$

$$2O_2^{\cdot -} + 2H^+ \rightarrow H_2O_2 + O_2 \tag{4}$$

In the presence of "free" or "catalytic" iron, as indicated by Equation 1, ferric iron can be reduced by superoxide anion to give ferrous iron which, in the celebrated Fenton reaction (Equation 2), can react with hydrogen peroxide to give the extremely reactive hydroxyl radical. That free iron — whatever *that* may be — is involved in hydroxyl-radical-mediated oxidative damage now seems well established (reviewed in References 3 and 5), and this undoubtedly represents another pressing reason for keeping iron, whether within cells or in extracellular fluids, in a protein-bound form.

II. IBPs IN IRON TRANSPORT

A. TRANSFERRINS (Tf) — STRUCTURE AND MOLECULAR BIOLOGY

The physiological fluids of many vertebrates (and indeed of some nonvertebrate species, as the recent isolation and cloning of a transferrin from the sphinx moth *Manduca sexta* shows[6]) contain a class of iron-binding proteins collectively known as transferrins. Serotransferrin, as the name implies, is found in serum and in other extracellular secretions, whereas ovotransferrin and lactotransferrin are found respectively in egg white and in milk. Lactotransferrin is also found in tears and is secreted as part of the host defense mechanism by neutrophils during bacterial infection. All three of these transferrins were first discovered because of their antibacterial properties, contributing to defense of the mammalian cell against infection by depriving bacteria of iron. In contrast, a cell-surface glycoprotein present on most human melanomas does not appear to have such a function, but has been identified

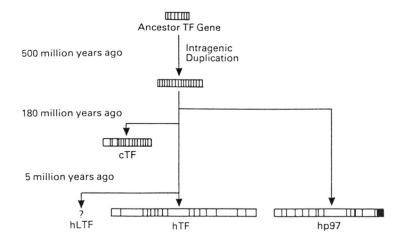

FIGURE 2. A scheme for the evolution of the genes encoding the transferrin family. The relative intron-exon lengths in the genes of chicken transferrin (cTF), human p97 (hp97), and human transferrin (hTF) are based on data discussed in the text. Exons and introns of the ancestor genes are not drawn to scale. The genomic structure for human lactoferrin (hLTF) is currently not known. (From Bowman, B. H., Yang, F., and Adrian, G. S., *Adv. Genet.*, 25, 1, 1988. With permission.)

as a member of the transferrin family by sequence homology and designated melanotransferrin.[7]

Mammalian transferrins consist of a single polypeptide chain of M_r around 80 kDa constituted from two very similar half molecules, disposed in space as two distinct lobes each capable of binding one atom of ferric iron together with a carbonate (or possibly bicarbonate) anion. The amino acid sequences of the two N- and C-terminal halves of vertebrate transferrin molecules, whether derived from direct protein sequencing or from cDNA studies, show extensive homologies and the exon-intron arrangements of the DNA are also homologous, (reviewed in References 3 and 8). This confirms that transferrins originated by a gene duplication event, which is thought to have occurred some 500 million years ago. Each transferrin gene contains 17 exons separated by 16 introns. During evolution of the transferrin family, elongation of the genes occurred, not only by intragenic duplication, but also by increases in the lengths of their introns (Figure 2). Thus, while the coding regions of ovotransferrin and human serotransferrin are both about the same length, 2.3 kb, the mammalian gene is 33.5 kb compared to only 10.5 kb for the chicken gene. This is due to the expansion of several introns in the mammalian transferrin gene. Of the 17 exons, 14 constitute 7 homologous pairs which code for corresponding regions in the N and C lobes of the protein. The first exon codes for a signal peptide, necessary for the secretion of the transferrin molecule, while the last two exons encode a sequence which is unique to the C-terminal lobe.

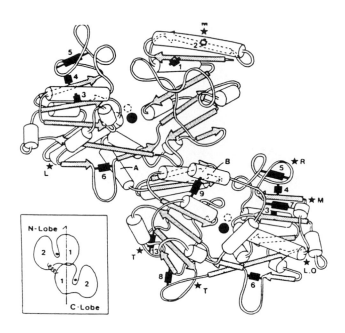

FIGURE 3. Schematic diagram of the complete human lactoferrin molecule. The positions of carbohydrate attachment are marked: O, ovotransferrin; T, human serotransferrin; L, human lactotransferrin; R, rabbit serotransferrin; M, melanotransferrin; A, the connecting helix; B, the C-terminal helix. The disulfide bridges are indicated by solid lines, and the iron- and bicarbonate- (or carbonate) binding sites are indicated by filled or open circles, respectively. (From Baker, E. N., Rumball, V., and Anderson, B. F., *TIBS*, 12, 350, 1987. With permission.)

We now turn to the three-dimensional structure of transferrins in order to better interpret the data presented above. The X-ray crystallographic studies of the diferric forms of human lactotransferrin,[9,10] rabbit serotransferrin,[11] and the apo-form of human lactotransferrin[12] have recently led to the determination of their structures at near to atomic resolution. As was suggested by earlier low-resolution data,[13] the transferrin molecule is bilobal, and closer examination reveals that both lobes have a remarkably similar peptide conformation (Figure 3), reflecting the sequence homology of the two halves of all vertebrate transferrin molecules and their origins from a gene duplication event. Indeed, the insect transferrin recently sequenced from *M. sexta* also shows evidence of gene duplication. The human lactotransferrin molecule has a general organization essentially the same as rabbit serotransferrin. Residues 1 to 333 constitute the N-terminal lobe and residues 345 to 691 the C-terminal lobe. They are connected by a three-turn α-helix, composed of residues 334 to 344, which is indicated as A in Figure 3. The two lobes have very similar structures, essentially constituted by a network of parallel and (occasionally) antiparallel β-sheets connected by α-helices with non-α-helical, non-β-sheet structures joining the two structural elements (Figures 3 and 4). This is con-

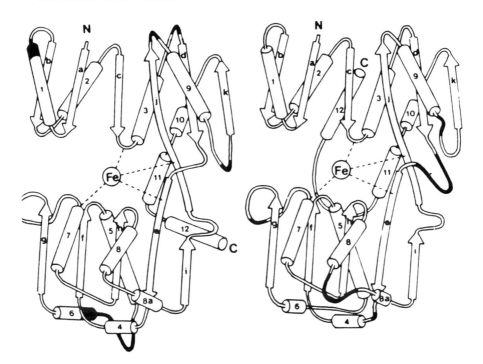

FIGURE 4. Schematic representation of the folding pattern for the N-lobe (top) and C-lobe (bottom) of human lactoferrin. Helices are shown as cylinders; b-strands as arrows. (From Anderson, B. F., Baker, H. M., Norris, G. E., Rice, D. W., and Baker, E. N., *J. Mol. Biol.*, 209, 711, 1989. With permission.)

sistent with their high degree of sequence homology (around 40% when their sequences are aligned and compared), with a small number of differences mostly localized in external loops. In Figure 3 the N lobe is on top and the C lobe below, with the twofold screw axis which relates them localized approximately in the plane of the paper. Disulfide bridges, six in the N and ten in the C lobe, are indicated as heavy bars, and glycosylation sites in lactotransferrin (one in each lobe designated L) by stars. The glycosylation sites in other transferrins are also indicated by stars with the appropriate letter: O — ovotransferrin, T — human serotransferrin, R — rabbit serotransferrin, M — melanotransferrin. Further (Figure 4), the two lobes can be subdivided into two domains, each of approximately 160 amino acid residues, which have a rather similar supersecondary structure consisting of a central core of five or six irregular twisted β-sheets of similar topology with helices packed on either side. The N-terminal β-sheet a is linked (Figure 4) by helix 1 to β-sheet b, which connects to helix 2 and continues through β-sheet c, helix 3, and β-sheet d. This ensemble constitutes the first part of domain 1. Then, a long β-sheet e crosses from the upper domain of the molecule (N 1 and C 1) to enter into the lower domain (N 2 and C 2) of the lobe. This domain is made up of some 160 residues, comprising in order, helix 4 β-sheet f, helices 5 and 6, β-sheet g, which leads after a variable turn into helix 7, through β-sheet h to terminate in helices 8 and 8a. The β-sheets i and j then traverse the lobe from the lower to the upper domains where domain 1 is completed by helix 9, β-sheet k, and helices 10 and 11. Helix 12 of the N-lobe then connects with the C lobe (indicated as A in Figure 3). In contrast, helix 12 in the C lobe is positioned in a quite different position with regard to helices 10 and 11. It is indicated by B in Figure 3, and contains the C terminus of the protein.

Thus, we can summarize the transferrin molecules as being derived from four closely similar domain structures which are organized into two lobes. Each lobe within the structure is constituted by two domains which are connected by two potentially flexible connections, the β-sheets e, i, and j, and the helices 10 and 11. As we will see shortly, this may allow movements of the two domains with respect to one another, resulting in opening and closing of an iron-binding cavity.

The two iron-binding sites in the lactotransferrin molecule are about 4.2 nm apart and are buried at the inner end of the deep interdomain cleft (Figure 3), with the iron atoms at least 1.0 nm from the exterior of the molecule. The coordination sphere of the iron atoms is the same for both lobes (Figure 5) and involves four ligands from the protein, namely one carboxylate oxygen, two phenolate oxygens, one imidazole nitrogen, and two bidentate oxygen ligands from the anion (carbonate or bicarbonate). The four protein ligands occupy four octahedral positions about the iron atom: in the N lobe, Asp 60 and Tyr 192 are *trans* to one another while Tyr 92 and His 253 occupy *cis* positions. In the C-lobe the corresponding residues are Asp 395, Tyr 528, Tyr 435, and His 597. The two remaining *cis*-octahedral positions are left vacant for the two nonprotein ligands. The protein ligands are widely spaced along the polypeptide backbone; Asp 60 is located in the main part of domain N 1, at the junction of β-sheet c and helix 3; Tyr 192 in domain N 2 at the N-terminal extremity of helix 7, pointing toward the middle of the cleft; Tyr 92 and His 253 come from the interconnecting backbone strands which cross between the two domains at the back of the iron site. Tyr 92 is at the beginning of β-sheet e, which crosses from domain N 1 to N 2 at the bottom of the cleft, while His 253 is situated in the middle of β-sheet j, which, with β-sheet j, again crosses the two domains this time from N 2 to N 1 (Figure 5). Unlike many other metal-binding proteins, the essential metal-binding ligands are distributed among several exons — for the N lobe His 61 is on exon 3, Tyr 93 on exon 4 (with Arg 121 and the N terminus of helix 5, both necessary for anion binding), Tyr 191 on exon 5, and His 252 on exon 7. This may reflect the fact that iron is not necessary for the correct folding of the apo-transferrin polypeptide chain, whereas in many other metal-binding proteins the metal-binding site may facilitate protein folding.

The anion site appears to involve most probably carbonate, which binds as a bidentate ligand to the iron atom, fitting perfectly between the iron atom,

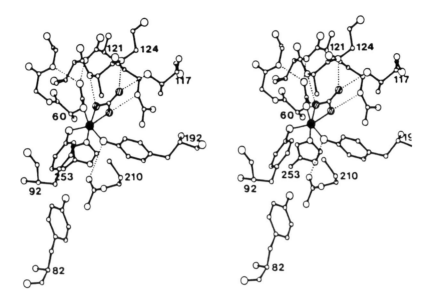

FIGURE 5. Stereo diagram of the metal and anion binding site in lactoferrin (shown for the N-lobe). The iron atom is shown by a filled circle; the CO_3^{2-} anion by hatched circles. Hydrogen bonds to the anion and the iron ligands are indicated by dotted lines. The nearby side-chains of Tyr 82 and Arg 210 are also shown. (From Anderson, B. F., Baker, H. M., Norris, G. E., Rice, D. W., and Baker, E. N., *J. Mol. Biol.*, 209, 711, 1989. With permission.)

the side chain of Arg 121, and the N terminus of helix 5, residues 121 to 136 (Figure 5). One oxygen is bound to iron and forms a hydrogen bond with Arg 121, the second also binds to iron and forms a hydrogen bond with the NH of residue 123, while the third oxygen makes two hydrogen bonds with NH(124) and the side chain of Thr 117. The importance of helix 5 in defining this anion-binding site in the pocket created by the side chain of Arg 121 and the main-chain atoms of residues 122 to 125 (and of the corresponding residues 465 to 469 in the C lobe) is underlined by its invariance in all transferrins so far sequenced (except the C lobe of melanotransferrin). Residues 121, 123, 124, and 125 are totally invariant in both halves of each transferrin, and 122 is always either Thr or Ser. The first turn of helix 5 is unusually wide with two π-type (1 to 6) hydrogen bonds (O121-N126 and O122-N127), and this may have functional importance in presenting the NH groups of the helix N terminus in the right geometry for anion binding.

The structure of human apolactotransferrin determined by X-ray diffraction[12] reveals interesting differences compared to the diferri-protein (Figure 6). Whereas the C lobe is still in its closed configuration, as in the iron-bound structure, the N lobe is in an open configuration, with the two domains largely separated one from the other. The N 2 domain has undergone a rotation of about 53° relative to the N 1 domain. This appears to involve

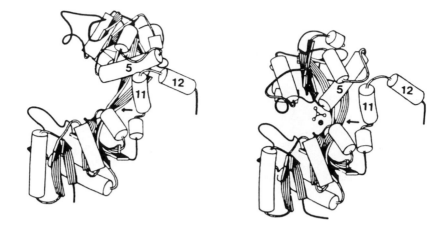

FIGURE 6. Schematic representation of the N-lobe polypeptide chain fold showing the conformational change between open (left) and closed (right) forms. An arrow marks the approximate hinge point in the two antiparallel b-strands (backbone strands) connecting the two domains. In the domain rotation, helix 5, which is an integral part of domain N2, pivots on helix 11, which remains associated with domain N1. Helix 12 is the connecting peptide to the C-lobe. Disulfide bridges may modify this conformational change in detail; in the C-lobe of lactoferrin (and other transferrins) the C-termini of helices 5 and 11 are joined; in serum transferrin the C-terminus of helix 5 is joined to the connecting peptide, which also differs structurally from that in lactoferrin. (From Anderson, B. F., Baker, H. M., Norris, G. E., Rumball, S. V., and Baker, E. N., *Nature,* 281, 157, 1979. With permission.)

mutual displacement (flexing) of the two antiparallel β-sheets which connect the two domains (e, i, and j), accompanied by the pivotal movement of helix 5 on helix 11, effectively moving the N 2 domain away from the N 1 domain (Figure 6). The open configuration of the binding cleft which is formed exposes three basic amino acid residues which were buried in the closed configuration, namely Arg 121, Arg 210, and Lys 301 (this latter is replaced by Asn in the C-lobe). If we assume, as seems likely from chemical and kinetic arguments,[14,15] that carbonate binds first, it would be attracted into the bottom of the open interdomain cleft by the positive charges on Arg 121 and Arg 210 (the latter near the end of β-sheet h, pointing into the bottom of the cleft), and bind to the N 2 domain at the N terminus of helix 5. Four of the iron-binding ligands are now in place (Tyr 92, Tyr 192, and the two carbonate oxygens), and the iron could then bind to the N 2 domain. Binding would be completed by rotation of N 2, closing the cleft with Asp 60 and His 253 completing the iron coordination and Asp 60 further linking the two domains by hydrogen bonding.[10] It was previously shown[9] that each lobe of lactotransferrin (and the other transferrins) bears a striking resemblance to the group of periplasmic binding proteins characterized by Quiocho and co-workers.[16] These proteins can exist in three structural forms — liganded closed, liganded open and unliganded open. A comparison of the N lobes of apolactotransferrin and iron-lactotransferrin indicates the same hinge-bending, ligand-induced conformational change as in the bacterial periplasmic binding proteins. In this respect lactotransferrin can be justifiably likened to a Venus fly trap. It is interesting to reflect that the transport of ferri-siderophores across the periplasmic space in bacteria is also assured by a periplasmic-binding protein (see above). Perhaps this is the bacterial equivalent of transferrin.

Binding of iron as Fe(III) to the N and C lobes of transferrin involves the release of three protons concomitant with the binding of the carbonate (or bicarbonate) ion. Thus, after iron and anion binding, the negative charge of the molecule increases by one unit for each atom bound.[17] The two iron-binding sites in human serotransferrin have an affinity for iron under physiological conditions of the order of 10^{22} M^{-1}; although the C-lobe site has a somewhat higher affinity than the N-lobe site, in serum it is the weaker and more acid-labile N-site which is predominantly occupied (reviewed in Reference 3).

Iron release from transferrin *in vitro* can be achieved by a number of means — the routine method for apotransferrin preparation involves dialysis at pH 5.5 in the presence of a chelator of Fe^{3+}. Spontaneous release of iron from transferrin at acidic pH is very slow in the absence of chelators. However, naturally occurring chelators such as amino acids, nucleotides, phosphoglycerates, low-molecular-weight iron binding proteins or other components of the low-molecular-weight iron pool could, under these circumstances, have high affinity for Fe^{3+}. Alternatively, reduction of acid-labile Fe(III) followed by its chelation (reviewed in Reference 3) could occur. However, diferric-transferrin has been shown incapable of promoting hydroxyl radical formation via the Haber-Weiss reaction *in vitro* under conditions found within the cell.[18] Although we know that the iron and anion-binding sites in human lactotransferrin and rabbit serotransferrin are identical for both lobes, this does not explain the significantly greater stability toward acidic pH of lactotransferrin compared to serotransferrin.

B. TRANSFERRIN RECEPTOR (TfR) — STRUCTURE AND MOLECULAR BIOLOGY

Iron uptake from transferrin by reticulocytes is abolished by trypsin,[19] suggesting the presence of a membrane receptor for transferrin. Further, studies with doubly labeled transferrin show that whereas the iron is rapidly removed from the circulation, transferrin protein recycles many times.[20] This led to the proposal[21] of a transferrin-to-cell cycle in which iron is released from transferrin and remains within the cell, while the protein part, apotransferrin, is released back into the circulation where it can go off in search of more iron. Where it finds this iron is not known.

The iron uptake of a great many mammalian cell types seems to be mediated by the transferrin receptor. It is present on virtually all dividing cells, suggesting that its expression is coordinated with cell proliferation, and specific anti-receptor monoclonal antibodies are employed in a standard procedure which uses transferrin receptor expression as a measure of the growth potential of tumors. The level of TfR seems to be the major factor in determining the rate of iron uptake during the development of erythroid cells. Further, the expression of TfR on cultured cells is regulated by the availability of iron. TfR expression increases two- to fivefold in the presence of desferrioxamine B, a permeable iron chelator, and decreases by the same order of magnitude in the presence of sources of exogenous iron such as hemin or ferric salts (reviewed in Reference 3). The concentration of transferrin in the circulation is 30 to 40 μM, with an iron saturation level in normal humans of 30% and the dissociation constant of the receptor for diferric transferrin typically 0.01 to 1 NM. Thus, there is always a saturating concentration of transferrin with regard to its receptor, and so if a particular cell wishes to increase its iron uptake, it must increase the number of transferrin receptors that it expresses — which is precisely what tumor cells do (reviewed in Reference 22).

The major structural features of the transferrin receptor, based on studies in human, mouse, rat, and chicken cells, are very similar (reviewed in Reference 3). They are all disulfide-linked dimers, consisting of two identical transmembrane subunits of some 760 amino acid residues with an apparent molecular weight of 95,000. A schematic representation of the human TfR is presented in Figure 7. The receptor, which lacks a cleavable signal peptide, is inserted into the membrane of the rough endoplasmic reticulum during its synthesis with the N-terminus facing the cytoplasm.[23] The N-terminal domain consists of 61 amino acid residues and can be phosphorylated by protein kinase C at residue Ser 24. The hydrophobic transmembrane region of 28 amino acid residues presumably contains the signal for translocation of the receptor across the membrane. It contains two cysteine residues. Cys 62, at the internal face of the cytoplasmic membrane, is acylated by a palmitate residue, whereas Cys 89, located at the external face of the membrane, is involved in an intersubunit disulphide bond with its corresponding homologue in the dimer, as is Cys 98 in the external domain. Acylation of the TfR is not necessary for rapid internalization nor for iron uptake.[24] The external domain of 671 residues can be isolated almost intact by trypsin digestion as a 70 kDa fragment which is not disulphide bridged but can still bind transferrin and antireceptor antibodies. A soluble tryptic fragment of human TfR (residues 121 to 760) has recently been crystallized: it retains the transferrin-binding activity of the intact receptor, and, although lacking the intermolecular disulfide bonds, the receptor fragment is dimeric both under physiological conditions and at the high salt concentrations used for crystallization.[25] A structure determination is in progress. The intermolecular disulfide bonds do not appear to be required for the expression of the dimeric state nor for the functional activity of the human TfR.[26] The external domain is N-glycosylated

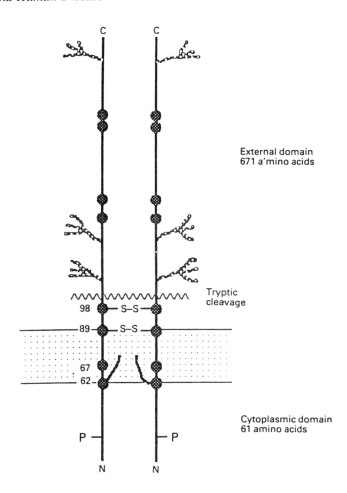

FIGURE 7. Schematic representation of the human transferrin receptor. Shown are the position of the eight cysteine residues (●) and the three potential N-linked glycosylation sites in each peptide chain. The intermolecular disulfide bonds between cysteines 89 and 98 of the two subunits are also indicated, as is the localization of the fatty acid chain on cysteine 62 and the position at which the cytoplasmic domain can be phosphorylated. (From Trowbridge, I. S. and Shackelford, D. E., *Biochem. Soc. Symp.*, 51, 117, 1986. With permission.)

by complex-type oligosaccharides at Asn 251 and 317, and by a high mannose-type glycan at Asn 727. Inhibition of N-glycosylation of the human TfR blocks the translocation of the receptor to the plasma membrane, interferes with the formation of disulphide-bound dimers, and prevents transferrin binding.[27] In contrast, neither the absence of N-glycosylation nor modification of the N-glycan structures of the murine TfR significantly affects dimer formation or its ability to bind transferrin.[28]

Functional studies of mutant receptors have established that the cytoplasmic tails of a number of different receptors contain the structural deter-

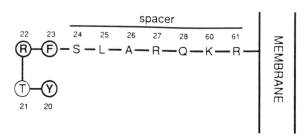

FIGURE 8. Schematic representation of the structural and chemical requirements for efficient endocytosis. The tetrapeptide forming the proposed tight turn is shown inside a stippled rectangle. The spacer region must be a minimum of seven residues. (From Collawn, J. F., Stangel, M., Kuhn, L. A., Esekogwu, V., Jing, S., Trowbridge, I. S., and Tainer, J. A., *Cell,* 63, 1061, 1990. With permission.)

minants required for clustering in coated pits (reviewed in Reference 29). Deletion of 57 of the 61 residues (3 to 59) results in a tenfold reduction of internalization efficiency compared to the wild-type receptor. Further, the recognition signal for rapid endocytosis of human TfR was localized to a 10-residue region (residues 19 to 28) of the cytoplasmic domain and Ty20 was identified as an important element of the signal.[30] From functional studies on 24 human TfR mutants the internalization signal was identified as YXRF, and it was shown that this tetrapeptide must be separated from the transmembrane region by at least 7 residues.[29] Computational analyses showed that most of the tetrapeptide sequences in proteins of known three-dimensional structures which were closely similar to either YXRF or NPXY, the corresponding tetrapeptide motif related to internalization of the low density lipoprotein receptor, significantly favored tight turns similar to a type-1 turn (Figure 8). The internalization sequences of both receptors contain aromatic residues with intervening hydrogen bonding residues. The implication seems clear that an exposed tight turn is the recognition motif for high efficiency endocytosis.

The transferrin-to-cell cycle has been well established in erythroid cells and in many transformed cell lines and involves receptor-mediated endocytosis of transferrin, iron release from transferrin within the cell, and recycling of the apotransferrin-TfR complex back to the plasma membrane where the apotransferrin is released into the extracellular medium. In the initial stages, the transferrin-to-cell cycle follows the general pathway of receptor-mediated uptake of extracellular ligands by endocytosis (reviewed in Reference 31). As we pointed out earlier, all growing cells contain surface transferrin receptors which bind ferritransferrin with high affinity ($K_M = 6 \times 10^{-9} M$) at neutral pH. Once the transferrin has bound to its receptor the Tf-TfR complexes accumulate in clathrin-coated pits, which, within 1 to 2 min pinch off from the outer surface of the cell to be internalized as clathrin-coated vesicles. These vesicles lose their clathrin coats after endocytosis in a process that requires hydrolysis of ATP to ADP and P_i, forming smooth-surfaced vesicles called endosomes. The endosome then fuses with an uncoupling vesicle, called the compartment of uncoupling of receptor and ligand (CURL), which is characterized by an internal pH of around 5.0. For most ligands, such as low-density lipoproteins, asialoglycoproteins, and insulin, the acidic pH causes the dissociation of the ligand from its receptor. The free receptors congregate in one membrane section of the uncoupling vesicle, which ultimately buds off to form a separate elongated vesicle in which the receptors are recycled back to the plasma membrane, where they may function in further cycles of ligand binding. In contrast, the ligand is segregated into a different type of vesicle which ends up by fusing with a lysosome, wherein the ligand is degraded by lysosomal hydrolases. However, in the transferrin receptor-mediated endocytosis (in contrast) we know from the early double labeling experiments[20] that, whereas the two bound Fe^{3+} atoms remain within the cell, the apotransferrin molecule is secreted from the cell within minutes to go off in the circulation in search of more iron. The properties of the receptor-ligand complex which explain the difference between other endocytosed ligands and transferrin reside in the affinities of transferrin and apotransferrin for the transferrin receptor as a function of pH. Within the acidic environment of the endosome or CURL, it is assumed that iron is released from ferritransferrin (we discuss the possible mechanisms shortly). The apotransferrin thus formed retains a high affinity for the transferrin receptor ($K_M = 6 \times 10^{-9} M$) at pH 5.0 and remains bound to the receptor. While the iron remains in the endocytic vesicle or in the CURL, and is subsequently transported into the cytoplasm, the apotransferrin remains bound to the transferrin receptor at the pH of these vesicles and, when the transferrin receptor is recycled back to the surface of the cell, the apotransferrin remains bound. Although apotransferrin binds tightly to its receptor at pH 5.0, at neutral pH it binds only weakly. Thus, when the recycling vesicles fuse with the plasma membrane and the receptor-ligand complex encounters the neutral or slightly alkaline pH of the extracellular fluid or of the growth medium, the apotransferrin dissociates from its receptor to go off in search of iron, liberating the receptor to bind another molecule of ferritransferrin. The transferrin-to-cell cycle is outlined in Figure 9.

We may now pose the question of the mechanism of iron release from ferritransferrin, which we assume takes place in the endosome or CURL at a pH value of 5.0 to 5.5. We know from *in vitro* studies that the rate of spontaneous dissociation of iron from transferrin at this pH is much too slow to account for the observed rate of iron release, suggesting that some other factors such as chelation and/or reduction are necessary to ensure that iron is effectively released during the relatively short dwell time that the ferritransferrin molecule remains within the endosome/CURL (a matter of a few minutes at most). Recent *in vitro* results indicate that iron release from ferritransferrin at mildly acidic pH values (5.6 to 6.0) is substantially increased when it is bound to its receptor compared to release from free ferritransferrin,[32,33] suggesting that within the endosome/CURL the transferrin receptor facilitates iron release from transferrin. It has been further suggested that by considering

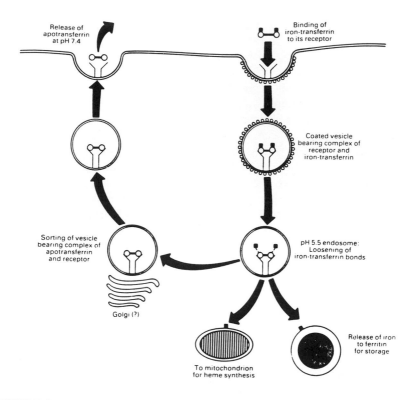

FIGURE 9. The receptor-mediated transferrin-to-cell cycle in iron metabolism. (From Theil, E. C. and Aisen, P., *Iron Transport in Microbes, Plants and Animals*, VCH Publishers, Weinheim, Germany, 1987, 491. With permission.)

slowing iron release from transferrin at extracellular pH[32] the receptor could minimize non-specific release of iron from transferrin at the cell surface. It has also been argued recently, from studies on preparations of endocytic vesicles from reticulocytes enriched in transferrin-transferrin receptor complexes, that an NADH-ferricyanide reductase activity might be involved in iron release from ferritransferrin.[34] The authors propose, in addition, a translocation system that would move Fe(II) to the *trans* side of the vesicular membrane, and which would subsequently deliver the reduced iron to the low-molecular-weight iron pool. A similar NADH-ferricyanide reductase system has been proposed to be involved in the release of transferrin iron at the plasma membrane,[35] although its precise relevance to cellular iron uptake remains controversial.[36,37] All of these possibilities are summarized in Figure 10.

It has been suggested that mechanisms other than the transferrin/transferrin receptor cell cycle described above might be involved in iron uptake by mammalian cells. As was pointed out above, the Tf/TfR cycle seems to be the major if not only pathway of iron uptake by human erythroid cells and by many human tumor cell lines in culture. However, the case of the hepatocyte is particularly controversial (reviewed in Reference 38). The number

Iron Metabolism in Iron-Loaded Cells

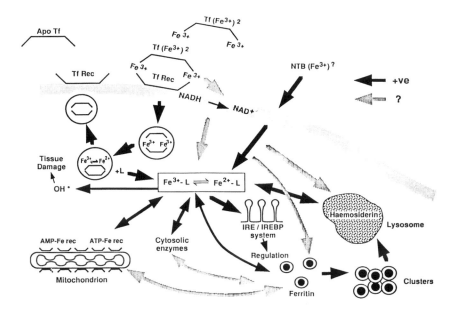

FIGURE 10. Iron metabolism in iron-loaded cells. Abbreviations: Tf-Fe$_2^{3+}$, Diferric transferrin; Tf-Rec, Transferrin receptor; Apo-Tf, Apoferritin; NTB(Fe^{3+}), nontransferrin bound serum iron; IRE/IRE-BP system, Iron regulatory elements (in ferritin, transferrin receptor, and 5-aminolevulinate synthase regulation): IRE-BP-IRE-binding protein, NADPH→NADP+ in plasma membrane NAD(P)H - ferricyanide reductase activity. Black arrows represent well-established pathways; gray arrows more speculative pathways.

of transferrin receptors on hepatocyte plasma membranes is relatively small, and *in vitro* studies show that at 37°C cellular uptake of iron increases continuously when the extracellular concentration of transferrin is increased to levels far above that needed to saturate hepatocyte TfR receptors. It has been concluded that adsorptive or fluid phase endocytosis is the main pathway of hepatocyte iron uptake from transferrin (although no evidence was found for the release of degradation products of transferrin into the extracellular medium). This might be due to fusion of pinocytic vesicles containing transferrin with endocytic vesicles containing unoccupied transferrin receptors,[39] which would ensure that the apotransferrin-transferrin receptor complex escapes lysosomal degradation by virtue of its high affinity and that the apotransferrin is then returned intact to the plasma membrane. The uptake of iron by hepatocytes from nontransferrin sources, particularly in iron overload, where the iron-binding capacity of serotransferrin is saturated, is briefly discussed later (see Section IV), but it is clear from *in vitro* studies that hepatocytes take up iron from, for example, ferric citrate much better than they do from ferric transferrin. However, we must emphasize that results from *in vitro* studies on rat hepatocyte cultures do not necessarily reflect the situation *in vivo* in the human liver. It can be reasonably concluded that in normal human subjects with a transferrin saturation level of 30%, uptake of iron from non-transferrin forms is unlikely to play an important role. An interesting exception to this premise (again from *in vitro* studies) is furnished by the results of Aisen et al.,[40,41] which indicate that iron taken up by hepatic Kupffer cells from effete erythrocytes can be released from the Kupffer cells as ferritin into the extracellular medium. Thereafter, the iron present in this neosynthesized Kupffer cell ferritin can either be transferred to apotransferrin or, alternatively, be assimilated by hepatocytes if they are co-cultured with the Kupffer cells via a specific receptor. In the latter case, the ferritin is internalized by the hepatocytes and follows the endocytic pathway to the CURL and thence to the lysosomal compartment where the protein is degraded and the iron released, either for incorporation into lysosomal hemosiderin or into the cytosolic ferritin pool. Whereas the rate of ferritin endocytosis is modest compared with that of transferrin, the amount of iron delivered per protein molecule (the Kupffer cell ferritin contains about 2500 atoms of iron per molecule compared with the two ferric iron atoms per transferrin molecule) by ferritin is at least one if not two orders of magnitude greater than that delivered by transferrin. Once again, we are in the realm of speculation between what can be observed in an *in vitro* situation (co-culture of hepatocytes and iron-loaded Kupffer cells) and what is actually taking place in the human liver *in vivo*.

The important question of regulation of the expression of the transferrin receptor will be dealt with later in Section III.B.

III. IBPs IN IRON STORAGE

A. FERRITIN

Inside the cell, iron is stored in two major components: ferritin, which is a soluble protein located in the cytosol, and hemosiderin, which is a water-insoluble storage form found essentially in the lysosomes. In normal humans it seems probable that there is some ferritin in every cell in the body, with the largest amounts in the liver parenchyma and the bulk of the remainder divided between the muscle mass and reticuloendothelial cells.[42] During normal iron metabolism the liver contains 95% of the total hepatic ferritin, which is located to the parenchymal cell, while hemosiderin, if present, is visible by electron microscopy in the Kupffer cells.

Ferritin is a molecule of considerable heterogeneity — it consists of a hollow protein shell of about 13 nm diameter composed of 24 subunits each of M_r around 20 kDa which enclose a cavity of about 7 nm diameter. Iron is deposited within this cavity in amounts which vary from zero to a maximum of 4500 atoms of iron (III) in a hydrolyzed and polymerized form, which in normal human ferritin resembles the mineral phase known as ferrihydrite. The structure of this product of biomineralization is represented in Figure 11.

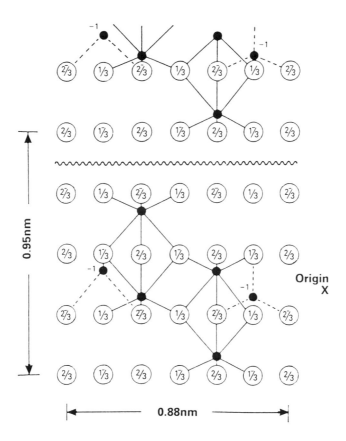

FIGURE 11. The structure of ferrihydrite (after Towe and Bradley, 1967). The figure shows an idealized detail of four Fe octahedra with fragments of adjacent units. Full circles are Fe in (1120) and one level below. Open circles are oxygens above and below (1120) as indicated. The wavy line indicates a level at which lateral displacements are optional. This level accommodates additional Fe^{3+} or protons. The *c*-period consists of only four oxygen layers. (From St. Pierre, T. G., Webb, J., and Mann, S., *Biomineralisation*, VCH Publishers, Weinheim, Germany, 1989, 295. With permission.)

The ferrihydrite core structure of human and other mammalian ferritins can perhaps best be described as a hydrous ferric oxide containing small amounts of phosphate with a semi-random structure. The mineral in well-ordered cores gives X-ray and electron diffraction patterns similar to ferri-hydrite, although the crystallinity of ferritin cores can differ widely from molecule to molecule. Some have well-ordered single crystals that occupy much of the internal cavity, whereas others contain mixtures of small crystals and poorly crystalline or amorphous regions. Ferrihydrite has the composition $5Fe_2O_3.9H_2O$,[43] and the electron diffraction data indicate that many mammalian ferritins have similar interplanar D-spacings to ferrihdrite (reviewed in Reference 44).

Human ferritins are not only heterogenous with respect to their iron content, but also with respect to the subunit composition of their protein shell. Thus, different tissue ferritins have a content of L subunits (M_r around 20 kDa) and H subunits (M_r around 22 kDa) which vary from tissue to tissue: ferritins from human liver and spleen have a higher content of the L subunit, whereas ferritins from heart, for example, have an increased content in H subunits. They are all heteropolymers of variable composition ranging in principle from $L_{24}H_0$ to L_0H_{24} with all of the other 23 combinations present in proportions that correspond to the preponderence of one or the other subunit type in the tissue in question. It is as if nature had constructed a set of variations based upon two themes, both of which have the same (or almost the same) three-dimensional architecture, but with salient features which are particular to each of the individual subunit types. Without indulging in a reflection as to what Bach or Vivaldi could have done with such a melodic line so rich in inherent variations, we can suggest that the juxaposition of two such similar tertiary structural building blocks in the quaternary structure of the apoferritin molecule in variable proportions would have had considerable effects on the biochemical and metabolic properties of the heteropolymers that resulted.

Figure 12 presents the amino acid sequences of human H and L subunits. They show about 55% identity, whereas H subunits from different species are much more similar (greater than 90% identity), as are L subunits from different species (greater than 80% identity). For a more detailed discussion of the differences between these two subunit classes from different species see Reference 3. Although the figure underlines the differences in amino acid sequence, the reality at the level of the three-dimensional structure of the individual H and L subunits within the 24-subunit shell of human, horse and, rat apoferritin indicates a much greater similarity of the tertiary fold of the individual subunits within the apoferritin molecule.

Horse spleen apoferritin crystallizes in a face-centered cubic form in the space group F 432, with $a = 18.4$ nm containing four molecules per unit cell.[45] The three-dimensional structures of horse spleen apoferritin (nearly 90% L) rat liver apoferritin (66% L) recombinant L-chain apoferritin (100% L) and recombinant human H-chain apoferritin (100% H) have been determined at atomic resolution by Harrison et al. at the University of Sheffield (reviewed in Reference 46). We shall consider here the structure of horse spleen apoferritin; the structure of human apoferritins, whether of H or L subunit composition, are essentially similar, and the subtle differences between the different apoferritins will be commented on later.

The apoferritin subunit contains 174 amino acid residues of which 129 are found in 5 α-helices. These are organized in a parallel/antiparallel α-helix bundle of four long α-helices A to D, together with a shorter helix E. (Figure 13 presents the subunit conformation of horse spleen apoferritin.) The helical bundle has obvious structural similarities with a number of other proteins, including hemerythrin, cytochrome b_{562}, cytochrome c', tobacco mosaic virus protein, uteroglobin, and cytochrome b_5.

```
         1    5    10        20        30        40
HuL    SSQIRQNYSTEVDAAVNSLVNLYLQASYTYLSLGFYFDRD
HuH    T--V----HQDSE--I-RQI--E-Y---V---MSY-----
```

```
         41        50        60        70        80
Hul    DVALEGVSHFFRELAEEKREGYERLLKMQNQRGGRALFQD
HuH    ----KNFAKY-LHQSH-E--HA-K-M-L-------IFL--
```

```
         81        90        100       110       120
HuL    IKKPAEDEWGKTPDAMKAA MALEKKLNQALLDLHALGSAR
HuH    ----DC-D-ESGLN--EC-LH---NV--S--E--K-ATDK
```

```
         121       130       140       150       160
HuL    TDPHLCDFLETHFLDEEVKLIKKMGDHLTNLHRLGGPEAG
HuH    N-------I---Y-N-Q--A--EL---V---RKM-A--S-
```

```
         161       170 174 178
HuL    LGEYLFERLTLKHD
HuH    -A----DKH--GDSDNES
```

HuH   N-terminal TTAS not shown

FIGURE 12. Amino acid sequences of human L and H ferritins. Where the sequence is identical, a continuous line is indicated.

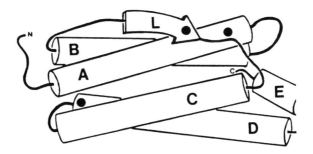

FIGURE 13. Subunit conformation of horse spleen apoferritin, showing four long helices A, B, C, D (cylinders), a short helix E and a long loop L. Helices correspond to sequence numbers: A, 9 to 39; B, 44 to 73; C, 91 to 121; D, 122 to 154; E, 158 to 172, and loop, L, 74 to 90 inclusive. Genomic exons correspond to residues 1 to 33, 34 to 82, 83 to 124, and 125 to 174. Intron positions are indicated by filled circles (between residues 33 to 34, 82 to 83, and 124 to 125). (From Harrison, P. M., Artymiuk, P. J., Ford, G. C., et al., *Biomineralization,* VCH Publishers, Weinheim, Germany, 1989, 258. With permission.)

The 8 N-terminal residues of the protein project toward the outside of the protein shell (this is extended by 4 residues in human H apoferritin) and then form an α-helix A which runs from residue 9 to 39 along the outer surface of the cylindrical subunit structure. A short turn (residues 40 to 43) leads into helix B (residues 44 to 73), which is disposed on the inner surface of the helical bundle, turned toward the internal cavity of the protein shell. The polypeptide chain then crosses from the interior of the molecule to the exterior via the loop L, composed of residues 74 to 90, which includes a short β-sheet structure: this β-sheet is involved in a hydrogen-bonded interaction with the corresponding β-sheet of the L loop of a neighboring subunit to form an antiparallel β-structure at the external surface of the protein shell. The helix C, like the helix A, is again at the surface of the protein shell, (residues 91 to 121) and helix D (residues 122 to 154) returns toward the interior of the protein where with helix B it forms the internal surface of the protein shell. It is noteworthy that both helix B and D have a high content of polar amino acids (see the sequences in Figure 12), including both carboxylate functions, which may participate in iron binding and oxidation and positively charged Lys and Arg residues, which may interact with the phosphate found in the micellar cores of mammalian ferritins. The D helix extends a little beyond the four α-helical bundle, culminating in a short turn (residues 155 to 157) leading to the final helix E (residues 158 to 172) which lies almost perpendicular to the principal helix bundle. The C-terminal dipeptide (hexapeptide in human H ferritin) projects into the internal cavity of the protein shell.

The folded subunits form a very stable and compact quaternary structure which is illustrated in Figure 14. The association of pairs of subunits enables the formation of many intersubunit contacts along their long surface involving both hydrophobic and electrostatic interactions. Toward the opposite ends of the helical bundle of the subunits two types of intersubunit spaces develop, corresponding respectively to the threefold and fourfold axes of symmetry. These intersubunit spaces pass through the protein shell forming channels 0.3 to 0.4 nm wide. Figure 14a and b show a view of the apoferritin molecule down the threefold and fourfold axes, respectively. The long extended loops L lie on the outside of the protein shell and interact in antiparallel fashion in pairs. One hydrophilic side of the 4-helical bundle lies on the outside of the shell, while the other side faces inside, giving the inside surface of the protein shell a high concentration of polar residues, as mentioned earlier. Along the A helices, on one edge of the bundle, there are a number of hydrophobic residues which come together with the hydrophobic residues of the corresponding antiparallel neighbor in the subunit dimer A', as well as the inward-pointing residues of the loops L and L'. Not only is the formation of this apolar interface a powerful driving force in shell assembly, it also prevents the B helices which lie on the cavity surface from approaching closely to one another, such that there are relatively few interactions between them and that

a)

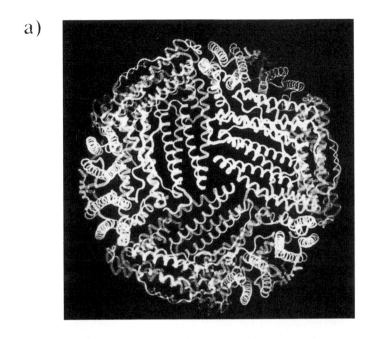

b)

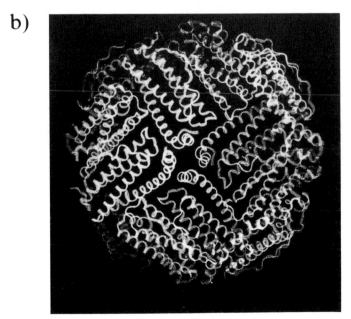

FIGURE 14. Computer-graphics representation of the horse spleen apoferritin structure viewed approximately down the threefold and fourfold axes, respectively. (From Harrison, P. M., Artymiuk, P. J., Ford, G. C., et al., *Biomineralisation,* VCH Publishers, Weinheim, Germany, 1989, 258. With permission.)

a groove is formed which has both the space and the electron density for water, two metal ions, and possibly other small molecules. For a more detailed analysis of apoferritin three-dimensional structure see References 3 and 47.

The dimer is the first assembly intermediate found in cross-linking and self-assembly experiments[48,49] and appears to be followed by trimers, transient hexamers, and dodecamers before formation of the intact tetracosamer. The intact apoferritin molecule is approximately spherical, but its basic architecture can best be represented by a rhombic dodecahedron. The 12 dimers, composed of pairs of antiparallel subunits, each lie on 1 of the 12 rhomb faces of the dedecahedron related by a twofold symmetry axis perpendicular to that face and passing through its center. At six apices of the rhombic dodecahedron the protein subunits are related by fourfold symmetry, while at another eight apices they are related by threefold symmetry. Many of the subunit-subunit interactions, including hydrogen bonds, salt bridges, and hydrophobic interactions which stabilize both the complete shell as well as its intermediates are conserved, or conservatively replaced when H and L subunits are compared: this probably explains the formation of heteropolymers. A notable exception is the salt bridge between Lys-58 and Glu-103 within the L subunit, which is absent in the H subunit (where Lys 58 is replaced by Glu). This no doubt explains, at least in part, why L-rich ferritins are more thermostable than H-rich ferritins. The oligomeric apoferritin structure is not only compact, but is extremely stable — horse spleen apoferritin resists temperatures of 80°C or more, is stable in $10\,M$ urea, does not dissociate into subunits between pH 3 to 11, and even resists $7\,M$ guanidine at pH values above 6.

The apoferritin shell formed in human cells is then an amalgam of the two subunits H and L in variable proportions in different tissues. We now concentrate our attention on the way in which these heteropolymers can influence the role of ferritin with the cell. The fundamental role of ferritin is to assimilate iron and to prevent it from either becoming inaccessible by hydrolysis, polymerization and precipitation, or to become ''aggressive'' as a ''LMW-Fe pool'' (see below). So we could consider ferritin as a soluble, nontoxic yet bio-available form of iron. We can then pose two questions of major importance — how is iron deposited in ferritin, and how is it mobilized from ferritin?

However, before addressing either of these two questions we should first consider how iron might pass from the outside of the protein shell to the inside and vice versa. The ports of entry of iron would seem most likely to involve one or other of the channels lying on the molecular threefold and fourfold symmetry axes. The channels in question are illustrated in Figure 15. The threefold channel (Figure 15a) is funnel-shaped, wider at the outside of the molecule and then narrowing to a passage 0.34 nm wide and 0.6 nm long. The amino acids which either line these channels or are neighbors are near one end of the subunit, including the C terminus of the C helix, the sharp CD turn, and the N terminus of the D helix. In L subunits these residues

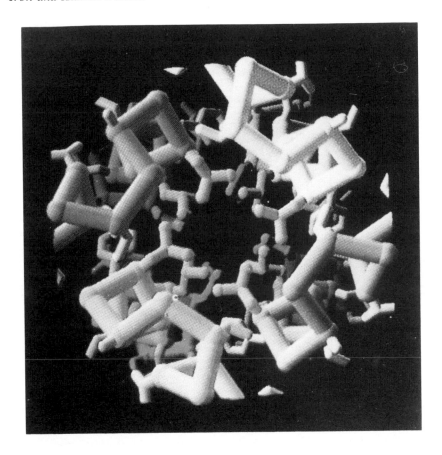

A

FIGURE 15. (A) Solid model of the fourfold channel region of an apoferritin molecule; (B) Solid model of the threefold channel region of an apoferritin molecule. (From Harrison, P. M., Artymiuk, P. J., Ford, G. C., et al., *Biomineralisation,* VCH Publishers, Weinheim, Germany, 1989, 258. With permission.)

(113 to 133) are highly conserved (only three positions containing substitutions). The same is true for residues 113 to 133 in H subunits, but when H and L chains are compared there are nine positions of substitution. The narrow region toward the interior of the channel is highly conserved in all species, with three glutamate carboxylates toward the outside and three aspartate carboxylates toward the inside. The threefold channels are hydrophilic in this narrow region and quite extensively hydrophilic at the wide external end of the funnel-like channel.

The fourfold channels are quite different. The channel is essentially constituted in horse spleen apoferritin by the E helix plus the C-terminal dipeptide (residues 158 to 174). It is 0.3 to 0.4 nm wide and about 1.25 nm long and,

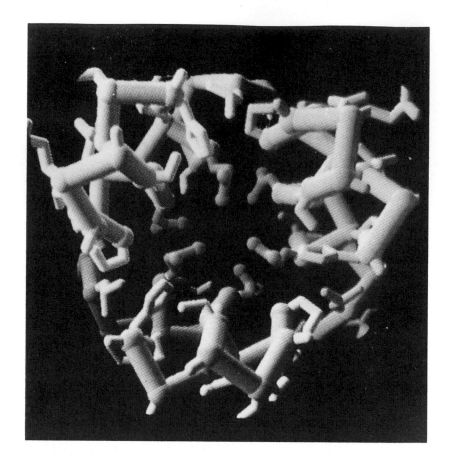

FIGURE 15B.

as in most L chain ferritins, it is lined by 12 leucine residues, Leu 161, Leu 165, and Leu 169 from each of the 4 subunits which form this apex of the rhombic dodecahedron. The inner end of the channel, at the C terminus of the subunit is hydrophilic — Lys-His-Asp, the latter two residues being disordered in the crystal structure. The entire channel region is conserved in most L subunit sequences. Although human H conserves Leu 161, most other H subunit have the rather conservative replacement Met 161, which maintains the hydrophobic nature of the channel, as does the retention of Leu 165 in all H subunits. However, Leu 169 is replaced by His in almost all H subunits, most often preceded by the sequence Asp 167-Lys 168 (Glu 167-Arg 168 in L subunits). In human H subunits the C-terminal sequence is longer, extends farther into the protein shell, and terminates with the quite hydrophilic sequence Gly-Asp-Ser-Asp-Asn-Glu-Ser. In view of the rather hydrophobic nature of the fourfold channel (His 169 notwithstanding in H subunits) it would seem to represent a formidable obstacle to the entry of charged metal ions of high-charge density, but perhaps not to metal ions surrounded by a hydration shell, nor to metal ions bound to neutral chelators.

The hydrophilic threefold channels and the hydrophobic fourfold channels remain the most obvious ways for iron to enter or leave the ferritin protein shell. The recent X-ray structure of human H ferritin[46] suggests that there may be a third possibility. In the human H subunit a Connolly surface representation (an indication of the molecular surfaces accessible to a spherical probe size set at 0.1 nm) shows the presence of a 0.1-nm channel leading through the 4-helix bundle from the outside surface of the protein through the subunit to the cavity surface on the inside by way of a metal binding site. This metal binding site is proposed as the ferroxidase center of the H-subunit (discussed in more detail below) and is located 1.0 to 1.2 nm from the outside surface of the protein and 0.7 to 0.8 nm from the inside. These channels could perhaps provide a means of access from the outside of the molecule for iron and dioxygen. The channel is blocked in L ferritin subunits by the salt bridge Lys 58-Glu 103.

In all of these discussions concerning access to the interior of the ferritin molecule there is one troubling aspect. Although none of the channels we have described above have a diameter greater than 0.4 nm, it is clear from X-ray and neutron scattering studies in solution that sugars and other small molecules of considerably larger diameter (0.7 to 1.0 nm) can penetrate into the interior of the protein shell.[50,51] In the crystalline state a large number of heavy metal salts can penetrate into the interior of the protein shell where they can be localized to the interior surface by X-ray crystallography (reviewed in Reference 47). This illustrates, as we have pointed out before, that even sleeping giants must breathe and should serve as a salutory reminder that crystallographic structures are not cast in blocks of granite descended with reverence from the mountain of "Absolute Truth", but are snapshots of the average conformation of a protein molecule reposing in a local free-energy minimum.

The process of ferrihydrate mineralization must take place within the protein shell and not outside of it, otherwise the mineral will precipitate. The protein must provide a means of easy access to the interior of the protein shell for either the ferrous aqua ion $Fe(H_2O)_6^{2+}$ or eventually for some liganded form of Fe^{2+} or Fe^{3+}. It must provide an internal surface which can catalyze the growth of the iron core, and in view of the evidence that the initial phase of iron deposition requires divalent iron, the protein must also possess a catalytic center for Fe(II) oxidation. The formation of the iron core of ferritin can be initiated when Fe^{2+} is added to apoferritin in the presence of an appropriate oxidant such as molecular oxygen. Thereafter, the role of the protein seems to be to provide a surface, at the interior of the protein shell, which supplies ligands that can partially coordinate iron (and perhaps catalyze its oxidation), but which leaves some coordination spheres available for mineral-phase anions. This allows biomineralization to proceed with the formation of one or more polynuclear ferrihydrite crystallites. The role of the protein increasingly becomes that of a template on which the insoluble fer-rihydrite mineral phase can grow, maintained in solution within the confines of the soluble apoferritin protein shell.

The initial phase of iron deposition, at least as far as *in vitro* studies go, seems to involve uptake of Fe(II) by apoferritin, followed by the binding of Fe(II) to specific sites on the protein, and its subsequent oxidation, catalyzed in the initial phase by the protein. As we pointed out some considerable time ago (reviewed in Reference 52) the kinetics plead in favor of this initial phase being at least second order with regard to iron concentration, and a model was developed involving the sequence of events presented in what follows. The initial binding site for Fe(II) was assumed to be at a binuclear site where two ferrous ions would be bound: then, molecular oxygen would bind between the two iron atoms forming what is formally a diferric-peroxo complex. This complex would then be converted to two diferric-μ-oxo complexes which would hydrolyze to form FeO·OH with concomitant proton release (reviewed in Reference 52). As has been recently pointed out:[53] "That the process of iron oxidation in apoferritin involves a binuclear center bridging two poly-peptide chains has already been proposed from kinetic studies."

We can now consider the questions that we posed before. (i) What is the likely port of entry for iron to gain access to the interior of the protein? It appears likely that the hydrophilic threefold channels play this role (reviewed in Reference 3). Although many studies concur in underlining the potential role of the threefold channels as the sites of entry of iron into the interior of the protein shell (for a recent discussion see Reference 54), it is unlikely that these are the sites of iron oxidation. Further, site-directed mutagenesis of one or both of the three glutamates and aspartates of the threefold channels to histidine or alanine[55] does not prevent formation of the initial Fe(II) apoferritin complex nor of the iron-core ferrihydrite, although they form at somewhat reduced rates. The conclusion is that the glutamates and aspartates of the threefold channel are neither required for iron entry nor for iron-core nu-cleation. (ii) Where is the Fe(II) oxidized, i.e., are there specific ferroxidase sites within the apoferritin molecule? The polemic on this subject has been sparked recently by the identification of a "ferroxidase" site in human H ferritin, which communicates both with the outside and the inside of the protein shell via 0.1-nm-large channels: this ferroxidase site comprises the amino acid residues Glu 23, Glu 58, and His 61 and Glu 103,[46] and is replaced in L subunit ferritins by a salt bridge between Lys 58 (replacing Glu 58) and Glu 103. Mutation of Glu 58 to Lys and of His 61 to Gly (H to L subunit changes) results in an altered protein which has lost its ferroxidase activity.[56] In earlier studies it was shown that human recombinant L ferritin was able to incorporate and retain iron at physiological pH values but did not take up iron at acidic pH values and did not show detectable ferroxidase activity.[57]

However, it would be a trifle hasty to attribute the exclusivity of ferrox-idase activity to H subunits for several reasons: If human L chain recombinant ferritin can assimilate iron at physiological pH values, how can it do so if it is incapable of catalyzing ferrous iron oxidation? How does one explain that in iron overload both in humans and in animals the excess iron is stored in ferritins which contain exclusively L subunits? Yet again, the answer is prob-ably that one has too quickly extrapolated to *in vivo* the results of elegant, but none the less distinctly *in vitro*, experimentation. Since recombinant human L-chain ferritin can assimilate iron at physiological pH values, we may exclude the hypothesis that the ferroxidase site of a small number of H subunits in ferritins from a number of tissues with a high L-subunit content (such as horse spleen and human liver ferritins) is responsible for the initial phase of iron deposition in these ferritins. If recombinant L-chain ferritin can assimilate iron, is it not logical to conclude that it must also have a ferroxidase center, albeit less active in the *in vitro* assays that have been used up until now? Of the metal-binding sites that have been observed by X-ray crystal-lography (reviewed in Reference 47) one springs immediately to mind — that composed of Glu 53 and Glu 56, located inside the protein shell in the twofold groove. From chemical modification studies on horse spleen apo-ferritin with glycineamide[58] it was shown that whereas seven carboxyl func-tions could be modified per subunit without any effect on iron uptake capacity, the modification of four additional carboxyls totally blocked iron assimilation. Using ^{14}C-glycineamide to specifically label the essential carboxy functions,[59] a radioactive tryptic peptide was obtained which contained residues 53 to 59, i.e., which contained both Glu 53 and Glu 56. We have carried out the same modification this time using taurine instead of glycineamide, and are at present awaiting the results of MS/MS spectrometry. This metal-binding site seems to be unique to L-chain ferritins since most H-chain ferritins have His at positions 53 and 56. Perhaps the lesson to be drawn from this amusing contretemps is that if H-chain ferritins have their ferroxidase center, why should L-chain ferritins not have theirs (not necessarily at the same place in the subunit — as we would say in french "vive la différence"!)?

The third question we should address is to understand, once the initial iron oxidation phase has been catalyzed by the protein, how does the iron core grow; i.e., after the nucleation phase? What happens in the crystal growth phase? For human ferritins, analysis by HRTEM (high resolution transmission electron microscopy) indicates that the cores are essentially single crystals with extensive structural and stoichiometric irregularities (reviewed in Ref-erence 44), and this implies that the crystal growth must have taken place at one specific site on the protein interface. This suggests that nucleation sites (and oxidation sites) are probably carboxylate functions situated close to the subunit dimer interface. Though oxidation can occur at one specific site on the internal surface of the protein, it is a necessary prerequisite for crystal growth that a critical cluster of Fe(III) be formed. The clustering of glutamate

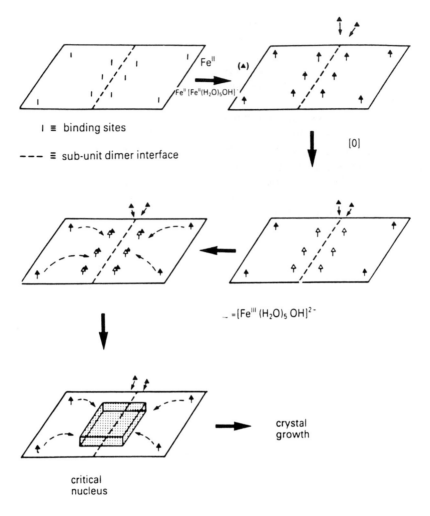

FIGURE 16. Diagrammatic representation of a possible mechanism of crystal growth of the mineral core in ferritin. The subunit dimer interface contains a cluster of possible binding sites at which Fe^{2+} is located. Oxidation of Fe^{2+} at specific sites at the interface creates a localized zone of Fe^{3+} species. This region is now energized with respect to further oxidation such that it becomes the focus for further Fe^{2+} diffusion and oxidation. The activation energy for the nucleation is overcome when the number of localized Fe^{3+} species attains a critical size. Crystal growth continues by further addition and oxidation of Fe^{2+} to the nucleation zone. (From St. Pierre, T. G., Webb, J., and Mann, S., *Biomineralisation,* VCH Publishers, Weinheim, Germany, 1989, 295. With permission.)

residues at the B-helix interface could favor such a nucleation zone. Once such a critical nucleus has been established, the growth process would then become auto-catalytic and spatially localized. Figure 16 summarizes possible mechanisms for iron-core formation.

We can conclude that the initial steps in iron deposition in ferritin necessitate the participation of the protein and that it probably involves a di-iron center which may have a μ-oxo bridge. The most recent studies suggest that the mixed valence Fe^{2+}-Fe^{3+} complex implicated in iron-core formation may contain a μ-oxo bridge.[53] Thereafter we enter into the world of speculation!

Iron can be mobilized from ferritin *in vitro* in several ways. Direct chelation of Fe(III) by a number of chelators normally present in cells, such as citrate, various sugars, thiols, including dihydrolipoate and dihydrolipoamide, as well as by synthetic chelators and microbial siderophores (reviewed in Reference 60), has been observed, although in general at rather slow rates. In those cases that have been studied in detail, iron release rates increase with decreasing pH values. Since we do not have any clear idea of what sorts of rates are required for ferritin iron release within cells, it may be premature to exclude such mechanisms, particularly from ferritins that have been recently transferred to the acidic lysosomal compartment. What we can say with some degree of certainty is that *in vitro* ferritin iron can be mobilized much more rapidly by the addition of electrons and protons, particularly in the presence of appropriate chelators of Fe(II). *In vitro* reduction can be achieved by thiols, such as thioglycollic acid, dithionite, and dihydrolipoate (the latter can also mobilize iron as Fe(III) without reduction), Cu(II) plus ascorbate, superoxide or methylviologen, and in the absence of oxygen by dihydroflavins. In the absence of a chelator, upon reduction a midpoint potential of -190 mV was observed at pH 7.0, and the iron was found to remain within the protein shell: from the variation of the midpoint potential as a function of pH, it was calculated that 2 H^+ were transferred to the core for each Fe(III) reduced to Fe(II).[61] This suggests that Fe(II) mobilization necessitates chelation and that iron is exported from the interior of the molecule as an Fe(II) chelate, perhaps via the apolar fourfold channels. Two general schemes for reductive iron mobilization can be envisaged. In the first, the reductant enters the core and reduces the Fe(III) at short range, perhaps at the same time chelating the Fe^{2+} produced. It was originally suggested that dihydroflavins mobilize iron in this way,[62] but studies with dihydroflavins, thioglycollic acid, and dithionite indicate that there is no penetration barrier to the core for either reductants or chelators.[63] This would be consistent with a mechanism where the reductant remains outside the protein shell and passes its electrons into the core, involving electron transfer over a distance of 2 to 2.5 nm. This is in accord with results that convincingly demonstrate long-range electron transfer by cytochrome C, flavodoxin, and blue copper proteins to produce oxidized ferritin from Fe^{2+}-containing ferritin.[64] More recently, similar results have been obtained for ferrihemoprotein reduction by reduced ferritin involving long-range transfer of electrons through the ferritin coat.[65]

Ferritin iron can also be mobilized by superoxide and by a number of flavoprotein oxidases and dehydrogenases including xanthine oxidase, an NADH oxido-reductase, NADH-lipoamide dehydrogenase (reviewed in Reference 3). In many of these cases it seems likely that ferritin iron mobilization is dependent upon superoxide, since superoxide dismutase inhibits, although it has been suggested that a flavin serves to shuttle electrons between flavoenzymes and ferritin iron.[66] The xanthine oxidase system can also mediate superoxide-dependent iron transfer from ferritin to transferrins.[67]

We have very little information concerning ferritin iron mobilization *in vivo*, as we have pointed out before.[3] There is, however, little credible evidence that dihydroflavins, superoxide anion, dihydrolipoate, reduced vitamin C, etc., participate in the release of ferritin iron within cells. Indeed, we are not even sure that iron release must take place at rapid rates — perhaps even slow release of iron from the ferrihydrite cores of hemosiderin within the acidic environment of the lysosomal compartment would be sufficient to ensure the intracellular homeostasis that will be developed in the next section.

B. CELLULAR IRON HOMEOSTASIS

It would clearly be in the interest of the cell, when it required iron, to increase its iron uptake capacity while at the same time down-regulating its intracellular iron-utilizing pathways. In contrast, when the cell is iron replete (or for that matter subjected to an excess of iron accumulation) it would be advantageous to down-regulate iron uptake and to stimulate iron-utilization pathways within the cell. That this is in fact the case has become apparent from a number of detailed studies of the regulation of ferritin mRNA translation, of transferrin receptor mRNA expression, and most recently of the genes of the heme biosynthesis pathway, at the level of the first enzyme of this pathway, 5-aminolevulinate synthase. It was clearly established in pioneering studies by Drysdale and Munro[66] that the regulation of ferritin synthesis was operational at the level of translation of the ferritin mRNA by iron and not, or at least to a much lesser extent, at the level of mRNA synthesis from DNA. The presence of a pool of ferritin mRNA within the cell was established, and it was shown that in the absence of iron within the cell much of this mRNA pool was inactive in ferritin protein synthesis. It had been suggested that the translation control of specific mRNAs might be regulated by specific proteins. We shall summarize much of the literature of the last four years (also reviewed in Chapter 2 of this book and Reference 3) by affirming that ferritin mRNA has a stem loop in the 5′ untranslated region (5′UTR) which binds a specific binding protein. The protagonists in this scenario are referred to, respectively, as IREs (iron responsive elements) and IRE-BPs (iron responsive element binding proteins). The IRE-BPs are cytosolic proteins of M_r 90 kDa. They bind not only to the 5′IRE of the ferritin mRNA, but also to a number of IREs (there are five in total) on the 3′UTR of transferrin receptor mRNAs. The effect of this binding is different with regard to the expression of the two mRNAs in question. However, before discussing their effect on ferritin and transferrin receptors in mRNA expression, we must insist on one property of cytosolic IRE-BPs. They can exist

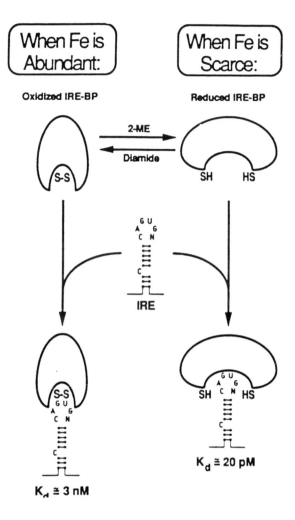

FIGURE 17. Schematic representation of a proposed model for IRE/IRE-BP interaction. (From Haile, D. J., Hentze, M. W., Roualt, T. A., Harford, J. B., and Klausner, R. D., *Mol. Cell. Biol.*, 9, 5055, 1989. With permission.)

in two forms, one of high affinity for the IREs (with a dissociation constant in the picomolar range) and one with a much lower dissociation constant (in the nanomolar range).[69] The two forms can be interconverted by thiols and oxidation. It is postulated that the high affinity form can be converted to the low affinity form by Fe^{2+} in the presence of a reductant. We summarize the proposed model for IRE/IRE-BP interaction in Figure 17. When the IRE-BP is in its high affinity form, it binds to the IRE in the 5'UTR of ferritin mRNA and prevents its translation into ferritin protein. In contrast, the high affinity form of the IRE-BP binds strongly to some (at least three) of the IREs of the transferrin receptor and protects the mRNA from nuclease attack, thus ensuring that transferrin receptor is expressed at high levels. When the IRE-BP is in its low affinity state, it dissociates from the 5'UTR of ferritin mRNA (and, from recent data from the 5'UTR which is also present in the mRNA for 5-aminolevulinate synthase, regulating heme synthesis) thus enabling the translation of the mRNA into protein. We may ask, what happens to transferrin receptor mRNA? In its low affinity state, the IRE-BP binds poorly to transferrin receptor mRNAs in the multiple UTR-IRE stem loops. The result is that they are no longer protected against nuclease attack; the transferrin receptor mRNA is degraded and can no longer assure the production of transferrin receptors. The result is that the cell assimilates intracellular iron and shuts off its supply in extracellular iron.

What could be the molecular trigger which tells the cell which way to go — i.e., either to increase its iron uptake, or to concentrate its efforts on increasing its intracellular utilization of the metal? One indicator has been that in going from its high affinity to the low affinity form, the IRE-BP requires iron in the Fe(II) form in the presence of a reducing agent. This recalls almost the inverse situation, namely that of aconitase (the Kreb's cycle enzyme which transforms citrate to isocitrate in a reaction which involves respective dehydration and hydration steps). As purified, mitochondrial aconitase is in an enzymatically inactive form which contains a 3Fe4S center and which can be transformed into a 4Fe4S center in the presence of Fe^{2+} and a reductant which is then catalytically active.[70] The human IRE-BP has been cloned and the corresponding cDNA sequenced,[71] and it was noted that the IRE-BP contains cysteine residues in sequence motifs that are reminiscent of those contained in iron sulfur proteins. Computer-based analysis of available data banks reveals a striking homology between IRE-BP and the Fe-S-protein aconitase from either pig heart or yeast.[72] There is 30 to 33% sequence identity and 53 to 56% homology. The IRE-BP has an extraordinary conservation of residues in the active site region of aconitase. The only three cysteines shared by each of yeast aconitase, pig heart aconitase, bovine heart aconitase, and IRE-BP are the three of the FeS center.[72] Whereas there is no fourth cysteine for the fourth iron atom in active aconitase, and this atom is liganded by solvent,[73] in contrast there is a fourth cysteine in IRE-BP close to the cleft which could perhaps serve as ligand for the fourth iron atom. It is proposed that IRE-BP possesses a dynamic Fe-S center which would sense alterations in iron availability, passing from a 3Fe4S form of high-binding affinity for IREs to a 4Fe4S form of low-binding affinity. This would explain the basis of cellular iron homeostasis.

C. HEMOSIDERIN

During normal cellular metabolism it is clear that the uptake, transfer, and storage of iron is carefully controlled. However, in various clinical conditions such controls are overwhelmed. This may be due to a variety of defects which include increased iron uptake at the intestinal mucosa due to an as yet

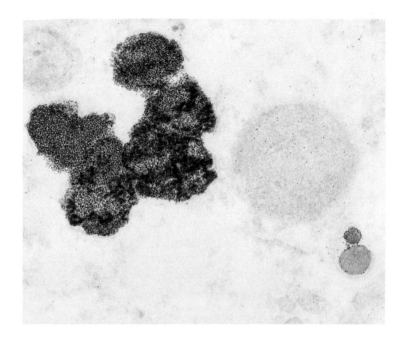

FIGURE 18. Electron micrograph of iron-loaded liver cell. Ferritin can be observed in the cytosol and accumulating into the cluster where ferritin molecules can be clearly seen. A lysosome containing hemosiderin is clearly distinguishable. (Magnification × 100,000.)

unidentified gene defect (primary hemochromatosis), excessive breakdown of erythrocytes due to abnormal globin synthesis enhanced by multiple blood transfusion (beta-thalassemia), a defect in heme synthesis pathway (porphyria cutanea tarda), excessive intake of iron from the diet (e.g., Bantu siderosis), and chronic alcohol consumption where stimulation of gastric acid secretion will increase the solubility of ferric ions and hence its availability for absorption.[74] Even though transferrin receptors are down-regulated and ferritin synthesis increased at the molecular level (See Section III.B), the cell is still unable to limit its uptake. This has been attributed in part to the unregulated and rapid uptake of the nontransferrin bound iron which is possibly increased in the plasma of hemochromatotic patients (see Section IV), whose fate is presumably to be incorporated either into the low-molecular-weight pool, into ferritin, or directly into lysosomes to contribute to the hemosiderin pool (Figure 10). Although ferritin synthesis is able to respond initially to this excessive intake of iron, eventually the cytosol becomes filled with ferritin which is heavily iron loaded, i.e., approximately 4000 atoms of iron per molecule. These iron-rich ferritin molecules accumulate in the cytosol and will eventually form into clusters (Figure 18), possibly due to the polymerization of the ferritin protein.[75] These clusters will be engulfed by secondary vacuoles to be taken up by lysosomes, where hydrolytic enzymes will degrade

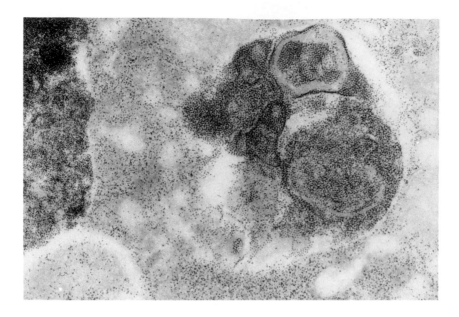

FIGURE 19. Electron micrograph of an iron-loaded lysosome: an arrow indicates the presence of a paracrystalline array. (Magnification × 100,000.)

the protein shell. The undegraded iron cores, partially divested of the protein shells, are referred to as hemosiderin.[76,77] The relatively low abundance of aromatic and thiol residues in hemosiderin protein compared to those in ferritin[78] may implicate iron catalyzed free radical mediated oxidation of the protein shell, in combination with proteolysis.

In all clinical conditions of iron overload the major storage protein is hemosiderin, which is increased approximately a hundredfold in comparison to that of ferritin, which only increases tenfold.[79] The excessive iron is localized to membrane bodies termed siderosomes or lysosomes.[76] By electron microscopy, clumps of the insoluble material are clearly visible, while at higher magnification paracrystalline arrays of ferritin can be seen within the lysosomes (Figure 19). Hemosiderin is characterized by its water insolubility and the fact that during its isolation from iron-loaded tissues it will sediment during ultracentrifugation through chaotropic solutions of high ionic densities, i.e., potassium iodide, 4.1 M.

It was initially assumed that since ferritin was the precursor of hemosiderin that the iron cores would be of a similar composition to that of ferritin, i.e., ferrihydrite. However, it has become increasingly apparent in our research over the past few years that hemosiderins isolated from tissues of differing iron-loading syndromes show important differences with regard to their morphological appearance by electron microscopy, the biomineralization of their iron cores, and in the structure of their associated proteins. Two of the major difficulties in the characterization and identification of these different hemosiderins has been the availability of biological samples (invariably only a limited number of specimens are available for such studies), and the gross insolubility of the hemosiderin molecule (which has been overcome by the use of tetramethyl ammonium hydroxide).[80] However, despite such limitations there is good agreement of the results for each of the various hemosiderin types identified.

The hemosiderins can be grouped into three different classes according to their iron core mineralization product. (1) The hemosiderins isolated from the tissues either of patients who have died of natural causes with no indication of excessive iron overload, patients with untreated primary hemochromatosis, or a variety of animal species whether loaded with iron either naturally (e.g., bird,[81,82] horse, Spitsbergen reindeer[83]) or experimentally (i.e., carbonyl iron,[84] nitrilotriacetic acid,[85] or ferrocene[86]). (2) The hemosiderin isolated from the livers of primary hemochromatosis patients at post-mortem who had been previously treated by venesection for their iron-loading condition. (3) The third type identified in the livers and spleens of secondary hemochromatosis patients who were treated by chelation with desferrioxamine.[87] Various biophysical and biochemical techniques have been used for the identification of these different hemosiderin types, the results of which are shown in Table 1. Electron micrographs of the three different hemosiderin iron cores are presented in Figure 20.

The cytoprotective advantage inferred upon the cell by the formation of hemosiderin is exemplified by the slower release of iron from these iron-storage proteins by comparison to ferritin.[89] The mobilization of iron from the hemosiderins will be dependent upon a variety of factors, including the nature of the iron core with regard to both its mineralization and phosphate content. Studies of the mobilization of iron from these different hemosiderin types show the release of iron to be relatively fast from amorphous ferric oxide, intermediate by the ferrihydrite iron cores, and strongly retarded in the goethite form when either weak,[90] or strong,[91] chelators were investigated for their ability to remove iron from the cores.

It is unclear how these different iron cores could be formed *in vivo* since the conditions shown necessary for the *in vitro* conversion of ferrihydrite to these different mineralization states would not be found under normal physiological conditions, e.g., high cysteine[92] and copper[93] content. It has therefore been hypothesized that there may be an alternative process in the formation of these different hemosiderin types which does not involve the normal degradation of ferritin via cluster formation and uptake by lysosomes. This could involve the direct uptake of the non-transferrin bound plasma fraction into the lysosomal pool (Figure 10). Alternatively, the etiology of the excess iron may be implicated in the formation of these different hemosiderin iron cores. However, the iron loading of animals with comparable sources of iron to that of the hemosiderin type (as seen in secondary hemochromatosis hemosiderin,

TABLE 1

Biophysical and Biochemical Characteristics of Ferritin and Hemosiderins

	Ferritin	Hd1	Hd2	Hd3
Fe/protein ratio	0.11	0.25	0.43	0.40
Size of iron core (nm)	7.22 ± 0.44	6.12 ± 0.51 5.8 ± 0.59	5.36[a]	5.49 ± 0.55 6.83 ± 0.36
Mossbauer blocking temperature (K)	40	28	<3	63
Electron diffraction lines (A)	2.47 2.22 1.93 1.71 1.51 1.46	2.50 1.99 1.71 1.51 1.46	2.49 2.12 1.53	4.25 2.68 2.45 2.20 1.99 1.71 1.54 1.47 1.48
Elemental composition (mmol element/mol Fe)	P 115	306	1454	98
Principal elements detected	Cu 0.15 Ca 3.2 Zn 12.4 Ba 0.86	0.88 13.6 1.39 0.02	50.4 n/d 45.8 1.21	0.07 1.8 0.17 0.004
Crystallinity	Good	Good	Poor	Good
Peptides identified after SDS/PAGE (kD)	20	20	14.5 20.0	14.5 20.0
Mineralization	Ferrihydrite	Ferrihydrite	Amorphous ferric oxide	Goethite

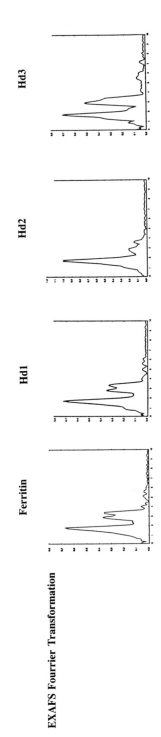

Note: Hd1 hemosiderin extracted from old age tissue and from untreated primary hemochromatosis patients; Hd2 hemosiderin from treated (i.e., venesected) primary hemochromatosis patients; and Hd3 hemosiderin from treated (i.e., by chelation with desferrioxamine) secondary hemochromatosis patients. n/d = no data. The results shown are taken from References 86 to 88 and 90.

[a] Too few cores to obtain statistical analysis: result is average of iron cores counted.

EXAFS Fourrier Transformation

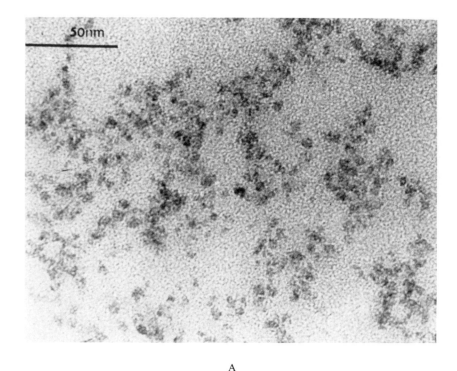

50nm

A

FIGURE 20. Electron micrographs of three different hemosiderin iron cores. (A) ferrihydrite iron core: the iron core particles are clearly resolved; (B) hemosiderin cores from a primary hemochromatosis patient which are of low electron density, extremely aggregated and irregular in morphology; (C) hemosiderin cores from the liver of a secondary hemochromatosis patient are well-defined angular particles. (Bar = 50 nm in (A); 100 nm in (B), (C).)

which is also observed in the horse or in rats overloaded orally with ferrocene) to hepatic levels comparable to that of primary hemochromatosis patients (i.e., 10,000 μ/g liver) have not as yet reproduced the changes identified in our different clinical groups, both of these animal species having hemosiderin with a ferrihydrite iron core. We would therefore conclude either that the duration of iron-loading may be important or that the clinical intervention in some way has altered the mineralization of the iron core. The changes that occur in the treated primary hemochromatosis hemosiderin, i.e., the amorphous ferric (III) oxide iron core which shows high phosphorus content, may be attributable to the fact that venesection induces iron mobilization from the lysosomes without concomittant release of the accompanying phosphorus. This results in a cummulative increase in the P:Fe content of the lysosomal environment. Spontaneous deposition of iron within the phosphate-rich lysosome, for example, via acidic dissolution of ferritin iron or direct entry of non-transferrin bound iron, would then result in an amorphous mineral due

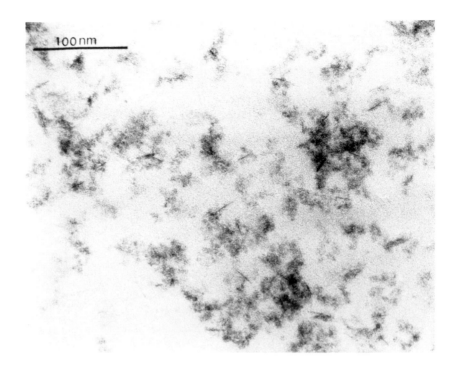

FIGURE 20B.

to phosphate bridging in the oxide framework. In the hemosiderins that have been isolated from the tissues of treated secondary hemochromatosis patients, the lower elemental content of the iron core may be of some importance in the formation of the goethite iron core, but the significance of such alterations in the elemental composition await further studies.

The hemosiderin peptides isolated from the tissues of each of the iron-loaded patients after SDS/PAGE analysis all show a band at 20 kDa, but, in addition, in all of the secondary hemochromatosis samples and one of the untreated primary hemochromatosis hemosiderin sample there was also a band at 14.5 kDa. The band at 20 kDa corresponds to the L subunit of ferritin. The 14.5 kDa band has been shown to be derived from ferritin by its positive reaction with both antiferritin antisera and specific monoclonals to ferritin sequences, 83 to 91, 116 to 125, and 151 to 162.[94] This is consistent with cleavage in the N-terminal part of the ferritin protein.[94,95]

IV. LOW-MOLECULAR-WEIGHT SPECIES

Iron is required by the cell for a variety of cellular functions and enzymes. It is transported to the tissues bound to transferrin where it is taken up by the transferrin receptors on the cellular membrane, internalized and endocytozed

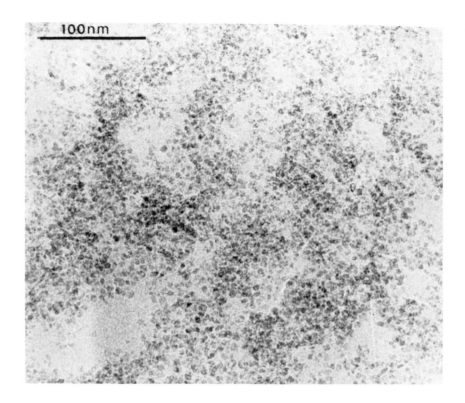

FIGURE 20C.

(as described above). The apotransferrin-receptor complex is recycled to the cell surface, while the iron remains within the acidic endosome. Such iron has then to be transported to the specific iron-requiring biosynthetic pathway, to iron storage proteins, or to an easily accessible pool of iron for cellular needs. However, its identification and quantification within the cells remains unclear, whether it increases during cellular injury or iron-overload similarly is unresolved, and the nature of its associated ligand is unknown. However, it would seem inappropriate that after such a sequence of highly specific reactions that the continuation of iron transport and its existence within this easily accessible pool would be ascribed to several aspecific amino acids or nucleotides. It is therefore probable that a specific iron-binding complex does exist, possibly within the interior of the endosome or its membrane, to transport iron to where it is required within the cell and maintain it within the LMW-Fe pool.

Although Fe^{3+} is initially present within the transferrin-receptor complex, the acidic nature of the endosome may reduce it to Fe^{2+}, associated with an NADH-NAD dependent ferri-reductase, a form which most iron-requiring systems would need (Figure 10). Furthermore, Fe^{2+} would be readily incorporated into apoferritin, the major iron-storage protein in normal mammalian tissue. Although it has been argued that to avoid toxicity the low molecular weight iron species are probably stable complexes of Fe(III),[96] there probably exists an equilibrium between Fe^{2+} and Fe^{3+} (possibly hexacoordinated high-spin Fe^{2+} and Fe^{3+} complexes) within the cell in a possible concentration of 10^{-8} and 10^{-16} M, respectively.

Attempts to quantify and identify the intracellular low-molecular-weight pool (LMW-Fe) are thwarted by a multitude of problems. Such a pool will be relatively small in order to minimize any toxic effect, and, consequently, will be difficult to detect. Its isolation and characterization within the cell invariably will involve a series of steps which will possibly include cell disruption, molecular sieve chromatography, and ultrafiltration which could invalidate the final result due to decompartmentalization and recombination of iron with other ligands, in addition to possibly changing the oxidation state of the iron. Therefore, the true *in vivo* situation may not be reflected. Quantification of the so-called chelatable iron pool in tissue extracts (believed to be equivalent to the LMW-Fe by some investigators) by its association with a variety of chelators may overestimate its size since other subcellular iron pools besides the cytosolic iron will be chelated, possibly lysosomal iron,[97] the latter being available to the chelator after a longer period of incubation.

A. SOURCES OF IRON FOR THE INTRACELLULAR IRON POOL

Normal cellular homeostasis — From cellular uptake of iron via transferrin-transferrin receptors, internalization and endocytosis occur as described above, and ferritin is the major iron storage protein in normal iron status (see Section III.A). Other sources include:

(a) Endogenous heme breakdown. During the breakdown of various heme proteins, e.g., hemoglobin and myoglobin, iron may be released into the cytoplasmic compartment.
(b) Breakdown of other iron-containing enzymes.
(c) Mitochondria play an important role in keeping the concentration of the low-molecular-weight iron pool constant. The Fe^{3+} receptors on the mitochondria have an unsaturated binding capacity for iron under normal circumstances and will therefore accept or donate iron to the LMW-Fe pool as required.

Pathological cells — During certain pathological conditions, there may be upregulation of transferrin receptors by the diseased cell which could increase the amount of iron taken up by the cell. However, such excess iron initially would be successfully sequestered into the iron storage proteins ferritin and hemosiderin and other iron proteins (see Section III), such that it remains doubtful as to whether the LMW-Fe pool will be increased (see Section IV.C). However, under certain conditions iron may be released from the two major iron storage proteins.

(a)   Ferritin — After cellular injury there may be perturbation of the normal cellular homeostasis such that there is decompartmentalization of various enzymes which could facilitate the release of iron from this iron storage protein; e.g., during ischemia-reperfusion damage, xanthine oxidase, formed from the degradation of xanthine dehydrogenase, which mobilizes iron from ferritin as Fe^{2+} and could increase the LMW-Fe pool.

(b)   Hemosiderin — Hemosiderin is the major iron storage protein in pathological conditions of iron overload (see Section III.C) Iron may be mobilized from hemosiderin under acidic conditions in the presence of suitable chelators such as citrite or ascorbate.[89]

B. IDENTIFICATION OF LIGANDS ASSOCIATED WITH LMW-FE POOL

Two principal approaches have been used to identify this pool. The first approach is to identify the nature of the iron which is nontransferrin bound in the extracellular fluid. It has been suggested that this may be equivalent in speciation to the LMW-Fe pool because of its rapid uptake by parenchymal cells, possibly to equilibrate directly with the intracellular LMW-Fe pool (Figure 10). The second approach is to identify the LMW-Fe pool in various tissue cells types either where there is a high uptake of iron, e.g., reticulocytes, or to which ^{59}Fe has been equilibrated and its intracellular distributed within the cytosol determined by a variety of chromatographic techniques.

Great interest has been focused on the nontransferrin-bound iron species in extracellular compartments, on both its nature and reactivity, as this may be of significance in determining the identity of the associated ligand intracellularly and the manner of tissue damage. Nontransferrin bound iron in the plasma is probably increased in the plasma of iron-loaded patients and is thought to bypass the normal transferrin-mediated iron uptake by the cell and enter directly into the LMW-Fe pool of parenchymal cells of the liver and possibly the pancreas. Brissot et al.[98] showed the presence of a clearance system for nontransferrin bound iron in perfused liver by the uptake of both ferrous and ferric ions in ultrafiltered human serum when complexed either to specific physiological chelators or not. This system was both highly efficient and effectively irreversible. Extracellularly, the presence of a low-molecular-weight iron species in plasma was first identified by Hershko,[99] who showed that diethylenetriamine pentacetic acid (DTPA), a water-soluble chelator, increased urinary excretion in hemochromatotic mice although it was unable to penetrate cells and interact directly with iron stores. Quantitation of this nontransferrin-bound iron pool in the plasma of either primary or secondary hemochromatosis patients has proved to be difficult since some of the published methods for its detection may be nonspecific for this pool of iron such that its concentration may be either over- or underestimated. Additionally, the concentration of this iron species in the plasma will be dependent upon a variety of biochemical factors including the degree of iron loading of the liver, the transferrin saturation, and the serum iron content. Values for the serum nontransferrin-bound iron pool of between 7.0 to 20 μmol/l have been determined in the plasma of primary hemochromatosis patients by the bleomycin assay,[100,101] approximately 5.0 to 10.0 μmol/l in plasma of untreated thalassemic patients either by a chelatable iron assay in which nitrilotriacetic acid complexes all low-molecular-weight iron and iron non-specifically bound to plasma proteins,[102] by ultrafiltration of the plasma sample after chelation of the nonspecifically bound iron with ethylenediamine tetraacetic acid,[103] or by the mathematical differences between the excess of iron present above the calculated transferrin-bound iron.[104] Lower values were measured in the serum of thalassemic patients, between 0.5 to 5.5 μmol/l, using a DEAE-Sephadex-catechol disulphonic acid column, while higher values, up to 21 μmol/l, were determined in splenectomized patients.[105] During iron chelation with desferrioxamine this nontransferrin bound iron fraction decreased significantly, although it returned to its original value rapidly at the end of the chelation period.[106] Homozygotic hypotransferrin mice, which have no detectable circulating transferrin, similarly show high levels for the nontransferrin bound species in plasma, and values of up to 29 μmol/l for LMW-Fe were determined for this fraction by the bleomycin iron assay.[107]

A multitude of associated ligands for this nontransferrin-bound iron in the plasma have been tentatively identified, ranging from citrate or a ternary iron-citrate-acetate complex[108] to ferritin.[104] A plausible alternative would seem to be albumin, although ultrafiltration studies have shown the molecular weight to be <24,000; other studies have indicated a molecular weight of <1000.[109,106]

Intracellularly, the nature of the associated ligand in the LMW-Fe pool has similarly eluded identification. Early studies by Barlett[110] and Konopka and Szotov,[111] indicated that this small iron pool was associated with nucleotides such as ATP and GTP, and confirmatory evidence for the importance of the nucleotides as ligands for LMW-Fe was furnished by the identification of receptors for ATP-Fe^{3+} and ATP-Fe^{2+} on mitochondria,[112] which would provide iron necessary for heme biosynthesis. These were of two types: the first accepts iron from ATP with relatively low efficiency and a second accepts Fe from AMP with high efficiency. It is unclear as to why AMP-Fe should exist in the cell since the higher affinity of ATP for iron and its higher concentration in the cytosol would make ATP a more plausible ligand than AMP. Pollack et al.[113] suggested that AMP-Fe was the major constituent of the LMW pool and showed *in vitro* that the AMP-Fe complex could exist even when excess ATP was added.[114] It was therefore hypothesized that ATP interacts with transferrin to effect the initial release of iron from the endosome and then continues as the principal ligand for iron in the cytosol. Because ATP-Fe^{3+} is more highly charged and bulkier than AMP-Fe^{3+}, it would be less available to both apoferritin and mitochondria.[114] Therefore, its degradation to AMP-Fe *in vivo* would make the iron more available for heme synthesis. Other ligands which have been suggested as possible ligands for iron in the LMW-Fe pool include pyrophosphates, which are generated in the cytosol during activation of acetate and biosynthesis of nucleic acids, lipids, and glycogen, which could transport iron from transferrin to protoporphyrin within the mitochondria,[115] amino acids, polypeptides, proteins, and uncharacterized growth factors.[116-119] However, none of these ligands, including AMP and ATP, have been universally accepted as being the principal binding ligand for iron in the LMW-Fe pool.

In other studies, a variety of cells have been radiolabeled with ^{59}Fe, e.g., intestinal mucosa,[120-122] heart,[123] bone marrow,[118,124] erythroid tissue,[125] and cultured Chang cells[126] in an attempt to locate and possibly identify the LMW-Fe pool. However, the preparation of the samples as previously discussed may cause decompartmentalization of the various iron-containing amino acids, peptides, and protein fractions which would explain the wide variation in the molecular weights determined in many of these studies (cytosolic peptides of molecular weight 13,000, 1400, and 350,[127] or of 1000[128]). In our opinion, it is difficult to verify any of these results for the reasons previously given, especially as ^{59}Fe would equilibrate, nonspecifically, with a wide number of peptides and proteins present in the cell, especially once the cell is disrupted, and will therefore not reflect the true *in vivo* situation.

C. REGULATION OF THE IRON POOL

Studies by Mulligan et al.[127] showed that the size of the LMW-Fe pool did not increase according to iron status but remained constant whether the cell was iron-deficient, iron-loaded, or of normal status. As has already been stated, the size of the LMW-Fe pool would be low (0.5 to 1.0 μmol/l) in the cell during normal iron metabolism and, therefore, there must be an alternative pathway to maintain this level of LMW-Fe. Although earlier *in vitro* studies identified the presence of certain cytosolic iron proteins of various molecular weights: e.g., 5500 mol wt,[124] and 400,000 and 68,000 mol wt,[129] while retaining a constant LMW-Fe pool, the recent work of the IRE-BP clearly shows that these play a pivoting role in the control of iron homeostasis. It may be that the situation in iron overload is that the *flux* through the LMW-Fe pool is increased, although the actual concentration of iron present at any given point is unchanged. If we assume, in agreement with a recent review,[130] that the bulk of the LMW-Fe pool is Fe^{2+}, this would force the IRE-BP toward its low affinity form, thus releasing ferritin and delta aminolevulinic acid synthetase mRNAs for synthesis and hence intracellular iron utilization.

In conclusion, the evidence from within the extensive literature cited above for the existence of an intracellular LMW-Fe pool would indicate that such a pool of iron does exist. This is somewhat contrary to the previous remarks of one of the authors which liken its existence to that of the Loch Ness monster.[131] However, in common with this Scottish creature, its identity remains uncharacterized, its size unknown, and extensive investigations will no doubt continue with more sophisticated instrumentation to clarify such imponderables.

ACKNOWLEDGMENTS

Much of the work cited in the hemosiderin section was carried out in collaboration with Dr. D. P. E. Dickson at Liverpool University, Prof. S. Mann at Bath University, Prof. C. O. Garner at Manchester University, Dr. M. Ramsey and Prof. T. J. Peters at the University of London.

REFERENCES

1. **Gordeuk, V. R., Bacon, B. R., and Brittenham, G. M.,** Iron overload: causes and consequences, *Annu. Rev. Nutr.,* 7, 485, 1987.
2. **Simon, M. and Brissot, P.,** The genetics of haemochromatosis, *J. Hepatol.,* 6, 116, 1988.
3. **Crichton, R. R.,** *Inorganic Biochemistry of Iron Metabolism,* Ellis Horwood, Chichester, 1991.
4. **Aust, S. D.,** Sources of iron for lipid peroxidation in biological systems, in *Upjohn Symposium/Oxygen Radicals,* 1987, 27.
5. **Floyd, R.,** Role of oxygen free radicals in carcinogenesis and brain ischemia, *FASEB J.,* 4, 2587, 1990.
6. **Bartfeld, N. S. and Law, J. H.,** Isolation and molecular cloning of transferrin from the tobacco hornworm, *Manduca sexta, J. Biol. Chem.,* 265, 21684, 1990.
7. **Rose, T. M., Plowman, G. D., Teplow, D. P., Dreyer, W. J., Hellström, K. H., and Brown, J. P.,** Primary structure of the human melanoma-associated antigen p97 (melanotransferrin) deduced from the mRNA sequence, *Proc. Natl. Acad. Sci. U.S.A.,* 83, 1261, 1986.
8. **Bowman, B. H., Yang, F., and Adrian, G. S.,** Transferrin, evolution and genetic regulation of expression, *Adv. Genet.,* 25, 1, 1988.
9. **Baker, E. N., Rumball, V., and Anderson, B. F.,** Transferrins: insights into structure and function from studies on lactotransferrin, *TIBS,* 12, 350, 1987.
10. **Anderson, B. F., Baker, H. M., Norris, G. E., Rice, D. W., and Baker, E. N.,** Structure of human lactoferrin:crystallographic structure analysis and refinement at 2.8 Å resolution, *J. Mol. Biol.,* 209, 711, 1989.
11. **Bailey, S., Evans, R. W., Garratt, R. C., Gorinsky, B., Hasnain, S., Horsburgh, C., Jhoti, H., Lindley, P. F., Mydin, A., Sarra, R., and Watson, J. L.,** Molecular structure of serum transferrin at 3.3 Å resolution, *Biochemistry,* 27, 5804, 1988.
12. **Anderson, B. F., Baker, H. M., Norris, G. E., Rumball, S. V., and Baker, E. N.,** Apolactoferrin structure demonstrates ligand-induced conformational change in transferrins, *Nature,* 344, 784, 1990.
13. **Gorinsky, B., Horsburgh, C., Lindley, P. F., Moss, D. S., Parker, M., and Watson, J. L.,** Evidence for the bilobal nature of diferric rabbit plasma transferrin, *Nature,* 281, 157, 1979.
14. **Kojima, N. and Bates, G. W.,** The formation of Fe^{3+}-transferrin-CO_3^{2-} via the binding and oxidation of Fe^{2+}, *J. Biol. Chem.,* 256, 12034, 1981.

15. **Cowart, R. E., Kojima, N., and Bates, G. W.,** The exchange of Fe^{3+} between ace-tohydroxamic acid and transferrin, *J. Biol. Chem.,* 257, 7560, 1982.
16. **Sack, J. C., Saper, M. A., and Quiocho, F. A.,** Periplasmic binding protein structure and function, *J. Mol. Biol.,* 206, 171, 1989.
17. **Warner, R. G. and Weber, I.,** The metal combining properties of conalbumin, *J. Am. Chem. Soc.,* 75, 5094, 1953.
18. **Baldwin, D. A., Jenny, E. R., and Aisen, P.,** The effect of human serum transferrin and milk lactoferrin on hydroxyl radical formation from superoxide and hydrogen per-oxide, *J. Biol. Chem.,* 259, 13391, 1984.
19. **Jandl, J. H., Inman, J. K., Simmons, R. L., and Allen, D. W.,** Transfer of iron from serum iron-binding protein to human reticulocytes, *J. Clin. Invest.,* 38, 161, 1959.
20. **Katz, J. H.,** Iron and protein kinetic studies by means of doubly labeled human crystalline transferrin, *J. Clin. Invest.,* 40, 2143, 1961.
21. **Jandl, J. H. and Katz, J. H.,** The plasma to cell cycle of transferrin, *J. Clin. Invest.,* 42, 314, 1963.
22. **Trowbridge, I. S. and Shackelford, D. E.,** Structure and function of transferrin receptors and their relationship to cell growth, *Biochem. Soc. Symp.,* 51, 117, 1986.
23. **Zerial, M., Malancon, P., Schneider, C., and Garoff, H.,** The transmembrane segment of the human transferrin receptor functions as a signal peptide, *EMBO J.,* 5, 1543, 1986.
24. **Jing, S. and Trowbridge, I. S.,** Nonacylated human transferrin receptors are rapidly internalized and mediate iron uptake, *J. Biol. Chem.,* 265, 11,555, 1990.
25. **Borhani, D. W. and Harrison, S. C.,** Crystallization and X-ray diffraction studies of a soluble form of the human transferrin receptor, *J. Mol. Biol.,* 218, 685, 1991.
26. **Alvarez, E., Gironès, N., and Davis, R. J.,** Intermolecular disulphide bonds are not required for the expression of the dimeric state and functional activity of the transferrin receptor, *EMBO J.,* 8, 2231, 1989.
27. **Reckhow, C. L. and Enns, C. A.,** Characterization of the transferrin receptor in tuni-camycin-treated A431 cells, *J. Biol. Chem.,* 263, 7297, 1988.
28. **Ralton, J. E., Jackson, H. J., Zanoni, M., and Gleeson, P. A.,** Effect of glycosylation inhibitors on the structure and function of the murine transferrin receptor, *Eur. J. Biochem.,* 186, 637, 1989.
29. **Collawa, J. F., Stangel, M., Kuhn, L. A., Esekogwu, V., Jing, S., Trowbridge, I. S., and Tainer, J. A.,** Transferrin receptor internalization sequence YXRF implicates a tight turn as the structural recognition motif for endocytosis, *Cell,* 63, 1061, 1990.
30. **Jing, S., Spencer, T., Miller, K., Hopkins, C., and Trowbridge, I. S.,** Role of the human transferrin receptor cytoplasmic domain in endocytosis: localization of a specific signal sequence for internalization, *J. Cell Biol.,* 110, 283, 1990.
31. **Kornfeld, S. and Mellman, I.,** The biogenesis of lysosomes, *Annu. Rev. Cell Biol.,* 5, 483, 1989.
32. **Bali, P. K., Zak, O., and Aisen, P.,** A new role for the transferrin receptor in the release of iron from transferrin, *Biochemistry,* 30, 324, 1991.
33. **Sipe, D. M. and Murphy, R. F.,** Binding to cellular receptors results in increased iron release from transferrin at mildly acidic pH, *J. Biol. Chem.,* 266, 8002, 1991.
34. **Nunez, M.-T., Gaete, V., Watkins, J. A., and Glass, J.,** Mobilization of iron from endocytic vesicles, *J. Biol. Chem.,* 265, 6688, 1990.
35. **Sun, I. L., Navas, P., Crane, F. L., Morré, D. J., and Löw, H.,** NADH diferric transferrin reductase in liver plasma membrane, *J. Biol. Chem.,* 262, 15,915, 1987.
36. **Thorstensen, K. and Aisen, P.,** Release of iron from diferic transferrin in the presence of rat liver plasma membranes: no evidence of a plasma membrane diferric transferrin reductase, *Biochim. Biophys. Acta,* 1052, 29, 1990.
37. **Toole-Simms, W., Sun, I. L., Faulk, W. P., Löw, H., Lindgren, A., Crane, F. L., and Morré, D. J.,** Inhibition of transplasma membrane electron transfer by monoclonal antibodies to the transferrin receptor, *Biochem. Biophys. Res. Commun.,* 176, 1437, 1991.

38. **Thorstensen, K. and Romslo, I.,** The role of transferrin in the mechanism of cellular iron uptake, *Biochem. J., 271,* 1, 1990.
39. **Quintart, J., Baudhuin, P., and Courtoy, P.,** Marker enzymes in rat liver vesicles involved in transcellular transport, *Eur. J. Biochem.,* 184, 32, 1989.
40. **Kondo, H., Saito, K., Grasso, J.P., and Aisen, P.,** Iron metabolism in the erythrophagocytosing Kupffer cell, *Hepatology,* 8, 32, 1988.
41. **Sibille, J. C., Kondo, H., and Aisen, P.,** Interactions between isolated hepatocytes and Kupffer cells in iron metabolism; a possible role for ferritin as an iron carrier protein, *Hepatology,* 8, 296, 1988.
42. **Bothwell, T. H., Charlton, R. W., Cook, J. D., and Finch, C. A.,** *Iron Metabolism in Man,* Blackwell, Edinburgh, 1979.
43. **Towe, K. M. and Bradley, W. F.,** Mineralogical constitution of colloidal 'hydrous ferric oxides', *J. Colloid Interface Sci.,* 24, 384, 1967.
44. **St. Pierre, T. G., Webb, J., and Mann, S.,** Ferritin and hemosiderin: structural and magnetic studies of the iron core, in *Biomineralisation,* Mann, S., Webb, J., and Williams, R. J. P., Eds., VCH Publishers, Weinheim, Germany, 1989, 295.
45. **Harrison, P. M.,** The structures of ferritin and apoferritin: some preliminary X-ray data, *J. Mol. Biol.,* 1, 69, 1959.
46. **Lawson, D. M., Artymiuk, P. J., Yewdall, S. J., Smith, J. M. A., Livingstone, J. C., Treffry, A., Luzzago, A., Levi, S., Arosio, P., Cesareni, G., Thomas, C. D., Shaw, W. V., and Harrison, P. M.,** Solving the structure of human H ferritin by genetically engineering intermolecular crystal contacts, *Nature,* 349, 541, 1991.
47. **Harrison, P. M., Artymiuk, P. J., Ford, G. C., Lawson, D. M., Smith, J. M. A., Treffry, A., and White, J. L.,** Ferritin: function and structural design of an iron-storage protein, in *Biomineralisation,* Mann, S., Webb, J., Williams, R. J. P., Eds., VCH Publishers, Weinheim, Germany, 1989, 258.
48. **Gerl, M. and Jaenicke, R.,** Self-assembly of apoferritin from horse spleen after reversible chemical modification with 2,3-dimethylmaleic anhydride, *Biochemistry,* 27, 4089, 1988.
49. **Gerl, M. and Jaenicke, R.,** Mechanism of the self-assembly of apoferritin from horse spleen, *Eur. Biophys. J.,* 15, 103, 1987.
50. **Fischbach, F. A. and Anderegg, J. W.,** An X-ray scattering study of ferritin and apoferritin, *J. Mol. Biol.,* 14, 458, 1965.
51. **Stuhrmann, H. B., Haas, J., Ibel, K., Koch, M. H. J., and Crichton, R. R.,** Low angle neutron scattering of ferritin studied by contrast variation, *J. Mol. Biol.,* 100, 399, 1976.
52. **Crichton, R. R., Roman, F., Roland, F., Pâques, E., Pâques, A., and Vandamme, E.,** Ferritin iron deposition and mobilisation, *J. Mol. Catal.,* 7, 267, 1980.
53. **Hanna, P. M., Chen, Y., and Chasteen, N. D.,** Initial iron oxidation in horse spleen apoferritin, *J. Biol. Chem.,* 266, 886, 1991.
54. **Stefanini, S., Desideri, A., Vecchini, P., Drakenberg, T., and Chiancone, E.,** Identification of the iron entry channels in apoferritin. Chemical modification and spectroscopic studies, *Biochemistry,* 28, 378, 1989.
55. **Treffry, A., Harrison, P. M., Luzzago, A., and Cesareni, G.,** Recombinant H-chain ferritins: effects of changes in the three-fold channels, *FEBS Lett.,* 247, 268, 1989.
56. **Lawson, D. M., Treffry, A., Artymiuk, P. J., Harrison, P. M., Yewdall, S. J., Luzzago, A., Cesareni, G., Levi, S., and Arosio, P.,** Identification of the ferroxidase centre in ferritin, *FEBS Lett.,* 254, 207, 1989.
57. **Levi, S., Franceschinelli, F., Cozzi, A., Dorner, M. H., and Arosio, P.,** Expression and structure and functional properties of human ferritin L-chain from *Escherichia coli, Biochemistry,* 28, 5179, 1989.
58. **Wetz, K. and Crichton, R. R.,** Chemical modification as a probe of the topography and reactivity of horse spleen apoferritin, *Eur. J. Biochem.,* 61, 545, 1976.
59. **Vandamme, E.,** Etude cinétique de la déposition du fer la ferritine, Thèse de Doctorat, Université Catholique de Louvain, 1980.

60. **Crichton, R. R. and Charloteaux-Wauters, M.,** Iron storage and transport, *Eur. J. Biochem.,* 164, 485, 1987.

61. **Watt, G. D., Frankel, R. B., and Papefthymiou, G. C.,** Reduction of mammalian ferritin, *Proc. Natl. Acad. Sci. U.S.A.,* 82, 3640, 1985.

62. **Jones, T., Spencer, R., and Walsh, C.,** Mechanisms and kinetics of iron release from ferritin by dihydroflavins and dihydroflavin analogues, *Biochemistry,* 17, 4011, 1978.

63. **Funk, F., Lenders, J. P., Crichton, R. R., and Schneider, W.,** Reductive mobilisation of ferritin iron, *Eur. J. Biochem.,* 152, 167, 1985.

64. **Watt, G. D., Jacobs, D., and Frankel, R. B.,** Redox reactivity of bacterial and mammalian ferritin: is reductant entry into the ferritin interior a necessary step for iron release?, *Proc. Natl. Acad. Sci. U.S.A.,* 85, 7457, 1988.

65. **Kadir, F. H. A., Al-Massad, F. K., Fatemi, S. J. A., Singh, H. K., Wilson, M. T., and Moore, G. R.,** Electron transfer between horse ferritin and ferrihaemoproteins, *Biochem. J.,* 278, 817, 1991.

66. **Topham, R., Goger, M., Pearce, K., and Schultz, P.,** The mobilization of ferritin iron by liver cytosol, *Biochem. J.,* 261, 137, 1989.

67. **Monteiro, H. P. and Winterbourn, C. C.,** The superoxide-dependent transfer of iron from ferritin to transferrin and lactoferrin, *Biochem. J.,* 256, 923, 1988.

68. **Drysdale, J. W. and Munro, H. N.,** Regulation of synthesis and turnover of ferritin in rat liver, *J. Biol. Chem.,* 241, 3630, 1966.

69. **Haile, D. J., Hentze, M. W., Roualt, T. A., Harford, J. B., and Klausner, R. D.,** Regulation of interaction of the iron-responsive element binding protein with iron-responsive RNA elements, *Mol. Cell. Biol.,* 9, 5055, 1989.

70. **Beinert, H. and Kennedy, M. C.,** Engineering of protein-bound iron-sulfur clusters, *Eur. J. Biochem.,* 186, 5, 1989.

71. **Roualt, T. A., Tang, C. K., Kaptain, S., Burgess, Haile, D. J., Samaniego, F., McBride, O. W., Harford, J. B., and Klausner, R. D.,** Cloning of the cDNA encoding an RNA regulatory protein — the human iron-responsive element-binding protein, *Proc. Natl. Acad. Sci. U.S.A.,* 87, 7958, 1990.

72. **Roualt, T. A., Stout, C. D., Kaptain, S., Harford, J. B., and Klausner, R. D.,** Structural relationship, between an iron-regulated RNA-binding protein (IRE-BP) and aconitase: functional implications, *Cell,* 64, 881, 1991.

73. **Robbins, A. H. and Stout, C. D.,** Structure of activated aconitase: formation of the (4Fe-4S) cluster in the crystal, *Proc. Natl. Acad. Sci. U.S.A.,* 86, 3639, 1989.

74. **Charlton, R., Jacobs, P., Seftel, H., and Bothwell, T.,** Effects of alcohol on iron absorption, *Br. Med. J.,* 1427, 1964.

75. **Hoy, T. G. and Jacobs, A.,** Ferritin polymers and the formation of haemosiderin, *Br. J. Haematol.,* 49, 593, 1981.

76. **Richter, G. W.,** The iron-loaded cell — the cytopathology of iron storage, *Am. J. Pathol.,* 91, 363, 1976.

77. **Richter, G. W.,** Studies of iron overload, *Lab. Invest.,* 50, 26, 1984.

78. **O'Connell, M. J., Ward, R. J., Baum, H., and Peters, T. J.,** In vitro and in vivo studies on the availability of iron from storage proteins to stimulate membrane lipid peroxidation, in *Free Radicals, Cell Damage and Disease,* Rice-Evans, C., Ed., Publ. Richelieu, London, 1986, 29.

79. **Selden, C., Owen, J. M. P., Hopkins, J. M. P., and Peters, T. J.,** Studies on the concentration and intracellular localization of iron proteins in liver biopsy specimens from patients with iron overload with special reference to their role in lysosomal disruption, *Br. J. Haematol.,* 44, 593, 1980.

80. **Weir, M. P., Gibson, J. F., and Peters, T. J.,** Biochemical studies on the isolation and characterisation of horse spleen haemosiderin, *Biochem. J.,* 223, 31, 1984.

81. **Ward, R. J., Iancu, T. C., Henderson, G. M., Kirkwood, J. R., and Peters, T. J.,** Hepatic iron overload in birds: analytical and morphological studies, *Avian Pathol.,* 17, 451, 1988.

82. **Ward, R. J., Smith, T., Henderson, G. M., and Peters, T. J.,** Investigation of the aetiology of haemosiderosis in the starling, *(Sturnus vulgaris) Avian Pathol.,* 20, 225, 1991.

83. **Dickson, D. P. E., Pollard, R. K., Borch-Iohnsen, B., Ward, R. J., and Peters, T. J.,** Mossbauer spectroscopic studies of haemosiderins from different sources, *Hyper. Inter.,* 42, 889, 1988.

84. **Peters, T. J., O'Connell, M. J., and Ward, R. J.,** Role of free-radical mediated lipid peroxidation in the pathogenesis of hepatic damage by lysosomal disruption, in *Free Radicals in Liver Injury,* Poli, G., Cheeseman, K. H., Dianzani, M. U., and Slater, T. F., Eds., IRL Press, London, 1986.

85. **O'Connell, M. J., Ward, R. J., Baum, H., and Peters, T. J.,** Iron overload, lysosomes and free radicals, in *Cells, Membranes and Disease, Including Renal,* Reid, E., Cook, G. M. W., and Luzio, J. P., Eds., Plenum Press, New York, 1987, 109.

86. **Ward, R. J., Florence, A. L., Baldwin, D., Abiaka, C., Roland, F., Ramsey, M. H., Dickson, D. P. E., Peters, T. J., and Crichton, R. R.,** Biochemical and biophysical investigations of the ferrocene-iron loaded rat: an animal model of primary haemochromatosis, *Eur. J. Biochem.,* 202, 405, 1991.

87. **Mann, S., Wade, V. J., Dickson, D. P. E., Reid, N. M. K., Ward, R. J., O'Connell, M., and Peters, T. J.,** Structural specificity of haemosiderin iron cores in iron-overload diseases, *FEBS,* 234, 68, 1988.

88. **Mackle, P., Garner, C. D., Ward, R. J., and Peters, T. J.,** Iron-K edge absorption spectroscopic investigations of the cores of ferritin and haemosiderins, *Biochim. Biophys. Acta,* 1115, 145, 1991.

89. **O'Connell, M. J., Ward, R. J., Baum, H., and Peters, T. J.,** The role of iron in ferritin- and haemosiderin-mediated lipid peroxidation in liposomes, *Biochem. J.,* 229, 135, 1985.

90. **Ward, R. J., O'Connell, M. J., Dickson, D. P. E., Reid, N. M. K., Wade, V. J., Mann, S., Bomford, A., and Peters, T. J.,** Biochemical studies of the iron cores and polypeptide shells of haemosiderin isolated from patients with primary or secondary haemochromatosis, *Biochim. Biophys. Acta,* 993, 131, 1989.

91. **O'Connell, M. J., Ward, R. J., Baum, H., and Peters, T. J.,** Iron release from haemosiderin and ferritin by therapeutic and physiological chelators, *Biochem. J.,* 260, 903, 1989.

92. **Cornell, R. M. and Schneider, W.,** Formation of goethite from ferrihydrite at physiological pH under the influence of cysteine, *Polyhedron,* 8, 149, 1989.

93. **Cornell, R. M. and Giovanoli, R.,** The influence of copper on the transformation of ferrihydrite ($5Fe_2O_3.9H_2O$) into crystalline products in alkaline media, *Polyhedron,* 7, 385, 1988.

94. **O'Connell, M. J., Ward, R. J., Baum, H., Treffry, A., and Peters, T. J.,** Evidence of a biosynthetic link between ferritin and haemosiderin, *Biochem. Soc. Trans.,* 17, 828, 1988.

95. **Wustefield, C. and Crichton, R. R.,** The amino acid sequence of human spleen apoferritin, 150, 43, 1982.

96. **Jacobs, A.,** Low molecular weight iron transport compounds, *Blood,* 50, 4331, 1977.

97. **Laub, R., Schneider, Y.-J., Octave, J. N., Trouet, A., and Crichton, R. R.,** Cellular pharmacology of desferrioxamine B and derivatives in cultured rat hepatocytes in relationship to iron mobilization, *Biochem. Pharmacol.,* 34, 1175, 1985.

98. **Brissot, P., Wright, T. L., Ma, W.-L., and Weissiger, R. A.,** Efficient clearance of non-transferrin-bound iron by rat liver. Implications for hepatic loading in iron overload states, *J. Clin. Invest.,* 76, 1463, 1985.

99. **Hershko, C.,** A study of the chelating agent diethylenetriamine pentaacetic acid using selective radio iron probes of reticulendothelical and parenchymal iron stores, *J. Lab. Clin. Med.,* 85, 913, 1975.

100. **Gutteridge, J. M. C., Rowley, D. A., Griffiths, E., and Halliwell, B.,** Low molecular-weight iron complexes and oxygen radical reactions in idiopathic haemochromatosis, *Clin. Sci.,* 68, 463, 1985.

101. **Aruoma, O. I., Bomford, A., Polson, R. J., and Halliwell, B.,** Non-transferrin-bound iron in plasma from haemochromatosis patients: effects of phlebotomy therapy, *Blood,* 72, 1416, 1988.

102. **Singh, S., Hider, R. C., and Porter, J. B.,** A direct method for quantification of non-transferrin-bound iron, *Anal. Biochem.,* 186, 320, 1990.

103. **Graham, G., Bates, G. W., Rachmilewitz, E. A., and Hershko, C.,** Nonspecific serum iron in thalassemia: quantitation and chemical reactivity, *Am. J. Hematol.,* 6, 207, 1979.

104. **Pootrakul, P., Josephson, B., Huebers, H. A., and Finch, C. A.,** Quantitation of ferritin iron in plasma, as explanation for non-transferrin iron, *Blood,* 71, 1120, 1988.

105. **Anuwatanakulchai, M., Pootrakul, P., Thuvasethakul, P., and Wasi, P.,** Non-transferrin plasma iron in thalassaemia/Hb E and haemoglobin H diseases, *Scand. J. Haematol.,* 32, 153, 1984.

106. **Batey, R. G., Fong, P. L. C., Shamir, S., and Sherlock, S.,** A non-transferrin serum iron in idiopathic haemochromatosis, *Dig. Dis. Sci.,* 25, 340, 1980.

107. **Simpson, R. J., Raja, K. B., Halliwell, B., Evans, P. J., Aruoma, O. I., Konijn, A. M., and Peters, T. J.,** Iron speciation in hypotransferrin mouse, *Biochem. Soc. Trans.,* 19, 316S, 1991.

108. **Grootveld, M., Bell, J. D., Halliwell, B., Aruoma, O. I., Bomford, and Sadler, P. J.,** Non-transferrin-bound iron in plasma or serum from patients with idiopathic hemochromatosis, *J. Biol. Chem.,* 264, 4417, 1989.

109. **Hershko, C., Graham, G., Bates, G. W., and Rachmilewitz, E. A.,** Non-specific serum iron in thalassemia: an abnormal serum iron fraction of potential toxicity, *Br. J. Haematol.,* 40, 255, 1978.

110. **Bartlett, G. R.,** Iron nucleotides in human and rat red cells, *Biochem. Biophys. Res. Commun.,* 70, 1063, 1976.

111. **Konopka, K. and Szotor, M.,** Determination of iron in the acid soluble fraction of human erythrocytes, *Acta Haematol.,* 47, 157, 1972.

112. **Weaver, J. and Pollack, S.,** Two types of receptors for iron on mitochondria, *Biochem. J.,* 271, 463, 1990.

113. **Pollack, S. and Weaver, J.,** Guinea pig and human red cell haemolysate release iron from transferrin, *J. Lab. Clin. Med.,* 105, 629, 1985.

114. **Weaver, J. and Pollack, S.,** Low molecular weight isolated from guinea pig reticulocytes as AMP-iron and ATP-iron complexes, *Biochem. J.,* 261, 787, 1989.

115. **Nilsen, T. and Romslo, I.,** Iron uptake and heme synthesis by isolated rat liver mitochondria. Diferric transferrin as iron donor and effect of pyrophosphate, *Biochim. Biophys. Acta,* 842, 162, 1985.

116. **Boulard, M., Delin, M., and Nafean, Y.,** Identification and purification of a new non-haem, non-ferritin iron protein, *Proc. Soc. Exp. Biol. Med.,* 139, 1379, 197.

117. **Fernandez-Pol, J. A.,** Isolation and characterisation of a siderophore like growth factor from mutants of SV-40 transformed cells adapted to picolinic acid, *Cell,* 14, 489, 1978.

118. **Bakkeren, D. L., Jeu-Jaspars, C. M., Heul, C., and Van Eijk, H. G.,** Analysis of iron binding components in the low molecular weight fraction of the reticulocyte cytosol, *Int. J. Biochem.,* 17, 925, 1985.

119. **Jones, R. L., Grady, R. W., Sorette, M. P., and Cerami, A.,** Host associated iron transfer factor in normal humans and patients with transfusion siderosis, *J. Lab. Clin. Med.,* 107, 431, 1986.

120. **Sheehan, R. G. and Frenkel, E. P.,** The control of iron absorption by the gastrointestinal mucosal cell, *J. Clin. Invest.,* 51, 2241, 1972.

121. **Linder, M. C., Dunn, V., Issac, E., Jones, D., Lim, S., and Munro, H. N.,** Ferritins and intestinal iron absorption: pancreatic enzymes and free iron, *Am. J. Physiol.,* 228, 196, 1975.

122. **Halliday, J. W., Powell, L. W., and Mack, U.,** Intestinal iron binding complexes in iron absorption, in *Proteins of Iron Storage and Transport in Biochemistry and Medicine,* Crichton, R. R., Ed., North-Holland, Amsterdam, 1975, 405.

123. **LaCross, D. and Linder, M. C.,** Synthesis of rat muscle ferritins and function in iron metabolism of heart and diaphragm, *Biochim. Biophys. Acta,* 633, 45, 1980.

124. **Primosigh, J. V. and Thomas, E. D.,** Studies on the partition of iron in bone marrow cells, *J. Clin. Invest.,* 47, 1473, 1968.

125. **Blackburn, G. W. and Morgan, E. H.,** Factors affecting iron and transferrin release from rabbit reticulocyte ghosts to cytosol, *Biochim. Biophys. Acta,* 497, 728, 1977.

126. **Bailey-Wood, R., White, G. P., and Jacobs, A.,** The use of Chang cells *in vitro* for the investigation of cellular iron metabolism, *Br. J. Exp. Pathol.,* 56, 358, 1975.

127. **Mulligan, M., Althaus, B., and Linder, M. C.,** Non-ferritin, non-heme iron pools in rat tissues, *Int. J. Biochem.,* 18, 791, 1986.

128. **Deighton, N. and Hider, R. C.,** Intracellular low molecular weight iron, *Biochem. Soc. Trans.,* 17, 490, 1989.

129. **Nunez, N. T., Coles, E. S., and Glass, J.,** Cytosol intermediates in the transport of iron, *Blood,* 55, 1051, 1980.

130. **Fontcave, M. and Pierre, J. L.,** Iron metabolism: the low-molecular-mass iron pool, *Biol. Metals,* 4, 133, 1991.

131. **Crichton, R. R.,** Iron uptake and utilization by mammalian cells. II. Intracellular iron utilization, *TIBS,* 9, 283, 1984.

132. **Theil, E. C. and Aisen, P.,** The storage and transport of iron in animal cells, in *Iron Transport in Microbes, Plants and Animals,* Winkelmann, G., van der Helm, D., and Neilands, J. B., Eds., VCH Publishers, Weinheim, Germany, 1987, 491.

2. Genetic Regulation of the Iron Transport and Storage Genes: Links with the Acute Phase Response

JACK T. ROGERS

Department of Medicine, Division of Hematology-Oncology, Brigham and Women's Hospital, Harvard Medical School, Boston, Massachusetts

78

I. INTRODUCTION

The transport, safe storage, and metabolism of iron are each necessary for the survival of both eukaryotic and prokaryotic cells. The active site of many cytoplasmic enzymes requires iron either as part of heme or in a form directly associated with the protein. Ribonucleotide reductase, for example, uses nonheme iron within its active site to reduce ribonucleotides to deoxy-nucleotides,[1,2] a step which regulates DNA synthesis during cell proliferation and during development.[3,4] Heme is formed by the chelation of iron into protoporphyrin IX by ferrochelatase.[5] In this form iron is the active moeity of the respiratory cytochromes during oxidative phosphorylation and is therefore vital for the generation of the energy-rich phosphate ATP bonds in all cells.[6] Erythrocytes are specialized to make even larger quantities of heme for hemoglobin synthesis.[7]

In multicellular organisms, iron delivery to individual cells within the tissues is carried out by three proteins. Transferrin (Tf) is required for serum iron transport.[8] Iron-charged *transferrin* binds to *transferrin receptors* (TfRs) on the cell surface and delivers iron into the cytoplasm where it is stored within the cavity of the large, 450,000 Da multimeric protein, *ferritin*.[9] The transferrin receptor and ferritin are crucial cellular proteins because iron is both an essential component of metabolism and at the same time is highly toxic. The safe storage and sequestration of intracellular ferric [Fe(III)] iron within ferritin is particularly important for survival since cytoplasmic ferrous [Fe(II)] iron can form dangerous hydroxy radicals which cause cell death by lipid peroxidation.[9-11] The metal is also known to bind to the phosphate backbone of DNA and at this site can generate hydroxyl radicals capable of causing extensive genetic damage to cells.[12]

The genetic regulation of the transferrin receptor for acquiring iron and the ferritin subunits for its safe storage are each highly coordinated as a part of the cellular response to adapt to iron levels. Sections II to V of this review describe the physiological control of iron homeostasis and detail how it represents a novel post-transcriptional system of genetic regulation in eukaryotes. These sections discuss how the cellular expression of the genes encoding the ferritin subunits, the TfR, and the erythroid heme biosynthetic enzyme, 5-

aminolevulinate synthase (eALAS), are each controlled by iron at the post-transcriptional level. Section VI will describe aspects of the regulation of the ferritin genes to control iron utilization at the organismal level during the acute phase response. Inflammatory cytokines, such as interleukin-1β (IL-1β), IL-6, and tumor necrosis factor (TNF-α), influence ferritin gene expression at both the transcriptional and post-transcriptional levels.

II. IRON UPTAKE AND STORAGE

A. THE TRANSFERRIN RECEPTOR (TfR)

Cells within tissues obtain iron from serum transferrin.[8,9] Circulating transferrin is a glycoprotein with a molecular weight of 80,000 Da that has two iron-binding sites.[8,13] The pathway by which iron is delivered from circulating transferrin to cells is mediated by the passage of the transferrin receptor and its bound ligand, ferrotransferrin, from the cell surface to sites within the cell (see also Chapter 1). In this regard, iron-loaded transferrin is known to bind to its receptor at a higher affinity than uncharged apo-transferrin in erythrocytes.[14] The sequence of the human transferrin receptor cDNA indicates that the receptor is a 95,000-Da protein inserted into the cell membrane.[15] The receptor is predicted to be anchored as a dimer within the lipid bilayer by a 61-amino-acid hydrophobic domain near the amino terminus. Therefore, the transferrin receptor and the asialoglycoprotein receptor share the common feature among membrane receptors of both having their C termini face outward from the cell.[15] Iron-charged transferrin first binds to the receptor C terminus, and the liganded complex migrates toward clathrin-coated pits.[16] Membrane folding occurs at these sites to form vesicles which are rapidly internalized and transported into the cytoplasm. Occupied and free receptors remain attached to the inside surface of the transiting vesicles (endosomes).[17,18] Iron is released from the receptor-bound transferrin within the acid environment of the endosomes.[19] This process is highly energy expensive because the cell must actively form endosomes for internalizing ferro-transferrin and then maintain a proton pump to generate its acid environment.[20] Iron is probably delivered to the lumen of cytoplasm across the endosome membrane by a ferroreductase, after which it enters a chelatable iron pool and is delivered to ferritin for storage or to other sites for metabolism.[13] The apo-transferrin remains attached to the receptor and is recycled out of the cell with the endosome such that the complete transit time for transferrin and its receptor has been estimated to be 7.5 min.[16,21-23] There is a continuous exchange of transferrin receptors from within endocytic vesicles and the cell surface. At any given time, one-third of the transferrin receptors are estimated to reside at the cell surface while the remainder are being shuttled through the cell within the recycling endosomes.[24] The outcome of this process is the delivery of iron to the cell and a recycling of apo-transferrin to the bloodstream where it is available to be recharged with iron.

B. FERRITIN

Cellular ferritin is the iron storage protein of all cells within which iron is oxidized to the ferric state as ferric oxyhydroxide [Fe(III)O·OH].[9] Ferritin consists of a mixture of 24 heavy (H, 21 kDa) and light (L, 19 kDa) subunits which co-assemble to form a heteropolymeric shell.[9,25-27] The structure of L-subunit-rich horse spleen ferritin was derived by Harrison et al. using X-ray crystallography.[28,29] Each of the L subunits within horse spleen ferritin is comprised of five α-helices (NH2-A,B,C,D,E-COOH). The ferritin shell allows the oxidative transfer of iron through channels into an internal cavity.[9] These pores are present both as a result of interactions of four subunits at their E-helices (six channels from a fourfold axis of symmetry) and via interactions between three subunits near their amino-termini (eight channels from a threefold axis of symmetry — see also Chapter 1).

Drysdale et al. demonstrated that the representation of each subunit (H/L ratio) incorporated into the ferritin shell varies between tissues.[25] Rat heart cells, for example, contain H-subunit-rich ferritins whereas liver cells possess shells with a higher L-subunit content.[25,27] This ratio is probably set by the steady-state levels of H-subunit mRNA (H-mRNA) relative to the L-subunit transcript (L-mRNA). Long-term exposure of hepatic cells to iron increases the amount of L subunit relative to H subunit, suggesting that L-rich shells may be better adapted for long-term iron storage.[27] Transcription of the liver L gene is selectively elevated after administration of iron to rats, an effect which resets the ratio of H- and L-mRNAs and therefore increases the relative abundance of L subunit within liver cells.[30] In contrast, the H/L ratio increases in a number of cell types during differentiation by means of a selective increase in the transcription of the H gene. There are two well-known developmental situations which illustrate how the proportion of H subunit increases relative to the L subunit as a consequence of higher H-mRNA accumulation. Dimethylsulfoxide (DMSO)-induced differentiation of the human promyelocytic cell line, HL60, to either macrophage or neutrophil macrophages is associated with a pattern of H- and L-gene expression that favors accumulation of H-mRNA.[31] Similarly, the increase in H-mRNA levels in Friend cells during erythroid development results from both increased transcription of the H gene and selective message stabilization.[32]

The ratio of heavy and light subunits contributes to the pI of ferritin isolated from different tissues as determined by isoelectric focusing.[27] The H subunit contributes more acidic surface charges than the L subunit. In recent years the amino-acid sequences of the two subunits have been determined from recombinant cDNAs and genomic clones encoding the human, rat, frog, mouse, and rabbit ferritin genes.[33-36] The human H subunit exhibits a 55% amino-acid similarity to its L-subunit counterpart.[37] On the other hand, the genes encoding the same subunits in different species are less diverged. The human and rat L-subunit genes are 85% identical at the level of their primary amino acid sequences, suggesting that the genes encoding the two subunits duplicated from a single ancestral sequence and began diverging about 300 million years ago. The genes coding for both the H and L subunits contain three introns which separate the four exons, each of which contains at least one α-helix.[34,35]

A 22-base sequence adjacent to the 5′ cap site within the untranslated (5′UTR) region of the genes for both the H and L subunits has been remarkably conserved throughout evolution.[38] This sequence is capable of forming highly related stem-loop structures within human, rat, mouse, and bullfrog H- and L-mRNAs. These stem loops have been the focus of considerable attention over the past five years (as discussed in Sections III.A and B). The stem loops have been identified as the *cis*-acting structures that regulate iron-induced, post-transcriptional control of both the ferritin and transferrin receptor genes.

III. THE IRON-RESPONSIVE ELEMENT (IRE) AND POST-TRANSCRIPTIONAL REGULATION

The cellular influx of iron downregulates the display of transferrin receptors on the cell surface by decreasing TfR protein synthesis.[40,41] At the same time, ferritin synthesis increases when iron is delivered to cells either as iron salts, diferric transferrin, or as hemin.[42,43] The levels of 5-amino-levulinate synthase (ALAS) within erythroid cells are also increased by an iron influx, thereby controlling heme biosynthesis for hemoglobin synthesis.[44] This section describes how the expression of these genes by iron is regulated without large-scale effects in their transcription. Specifically, TfR mRNA stability and the translational efficiency of ferritin subunit mRNAs is each regulated by iron, an example of post-transcriptional control that may be seen to serve two functions. First, the cell exerts a more rapid control of its iron levels than would be afforded if transcription were the only means to change transferrin receptor and ferritin levels. Second, the presence of iron in the nucleus might generate hydroxyl radicals capable of causing DNA strand-sissions and dangerous modification of the bases within DNA. The maintenance of cellular iron homeostasis by post-transcriptional mechansims within the cytoplasm may preclude entry of the potentially dangerous metal into the nucleus.

A. TRANSLATIONAL REGULATION OF FERRITIN GENE EXPRESSION BY IRON

The storage and oxidation of iron within ferritin decreases cellular levels of the more soluble ferrous [Fe(II)],[9] which otherwise would catalyze the formation of dangerous hydroxyl radicals.[10-12] The large transient elevation in ferritin production which occurs within tissues in order to cope with a potentially dangerous influx of iron has been described for many years.[45] Furthermore, much evidence indicated that acute iron administration to animals induces ferritin synthesis at the translational level.[45-48] However, the availability of recombinant ferritin cDNAs confirmed that the levels of Hand L-mRNAs within rat liver cells are largely unchanged by iron while subunit synthesis is elevated.[49] Polyribosome gradients demonstrated that H- and L-mRNAs are largely dissociated from ribosomes and are stored in the cytoplasm.[43,49] However, cellular exposure to iron results in translational recruitment of H-mRNA and L-mRNAs onto polyribosomes. This effect has been shown to occur both in rat liver cells *in vivo* and within hepatoma cells grown in tissue culture.[43,49] Transcription of the L gene is elevated threefold in rat liver after iron overload, although this enhancement is small compared to the fifty-to-one hundredfold increase observed for ferritin protein levels seen in iron excess.[30] Therefore, H- and L-mRNAs are expressed constitutively at high levels within the cytoplasm of most cell types, and ferritin gene expression is translationally regulated by iron in eukaryotic cells.

The 5′ untranslated regions of the rat L-mRNA, the human H-mRNA, and the rabbit L-mRNA were each shown to contain *cis*-acting elements which regulate ferritin translation in response to iron.[50-52] A region within 76 bases of the 5′ cap site of each ferritin message is sufficient to confer iron induction on transfected CAT and human growth hormone (HGH) genes.[50,51] *In vitro* transcripts of this region also prevent repression of ferritin mRNA translation in reticulocyte lysates.[52] This region is predicted to be capable of forming a stem-loop structure on the basis of intramolecular base pairing within RNA (Figure 1; Gibbs free energy, $\Delta G = -46.1$ kcal/mol for the first 76 bases of the rat L-mRNA).[38,50,53] In fact, a minimal 26-base oligonucleotide encoding this RNA hairpin controls the translation of a chimeric HGH transcript in an iron-dependent fashion when inserted in front of its coding sequence.[54] The stem-loop has been termed as the iron responsive element (IRE) and contains a 5-nucleotide loop sequence [5′-CAGUGN-3′] with a 5′ upstream unpaired cytosine within the stem (Figure 1).

The IRE is conserved at the level of primary sequence and is capable of forming stem loops in both H- and L-subunit mRNAs from species as divergent as humans and bullfrogs.[38] Translational repression depends upon the position of the IRE within the 5′UTR of transcripts (Section IV.B). The IRE does not repress translation at sites downstream from its usual position, which is within 60 bases from the 5′ terminus ferritin mRNAs.[55] However, *Xenopus laevis* ferritin mRNA possesses and IRE 160 bases from the 5′ cap site. This is unusual in that the IRE would not be predicted to influence translation from this position.[56]

B. REGULATION OF TRANSFERRIN RECEPTOR mRNA STABILITY BY IRON

The rate of transferrin receptor synthesis is regulated in the opposite direction to the ferritin subunits.[39,57] Expression of transferrin receptors is increased at the surface of cells growing in a shortage of iron and is diminished by an iron influx.[41,58] This change in receptor display is reflected in the biosynthesis of the protein, which is downregulated when iron is abundant

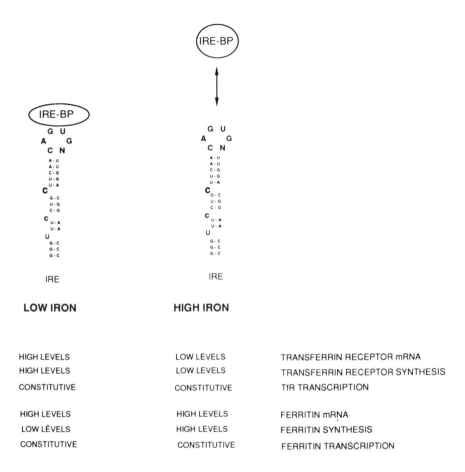

FIGURE 1. The post-transcriptional regulation of the ferritin and transferrin receptor genes by iron as adapted from References 50, 52, 54, and 78. The IRE within H-ferritin mRNA is shown to bind to the IRE-BP in an iron-dependent manner.

and increased when iron is scarce.[59] However, unlike ferritin mRNAs, the TfR mRNA levels reflect protein biosynthesis.[60]

Two lines of evidence suggested that iron influences the expression of the transferrin receptor gene by regulating the stability of its message in the cytoplasm after transcription. First, the transcription rate of the TfR promoter increases threefold in cells starved of iron by administration of the intracellular iron chelator, desferrioxamine.[60] At the same time, levels of TfR mRNA are elevated 20- to 30-fold in iron-depleted cells.[60,61] Therefore, changes in transcription rate cannot account for the observed modulation of receptor mRNA levels observed with iron deprivation.[61] Second, transfection experiments showed that the regulation of TfR mRNA levels by iron persisted even if the message is transcribed from a cloned cDNA downstream of an SV40 promoter which is unaffected by the metal.[61]

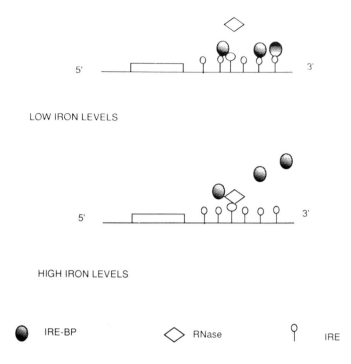

LOW IRON LEVELS

HIGH IRON LEVELS

● IRE-BP   ◇ RNase   ♀ IRE

FIGURE 2. The iron-dependent regulation of transferrin receptor mRNA stability based on models proposed in References 39 and 66. The RNAse can only gain access to the transferrin receptor transcript in a high intracellular iron environment. In this situation there is no steric hindrance from the IRE-BPs, which bind to a combination of the IREs within the 3'UTR of the TfR transcript in the absence of iron.

Mullner and Kuhn (1988) and Casey et al. (1988) showed that exchange of the TfR gene 3'UTR for the corresponding regions within the HGH and HLA-A2 genes confers iron-dependent stability to the chimeric transcripts.[62-64] Deletion analysis confirms that a 680-base region within the 3'UTR of the TfR mRNA contains sequences responsible for iron regulation of receptor transcript levels.[62,63] Computer-assisted sequence analysis of the RNA within this *cis*-acting region predicts the presence of five stem-loop structures between bases 3429 to 4026 of the TfR gene 3' non-coding region.[65] Furthermore, each of the potential TfR mRNA stem loops were seen to be identical to the single IRE within the 5'UTR of ferritin mRNAs suggesting that the receptor mRNA contains IREs within its 3'UTR (IREs 5'-A,B,C,D,E-3').[64-66] The IREs within the TfR transcript exhibit the same loop sequence 5'CAGUGN3' and a similar 5' upstream unpaired cytosine within the stem that is found in ferritin transcripts[64] (Figures 1 and 2). Single-base mutations within the TfR mRNA IRE-B, IRE-C, and IRE-D result in low levels of receptor mRNA even in the absence of iron. Another large stem loop is also predicted to exist between IRE-B and IRE-C within 3'UTR of the human and chicken TfR genes.[65] Its presence among the IREs is consistent with a model for iron-dependent regulation of transferrin receptor mRNA stability, which is described in Section IV.C (Figure 2).[39,67] The IREs within ferritin and TfR transcripts are functionally equivalent. Two of the five TfR mRNA IREs confer translational regulation on a reporter gene in response to iron when inserted in front of its coding block.[64] Therefore, the IRE regulates iron-dependent translation when placed in front of a functional open reading frame, as in the case for ferritin mRNAs, and modulates iron-dependent message stability when placed in a context downstream of a coding block, as is the case for the transferrin receptor.

C. ERYTHROID 5-AMINOLEVULINATE SYNTHASE (eALAS) IS REGULATED BY IRON

Heme biosynthesis is catalyzed by several enzymes in a pathway which is rate-limited at the first step of protoporphyrin IX synthesis by the levels of the mitochondrial matrix enzyme, 5-aminolevulinate synthase (ALAS).[68-70] ALAS is required for the biosynthesis of heme for the respiratory cytochromes present in all cells.[6] The production of heme is completed by the insertion of ferrous iron into the porphyrin ring by ferrochetalase on the inner mitochondrial membrane.[5] The levels of hepatic ALAS are inhibited by a feedback mechanism where the end product, heme, represses enzyme synthesis.[70] Heme downregulates transcription of the ALAS gene in rat liver cells.[71]

The expression of an erythroid-specific ALAS gene (eALAS) is required to supply heme for hemoglobin synthesis.[70,72] Approximately 80% of the iron that is absorbed from the gut is directed to the bone marrow for heme production.[7] As such, erythrocyte precursors might be expected to have different heme requirements than other cells. This viewpoint is consistent with the regulation of the erythroid enzyme which differs from its liver counterpart. Iron, rather than levels of eALAS, limits the rate of heme biosynthesis in cells committed toward erythroid differentiation.[44] Translational mechanisms appear to upregulate the rate of eALAS gene expression after the induction of differentiated MEL cells with succinylacetone, a potent inhibitor of heme biosynthesis.[72] Recently, a recombinant eALAS gene has been cloned to reveal the amino acid sequence of an erythroid specific gene.[73] This eALAS mRNA was discovered to contain a functional IRE within its 5'UTR. The presence of an IRE in eALAS mRNAs confirms the importance of translational mechanisms involved in the regulation of the eALAS gene in erythroid cells. Like ferritin mRNAs, the eALAS mRNA is probably regulated at the translational level in erythroid cells via iron-dependent release of IRE-BP from the IRE (Section IV.B).[73] However, the role of a cellular iron influx controlling heme biosynthesis via the IRE of eALAS mRNAs during erythropoeisis is yet to be determined.

IV. THE IRE-BINDING PROTEIN AND POST-TRANSCRIPTIONAL REGULATION

A. THE IRE-BP, A COMMON *TRANS*-ACTING RNA BINDING PROTEIN

The previous section showed that iron can regulate the translation of ferritin, and possibly eALAS mRNAs, by a single IRE positioned upstream of the coding sequence. At the same time, increased levels of the metal reduce TfR mRNA stability through *cis*-acting IREs downstream of the receptor coding block.[39] How does the position of IRE within each transcript lead to this inverse but coordinate control of gene expression?

The use of an RNA electrophoretic mobility shift technique has demonstrated that a specific protein within rat liver and human K562 cell extracts interacts with IRE-containing transcripts.[74,75] A 90 kDa protein binds to IRE-containing transcripts to form a complex which migrates more slowly than the same RNA in an uncomplexed form. This RNA binding protein has been designated as either the IRE-binding protein (IRE-BP),[75] the ferritin repressor protein (FRP),[76,77] or the iron regulatory factor (IRF).[66] The IRE-BP represses *in vitro* translation of ferritin mRNAs by virtue of its affinity for the IRE adjacent to the 5′ cap site (Section IV.B).[52,76] The same interaction with IREs in the 3′UTR of TfR mRNA protects receptor mRNA from degradation in a low iron environment (Section IV.C).[66]

B. THE IRE-BP AND FERRITIN TRANSLATION

The current model for ferritin translational repression is depicted in Figure 3. It proposes that the IRE-BP limits access of the 43S ribosome subunit to the 5′ cap site of the H- and L-mRNAs. The IRE-BP has a high affinity for the IRE in the absence of iron, an event which represses translation by preventing the first stage of 43S ribosome engagement with the 5′ cap structure. Haile et al. demonstrated that the affinity of the IRE-BP for the IRE is reduced in the event of an increase in intracellular iron levels.[78] This step releases the IRE-BP from its cognate RNA and induces ferritin translation by permitting 43S ribosome access to the H- and L-mRNA 5′ cap sites. Ferritin translation is also derepressed by hemin *in vitro*, suggesting that free iron may not be the only activator of IRE-BP binding to the IRE.[88] The mechanism by which iron changes the allosteric configuration of the IRE-BP has become clearer since the protein has been cloned.[79,80] Oligonucleotides designed from protein sequence of affinity purified IRE-BP were used to identify an appropriate recombinant cDNA which has generated the amino acid sequence of the IRE-BP.[79,80]

These analyses have identified the IRE-BP as being related to *cis*-aconitase.[81] This enzyme would seem unlikely to be related to an RNA-binding protein since it is a mitochondrial isomerase of the citric-acid cycle. However, the human IRE-BP shares a large structural similarity with mitochondrial

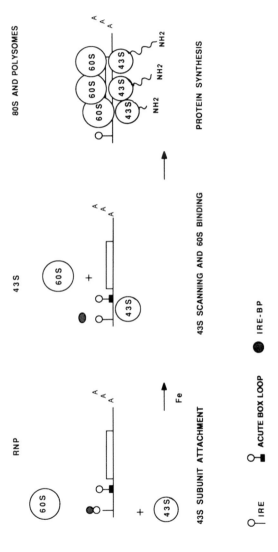

FIGURE 3. H-ferritin translational regulation. The IRE-BP binds to the IRE stem loop in cells depleted of intracellular iron, an event which represses ferritin translation because the 43S ribosomal subunit can no longer attach to the 5' cap site. The IRE-BP is released from its cognate IRE when iron levels increase within the cell. In this situation the 43S ribosome binds to the 5' cap and commences scanning the noncoding region in a 5'-to-3' direction. The 60S ribosome subunit begins polypeptide synthesis after it recognizes this scanning complex. Another downstream stem loop is predicted within a G+C-rich segment of the noncoding region. The contribution of this secondary structure in ferritin translation is unknown. IL-1β accelerates ferritin translation in the presence of iron and may act at either of these stages of translation.

aconitase isolated from pig heart and *Saccharomyces cerevisiae* (30% and 56% homologous at the primary sequence level). Inspection of the protein structure of *cis*-aconitase gives clues as to exactly how the IRE-BP is converted by the presence of cytosolic iron to a configuration wherein it is no longer attached to the IRE (Figure 1). Aconitase possesses an iron sulfur cluster which can be converted from a configuration with four iron atoms linked to four cysteines (4Fe-4S) to a 3Fe-4S state. These cysteine residues are located in the same relative position within the IRE-BP, suggesting that this RNA-binding protein also has an iron-sulfur cluster. It is possible that the IRE-BP may change conformation and be released from the IRE by an alteration in the number of iron atoms within its iron-sulfur cluster in the same way as occurs in aconitase. Recently, the purified IRE-BP has been demonstrated to exhibit aconitase activity *in vitro* and may answer questions as to the role of a previously described cytoplasmic aconitase.[81a] These recent observations lend weight to the suggestion that the IRE-BP is an aconitase which has been adapted to become an RNA-binding protein throughout evolution.[81] The possible contribution of hemin as an IRE-BP activator is discussed (Section V).

The characteristics of ferritin translational regulation are consistent with many of the properties of the Kozak scanning model for translational initiation.[82] The first step in the translational initiation of most mRNAs occurs when a 43S ribosome preinitiation complex, composed of the 40S ribosome subunit and a ternary complex of the initiation factor (Eif-2), GTP and met-tRNA, binds to the $m^7G(5')ppp(5')$ structure at the 5' cap structure of mRNA.[83,84] According to the scanning model, the 43S ribosome migrates in a 3' direction toward the first optimal start codon after attaching to the 5' cap site.[82,85] An important feature of this model is that the insertion of an artificial stem loop ($\Delta G = -30$ kcal/mol) 12 bases from the cap site of a reporter gene transcript prevents the 43S ribosomal subunit from engaging with the 5' terminus. This action represses translation.[86] However, the same stem loop situated farther downstream of the 5'-terminus is melted by the advancing 43S scanning ribosome subunit and therefore does not inhibit translation. In this regard, the proximity of the IRE to the 5' cap site is vital for its action in repressing ferritin translation. IREs located 67 bases from the 5' terminus of transcripts no longer inhibit translation.[55] Therefore, IRE-BP-dependent repression of ferritin translation is only effective when it attaches to a 5'-proximal IRE to prevent the 43S ribosomal subunit from binding to the 5'-terminus. The interaction between the IRE and its cognate IRE-BP is not sufficiently stable to prevent scanning by the small ribosome subunit after it has attached to the 5' cap site (Figure 3).

C. THE IRE-BP AND TfR mRNA STABILITY

The IREs which control iron-induced ferritin mRNA translation and transferrin receptor transcript stability each interact with the same *trans*-acting protein. RNA gel shift criteria has demonstrated that the 3' UTR of transferrin receptor mRNA interacts with the IRE-BP.[64-67] Koeller et al. showed that a large, 1059-base region of the TfR gene 3'UTR, which is predicted to contain five IREs, binds to protein(s) within human K562 erythroleukemic cytoplasmic extracts.[65] This complexed RNA generates an RNase T1 digestion pattern revealing that two of the IREs within the 3'UTR of the TfR transcript interact with a protein within a K562 lysate.[65] Gel mobility assays confirmed that this protein is the IRE-BP by showing that *in vitro* transcripts encoding for individual TfR IREs can compete for lysate binding with a labeled H-ferritin gene IRE. Competition between each of the five unlabeled TfR IREs (A,B,C,D,E) with a labeled ferritin IRE transcript showed that IRE-B and IRE-E have the highest affinity for the IRE-BP and that IRE-C interacts weakly with the IRE-BP.[65] These data are consistent with the capacity of TfR transcript IREs to confer iron-dependent translational regulation to a reporter gene when placed in a 5' context.[64] They confirm the biological equivalence of iron-dependent ferritin mRNA translation and TfR mRNA stability. It is interesting to note that several IRE-binding proteins may exist as members of a multigene family, each of which has a different affinity for the related IREs presented to them in different cells. The DNA sequencing of the H-ferritin IRE-BP clones revealed a related but different cDNA which is another member of a new multigene family.[80]

Mullner et al.[66] and Casey et al.[67] have proposed that IRE-BP (IRF) represses TfR transcript degradation by steric hinderance of an RNase to prevent it from gaining access to secondary structures within the RNA, possibly between IRE-B (3479 to 3511) and IRE-C (3882 to 3914) in the 3'UTR of TfR mRNA. At least four IRE-BP molecules are capable of concurrently binding to the 3'UTR of the transferrin receptor transcript.[66] This model accounts for iron regulation of transferrin receptor synthesis and display on the cell surface. It states that receptor mRNA levels are modulated by changes in message stability operating through binding of the TfR mRNA IREs with the IRE-BP in an iron-dependent manner. Two lines of genetic data support the steric hinderance model of TfR mRNA stabilization via IRE-BP binding (Figure 2):

1. Mutations within the TfR mRNA IREs inhibit both IRE-BP binding and result in low iron-independent TfR mRNA expression.
2. There are mutations that abolish regulation of TfR mRNA stability by iron without influencing the interaction of the IRE-BP with the 3'UTR IREs.[67] Deletions introduced into sites within the 3'UTR of the receptor cDNA permit constitutive expression of TfR mRNA at high levels irrespectively of the iron status of the transfected cells. These mutations may alter secondary structures within the TfR mRNA which represent a target for RNase action mRNA in the event of iron-induced IRE-BP dissociation from the IREs. It should be noted that no specific RNase capable of digesting TfR mRNAs has been detected, although such

enzymes may be associated with the ribosomes, as has been demonstrated for histone H4 mRNA degradation.[66,87]

V. FREE IRON AND HEME IRON AS POSSIBLE INDUCERS OF FERRITIN mRNA TRANSLATION AND TfR mRNA STABILITY

Both iron and heme have been hypothesized to be the active agents in translational derepression of ferritin mRNAs.[43,88,89] Hemin has been proposed as the active inducer of ferritin translation *in vitro*.[88] In this situation heme was shown to release IRE-BP repression of ferritin transcripts applied to a wheat germ lysate.[88] However, chelatable iron appears to be the important agent required to induce ferritin synthesis in intact cells.[43,89] The intracellular iron chelator, desferrioxamine, suppresses the ability of hemin to induce ferritin translation, suggesting that free iron must first be released from heme by the enzyme heme oxygenase within the cytoplasm to be effective (desferrioxamine is not able to remove iron from heme when the two compounds are mixed *in vitro*).[40,43] Tin mesoporphyrin IX, an inhibitor of heme degradation by heme oxygenase, reduces the ability of hemin to induce ferritin synthesis and provides further evidence that free iron is the active regulator of IRE-BP translational derepression.[89] Eisenstein et al. provide other evidence for free iron as the inducer of ferritin translation.[89] On the other hand, there is evidence that hemin dramatically reduces the half-life of the IRE-BP within the cell (R. Thach, personal communication).

The administration of heme and 5-aminolevulinic acid, an agent which stimulates intracellular heme accumulation, each downregulate HeLa cell surface display of transferrin receptors.[90] This provides some support for heme as the active agent for destabilizing TfR mRNA in an iron-rich environment.[90] However, more direct measurement of TfR biosynthesis shows that synthesis of the receptor protein is regulated by chelatable iron and not by heme.[40] The recent demonstration that the IRE-BP is related to *cis*-aconistase will soon provide conclusive molecular evidence as to whether iron or heme controls TfR mRNA stability and ferritin translation.[81] The possibility of converting the mitochondrial aconitase 3Fe-4S iron-sulfur cluster to a 4Fe-4S center aconitase may have implications for potential iron-induced allosteric changes bestowed upon the IRE-BP in an iron-rich environment.

VI. GENETIC REGULATION DURING THE ACUTE PHASE RESPONSE

A. INTRODUCTION
The acute phase response (APR) is a systemic reaction to infection and other inflammatory assaults during which time activated macrophages invade damaged tissues and, with T-lymphocytes, release a number of inflammatory

cytokines into the bloodstream.[91] These include interleukin 1 (IL-1β and IL-1α),[92] interleukin-6 (IL-6),[93] and tumor necrosis factor (TNF).[94-96] Each cytokine is recognized by a different receptor, although they appear to overlap in the responses they elicit.[97] Hepatic cells respond by increasing the transcription of the mRNAs, coding for many plasma proteins which are subsequently secreted into the bloodstream during the acute phase response.[98] These include the major acute phase reactants such as serum amyloid A (SAA)[99] and C-reactive protein (CRP).[100] Other acute phase reactant proteins, such as α_1-acid glycoprotein (AGP)[101] and α_1-antitrypsin inhibitor ($\alpha1AT$)[102] appear in the serum at slightly elevated levels during inflammation. Individual inflammatory cytokines, particularly IL-6, increase the hepatic transcription of many serum acute phase reactant genes.[103] Reduction of serum iron levels also occurs during acute and chronic inflammatory reactions in humans and in animals.[104] The next section describes how serum iron levels are lowered during the acute phase response as a result of sequestration into tissues where ferritin synthesis is elevated. The role of the inflammatory cytokines, IL-1β and TNF, to enhance ferritin gene expression at both the transcriptional and translational levels will be discussed.

B. SERUM IRON LEVELS AND THE ACUTE PHASE RESPONSE

Chronic disease and experimentally induced fever lower serum iron levels.[105] This effect can be partially attributed to individual inflammatory cytokines since IL-1β reduces serum iron levels when administered to mice and chickens.[106,107] This phenomenon is thought to serve as a protective role in animals undergoing a stress reaction to disease or trauma (see also Chapter 6). A reduction in serum iron levels has also been proposed to be one of the preventive benefits of exercise.[108] Serum iron reductions are thought to be adaptive by causing the following events:

1. A reduction in serum iron levels withholds the metal from the siderophores of opportunistic bacteria or parasites.[109] As an example, the intensity of infection by the parasite *Trypanosoma cruzi* was lowered by reducing hepatic iron stores in mice with the intracellular iron chelator desferrioxamine.[110] In this instance, all of the mice whose iron burden had been lowered survived, while 23% of control and 50% of iron-loaded animals died during the infection. Other experiments show that endotoxin injected into mice before inoculation with the fungus *Candida albicans* enhances host survival and that the restoration of plasma iron to normal levels neutralized the effect.[111]

2. A reduction in the bioavailability of iron may also provide protection against cell injury by hydroxyl radicals that are generated from superoxide and hydrogen peroxide released by phagocytic neutrophils.[112,113] Superoxide ions (O_2^-) are thought to reduce Fe^{3+} to Fe^{2+} within living systems. The resulting ferrous iron (Fe^{2+}) is a powerful catalyst which

produces damaging hydroxyl radicals from hydrogen peroxide by the well-known Fenton reaction[113] (see Chapter 7). This sequence of events is referred to as the iron-catalyzed Haber-Weiss reaction ($H_2O_2 + O_2^- \rightarrow O_2 + OH^{\cdot} + OH^-$). Ferrous iron catalyzes the formation of hydroxyl radicals within lipids to peroxidize fatty acids and release ethane.[10,11] This lipid peroxidation causes membrane injury and cell death.[11] The central deleterious role of iron in causing lipid peroxidation in HepG2 cells was demonstrated by the reduction in cellular toxicity of ferric iron by the presence of the iron chelator, desferrioxamine.[113] Damage to DNA by single-strand breaks and base modifications is also associated with hydroxyl radicals catalyzed by iron when complexed to the phosphate backbone of nuclear DNA.[12] The increased appearance of sister-chromatid exchanges in H_2O_2 or $O_2^{\cdot-}$-treated Chinese hamster fibroblasts is also created by iron-catalyzed hydroxyl radical production.[114] Removal of iron by the intracellular iron chelators desferrioxamine and o-phenanthroline prevents both the appearance of sister chromatid exchanges and prokaryotic cell death from single-stranded DNA breaks, as was previously described for lipid peroxidation.[12] The lowering of serum iron levels, therefore, may be seen as an adaptation to prevent the excessive release of dangerous hydroxyl radicals which cause damage to DNA and membranes during the acute phase response.

C. FERRITIN mRNA TRANSLATION AND INFLAMMATION

Several lines of evidence indicate that the fall in serum iron concentration during inflammation is the result of an enlarging of the ferritin pool in tissues. Konijn and Hershko (1977) demonstrated that increased ferritin synthesis precedes a fall in blood iron levels and proposed that this induction is an acute phase response designed to trap iron within the tissues and make it unavailable for release to the serum.[115] The liver has an iron-storage capacity of 195 μg Fe/g of tissue, which implies that hepatic ferritin synthesis is a significant component of the host response to sequester serum iron during the acute phase response.[116-118]

The onset of increased liver ferritin gene expression occurs as early as 6 h after the onset of an inflammatory response in rats.[116] This initial wave of synthesis is the result of a translational enhancement of ferritin mRNAs as demonstrated by a cell-free protein-synthesizing system isolated from rat liver and spleen lysates. Therefore, the enhancement of ferritin synthesis during inflammation is an important example of adaptation to cytokines at the translational level. Campbell et al. confirmed that rat L-mRNA is recruited by polyribosomes in liver and spleen cells responding to turpentine-induced inflammation.[117]

Individual inflammatory cytokines stimulate increased translation of ferritin mRNAs in hepatoma cells grown in culture.[118] In this model system IL-1β increases the synthesis of both H- and L-ferritin subunits in a time frame during which no changes in H- or L-mRNA levels occurs. Translational induction coincides with an increased association of the H- and L-mRNAs with polyribosomes. The induction of ferritin translation by IL-1β is not the indirect effect of an increase in iron uptake by the transferrin receptor. IL-1β has little effect on iron uptake into HepG2 cells from $^{59}Fe_2Tf$ (10% increase). Neither receptor receptor mRNA levels nor the number of Tfr receptors displayed on the cell surface increases in HepG2 cells after exposure to IL-1β.

Serum ferritin, like liver ferritin, is modulated during inflammation possibly in response to cytokines.[105,119] The tissue source of serum ferritin is unknown and there is still controversy as to whether it is actively exported from any tissue or whether it leaks from damaged tissue into the bloodstream. Serum ferritin is L-rich and glycosylated, suggesting that it may be encoded by a different gene from those of tissue H or L ferritins.[120,121] The amount of serum ferritin and L-subunit mRNA on membrane-bound polysomes is increased in the liver cells taken from rats after an experimentally induced inflammatory response, suggesting that this transcript may encode a serum ferritin mRNA. However, liver tissue slices from rats experimentally induced into an inflammatory reaction show no signs of exporting ferritin.[122]

D. IL-1β REGULATES FERRITIN TRANSLATION IN HEPATOCYTES: THE ROLE OF ANOTHER RNA STEM LOOP

The question of how IL-1β regulates ferritin translation carries implications for the translation of other hepatic acute phase mRNAs after their increased transcription. Levels of C-reactive protein (CRP) increase up to 1000-fold during inflammation, an induction that places it among the major acute phase reactants in man.[91] IL-6 enhances hepatic transcription of the CRP gene through sequences upstream of the 5′ cap site, as is the case for many other acute phase genes.[103,123,124] However, IL-1β increases CRP expression from a transfected gene without affecting transcription, suggesting that, like ferritin mRNAs, CRP is regulated by IL-1β by changing the translation of its mRNA. Translational enhancement of CRP mRNAs appears to operate through sequences within the first 15 bases of the CRP transcript.[124] This regulation of CRP mRNA translation implies that the influence of IL-1β may not be limited to the ferritin mRNAs among acute phase mRNAs.

Translation begins when the 43S small ribosome subunit attaches to the $m^7G(5′)ppp(5′)$ structure uniquely present at the 5′ termini of eukaryotic mRNAs.[83,84] Several initiation factors, including eIF-4E, eIF-4A, eIF-4B, and p220, facilitate the first ATP-dependent binding of the 43S ribosome to the 5′ cap structure and unwind RNA secondary structure within 5′ untranslated sequences.[125-127] Iron-induced ferritin translational repression operates when the IRE-BP limits access of the 40S ribosome subunit to the 5′ cap site of the H- and L-mRNAs (Figures 1 and 3). As previously discussed, the IRE-BP binds to the IRE stem loop and represses translation by preventing the first stage of 43S ribosome attachment. However, the IRE appears not to mediate IL-1β-stimulated ferritin translation.[118] There is a two-to-threefold increase in overall protein synthesis within hepatoma cells stimulated by IL-1β. Such an effect may be induced by phosphorylation of eIF-4E as occurs when cells are stimulated by TNF.[128] However, this enhancement is insufficient to account for the 20-fold increase in ferritin translation seen in hepatoma cells stimulated by IL-1β.

Recent data has revealed that a 60-base subregion of the H-mRNA 5′ noncoding block confers IL-1β-inducible translation regulation to a CAT reporter in HepG2 cells (J. Rogers and K. Bridges, unpublished data). Computer-assisted analysis of the sequence within this fragment has demonstrated that it contains a 20-base motif which is also present in the same position and orientation within the 5′UTRs of the transcripts coding for the L subunit and within the mRNAs encoding other acute phase reactant proteins.[129] This "acute box" region is predicted to form RNA stem-loop structures which are unique to their 5′ noncoding regions within each of these mRNAs. The stem loops are not found in either the coding sequences or in the 3′UTRs of the messages. Figure 4 shows the acute-box stem loops predicted for H- and L-mRNAs (16.7 kcal/mol for the H-mRNA acute-box stem loop). The free energy implies that this stem loop is only a moderately stable structure that would not be predicted to hinder 43S ribosome scanning (Figure 1).[86]

The exact role of the stem loop formed from the acute box region is yet to be determined, but it might present a target for 60S recognition of the preformed 43S scanning complex. The second step of translation starts after the 43S preinitiation complex migrates in the 3′ direction until it reaches the first appropriate initiation codon.[82,85] The components of this structure include the 40S ribosome subunit and the ternary complex which consists of the initiation factor eIF-2, GTP, and Met-tRNA. Polypeptide synthesis occurs as the 60S ribosome subunit attaches to the scanning complex at the translational start codon within an optimal surrounding sequence context ("Kozak consensus" CCPuCCATGG).[82,85] IL-1β may play a role in modulating the 60S joining step of H-mRNA translation to facilitate peptide synthesis at the initiation codon. Direct base pairing may be important in ribosome recognition of H-mRNA, since its acute box region is G + C rich and complementary to the variable regions of 28S mRNA.[130] However, the mechanism of IL-1β in regulating ferritin acute phase translation is as yet unclear.

E. TRANSCRIPTIONAL REGULATION OF THE FERRITIN H-SUBUNIT GENE DURING INFLAMMATION

Transcription of the rat liver ferritin genes is elevated during the later stages of an experimentally induced inflammatory response. Konijn et al. measured ferritin mRNA levels indirectly by *in vitro* translation of liver cell sap and polyribosomes.[116] The steady-state levels of the ferritin subunit mRNAs are increased in liver cells beginning 24 h after the injection of rats with turpentine.[116] The use of recombinant ferritin cDNAs and individual inflam-

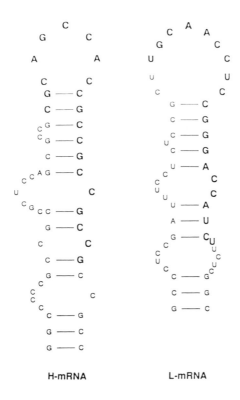

H-mRNA   L-mRNA

FIGURE 4. The RNA stem loops predicted to be present within the acute box regions in the 5′ untranslated regions of the human ferritin mRNAs. The nucleotides which are most similar for the secondary structure elements within the 5′ UTRs of both genes are represented in bold letters.

matory cytokines has demonstrated that ferritin gene expression is regulated at the transcriptional as well as translational mechanisms during the acute phase response. The inflammatory cytokines IL-1β, IL-6, and TNF-α each enhance ferritin subunit gene expression at the transcriptional level. Cell lines from several sources, including mouse adipocytes and human muscle cells, exhibit a four-to-sixfold increase in levels of H-subunit mRNA after 48 h exposure to TNF-α.[96] Furthermore, the induction of the H-subunit mRNA by TNF in primary myoblasts is iron-dependent and sensitive to actinomycin-D.[131] Like TNF, IL-1α increases the levels of H-ferritin mRNA in human myoblasts and myotubules without affecting the steady-state levels of the L-subunit mRNA.[132] These results suggest that TNF-α specifically increases H-subunit gene transcription since L-subunit synthesis is unaffected by the cytokine. As discussed previously, an increase in plasma ferritins, enriched in L subunits, occurs during an inflammatory response.[119,120] The specific induction of H-subunit mRNAs by individual cytokines in several tissues grown *in vitro* is inconsistent with these clinical and experimental observations. However, the tissue source of serum ferritin is still unknown. The lack of a specific induction in the steady-state levels of L-subunit mRNA by TNF, IL-1β and IL-1α within fibroblasts, myoblasts, and hepatoma cell lines suggests that an alternative tissue source for serum ferritin exists.[96,118,131]

An indirect consequence of the increase in H-mRNA levels was observed as a decrease in the translation of both H- and L-ferritin subunits in cells after prolonged (8 h) exposure to TNF-α.[131] This effect occurs because the induction of H-subunit mRNA levels by TNF elevates the proportion of ferritin shells rich in H subunits within the cell. Current evidence suggests that H-rich ferritin shells readily store free iron.[133] These circumstances would indirectly repress ferritin translation since the increased presence of H-rich ferritin shells would diminish intracellular iron levels during an inflammatory response. Transferrin receptor message and protein synthesis is enhanced three- to fourfold after 24 h of TNF and IL-1α stimulus of MRC5 fibroblasts without a concomitant increase in cell growth.[134] However, as in the case for ferritin translation, TNF-α appears to regulate transferrin receptor expression as an indirect consequence of increased H-subunit transcription and rapid iron sequestration into newly synthesized H-subunit-rich ferritin shells.[134] In summary, TNF and IL-α seem to elevate cellular levels of ferritins which are enriched with H subunits by increasing the H-mRNA levels. This reduces the amount of iron within the cell and regulates the IRE-BP and IRE interaction to change TfR mRNA stability and ferritin translation.

VII. CONCLUSIONS

The genetic control of iron homeostasis provides many insights into post-transcriptional regulation. TfR and ferritin gene expression is extremely sensitive to changes in iron levels at the cellular level. These genes are coordinately regulated at the post-transcriptional level by the affinity of the IRE-BP for its cognate IRE present within either 3'UTR of the transferrin receptor message or the 5'UTR of the ferritin transcript. Both genes are transcribed at a constitutively high level. A more complex response occurs at the level of the organism. Different tissues respond to the inflammatory cytokines TNF, IL-1α, IL-1β, and IL-6 at both transcriptional and translational levels. Both of these levels of regulation have been observed for ferritin gene expression during inflammation. Transferrin receptor message levels appear to change only as an indirect response to increased TNF and IL-1α-induced H-subunit synthesis. These events can be seen as a part of an integrated response between tissues and cytokines to regulate iron homeostasis during the acute phase response.

VIII. ACKNOWLEDGMENTS

The author would like to thank Teresa O'Neil, Nazneen Aziz, and Kristin Kasschau for reviewing this manuscript. I am particularly grateful to Dr.

Kenneth Bridges for support, encouragement, and for reviewing the manuscript.

REFERENCES

1. **Graslund, A., Ehrenberg, A., and Thelander, C.,** Characterization of the free radical of mammalian ribonucleotide reductase, *J. Biol. Chem.,* 257, 5711, 1982.
2. **Thelander, L., Graslund, A., and Thelander, M.,** Continual presence of oxygen and iron required for mammalian ribonucleotide reductase: possible regulation mechanism, *Biochem. Biophys. Res. Commun.,* 110, 859, 1983.
3. **Reichard, P. and Ehrenberg, A.,** Ribonuclease reductase — a radical enzyme, *Science,* 221, 514, 1983.
4. **Standart, N., Hunt, T., and Ruderman, J. V.,** Differential accumulation of ribonucleotide reductase subunits in clam oocytes: the large subunit is stored as a polypeptide, the small subunit as untranslated mRNA, *J. Cell Biol.,* 103, 2129, 1986.
5. **Ferriera, G. C., Andrew, T. L., Karr, S. W., and Dailey, H. A.,** Organization of the terminal two enzymes of the heme biosynthetic pathway, *J. Biol. Chem.,* 263, 3835, 1988.
6. **Lehninger, A.,** *Biochemistry,* Worth Publishers, New York, 1975, chap. 18.
7. **Worwood, M.,** Aberrations of iron and porphyrin metabolism, in *Iron Excess,* Muller-Eberhard, U., Miescher, P. A., and Jaffe, E. R., Eds., Grune & Stratton, New York, 1977, 3.
8. **Aisen, P.,** The transferrins, in *Iron Biochemistry and Medicine,* Vol. 2, Jacobs, A. and Worwood, M., Eds., Academic Press, New York, 1980, 87.
9. **Theil, E. C.,** Ferritin: structure, gene regulation, and cellular function in animals, plants, and microorganisms, *Annu. Rev. Biochem.,* 56, 289, 1987.
10. **Munro, H. N., Aziz, N., Leibold, E. A., Murray, M., Rogers, J., Vass, J. K., and White, K.,** The ferritin genes: structure, expression, and regulation, *Ann. N.Y. Acad. Sci.,* 526, 113, 1988.
11. **Halliwell, B. and Gutteridge, J. M. C.,** Oxygen toxicity, oxygen radicals, transition metals and disease, *Biochem. J.,* 219, 1, 1984.
12. **Imlay, J. A. and Linn, S.,** DNA damage and oxygen radical toxicity, *Science,* 240, 1302, 1988.
13. **Nunez, M., Gaete, V., Watkins, J. A., and Glass, J.,** Mobilization of iron from endocytic vesicles: the effects of acidification and reduction, *J. Biol. Chem.,* 265, 6688, 1990.
14. **Heubers, H. A., Csiba, E., and Heubers, E., et al.,** Competitive advantage of diferric transferrin in delivering iron to reticulocytes, *Proc. Natl. Acad. Sci. U.S.A.,* 80, 300, 1983.
15. **McClelland, A., Kuhn, L. C., and Ruddle, F. H.,** The human transferrin receptor gene: genomic organization and the complete primary structure of the receptor deduced from a cDNA sequence, *Cell,* 39, 267, 1984.
16. **Hopkins, C. R.,** The appearance and internalization of transferrin receptors at the margins of spreading cells, *Cell,* 40, 199, 1985.
17. **Klausner, R. D., van Renswoude, J., Ashwell, G., Kempf, C., Schechter, A. N., Dean, A., and Bridges, K. R.,** Receptor-mediated endocytosis of transferrin in K562 cells, *J. Biol. Chem.,* 258, 4715, 1983.

18. **Karin, M. and Mintz, B.,** Receptor-mediated endocytosis of transferrin in developmentally totipotent mouse teratocarcinoma stem cells, *J. Biol. Chem.,* 256, 3245, 1981.

19. **van Renswoude, J., Bridges, K. R., Harford, J. B., and Klausner, R. D.,** Receptor-mediated endocytosis of transferrin and the uptake of Fe in K562 cells: identification of a non-lysosomal acidic compartment, *Proc. Natl. Acad. Sci. U.S.A.,* 79, 6186, 1982.

20. **Tycko, B. and Maxfield, F. R.,** Rapid acidification of endocytic vesicles containing α_2-macroglobulin, *Cell,* 28, 643, 1982.

21. **Klausner, R. D., Ashwell, G., van Renswoude, J., Harford, J. B., and Bridges, K. R.,** Binding of apo-transferrin to K562 cells: explanation of the transferrin cycle, *Proc. Natl. Acad. Sci. U.S.A.,* 80, 2263, 1983.

22. **Dautry-Varsat, A., Ciechanover, A., and Lodish, H. F.,** pH and the recycling of transferrin during receptor-mediated endocytosis, *Proc. Natl. Acad. Sci. U.S.A.,* 80, 2258, 1983.

23. **Hopkins, C. R. and Trowbridge, I. S.,** Internalization and processing of transferrin and the transferrin receptor in human carcinoma A431 cells, *J. Cell Biol.,* 97, 508, 1983.

24. **Bleil, J. D. and Bretscher, M.,** Transferrin receptor and its recycling in HeLa cell, *EMBO J.,* 1, 351, 1982.

25. **Arosio, P., Adelman, T. G., and Drysdale, J. W.,** On ferritin heterogeneity (further evidence for heteropolymers), *J. Biol. Chem.,* 253, 4451, 1978.

26. **Watanabe, N. and Drysdale, J. W.,** Evidence for distinct mRNAs for ferritin subunits, *Biochem. Biophys. Res. Commun.,* 98, 507, 1981.

27. **Bomford, A., Conlon-Hollingshead, C., and Munro, H. N.,** Adaptive responses of rat tissue isoferritins to iron administration, *J. Biol. Chem.,* 256, 948, 1981.

28. **Clegg, G. A., Stansfield, R. F. D., Bourne, P. E., and Harrison, P. M.,** Helix packing and subunit conformation in horse spleen apoferritin, *Nature,* 288, 298, 1980.

29. **Ford, G. C., Harrison, P. M., Rice, D. W., Smith, T. M., White, J. L., and Yariv, J.,** *Philos. Trans. R. Soc. London Ser. B,* 304, 551, 1984.

30. **White, K. and Munro, H. N.,** Induction of ferritin subunit synthesis by iron is regulated at both the transcriptional and translational levels, *J. Biol. Chem.,* 263, 8938, 1988.

31. **Chou, C. C., Gatti, R. A., Fuller, M. L., Concannon, P., Wong, A., Chada, S., Davis, R. C., and Salser, W. A.,** Structure and expression of ferritin genes in a human promyelocytic line that differentiates *in vitro, Mol. Cell. Biol.,* 6, 566, 1986.

32. **Beaumont, C., Dugast, I., Renaudie, F., Souroujou, M., and Grandchamp, B.,** Transcriptional regulation of Ferritin H and L subunits in adult erythroid and liver cells from the mouse, *J. Biol. Chem.,* 264, 7498, 1989.

33. **Brown, A. J. P., Leibold, E. A., and Munro, H. N.,** Isolation of cDNA clones for the light subunit of rat liver ferritin: evidence that the light subunit is encoded by a multigene family, *Proc. Natl. Acad. Sci. U.S.A.,* 80, 1265, 1983.

34a. **Boyd, D., Vecoli, C., Belcher, D. M., Jain, S. K., and Drysdale, J. W.,** Structural and functional relationships of human ferritin H and L chains deduced from cDNA clones, *J. Biol. Chem.,* 260, 11755, 1985.

34b. **Jain, S. K., Barrett, K. J., Boyd, D., Favreau, M. F., Crampton, J., and Drysdale, J. W.,** Ferritin H and L chains are derived from different multigene families, *J. Biol. Chem.,* 260, 11762, 1985.

35a. **Santoro, C., Marone, M., Ferrone, M., Constanzo, F., Colombo, M., Minganti, C., Cortese, R., and Silengo, L.,** Cloning of the gene coding for human L apoferritin, *Nucleic Acids Res.,* 14, 2863, 1986.

35b. **Constanzo, F., Colombo, M., Staempfli, S., Santoro, C., Marone, M., Rainer, F., Delius, H., and Cortese, R.,** Structure of gene and pseudogenes of human apoferritin H, *Nucleic Acids Res.,* 14, 721, 1986.

36. **Didsbury, J. R., Theil, E. C., Kaufman, R. E., and Dickey, L. F.,** Multiple red cell ferritin mRNAs, which code for an abundant protein in the embryonic cell type, analyzed by primer extension of the 5′-untranslated regions, *J. Biol. Chem.,* 261, 949, 1985.

37. **Dorner, M. H., Salfeld, J., Leibold, E. A., Vass, J. K., and Munro, H. N.,** Structure of human ferritin light subunit mRNA: comparison with heavy subunit message and functional implications, *Proc. Natl. Acad. Sci. U.S.A.,* 82, 3139, 1985.

38. **Murray, M. T., White, K., and Munro, H. N.,** Conservation of ferritin heavy subunit gene structure: implications for the regulation of ferritin gene expression, *Proc. Natl. Acad. Sci. U.S.A.,* 84, 7438, 1987.

39. **Klausner, R. D. and Harford, J. B.,** *Cis-trans* models for post-transcription gene expression, *Science,* 246, 870, 1989.

40. **Rouault, T. A., Rao, K., Harford, J., Mattia, E., and Klausner, R. D.,** Hemin, chelatable iron, and the regulation of transferrin receptor biosynthesis, *J. Biol. Chem.,* 260, 14682, 1985.

41. **Rudolph, N. S., Ohlsson-Wilhelm, B. M., Leary, J. F., and Rowley, P. T.,** Regulation of K562 cell transferrin receptors by exogenous iron, *J. Cell. Physiol.,* 122, 441, 1985.

42. **Mattia, E., Josic, D., Ashwell, G., Klausner, R. D., and van Renswoude, J.,** Regulation of intracellular iron distribution in K562 human erythroleukemia cells, *J. Biol. Chem.,* 261, 4587, 1986.

43. **Rogers, J. T. and Munro, H. N.,** Translation of ferritin light and heavy subunit mRNAs is regulated by intracellular chelatable iron levels in rat hepatoma cells, *Proc. Natl. Acad. Sci. U.S.A.,* 84, 2277, 1987.

44. **Laskey, J. D., Ponka, P., and Schulman, H. M.,** Control of heme synthesis during Friend cell differentiation: role of iron and transferrin, *J. Cell. Physiol.,* 129, 185, 1986.

45. **Drysdale, J. W. and Munro, H. N.,** Regulation of synthesis and turnover of ferritin in rat liver, *J. Biol. Chem.,* 241, 3630, 1966.

46. **Schaefer, F. V. and Theil, E. C.,** The effect of iron on the synthesis and amount of ferritin in red blood cells during ontogeny, *J. Biol. Chem.,* 256, 1711, 1981.

47. **Schull, G. E. and Theil, E. C.,** Regulation of ferritin mRNA: a possible gene-sparing phenomenon, *J. Biol. Chem.,* 258, 7921, 1983.

48. **Zahringer, J., Baliga, B. S., and Munro, H. N.,** Novel mechanism for translational control in regulation of ferritin by iron, *Proc. Natl. Acad. Sci. U.S.A.,* 73, 857, 1976.

49. **Aziz, N. and Munro, H. N.,** Both subunits of rat liver ferritin are regulated at the translational level by iron induction, *Nucleic Acids Res.,* 14, 915, 1986.

50. **Aziz, N. and Munro, H. N.,** Iron regulates ferritin mRNA translation through a segment of its 5' untranslated region, *Proc. Natl. Acad. Sci. U.S.A.,* 84, 8478, 1987.

51. **Hentze, M. W., Rouault, T. A., Wright Caughman, S., Dancis, A., Harford, J. B., and Klausner, R. D.,** A *cis*-acting element is necessary and sufficient for translational regulation of human ferritin expression in response to iron, *Proc. Natl. Acad. Sci. U.S.A.,* 84, 6730, 1987.

52. **Walden, W. E., Daniels-McQueen, S., Brown, P. H., Gaffield, L., Russell, D. A., Bielser, D., Bailey, L. C., and Thach, R. E.,** Translational repression in eukaryotes: partial purification and repression of ferritin mRNA translation, *Proc. Natl. Acad. Sci. U.S.A.,* 85, 9503, 1988.

53. **Zuker, M. and Steigler, P.,** Optimal computer folding of large RNA sequences using thermodynamic and auxillary information, *Nucleic Acids Res.,* 9, 133, 1981.

54. **Hentze, M. W., Wright Caughman, S., Rouault, T. A., Barriocanal, J. G., Dancis, A., Harford, J. B., and Klausner, R. D.,** Identification of the iron-responsive element for the translational regulation of human ferritin mRNA, *Science,* 238, 1570, 1987.

55. **Goossen, B., Wright Caughman, S., Harford, J. B., Klausner, R. D., and Hentze, M. W.,** Translational repression by a complex between the iron responsive element of ferritin mRNA and its specific cytoplasmic binding protein is position-dependent *in vivo,* *EMBO J.,* 9, 4127, 1990.

56. **Moskaitis, J. E., Pastori, R. L., and Schoenberg, D. R.,** Sequence of *Xenopus laevis* ferritin mRNA, *Nucleic Acids Res.,* 18, 2184, 1990.

57. **Pelosi, E., Testa, U., Louache, F., Thomopoulos, P., Salvo, G., Samoggia, P., and Peschle, C.,** Expression of transferrin receptors in phytohemagglutinin-stimulated human T-lymphocytes (evidence for a three step model), *J. Biol. Chem.,* 261, 3036, 1986.

58. **Bridges, K. R. and Cudkowicz, A.,** Effect of iron chelators on the transferrin receptor in K562 cells, *J. Biol. Chem.,* 259, 12,970, 1984.

59. **Mattia, E., Rao, K., Shapiro, D. S., Sussman, H. H., and Klausner, R. D.,** Biosynthetic regulation of the human transferrin receptor by desferrioxamine in K562 cells, *J. Biol. Chem.,* 259, 2689, 1984.

60. **Rao, K., Harford, J. B., Rouault, T. A., McClelland, A., Ruddle, F. H., and Klausner, R. D.,** Transcriptional regulation by iron of the gene for the transferrin receptor, *Mol. Cell. Biol.,* 6, 236, 1986.

61. **Owen, D. and Kuhn, L. C.,** Noncoding 3′ sequences of the transferrin receptor gene are required for mRNA regulation by iron, *EMBO J.,* 6, 1287, 1987.

62. **Casey, J. L., Di Jeso, B., Rao, K., Klausner, R. D., and Harford, J. B.,** Two genetic loci participate in the regulation by iron of the gene for the human transferrin receptor, *Proc. Natl. Acad. Sci. U.S.A.,* 85, 1787, 1988.

63. **Mullner, E. W. and Kuhn, L. C.,** A stem-loop in the 3′ untranslated region mediates iron-dependent regulation of transferrin receptor mRNA stability in the cytoplasm, *Cell,* 53, 815, 1988.

64. **Casey, J. L., Hentze, M. W., Koeller, D. M., Wright Caughman, S., Rouault, T. A., Klausner, R. D., and Harford, J. B.,** Iron-responsive elements: regulatory RNA sequences that control mRNA levels and translation, *Science,* 240, 924, 1988.

65. **Koeller, D. M., Casey, J. L., Hentze, M. W., Gerhardt, E. M., Chan, L. L., Klausner, R. D., and Harford, J. B.,** A cytosolic protein binds to structural elements within the iron regulatory region of the transferrin receptor mRNA, *Proc. Natl. Acad. Sci. U.S.A.,* 86, 3574, 1989.

66. **Mullner, E. W., Neupert, B., and Kuhn, L. C.,** A specific mRNA binding factor regulates the iron-dependent stability of cytoplasmic transferrin receptor mRNA, *Cell,* 58, 373, 1989.

67. **Casey, J. L., Koeller, D. M., Ramin, V. C., Klausner, R. D., and Harford, J. B.,** Iron regulation of transferrin receptor mRNA levels requires iron-responsive elements and a rapid turnover determinant in the 3′ untranslated region of the mRNA, *EMBO J.,* 8, 3693, 1989.

68. **Levere, R. D. and Granick, S.,** Control of hemoglobin synthesis in the cultured chick blastoderm by δ-aminolevulinic acid synthetase: increase in the rate of hemoglobin formation with δ-aminolevulinic acid, *Proc. Natl. Acad. Sci. U.S.A.,* 54, 134, 1965.

69. **Volland, C. and Urban-Grimal, D.,** The presequence of yeast 5-aminolevulinate synthetase is not required for targeting to mitochondria, *J. Biol. Chem.,* 263, 8294, 1988.

70. **London, I. M., Bruns, G. P., and Karibian, D.,** The regulation of hemoglobin synthesis and the pathogenesis of some hypochromic anemias, *Medicine,* 43, 789, 1964.

71. **Srivastava, G., Borthwick, I. A., Maguire, D. J., Elferink, C. J., Bawden, M. J., Mercer, J. F. B., and May, B. K.,** Regulation of 5-aminolevulinate synthase mRNA in different rat tissues, *J. Biol. Chem.,* 263, 5202, 1988.

72. **Elferink, C. J., Sassa, S., and May, B. K.,** Regulation of 5-aminolevulinate synthase in mouse erythroleukemic cells is different from that in the liver, *J. Biol. Chem.,* 263, 13,012, 1988.

73a. **Cox, T. C., Bawden, M. J., Martin, A., and May, B. K.,** Human erythroid 5-aminolevulinate synthase identification of an iron-responsive element in the mRNA, *EMBO J.,* 10, 1891, 1991.

73b. **Dandekar, T., Stripecke, R., Gray, K. K., Goossen, B., Constable, A., Johansson, H. E., and Hentze, M. W.,** Identification of a novel iron-responsive element in murine and human erythroid δ-aminolevulinic acid synthase mRNA, *EMBO J.,* 10, 1903, 1991.

74. **Leibold, E. A. and Munro, H. N.**, A cytoplasmic protein binds *in vitro* to a highly conserved sequence in the 5' untranslated region of ferritin heavy- and light-subunit mRNAs, *Proc. Natl. Acad. Sci. U.S.A.*, 85, 2171, 1988.

75. **Rouault, T. A., Hentze, M. W., Wright Caughman, S., Harford, J. B., and Klausner, R. D.**, Binding of a cytosolic protein to the iron-responsive element of human ferritin mRNA, *Science*, 241, 1207, 1988.

76. **Walden, W. E., Patino, M. M., and Gaffield, L.**, Purification of a specific repressor of ferritin mRNA translation from rabbit liver, *J. Biol. Chem.*, 264, 13765, 1989.

77. **Brown, P. H., Daniels-McQueen, S., Walden, W. E., Patino, M. M., Gaffield, L., Bielser, D., and Thach, R. E.**, Requirements for the translational repression of ferritin transcripts in wheat germ extracts by a 90-kDa protein from rabbit liver, *J. Biol. Chem.*, 264, 13,383, 1989.

78. **Haile, D. J., Hentze, M. W., Rouault, T. A., Harford, J. B., and Klausner, R. D.**, Regulation of interaction of the iron-responsive element binding protein with iron-responsive RNA elements, *Mol. Cell. Biol.*, 9, 5055, 1989.

79. **Rouault, T. A., Hentze, M. W., Haile, D. J., Harford, J. B., and Klausner, R. D.**, The iron-responsive element binding protein: a method for affinity purification of a RNA binding protein, *Proc. Natl. Acad. Sci. U.S.A.*, 86, 5768, 1989.

80. **Rouault, T. A., Tang, C. K., Kaptain, S., Burgess, W. H., Haile, D. H., Samaniego, F., McBride, O. W., Harford, J. B., and Klausner, R. D.**, Cloning of the cDNA encoding an RNA regulatory protein — the human iron-responsive element binding protein, *Proc. Natl. Acad. Sci. U.S.A.*, 87, 7958, 1990.

81. **Rouault, T. A., Stout, C. D., Kaptain, S., Harford, J. B., and Klausner, R. D.**, Structural relationship between an iron-regulated RNA-binding protein (IRE-BP) and aconitase: functional implications, *Cell*, 64, 881, 1991.

81a. **Kaptain, S., Downey, W. E., Tang, C., Philpott, C., Haile, D., Orloff, D. G., Harford, J. B., Rouault, T. A., and Klausner, R. D.**, A regulated RNA binding protein also possesses aconitase activity, *Proc. Natl. Acad. Sci. U.S.A.*, 88, 10,109, 1991.

82. **Kozak, M.**, The scanning model for translation: an update, *J. Cell Biol.*, 108, 229, 1989.

83. **Lazaris-Karatzas, A., Montine, K. S., and Sonnenberg, N.**, Malignant transformation by a eukaryotic initiation factor subunit that binds to mRNA 5' cap, *Nature*, 345, 544, 1990.

84. **Shatkin, A. J.**, Capping of eucaryotic mRNAs, *Cell*, 9, 645, 1976.

85. **Kozak, M.**, Point mutations define a sequence flanking the AUG initiator codon that modulates translation by eukaryotic ribosomes, *Cell*, 44, 283, 1986.

86. **Kozak, M.**, Circumstances and mechanisms of inhibition of translation by secondary structure in eucaryotic mRNAs, *Mol. Cell. Biol.*, 9, 5134, 1989.

87. **Schumperli, D.**, Multilevel regulation of replication-dependent histone genes, *Trends Genet.*, 4, 187, 1988.

88. **Lin, J.-J., Daniels-McQueen, S., Patino, M. M., Gaffield, L., Walden, W. E., and Thach, R. E.**, Derepression of ferritin messenger RNA translation by hemin *in-vitro*, *Science*, 247, 74, 1990.

89. **Eisenstein, R. S., Garcia-Mayol, D., Pettingell, W., and Munro, H. N.**, Regulation of ferritin and heme oxygenase synthesis in rat fibroblasts by different forms of iron, *Proc. Natl. Acad. Sci. U.S.A.*, 88, 688, 1991.

90. **Ward, J. H., Jordan, I., Kushner, J. P., Kaplan, J.**, Heme regulation of HeLa cell transferrin receptor number, *J. Biol. Chem.*, 259, 13235, 1984.

91. **Kushner, I.**, The phenomenon of the acute phase response, *Ann. N.Y. Acad. Sci.*, 389, 39, 1982.

92. **Dinarello, C. A.**, The biology of interleukin-1, *FASEB J.*, 2, 108, 1988.

93. **Kishimoto, T.**, The biology of interleukin-6, *Blood*, 74, 1, 1989.

94. **Carswell, E. A., Old, L. J., Kassel, R. L., Green, S., Fiore, N., and Williamson, B.**, An endotoxin-induced serum factor that causes necrosis of tumors, *Proc. Natl. Acad. Sci. U.S.A.*, 72, 3666, 1975.

95. **Darlington, G. J., Wilson, D. R., and Lachman, L. B.**, Monocyte-conditioned medium, interleukin-1, and tumor necrosis factor stimulate the acute phase response in human hepatoma cells *in vitro, J. Cell Biol.*, 103, 787, 1986.

96. **Torti, S. V., Kwak, E. L., Miller, S. C., Miller, L. L., Ringold, G. M., Myambo, K. B., Young, A. P., and Torti, F. M.**, The molecular cloning and characterization of murine ferritin heavy chain, a tumor necrosis factor inducible gene, *J. Biol. Chem.*, 263, 12638, 1988.

97. **Akira, S., Hirano, T., Taga, T., and Kishimoto, T.**, Biology of multifunctional cytokines: Il-6 and related molecules (Il-1 and TNF), *FASEB J.*, 4, 2860, 1990.

98. **Ramadori, G., Sipe, J. D., Dinarello, C. A., Mizel, B., and Colten, H. R.**, Pretranslational modulation of acute phase hepatic protein synthesis by murine recombinant interleukin I (Il-1) and purified human Il-1, *J. Exp. Med.*, 162, 930, 1985.

99. **Lowell, C. A., Stearman, R. S., and Morrow, J. F.**, Transcriptional regulation of serum amyloid A gene expression, *J. Biol. Chem.*, 261, 8453, 1986.

100. **Arcone, R., Gualandi, G., and Ciliberto, G.**, Identification of sequences responsible for acute-phase induction of human C-reactive protein, *Nucleic Acids Res.*, 16, 3195, 1988.

101. **Dente, L., Pizza, M. G., Metspalu, A., and Cortese, R.**, Structure and expression of the genes coding for human α1-acid glycoprotein, *EMBO J.*, 6, 2289, 1987.

102. **Ciliberto, G., Dente, L., and Cortese, R.**, Cell-specific expression of a transfected human α_1-antitrypsin gene, *Cell*, 41, 531, 1985.

103. **Morrone, G., Cilliberto, G., Oliviero, S., Arcone, R., Dente, L., Content, J., and Cortese, R.**, Recombinant interleukin-6 regulates the transcriptional activation of a set of human acute phase response genes, *J. Biol. Chem.*, 263, 12554, 1988.

104. **Beissel, W. R.**, Magnitude of the host nutritional response to infection, *Am. J. Clin. Nutr.*, 30, 1236, 1977.

105. **Elin, R. J., Wolf, S. M., and Finch, C. A.**, Effect of induced fever on serum iron and ferritin concentrations in man, *Blood*, 49, 147, 1977.

106. **Westmacott, D., Hawkes, J. E., Hill, R. P., Clarke, L. E., and Bloxham, D. P.**, Comparison of the effects of recombinant murine and human interleukin-1 *in vitro* and *in vivo, Lymph. Res.*, 5, S87, 1986.

107. **Klassing, K. C.**, Effect of inflammatory agents and interleukin 1 on iron and zinc metabolism, *Am. J. Physiol.*, 247, R901, 1984.

108. **Lauffer, R. B.**, Exercise as prevention: do the health benefits derive in part from lower iron levels?, *Med. Hypoth.*, 35, 103, 1991.

109. **Weinberg, E. D.**, Iron, infection and neoplasia, *Clin. Physiol. Biochem.*, 4, 50, 1986.

110. **LaLonde, R. G. and Holbein, B. E.**, Role of iron in *trypanosoma cruzi* infection in mice, *J. Clin. Invest.*, 73, 470, 1984.

111. **Elin, R. J. and Wolf, S. M.**, The role of iron in non-specific resistance to infection induced by endotoxin, *J. Immunol.*, 112, 737, 1974.

112. **Babior, B. M.**, Oxidants from phagocytes: agents of defense and destruction, *Blood*, 64, 959, 1984.

113. **Starke, E. P. and Farber, J. L.**, Ferric iron and superoxide ions are required for the killing of cultured hepatocytes by hydrogen peroxide, *J. Biol. Chem.*, 260, 10099, 1985.

114. **Larramendy, M., Mello-Filho, A. C., Leme Martins, E. A., and Meneghini, R.**, Iron-mediated induction of sister-chromatid exchanges by hydrogen peroxide and superoxide anion, *Mutat. Res.*, 178, 57, 1987.

115. **Konijn, A. M. and Herskho, C.**, Ferritin synthesis in inflammation. I. Pathogenesis of impaired iron release, *Br. J. Haematol.*, 37, 7, 1977.

116. **Konijn, A. M., Carmel, N., Levy, R., and Hershko, C.**, Ferritin synthesis in inflammation. II. Mechanism of increased ferritin synthesis, *Br. J. Haematol.*, 49, 361, 1981.

117. **Campbell, C. H., Solgonick, R. M., and Linder, M. C.**, Translational regulation of ferritin synthesis in rat spleen: effect of iron and inflammation, *Biochem. Biophys. Res. Commun.*, 160, 453, 1989.

118. **Rogers, J. T., Bridges, K. B., Durmowicz, G., Glass, J., Auron, P. E., and Munro, H. N.**, Translational control during the acute phase response, *J. Biol. Chem.*, 265, 14572, 1990.

119. **Roesner, H. P.**, The increase in serum ferritin observed in acute inflammations and chronic infections, *Iron in Biochemistry and Medicine*, Vol. 2, Jacobs, A. and Worwood, M., Eds., Academic Press, New York, 1980, 605.

120. **Cragg, S. J., Wagstaff, M., and Worwood, M.**, Detection of a glycosylated subunit in human serum ferritin, *Biochem. J.*, 199, 565, 1981.

121. **Hentze, M. W., Keim, S., Papadopolous, P., O'Brien, S., Modi, W., Drysdale, J. W., Leonard, W. J., Harford, J. B., and Klausner, R. D.**, Cloning, characterization, expression, and chromosomal localization of a human ferritin heavy-chain gene, *Proc. Natl. Acad. Sci. U.S.A.*, 83, 7226, 1986.

122. **Schiaffonati, L., Rappacciolo, E., Tacchini, L., Bardella, L., Arosio, P., Cozzi, A., Cantu, G. B., and Cairo, G.**, Mechanisms of regulation of ferritin synthesis in rat liver during experimental inflammation, *Exp. Mol. Pathol.*, 48, 174, 1988.

123. **Ganapathi, M. K., May, L. T., Schultz, D., Brabenec, A., Weinstein, J., Seghal, P. B., and Kushner, I.**, Role of interleukin-6 in regulating synthesis of C-reactive protein and serum amyloid A in human hepatoma cell lines, *Biochem. Biophys. Res. Commun.*, 157, 271, 1988.

124. **Ganter, U., Arcone, R., Toniatti, C., Morrone, G., and Ciliberto, G.**, Dual control of C-reactive protein gene expression by interleukin-1 and interleukin-6, *EMBO J.*, 8, 3773, 1989.

125. **Rozen, F., Edery, I., Meerovitch, K., Dever, T. E., Merrick, W. C., and Sonnenberg, N.**, Bidirectional RNA helicase activity of eucaryotic translation initiation factors 4A and 4F, *Mol. Cell. Biol.*, 10, 1134, 1990.

126. **Ray, B. K., Lawson, T. G., Abramson, R. D., Merrick, W. C., and Thach, R. E.**, Recycling of messenger RNA cap-binding proteins mediated by eukaryotic initiation factor 4B, *J. Biol. Chem.*, 261, 11466, 1986.

127. **Etchinson, D., Milburn, S. C., Edery, I., Sonnenberg, N., and Hershey, J. W. B.**, Inhibition of Hela cell protein synthesis following poliovirus infection correlates with the proteolysis of a 220,000-dalton polypeptide associated with eucaryotic initiation factor 3 and a cap-binding protein complex, *J. Biol. Chem.*, 257, 14806, 1982.

128. **Marino, M. W., Pfeffer, L. M., Guidon, P. T., and Donner, D. B.**, Tumor necrosis factor induces phosphorylation of a 28-kDa mRNA cap-binding protein in human cervical carcinoma cells, *Proc. Natl. Acad. Sci. U.S.A.*, 86, 8417, 1989.

129. **Dente, L., Ciliberto, G., and Cortese, R.**, Structure of the human α1-acid glycoprotein gene: sequence homology with other human acute phase protein genes, *Nucleic Acids Res.*, 13, 3941, 1985.

130. **Jain, S. K., Crampton, J., Gonzalez, I. L., Schmickel, R. D., and Drysdale, J. W.**, Complementarity between ferritin H mRNA and 28S ribosomal RNA, *Biochem. Biophys. Res. Commun.*, 131, 863, 1985.

131. **Miller, L. L., Miller, S. C., Torti, S. V., Tsuji, Y., and Torti, F. M.**, Iron-independent induction of ferritin H chain by tumor necrosis factor, *Proc. Natl. Acad. Sci. U.S.A.*, 88, 4946, 1991.

132. **Wei, Y., Miller, S. C., Tsuji, Y., Torti, S. V., and Torti, F. M.**, Interleukin I induces ferritin heavy chain in human muscle cells, *Biochem. Biophys. Res. Commun.*, 169, 289, 1990.

133. **Levi, S., Luzzago, A., Cesareni, G., Cozzi, A., Franceschinelli, F., Albertini, A., and Arosio, P.**, Mechanism of ferritin iron uptake: activity of H-chain and deletion mapping of the ferro-oxidase site, *J. Biol. Chem.*, 263, 18,086, 1988.

134. **Tsuji, Y., Miller, L. L., Miller, S. C., Torti, S. V., Torti, F.,** Tumor necrosis factor-α and interleukin 1-α regulate transferrin receptor in human diploid fibroblasts, *J. Biol. Chem.,* 266, 7257, 1991.

Part II
Iron Accumulation and Metabolism in Humans

3. Iron Balance in Western Societies as Measured by Serum Ferritin

BARBARA A. LEGGETT* and JUNE W. HALLIDAY**

*Department of Gastroenterology, Royal Brisbane Hospital, and **Liver Unit, Queensland Institute of Medical Research, The Bancroft Centre, Herston, Brisbane, Australia*

108

I. INTRODUCTION

Iron is an essential element for all living organisms and appropriate iron balance is necessary for survival. Iron deficiency is a serious cause of morbidity and mortality in human populations.[1] On the other hand, excessive iron can be equally detrimental, as evidenced by the genetic disorder hemochromatosis, which leads to severe parenchymal damage of multiple organs, particularly the liver.[2] There is evidence that excessive concentrations of iron are injurious to the cell, probably as a result of peroxidative damage to the lipid membranes of cellular organelles.[3] Thus, the body must maintain a fine homeostatic control over iron input and output to ensure body iron stores are kept at the optimal level.

In Western societies, both iron overload and iron deficiency are significant problems, whereas in developing countries the problem of iron deficiency predominates. This review concentrates on iron balance in Western societies. The mechanisms by which iron balance is maintained by control of iron absorption are first briefly summarized. Studies which measured body iron stores directly by quantitative phlebotomy are then reviewed. It was not until the development of a sensitive radioimmunoassay for ferritin in normal serum[4] and the demonstration that its concentration was directly proportional to body iron stores[5] that it became feasible to assess body iron stores in large numbers of asymptomatic individuals in a population. The remainder of this review examines serum ferritin concentrations in Western populations and the factors which affect these.

II. IRON ABSORPTION

The absorption of iron by the small intestine is a process tightly linked to the body's iron needs. This tight linkage is necessary because the human has only very limited capacity to excrete iron.[6] Thus, control of body iron content must be achieved at the point of absorption. The uptake of iron is closely regulated to replace the small physiological losses in bile and urine and in shedding of skin and gastrointestinal (GI) cells. In healthy adult males approximately 1 mg of iron per day is absorbed. Healthy adult females must absorb 1.5 mg/day to balance the additional iron lost during menstruation.[1] When iron requirements rise for physiological or pathological reasons, iron absorption increases. However, the iron content of the diet and its bioavailability place a ceiling on the amount that can be absorbed. With typical Western diets, maximum absorption is between 3 and 4 mg per day.

III. IRON LOSS

In men and non-menstruating women, approximately 60% of the total iron loss is from the GI tract.[1] This is in the form of intracellular iron in shed epithelial cells and leaked red blood cells and extracellular iron in biliary secretions. Most of the remainder is lost from the skin as epithelial cells are sloughed, and only a small fraction is lost in the urine. Menstrual losses (expressed as a mean daily figure) usually range between 0.5 and 1 mg, thus approximately doubling iron requirements. During pregnancy, menstrual losses cease but the iron in the fetus and placenta together with blood loss at delivery amount to a mean loss of about 2 mg/d over the 280 d of gestation.[1]

IV. FACTORS CONTROLLING IRON ABSORPTION

The most important factors controlling absorption relate to changes in the two largest pools of iron within the body — storage iron and iron in the erythroid mass. If the body iron stores become low due to excessive iron loss, iron absorption is increased. It is also increased when the erythroietic rate is increased, usually but not always reflecting blood loss. Iron absorption is affected by a number of other factors including pregnancy, hypoxia, and the acute phase response.

A. BODY IRON STORES

A very strong inverse relationship has been demonstrated between body iron stores and absorption.[7-16] The increased iron absorption during pregnancy is associated with a decrease in maternal iron stores and serum ferritin concentration[17-19] and therefore may be simply a reflection of maternal iron status. Other factors, however, cannot be completely ruled out. A major exception to the rule that an increase in body iron stores leads to a decrease in iron absorption is found in hemochromatosis, where the pathological defect results in disproportionately high iron absorption relative to iron stores.[13,20]

B. ERYTHROPOIESIS

Iron absorption is enhanced when erythropoiesis is stimulated by bleeding or acute hemolysis.[7,21] or following androgen treatment.[22] It falls when the erythroietic rate is decreased by hypertransfusion,[7] radiation treatment,[23] or simulated descent from high altitudes to sea level.[24] However, in chronic hemolytic states in man, the iron absorption rate is usually normal.[1] It is only in anemias such as β-thalassemia major and sideroblastic anemia, where erythropoiesis is markedly ineffective that iron absorption remains persistently high.[1,25] Recent studies in mice[26] have indicated that changes in the erythropoietic rate exert their effects on the transfer phase of iron absorption.

C. HYPOXIA

Hypoxia is associated with an increase in iron absorption independent of changes in the rate of erythropoiesis.[23,26-29] The effect of hypoxia on iron absorption occurs before a response from the erythropoietic bone marrow.[30] Hypoxia appears to induce a brush border iron carrier leading to increased Fe^{3+} uptake.[26,31-34] Iron transfer from the enterocyte into the circulation also increases.[35]

D. IRON ABSORPTION IN THE NEONATE

Iron absorption is high during the neonatal period. This phenomenon has been most studied in experimental animals and appears to last from birth to about the time of weaning.[36-39] Up to 100% of a radioactively labeled dose of iron may be absorbed. The mechanism of the high neonatal absorption is unknown.

E. THE ACUTE PHASE RESPONSE

Iron absorption is rapidly decreased after the administration of bacterial endotoxin.[40] The mechanism of this response is not known. (See also Chapters 2 and 6.)

V. THE PROCESS OF IRON ABSORPTION

The process of intestinal iron absorption may be conveniently divided into several steps: (1) the luminal phase — the processing of iron in the intestinal lumen making it available or unavailable for absorption, (2) the uptake phase — the process of iron binding to and being transported across the brush border of the enterocyte, and (3) iron transfer — the handling of iron within the enterocyte and its passage out of the enterocyte into the circulation. Iron is absorbed as either inorganic iron (Fe^{2+} or Fe^{3+}) or as heme iron. Quantitatively, the most important site of absorption is the proximal small intestine.[41-43] Iron deficiency is associated with higher iron absorption along a greater length of the intestine.[41-43] Both heme and non-heme iron are absorbed in the small intestine, but the pathway of iron absorption is at least initially somewhat different.[44,45]

A. LUMINAL PHASE

A typical Western diet contains 15 to 20 mg of iron per day, but only 1 to 2 mg of this is absorbed.[1] Non-heme iron is absorbed from a common intraluminal pool,[46] and the ability of the iron to enter this pool is strongly influenced by dietary composition. The heme moiety is absorbed intact, and is absorbed more readily than non-heme iron and is less affected by dietary composition.[47] Although heme often constitutes only 5 to 10% of dietary iron, it may contribute over one third of the iron absorbed.[48]

Western diets usually contain 6 mg iron per 1000 kcal with surprisingly little variation.[49,50] Variations in the bioavailability of iron are usually of more importance than the total amount of iron ingested. When eaten alone, the iron in most cereals is poorly absorbed with geometric mean absorptions of between 0.8 and 5.7%.[51] Dietary factors which enhance iron absorption include ascorbic acid, citric acid, amino acids, and sugars.[52] These factors convert ferric iron to more soluble ferrous iron and also enhance solubility by forming stable complexes. Of these factors, ascorbic acid appears to be quantitatively the most important. Meat itself also enhances the absorption of non-heme iron.[51] Factors which reduce iron absorption include EDTA (a common food additive), phosphates, phytates and dietary fiber.[53,54] These factors either bind iron directly or cause precipitation, although these factors have minimal effects on the absorption of heme iron.[50]

B. IRON UPTAKE

At physiological concentrations, iron uptake has the features of an active, carrier-mediated transport process.[11,12,35,55,56] A higher rate of uptake is found in iron deficiency, suggesting the iron carriers are inducible and that the uptake step is a site at which iron absorption is regulated. However, it is not yet clear whether iron uptake or iron transfer is the rate-limiting step in iron absorption. The step which is rate-limiting in a particular situation may depend on the iron status of the individual.[57]

There are few studies on the mechanism of heme uptake. Studies with labeled heme have demonstrated specific binding to brush borders.[58] Once heme has entered the cell, it is localized in lysosomes where the iron is released.[45]

C. IRON TRANSFER

Incorporation of iron into mucosal ferritin is highest when body iron stores are high and lowest during iron deficiency.[59] This suggests recently absorbed mucosal iron not required for immediate transfer into the circulation is stored in ferritin and later lost when the enterocytes are shed into the lumen. Early studies showed that the transfer of iron from the mucosal cells to the body, like the uptake step across the brush border, was an active transport process.[60] However, much concerning the mechanisms of iron transfer (and the iron pathways within the cell) still remains unclear. A recent description of a 56,000 kDa iron-binding protein by Stremmel[61] is of interest as providing a possible new pathway in iron absorption.

D. MECHANISMS FOR THE CONTROL OF IRON ABSORPTION

Animal studies have provided some evidence of a circulating factor influencing iron absorption.[62-65] However, several studies have failed to show any consistent correlation between absorption and serum iron concentration.[16,26,66,67] It has been suggested that serum ferritin concentration may provide a signal regulating iron absorption,[62] but infusions of ferritin have no effect on iron absorption[68] and evidence to support this is lacking at the present time.

Probably the best current hypothesis explaining the regulation of iron absorption was proposed by Cavill et al. in 1975.[69] This hypothesis suggests that each tissue donates iron to a labile plasma pool in an amount proportional to the iron stores of the tissue. This iron is bound to transferrin and used by tissues such as bone marrow to meet their iron requirements. If the iron requirement increases, the amount of iron supplied by all tissues, including the gut, increases.

The mechanisms by which transcellular iron movement within the enterocyte are regulated are still unclear. Hahn et al.[70] suggested the "mucosal block" theory in which the mucosal cell was considered to contain a certain number of iron-binding sites which were saturated when body iron stores were high. Aspects of this model still seem valid. Granick[71] suggested that ferritin in the enterocyte could explain Hahn's mucosal block theory. Mucosal ferritin concentration varies directly with body iron stores and inversely with iron absorption.[72-74] The ferritin concentration probably reflects the quantity of iron available to mucosal cells when they are developing in the crypts. If the ferritin concentration is high, a high proportion of iron taken up will enter the ferritin compartment of the enterocyte and not be available for binding to transferrin and transfer into the circulation. The ferritin in the enterocyte is subsequently excreted from the body when the mucosal cell is shed into the lumen.

VI. TOTAL BODY IRON STORES IN NORMAL SUBJECTS

Normally, absorbed iron that is surplus to immediate metabolic requirements is stored in the tissues as ferritin and hemosiderin. These iron stores are predominantly located in the reticuloendothelial system and the hepatic parenchyma. The size of these iron stores depends on the rate of iron absorption and iron requirements. Low iron stores may be caused by lack of available iron in the diet, malabsorption, increased blood loss, blood donation, or frequent pregnancies. A modest increase in iron stores occurs with increased absorption associated with ineffective erythropoiesis or increased dietary in-

TABLE 1
Published Values for Iron Stores Determined by Quantitative Phlebotomy

Ref.	Iron stores (mg)		
	Males	Females	Blood donors
76	750 (11)[a]		110 (14)
77	687 (11)		
78	819 (3)	254 (10)	
75	844 (2)		93 (2)
79	600 (1)		
5	900 (7)	210 (10)	400 (5)
Mean of all series	767 (35)	232 (20)	

[a] Number of subjects studied given in brackets.

Adapted from Walters, G. O., Miller, F. M., and Worwood, M.,
J. Clin. Pathol., 26, 770, 1973.

take of bioavailable iron. Marked increases in iron stores are due to abnormal regulation of iron absorption as occurs in genetic hemochromatosis and to blood transfusions for refractory anemia not due to blood loss.

Quantitative phlebotomy is the standard reference measure for assessing iron stores, and it also measures the amount of mobilizable iron available for hemoglobin synthesis.[75] Because of the invasive nature of this investigation, large numbers of normal subjects have not been studied. Published values for iron stores determined by this method are as shown in Table 1. These studies have all been carried out on asymptomatic subjects in Western countries.

Other methods of estimating body iron stores must be used in the clinical setting. Clinically, iron deficiency can be confirmed by histological examination of bone marrow smears looking at the amount of hemosiderin in reticulum cells.[1] In iron deficiency, no stainable iron is present. Iron overload may be confirmed by histological examination of a liver biopsy specimen stained with Perls' Prussian Blue stain. Iron stores are graded from 1 to 4[80] according to the proportion of hepatocytes containing stainable iron, with grades 2 through 4 considered abnormally high.[80,81] Measurement of hepatic iron concentration further enhances the accuracy of this assessment,[82] and measurement of the hepatic iron index (HIC/age) is a useful diagnostic tool for hemochromatosis.[82,83]

VII. SERUM FERRITIN CONCENTRATION

A. RELATIONSHIP OF SERUM FERRITIN CONCENTRATION TO BODY IRON STORES

All the techniques discussed above are invasive and unsuitable for studies of large numbers of asymptomatic individuals in a population. Soon after the detection of ferritin in normal serum[4] it was realized that there was a close correlation between serum ferritin concentration and body iron stores. Serum ferritin concentration has since proved a most useful non-invasive test for estimating iron status. Quantitative phlebotomy on a group of 22 apparently healthy normal adult subjects (12 males and 10 females) showed there was a close correlation between serum ferritin concentration and mobilizable iron stores (r = 0.83, $p < 0.001$).[5] Data from this study suggested that 1 μg of ferritin per liter of serum represents about 8 mg of storage iron. The relationship between serum ferritin concentration and iron stores as measured by quantitative phlebotomy has been confirmed in subsequent studies.[84,85] A study in subjects with hemochromatosis undergoing phlebotomy also confirmed that 1 μg/l of serum ferritin correspondence to 7.5 mg of stored iron.[86]

Patients with uncomplicated iron deficiency almost always have serum ferritin concentrations of less than 15 μg/l.[87,88] Serum ferritin concentration is usually in the range of 1000 to 10,000 μg/l in the advanced stages of iron overload due to hemochromatosis.[87,89,90] Iron overload due to blood transfusions for severe chronic anemia also results in markedly elevated serum ferritin concentrations.[87,88] Serum ferritin concentration was closely correlated with the number of units of blood transfused up to a total of 100 units when serum ferritin concentration was approximately 4000 μg/l.[91]

Serum ferritin concentration has also been shown to be strongly correlated with iron absorption, which is another indicator of body iron stores.[9,92] In patients with iron overload and iron deficiency, as well as patients with apparently normal iron status, there is a significant correlation between bone marrow iron stores and serum ferritin concentration,[93] the exception being the genetic disease hemochromatosis.

B. CONCENTRATION OF SERUM FERRITIN IN NORMAL ADULT SUBJECTS

The earliest reported study of serum ferritin concentration in normal subjects was conducted by Addison et al.[4] and reported mean values of 29 and 52 μg/l in 18 female and 33 male subjects, respectively. The results of subsequent studies are summarized in Tables 2 and 3. It was apparent that serum ferritin concentration was lower in females than males, presumably reflecting the lower iron stores of females. There was, however, a skewed distribution for both sexes with a long tail stretching into the higher ranges. This distribution, which has been found in all studies, complicates comparisons between different studies because some give means, some geometric means, and some medians.

In Welsh male factory workers and female hospital staff, Jacobs et al.[87] found a mean serum ferritin concentration of 34.8 μg/l in females and 69.2 μg/l in males. Cook et al.[92] studied randomly selected non-anemic American subjects with no evidence of iron deficiency as determined by measurement

TABLE 2
Published Values of Serum Ferritin Concentration (SFC) in Male Populations

Number of subjects	Age	Population	Mean SFC (μg/l)	Range (μg/l)	Ref.
75	18-65	Cardiff (factory workers)	69.2	6-186	87
174	20-50	Washington State (nonanemic)	94[a]	27-329[b]	92
280	16-65	Cardiff (healthy nonanemic)	123	10-580	94
240	18-45	Washington State (low income)	94[c]	34-196[d]	95
95	20-39	Canada (random)	93[a]	14-618	96
120	20-79	Canada (healthy)	93[c]	20-330	97
803	18-45	Washington State (first-time donors)	127.3[a]	66-244[b]	99
118	18-45	Denmark (first-time donors)	67[a]	20-227[b]	93
134	18->65	England (university staff)	73.8	7.5-230[e]	98
60	Adult	Indian (urban)	58.9[a]	12-128	148

[a] Geometric mean.
[b] 95% confidence limits.
[c] Median.
[d] 10th to 90th percentile.
[e] 2nd to 98th percentile.

Adapted from Worwood, M., *Clin. Haematol.*, 11, 275, 1982.

of transferrin saturation and red cell protoporphyrin. The geometric mean for females was 34 μg/l (95% confidence limits 9 to 125 μg/l) and for males was 94 μg/l (27 to 329 μg/l). These values were higher than those found by Jacobs et al.,[87] possible because iron-deficient subjects had been excluded. A further study of the Welsh population examining non-anemic subjects found higher mean values of 56 μg/l for women and 123 μg/l for men.[94] Three further studies of randomly selected North American subjects found very consistent results.[95-97] These studies showed that levels in men increased in the latter part of the second decade and then either remained stable or rose only slowly until the age of 65 years.[95] In women, levels remained low until after the age of 45 years when they began to rise, although never reaching the same level as those of males. It is likely this rise parallels a rise in iron stores following the cessation of menstruation and childbearing. The preva-

TABLE 3
Published Values of Serum Ferritin Concentration (SFC) in Female Populations

Number of subjects	Age	Population	Mean SFC (μg/l)	Range (μg/l)	Ref.
44	?	Cardiff (hospital workers)	34.8	3-162	87
152	20-50	Washington State (nonanemic)	34[a]	9-125[b]	92
153	16-65	Cardiff (healthy, nonanemic)	56	10-400	94
370	18-45	Washington State (low income)	25[c]	7-140[d]	95
100	20-39	Canada (random)	23[a]	4-145[b]	96
60	21-50	Canada (healthy)	25	4-144[e]	97
812	18-45	Washington State (first-time donors)	46.0[a]	20-107[b]	99
113	18-45	Denmark (first-time donors)	23[c]	5-104[d]	93
168	18->65	England	35	3-115[e]	98
58	Adult	India (urban)	31.6[a]	6-109	148

[a] Geometric mean.
[b] 95% confidence limits.
[c] Median.
[d] 10th to 90th percentile.
[e] 2nd to 98th percentile.

Adapted from Worwood, M., *Clin. Haematol.*, 11, 275, 1982.

lence of iron deficiency ranged from 3% in males to 20% in menstruating women in the survey of Cook et al.[95] In the Canadian population studied by Valberg et al.[96] it was 3% in men and 30% in menstruating women.

More recent studies of asymptomatic university staff in the U.K.[98] and first-time Scandinavian blood donors[93] have shown somewhat lower serum ferritin concentrations. The highest levels of serum ferritin concentration have been found in American first-time blood donors[99] and South African men,[100] although the data in the latter study does not allow calculation of a mean or median value. Among the first-time blood donors geometric mean serum ferritin concentration was 46 μg/l in women and 127 μg/l in men, and it was suggested that this may have been related to the high socioeconomic class of this group of non-remunerated donors.[99] Blood donation markedly lowered serum ferritin concentration in both males and females. Donation of one unit per year halved the serum ferritin concentration in men. Finch et al.[99] concluded that men were able to donate 2 to 3 units per year without an appreciable incidence of iron deficiency even though their iron stores were lowered. Women were able to donate only about 1 to 2 units per year without developing iron deficiency. High serum ferritin concentrations were also found among 40- to 49-year-old males in the Faroe Islands,[101] and it has been postulated that this may be due to a high dietary intake of iron.

A recent, large Australian study[102] examined 1968 asymptomatic employees of two large corporations, a bank and an insurance company. The distribution of serum ferritin concentration according to age and sex is shown in Figure 1. There was close similarity between the results from the two populations in which serum ferritin concentration was measured by two different techniques. As in other studies,[95] median serum ferritin rose in young males to reach a plateau in the fourth decade and then varied little before the age of 65 years. In females, median serum ferritin rose slowly until the fifth decade when the rate of rise accelerated, although median levels never reached those of males. There was a wide spread of values which increased with age. The overall incidence of iron deficiency as estimated by a serum ferritin concentration less than or equal to 10 μg/l was 2.6% for males and 8.9% for females. The striking feature of these results was the high median ferritin concentrations observed. The causes for the variability in serum ferritin concentrations in different populations will be further discussed below.

C. SERUM FERRITIN CONCENTRATION IN CHILDREN

The serum ferritin concentration at birth as estimated from cord blood is relatively high. Siimes et al.[103] reported a median of 101 μg/l and Rios et al.[104] reported a geometric mean of 117 μg/l. Mean values of 245 μg/l[19] and 218 μg/l (Kelly et al. 1978) have been reported. Fenton et al.[19] and Kelly et al.[105] found significantly lower concentrations in babies of mothers with serum ferritin concentration <12 μg/l, but Rios et al.[104] did not. The results of studies on the effect of maternal iron supplements are also conflicting. Van Eijk et al.[106] found no significant correlation with serum ferritin concentration in the infant, whereas Kaneshige[107] did find one. Serum ferritin concentrations decreased in maternal blood during pregnancy,[19,106] and concentrations are lower from 35 weeks of pregnancy in women not receiving iron supplements.[90]

During the first few months of life serum ferritin concentration falls quickly as the infant grows rapidly and has a low oral intake of iron. At 12 months of age the mean serum ferritin concentration was found to be 31 μg/l.[108] During childhood the median value was 30 μg/l,[109] and during the second decade it was 18 μg/l.[96] Similarly, Milman and Ibsen[110] found geometric means of 29 μg/l in children aged 6 to 11 years and 26 μg/l in adolescents aged 12 to 15 years. There were no significant differences between males and females during childhood.

D. SERUM FERRITIN CONCENTRATION IN THE ELDERLY

Most but not all studies have found that serum ferritin concentration rises after the age of 65 years due to increasing iron stores and/or increasing

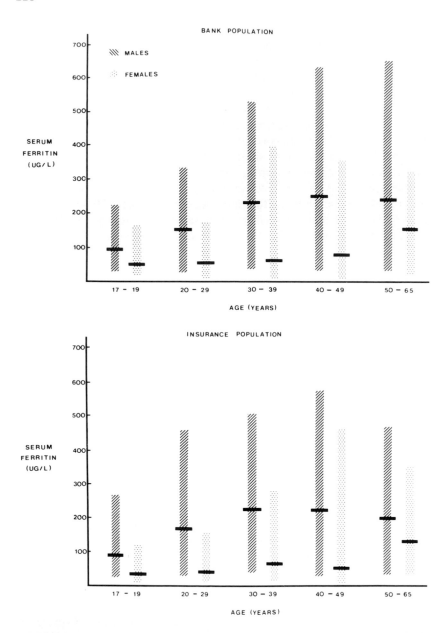

FIGURE 1. Median concentrations of ferritin in serum according to age and sex in a healthy Australian population. The horizontal bars represent the median concentrations of serum ferritin and the striped and stippled bars show the range from the 5th to the 95th percentiles in men and women, respectively. For this figure the bank population comprised 724 men and 643 women who were employees of a major banking corporation; the insurance population comprised 305 men and 277 women who were employees of a major insurance corporation. (Adapted from Leggett, B. A., Brown, N. N., Bryant, S., et al., *Clin. Chem.*, 36, 1350, 1990.)

incidence of diseases such as neoplasia and inflammatory conditions which tend to elevate serum ferritin concentration. Valberg et al.[96] found that the geometric mean serum ferritin concentration was unchanged with increasing age in men but rose from 29 μg/l in women aged 40 to 64 years to 52 μg/l in women over 65 years. Cook et al.[95] found the medium serum ferritin concentration to be 94 μg/l in men aged 18 to 45 years and 124 μg/l in men over 45 years. Similarly, a rise from 25 to 89 μg/l was noted in women. Other studies have also found a rise in both males and females with increasing age.[111,112] Loria et al.[113] showed a clear shift to higher values in subjects over 60 years of age. The increase was more marked in females, although elderly females still had a statistically lower mean than elderly males. The distribution of serum ferritin concentration in the elderly had a larger variance than in younger subjects. Of 55 elderly subjects with evidence of iron deficiency (response to oral iron therapy), 10 had normal or high serum ferritin levels, suggesting the rise in serum ferritin concentration in the elderly may not always reflect increased iron stores.

This question was further investigated by Touitou et al.[114] This large study of 776 unselected elderly patients aged 80.9 ± 9.7 years showed a marked shift toward higher serum ferritin concentration with persistence of the sex-related difference. Some 25% of subjects had levels greater than 220 μg/l, but 75% of these were thought to be explained by an association with diseases such as inflammatory syndromes, renal failure, and alcoholism. These workers concluded that the increase in serum ferritin concentration with age was related to associated pathology rather than being a normal physiological event. However, it should be noted that this study examined a very elderly population with a high burden of pathology. The balance of evidence seems to favor a rise in iron stores between the ages of 50 and 70 years, contributing to the rise in serum ferritin concentration at least in women. In a study by Milman et al.,[115] a rise in serum ferritin concentration in patients over 60 years compared to subjects aged 18 to 45 years was noted despite exclusion of all elderly patients with diseases known to be connected with inappropriately high serum ferritin levels. In addition, liver iron concentrations have been shown to rise with age.[116,117] It is possible that the rise with age may differ in different population groups as a result of environmental factors.

E. CAUSES OF THE VARIABILITY IN SERUM FERRITIN CONCENTRATION IN DIFFERENT POPULATIONS

There are two major possible causes for the variability in median serum ferritin concentrations reported in different populations. The serum ferritin concentration may (in some populations) be significantly altered by factors other than body iron stores. Secondly, there may be differences in the mean body iron stores in different populations. These two possibilities will be discussed in turn relative to the data presented above.

Despite the relationship of serum ferritin concentration to body iron stores, other factors which affect synthesis, cellular release, and clearance of ferritin have the potential to alter serum ferritin concentration. Studies in patients presenting with overt disease have shown the importance of the effect of inflammation,[88,118,119] liver disease,[88,91,120,121] and neoplasia.[122,123] It is possible that mild inflammation, subclinical liver disease, and, occasionally, occult malignancy contribute to the wide spread of values in apparently normal subjects. There is some evidence that other factors may also be involved, and these include smoking[98,114] and exercise.[124] Of the above factors, only liver disease evidenced by raised liver enzymes was found to significantly affect the median serum ferritin in a large symptomatic Australian population.[102]

Alcohol intake has been shown to be associated with high serum ferritin,[125-127] but it has been debated whether this effect is confined to subjects with evidence of liver disease. In the study of Leggett et al.,[102] heavy alcohol intake was found to be associated with significantly elevated serum ferritin concentration even in asymptomatic subjects with normal liver-function tests. It may be that serum ferritin is a more sensitive index of the effect of alcohol on the liver than serum gamma glutamyl-transferase. Alternatively, alcohol may have a specific effect on ferritin synthesis, release, or clearance. It is possible that the raised serum ferritin concentration in heavy drinkers is also partly related to the modest elevation of hepatic iron concentration observed in subjects with alcoholic liver disease.[128]

Alcohol intake in the Australian population is approximately twice that of the Swedish population.[129] Only 9% of American subjects drink 20 g or more of alcohol daily as compared to 32% of the Australian population.[102,130] Alcohol intake in the U.K. is similar to that in the Australian population, but its effect may be offset by the lower meat consumption of the British population.[129,131] Thus, it is not surprising that the effect of alcohol on serum ferritin concentration is clearer in the Australian population than in studies of populations with a much lower alcohol intake.

Despite the effects of the factors discussed above, it seems likely that most of the variation in median serum ferritin concentration between different populations is due to differences in iron stores. In support of this, most studies have usually found that the most important factors determining serum ferritin concentration within a population are obviously related to expected physiological changes in iron stores. Values tended to rise in all subjects with age, although the rate of rise is lower in women.[95,96,102] In all populations, values are lower in females due to iron loss during menstruation and pregnancy. Frequent blood donation causes a marked decrease in serum ferritin concentration in both men and women.[99,101] Thus, the percentage of blood donors within a studied population will have a significant effect on the median serum ferritin concentration.

Other possible causes for differences in iron stores between different Western populations studied include variations in socioeconomic status and diet. High socioeconomic status allows ready access to health care, thus reducing the incidence of diseases leading to iron loss. It may also be related to consumption of a diet high in available iron. The socioeconomic status of the Australian study subjects who demonstrated especially high iron stores was itself relatively high, as they were mostly clerical staff in large corporations. Interestingly, the American study showing the highest iron stores in that country examined first-time blood donors and suggested that this group of non-remunerated donors was of high socioeconomic class.[99] A study done in the same area of the U.S. but specifically examining members of low-income families showed a considerably lower median serum ferritin concentration.[95]

Diets high in meat provide a dietary iron content with a very high bioavailability. Within an individual population, ferritin concentration was higher in sera from nonvegetarians than from vegetarians.[102] It is likely that differences in the overall iron status of different populations reflect, in part, differences in diet, particularly meat intake. (See also Chapter 19.) The majority (81.2%) of the Australian population eat meat every day or on most days.[102] Meat consumption in the U.K. and Sweden, where median serum ferritin concentration is considerably lower, is only 68% (U.K.) and 54% (Sweden) that of Australia.[129] Meat consumption in Canada and the U.S. resembles that of the Australian population,[129] although median serum ferritin concentration in most studies from these countries is lower than the Australian study. However, it is of interest that the population with ferritin levels most closely approximating the Australian one was American.[99,102] This suggests not only that a high content of available iron in the diet is a necessary factor for a population to have high iron stores, but that other factors such as socioeconomic class may also be important in determining the overall iron status. Genetic differences between populations may also be important. For example, in Caucasian populations, about one in ten individuals may be heterozygous for genetic hemochromatosis[132,133] and thus have higher rates of iron absorption.

VIII. PREVALENCE OF IRON DEFICIENCY IN WESTERN COUNTRIES

There are particular groups within any human population which are especially susceptible to iron deficiency. Infants and adolescents require extra iron because of their rapid growth. Menstruating females must on average absorb an extra 0.5 to 1 mg of iron daily to account for iron lost during menstruation. Pregnant women are the most vulnerable group of all. The net requirement for the pregnancy is about 740 mg, and most of this is required in the latter stages.[1] During the third trimester, approximately 6 mg/day is required — more than can be absorbed from the unfortified diet. Iron deficiency is unavoidable unless the mother had at least 200 mg of iron stores prior to the pregnancy. This corresponds to a serum ferritin concentration of approximately 25 μg/l. From the data already presented, it is apparent that a substantial proportion of the females in Western populations have iron stores below this level.

There are many pathological causes of increased blood loss affecting individuals in Western societies, but the overall prevalence of these conditions is not high. Malabsorption is a relatively unusual cause of iron deficiency in Western societies. This is in contrast to developing societies where conditions such as hookworm infestation and tropical sprue make an important contribution to the prevalence of iron deficiency. In these countires, diets low in bioavailable iron exacerbate the problem, though diet alone is a rare cause of iron deficiency. Nonetheless, iron deficiency is still a significant problem in Western populations. Among low-income American families, 9.6% of children have iron deficiency. The prevalence was even greater among low-income menstruating women, with 20% being iron deficient. Once the iron loss associated with menstruation and childbearing ceased, the prevalence fell to 5.6% in elderly women. The lowest prevalence was among adolescent and adult males (2.4 and 3.3%, respectively). Clearly, socioeconomic factors are important in determining these prevalence rates. When the same investigators studied individuals from the same area but of higher income, only 6% of women and no men were iron deficient.[99] Similarly, the prevalence of iron deficiency in the Australian study was relatively low, with 8.9% of women and 2.6% of men being affected.[102] In a random sample of the Canadian population, 3% of men and 30% of women were affected.[96]

IX. PREVALENCE OF IRON OVERLOAD IN WESTERN COUNTRIES

Iron overload, while not as prevalent as iron deficiency, is nontheless frequent enough to constitute a significant medical problem in Western countries. This is largely due to the high prevalence of the genetic disease hemochromatosis in Caucasian populations (Chapter 4). Untreated, iron overload due to hemochromatosis leads to death from cirrhosis, hepatocellular carcinoma, cardiomyopathy, or diabetes. Early diagnosis of subjects with hemochromatosis and phlebotomy therapy before the development of cirrhosis result in normal life expectancy.[134]

Studies based on genotyping determined by HLA typing within families have suggested that the prevalence of the disease is higher than previously supposed. In Brittany, Beaumont et al.[135] estimated a prevalence of 0.3%. Similar studies estimated the prevalence to be 0.5% in Utah,[132] 0.79% in Australia,[136] and 0.3% in Canada.[137] These studies suggest that hemochromatosis may be one of the most common autosomal recessive diseases in Caucasian populations.

Population studies screening asymptomatic subjects by measuring transferrin saturation and serum ferritin concentration have largely confirmed these predictions. A large survey of Utah blood donors found a relatively high prevalence of 0.45%.[137] In the U.K., Tanner et al.[139] found a prevalence of 0.3% among 1800 blood donors. An Australian study found a surprisingly high prevalence of 1.2% among 343 male World War II veterans over 58 years.[139] A larger study of 1968 asymptomatic Australian men and women aged 18 to 65 years found a prevalence of 0.36%.[133] In a recent report from South Africa, the prevalence of hemochromatosis was assessed in 1783 Afrikaner men over the age of 40 years, and high disease prevalence of 0.95% was found.[141]

A small study of 623 male Swedish government employees aged between 30 and 39 years found a prevalence of 0.5%.[142] However, other studies from urban regions of southern Sweden have found a much lower prevalence despite a very similar study design.[144] A Finnish study also found a low prevalence of 0.05%.[145] These studies suggest there are real differences in gene frequency at least in different areas of Scandinavia.

In conclusion, it appears that in many Caucasian populations living in Western countries where the overall level of iron stores is relatively high, the prevalence of iron overload due to genetic hemochromatosis is at least one in 300 individuals. Thus, proposals to fortify the diet by adding iron to foodstuffs such as bread have the potential to harm significant numbers of individuals as well as decreasing the incidence of iron deficiency. It has been proposed that hemochromatosis has such a high incidence in such populations because, in the past, when overall levels of iron nutrition were much poorer, it offered a survival advantage especially to women during their reproductive years.[146,147]

X. CONCLUSIONS

Iron stores in Western societies as estimated by serum ferritin concentration are generally adequate or even high. They are strongly influenced by age and gender, and even in these societies there is a significant incidence of iron deficiency among women of child-bearing age. Some of the Western populations examined appear to have particularly high iron stores, and reasons for this include high socioeconomic status with ready access to health care and diets high in meat providing iron of very high bioavailability. In these populations, iron overload due to expression of the genetic disease hemochromatosis is a significant problem. Serum ferritin concentration has proven a convenient and reliable measure of iron stores, although it may be inappropriately elevated by some other factors, including liver disease, alcohol intake and the acute phase response. On a population basis, alcohol intake is the most important of these and may account for some of the variations of serum ferritin concentration reported between different Western populations.

ACKNOWLEDGMENTS

The authors acknowledge the support of the National Health Medical Research Council of Australia, the Mayne Bequest Fund of the University of Queensland, the AMP Life Assurance Co., and the Commonwealth Banking Corporation of Australia and the assistance of Lynette Duplock, Linda Fletcher, and Gregory Anderson.

REFERENCES

1. **Bothwell, T. H., Charlton, R. W., Cook, J. D., and Finch, C. A.,** *Iron Metabolism in Man,* Blackwell Scientific, Oxford, 1979.
2. **Powell, L. W., Bassett, M. L., and Halliday, H. W.,** Hemochromatosis: 1980 update, *Gastroenterology,* 78, 374, 1980.
3. **Bacon, B. R., Tavill, A., Brittenham, G. M., Park, C. H., and Rocknagel, R. O.,** Hepatic lipid peroxidation *in vivo* in rats with chronic iron overload, *J. Clin. Invest.,* 71, 429, 1983.
4. **Addison, G. M., Beamish, M. R., Hales, C. N., Hodgkins, M., Jacobs, A., and Llewellyn, P.,** An immunoradiometric assay for ferritin in the serum of normal subjects and patients with iron deficiency and iron overload, *J. Clin. Pathol.,* 25, 326, 1972.
5. **Walters, G. O., Miller, F. M., and Worwood, M.,** Serum ferritin concentration and iron stores in normal subjects, *J. Clin. Path.,* 26, 770, 1973.
6. **McCance, R. A. and Widdowson, E. M.,** Absorption and excretion of iron, *Lancet,* 2, 680, 1937.
7. **Bothwell, T. H., Pirzio-Biroli, G., and Finch, C. A.,** Iron absorption. I. Factors influencing absorption in the normal subject, *J. Lab. Clin. Med.,* 51, 24, 1958.
8. **Pirzio-Biroli, G., and Finch, C. A.,** Iron absorption. III. The influence of iron stores on iron absorption in the normal subject, *J. Lab. Clin. Med.,* 55, 216, 1960.
9. **Walters, G. O., Jacobs, A., Worwood, M., Trevett, D., and Thomson, W.,** Iron absorption in normal subjects and patients with idiopathic hemochromatosis: relationship with serum ferritin concentration, *Gut,* 16, 188, 1975.
10. **Heinrich, H. C., Bruggemann, J., Gabbe, E. E., and Glaser, M.,** Correlation between diagnostic $^{59}Fe^{2+}$ absorption and serum ferritin concentration in man, *Z. Naturforsch.,* 32c, 1023, 1977.
11. **Cox, T. M. and Peters, T. J.,** The kinetics of iron uptake *in vitro* by human duodenal mucosa: studies in normal subjects, *J. Physiol.,* 289, 469, 1979.
12. **Cox, T. M. and Peters, T. J.,** Cellular mechanisms in the regulation of iron absorption by the human intestine: studies in patients with iron deficiency before and after treatment, *Br. J. Haematol.,* 44, 75, 1980a.
13. **Cox, T. M. and Peters, T. J.,** *In vitro* studies of duodenal iron uptake in patients with primary and secondary iron storage disease, *Q. J. Med.,* 49, 249, 1980b.
14. **Marx, J. J. M.,** Mucosal uptake, mucosal transfer and retention of iron, measured by whole body counting, *Scand. J. Haematol.,* 23, 293, 1979.
15. **Magnussen, B., Bjorn-Rasmussen, E., Hallberg, L., and Rossander, L.,** Iron absorption in relation to iron status, *Scand. J. Haematol.,* 27, 201, 1981.
16. **Taylor, P., Martinez-Torres, C., Leets, I., Ramirez, J., Garcia-Casal, M. N., and Layrisse, M.,** Relationships among iron absorption, percent saturation of plasma transferrin and serum ferritin concentration in humans, *J. Nutr.,* 118, 1110, 1988.

17. **Batey, R. G. and Gallagher, N. D.,** Study of the subcellular localization of ^{59}Fe and iron-binding proteins in the duodenal mucosa of pregnant and nonpregnant rats, *Gastroenterology,* 73, 267, 1977B.

18. **Batey, R. G. and Gallagher, N. D.,** Role of the placenta in intestinal absorption of iron in pregnant rats, *Gastroenterology,* 72, 255, 1977a.

19. **Fenton, V., Cavill, I., and Fisher, J.,** Iron stores in pregnancy, *Br. J. Haematol.,* 37, 145, 1977.

20. **Powell, L. W., Campbell, C. B., and Wilson, E.,** Intestinal mucosal uptake of iron and iron retension in idiopathic haemochromatosis as evidence for a mucosal abnormality, *Gut,* 11, 727, 1970.

21. **Erlandson, M. E., Walden, B., Stern, G., Hilgartner, M. W., Wehman, J., and Smith, C. H.,** Studies on congenital hemolytic syndromes. IV. Gastrointestinal absorption of iron, *Blood,* 19, 359, 1962.

22. **Murray, M. J. and Stein, N.,** The effect of administered oestrogens and androgens on the absorption of iron by rats, *Br. J. Haematol.,* 14, 407, 1968.

23. **Mendel, G. A.,** Studies of iron absorption. I. The relationships between the rate of erythropoiesis, hypoxia and iron absorption, *Blood,* 18, 727, 1961.

24. **Weintraub, L. R., Conrad, M. E., and Crosby, W. H.,** Regulation of the intestinal absorption of iron by the rate of erythropoiesis, *Br. J. Haematol.,* 11, 432, 1965a.

25. **Heinrich, H. C., Gabbe, E. E., Oppitz, K. H., Whang, D. H., Gotz, Ch. B., Schafer, K. H., Schroter, W., and Pfau, A. A.,** Absorption of inorganic and food iron in children with heterozygous and homozygous β-thalassemia, *Z. Kinderheilk,* 115, 1, 1973.

26. **Raja, K. B., Simpson, R. J., Pippard, M. J., and Peters, T. J.,** *In vivo* studies on the relationship between intestinal iron (Fe^{3+}) absorption, hypoxia and erythropoiesis in the mouse, *Br. J. Haematol.,* 68, 373, 1988.

27. **Reynafarje, C. and Ramos, J.,** Influence of altitude changes on intestinal iron absorption, *J. Lab. Clin. Med.,* 57, 848, 1961.

28. **Peschle, C., Jori, G. P., Marone, C., and Condorelli, M.,** Independence of iron absorption from the rate of erythropoiesis, *Blood,* 44, 353, 1974.

29. **Peters, T. J., Raja, K. B., Simpson, R. J., and Snape, S.,** Mechanisms and regulation of intestinal iron absorption, *Ann. N.Y. Acad. Sci.,* 526, 141, 1988.

30. **Hathorn, M. K. S.,** The influence of hypoxia on iron absorption in the rat, *Gastroenterology,* 60, 76, 1971.

31. **Simpson, R. J., Raja, K. B., and Peters, T. J.,** Fe^{3+} transport by brush-border membrane vesicles isolated from normal and hypoxic mouse duodenum and ileum, *Biochim. Biophys. Acta,* 814, 8, 1985.

32. **Simpson, R. J., Raja, K. B., and Peters, T. J.,** Evidence for distinct, separately regulated mechanisms for the uptake of Fe^{2+} and Fe^{3+} by mouse duodenum, *Biochim. Soc. Trans.,* 14, 142, 1986b.

33. **Simpson, R. J. and Peters, T. J.,** Fe^{2+} uptake by intestinal brush-border membrane vesicles from normal and hypoxic mice, *Biochim. Biophys. Acta,* 814, 381, 1985.

34. **Raja, K. B., Pippard, M. J., Simpson, R. J., and Peters, T. J.,** Relationship between erythropoiesis and the enhanced intestinal uptake of ferric iron in hypoxia in the mouse, *Br. J. Haematol.,* 64, 587, 1986.

35. **Raja, K. B., Simpson, R. J., and Peters, T. J.,** Comparison of ^{59}Fe^{3+} uptake in vitro and in vivo by mouse duodenum, *Biochim. Biophys. Acta,* 901, 52, 1987b.

36. **Ezekial, E.,** Intestinal iron absorption by neonates and some factors affecting it, *J. Lab. Clin. Med.,* 70, 138, 1967.

37. **Loh, T.-T. and Kaldor, I.,** Intestinal iron absorption in suckling rats, *Biol. Neonate,* 17, 173, 1971.

38. **Gallagher, N. D., Mason, R., and Foley, K. E.,** Mechanisms of iron absorption and transport in neonatal rat intestine, *Gastroenterology,* 64, 438, 1973.

126

39. **Srai, S. K. S., Debnam, E. S., Boss, M., and Epstein, O.**, Age-related changes in the kinetics of iron absorption across the guinea pig proximal intestine *in vivo, Biol. Neonate*, 53, 53, 1988.
40. **Cortell, S. and Conrad, M. E.**, Effect of endotoxin on iron absorption, *Am. J. Physiol.*, 213, 43, 1967.
41. **Duthie, H. L.**, The relative importance of the duodenum in the intestinal absorption of iron, *Br. J. Haematol.*, 10, 59, 1964.
42. **Wheby, M. S., Jones, L. G., and Crosby, W. H.**, Studies on iron absorption: intestinal regulatory mechanisms, *J. Clin. Invest.*, 43, 1433, 1964.
43. **Wheby, M. S., Suttle, G. E., and Ford, K. T.**, Intestinal absorption of hemoglobin iron, *Gastroenterology*, 58, 647, 1970.
44. **Parmley, R. T., Barton, J. C., Conrad, M. E., Austin, R. L., and Holland, R. M.**, Ultrastructural cytochemistry and radioautography of hemoglobin-iron absorption, *Exp. Mol. Pathol.*, 34, 131, 1981.
45. **Wyllie, J. C. and Kaufman, N.**, An electron microscopic study of heme uptake by rat duodenum, *Lab. Invest.*, 47, 471, 1982.
46. **Hallberg, L.**, Bioavailability of dietary iron in man, *Ann. Rev. Nutr.*, 1, 123, 1981.
47. **Cook, J. D.**, Determinants of nonheme iron absorption in man, *Food Technol.*, 37, 124, 1983.
48. **Bjorn-Rasmussen, E., Hallberg, L., Isaksson, B., and Arvidsson, B.**, Food iron absorption in man: applications of the two-pool extrinsic tag method to measure heme and non-heme iron absorption from the whole diet, *J. Clin. Invest.*, 53, 247, 1974.
49. United States Department of Health, Education and Welfare No. 72-8131, Ten-State Nutritional Survey, Atlanta, 1972.
50. **Hallberg, L. and Bjorn-Rasmussen, E.**, Measurement of iron absorption from meals contaminated with iron, *Am. J. Clin. Nutr.*, 31, 1403, 1981.
51. *Report of the INACG*. The effects of cereals and legumes on iron availability, 1982.
52. **Van Campen, D.**, Enhancement of iron absorption from ligated segments of rat intestine by histidine, cysteine, and lysine: effects of removing ionizing groups and of stereoisomerism, *J. Nutr.*, 103, 139, 1973.
53. **Cook, J. D. and Monsen, E. R.**, Food iron absorption in man. II. The effect of EDTA on absorption of dietary non-heme iron, *Am. J. Clin. Nutr.*, 29, 614, 1976.
54. **Phillips, S. F. and Fernandez, R.**, Components of dietary fibre reduce iron absorption, *Gut*, 21, A904, 1980.
55. **Levey, J. A., Barrand, M. A., Callingham, B. A., and Hider, R. C.**, Characteristics of iron. III. Uptake by isolated fragments of rat small intestine in the presence of the hydroxypyrones, maltol and ethyl maltol, *Biochem. Pharmacol.*, 37, 2051, 1988.
56. **Cox, T. M. and O'Donnell, M. W.**, Studies on the control of iron uptake by rabbit small intestine, *Br. J. Nutr.*, 47, 251, 1982.
57. **McLaren, G. D., Nathanson, M. H., Jacobs, A., Trevett, D., and Thomson, W.**, Control of iron absorption in hemochromatosis: mucosal iron kinetics *in vivo, Ann. N.Y. Acad. Sci.*, 526, 185, 1988.
58. **Grasbeck, R., Kouvonen, I., Lundberg, M., and Tenhunen, R.**, An intestinal receptor for heme, *Scand. J. Haematol.*, 23, 4, 1979.
59. **Topham, R. W., Joslin, S. A., and Prince, J. S.**, The effect of short-term exposure to low iron diets on the mucosal processing of ionic iron, *Biochem. Biophys. Res. Commun.*, 133, 1092, 1985.
60. **Manis, J. and Schachter, D.**, Active transport of iron by intestine: features of the two-step mechanism, *Am. J. Physiol.*, 203, 73, 1962.
61. **Teichman, R. and Stremmel, W.**, Iron uptake by human upper small intestine microvillous membrane vesicles: indication for a facilitated transport mechanism mediated by a membrane iron-binding protein, *J. Clin. Invest.*, 86, 2145, 1990.
62. **MacDermot, R. P. and Greenberger, N. J.**, Evidence for a humoral factor influencing iron absorption, *Gastroenterology*, 57, 117, 1969.

63. **Fischer, D. S. and Price, D. C.**, A possible humoral regulator of iron absorption, *Proc. Soc. Exp. Biol. Med.,* 112, 228, 1963.
64. **Brittin, G. M., Haley, J., and Brecher, G.**, Enhancement of intestinal iron absorption by a humoral effect of hypoxia in parabiotic rats, *Proc. Soc. Exp. Biol. Med.,* 128, 178, 1968.
65. **Apte, S. V. and Brown, E. B.**, Effects of plasma from pregnant women on iron absorption by the rat, *Gastroenterology,* 57, 126, 1969.
66. **Wheby, M. S. and Jones, L. G.**, Role of transferrin in iron absorption, *J. Clin. Invest.,* 42, 1007, 1963.
67. **Finch, C. A., Huebers, H., Eng, M., and Miller, L.**, Effect of transfused reticulocytes on iron exchange, *Blood,* 59, 364, 1982.
68. **Greenman, J. and Jacobs, A.**, The effect of iron stores on iron absorption in the rat: the possible role of circulating ferritin, *Gut,* 16, 613, 1975.
69. **Cavill, I., Worwood, M., and Jacobs, A.**, Internal regulation of iron absorption, *Nature,* 256, 328, 1975.
70. **Hahn, P. F., Bale, W. F., Ross, J. F., Balfour, W. M., and Whipple, G. H.**, Radioactive iron absorption by gastro-intestinal tract, *J. Exp. Med.,* 78, 169, 1943.
71. **Granick, S.**, Protein apoferritin and ferritin in iron feeding and absorption, *Science,* 103, 1946.
72. **Halliday, J. W., Mack, U., and Powell, L. W.**, Duodenal ferritin content and structure. Relationship with body iron stores in man, *Arch. Intern. Med.,* 138, 1109, 1978.
73. **Savin, M. A. and Cook, J. D.**, Mucosal iron transport by rat intestine, *Blood,* 56, 1029, 1980.
74. **Whittaker, P., Skikne, B. S., Covell, A. M., Flowers, C., Cooke, A., Lynch, S. R., and Cook, J. D.**, Duodenal iron proteins in idiopathic haemochromatosis, *J. Clin. Invest.,* 89, 261, 1989.
75. **Haskins, D., Stevens, A. R., Jr., Finch, S., and Finch, C. A.**, Iron metabolism: iron stores in man as measured by phlebotomy, *J. Clin. Invest.,* 31, 543, 1952.
76. **Olsson, K. S.**, Iron stores in normal men and male blood donors, *Acta Med. Scand.,* 192, 401, 1972.
77. **Balcerzak, S. P., Westerman, M. P., Heinle, E. W., and Taylor, F. H.**, Measurement of iron stores using desferrioxamine, *Ann. Intern. Med.,* 68, 518, 1968.
78. **Pritchard, J. and Mason, R. A.**, Iron stores in normal adults and replenishment with oral iron therapy, *J. Am. Med. Assoc.,* 19, 897, 1964.
79. **Hynes, M.**, The iron reserves of a normal man, *J. Clin. Pathol.,* 2, 99, 1949.
80. **Scheuer, P. J., Williams, R., and Muir, A. R.**, Hepatic pathology in relatives of patients with hemochromatosis, *J. Pathol. Bacteriol.,* 84, 53, 1962.
81. **Brissot, P., Bourle, M., Henry, D., Verger, J.-P., Messner, M., Beaumont, C., Regnouard, F., Ferrand, B., and Simon, M.**, Assessment of liver iron content in 271 patients: a re-evaluation of direct and indirect methods, *Gastroenterology,* 80, 557, 1981.
82. **Bassett, M. L., Halliday, J. W., and Powell, L. W.**, Value of hepatic iron measurements in early hemochromatosis and determination of the critical iron concentration associated with fibrosis, *Hepatology,* 6, 24, 1986.
83. **Summers, K. M., Halliday, J. W., and Powell, L. W.**, Identification of homozygous hemochromatosis subjects by measurements of hepatic iron index, *Hepatology,* 12, 20, 1990.
84. **Jacob, R. A., Sanstead, H. H., Klevay, L. M., and Johnson, L. K.**, Utility of serum ferritin as a measure of iron deficiency in normal males undergoing repetitive phlebotomy, *Blood,* 56, 786, 1980.
85. **Birgegard, G., Hogman, C., Kellander, A., Levander, H., Simmonsson, B., and Wide, L.**, Serum ferritin and erythrocyte 2,3-DPG during quantitated phlebotomy and iron treatment, *Scand. J. Haematol.,* 19, 327, 1977.

86. **Basset, M. L., Halliday, J. W., Ferris, R. A., and Powell, L. W.,** Diagnosis of hemochromatosis in young subjects: predictive accuracy of biochemical screening tests, *Gastroenterology*, 87, 628, 1984.

87. **Jacobs, A., Miller, F., Worwood, M., Beamish, M. R., and Wardrop, C. A.,** Ferritin in the serum of normal subjects and patients with iron deficiency and iron overload, *Br. J. Med.*, 4, 206, 1972.

88. **Lipschitz, D. A., Cook, J. D., and Finch, C. A.,** A clinical evaluation of serum ferritin as an index of iron stores, *N. Engl. J. Med.*, 290, 1213, 1974.

89. **Halliday, J. W., Russo, A. M., Cowlishaw, J. L., and Powell, L. W.,** Serum ferritin in the diagnosis of hemochromatosis, *Lancet*, 2, 621, 1977.

90. **Worwood, M.,** Ferritin in human tissues and serum, *Clin. Haematol.*, 11, 275, 1982.

91. **Worwood, M., Cragg, S. J., Jacobs, A., McLaren, C., Ricketts, C., and Economidou, J.,** Binding of serum ferritin to concanavalin A: patients with homozygous β thalassaemia and transfusional iron overload, *Br. J. Haematol.*, 46, 409, 1980.

92. **Cook, J. D., Lipschitz, D. A., Miles, L. E. M., and Finch, C. A.,** Serum ferritin as a measure of iron stores in normal subjects, *Am. J. Clin. Nutr.*, 27, 681, 1974.

93. **Milman, N., Pedersen, N. S., and Visfeldt, J.,** Serum ferritin in healthy Danes: relation to marrow haemosiderin iron stores, *Dan. Med. Bull.*, 30, 115, 1983.

94. **Jacobs, A. and Worwood, M.,** Ferritin in serum: clinical and biochemical implications, *N. Engl. J. Med.*, 292, 951, 1975.

95. **Cook, J. D., Finch, C. A., and Smith, N. J.,** Evaluation of the iron status of a population, *Blood*, 48, 449, 1976.

96. **Valberg, L. S., Scorbie, J., Ludwig, J., and Pelletier, D.,** Serum ferritin and the iron status of Canadians, *Can. Med. Assoc. J.*, 114, 417, 1976.

97. **Luxton, A. W., Walker, W. H. C., Gauldie, J., Ali, M. A. M., and Pelletier, C.,** A radioimmunoassay for serum ferritin, *Clin. Chem.*, 23, 683, 1977.

98. **Rodger, R. S. C., Fletcher, K., Fail, B. J., Rohman, H., Sviland, L., and Hamilton, P. J.,** Factors influencing haematological measurements in healthy adults, *J. Chron. Dis.*, 40, 943, 1987.

99. **Finch, C. A., Cook, J. D., Labbe, R. F., and Culala, M.,** Effect of blood donation on iron stores as evaluated by serum ferritin, *Blood*, 50, 441, 1977.

100. **Ballot, D., Meyer, T. E., Bothwell, T. H., Bezwoda, W. R., Green, A., Baynes, R. D., Joffe, M., and Jenkins, T.,** Idiopathic haemochromatosis, *S. Afr. Med. J.*, 71, 639, 1987.

101. **Milman, N., Thomsen, H., and Mathiassen, B.,** Serum ferritin, iron status and plasma ascorbic acid in 40- to 49-year old males in the Faroe Islands, *Scand. J. Clin. Lab. Invest.*, 50, 559, 1990.

102. **Leggett, B. A., Brown, N. N., Bryant, S., Duplock, L., Powell, L. W., and Halliday, J. W.,** Factors affecting the concentration of ferritin in serum in a healthy Australian population, *Clin. Chem.*, 36, 1350, 1990.

103. **Siimes, M. A. and Dallman, P. R.,** New kinetic role for serum ferritin in iron metabolism, *Br. J. Haematol.*, 28, 7, 1974.

104. **Rios, E., Lipschitz, D. A., Cook, J. D., and Smith, N. J.,** Relationship of maternal and infant iron stores as assessed by determination of plasma ferritin, *Pediatrics*, 55, 694, 1975.

105. **Kelly, A. M., MacDonald, D. J., McDougall, A. N.,** Observations on maternal and fetal ferritin concentrations at term, *Br. J. Obstet. Gyn.*, 85, 338, 1978.

106. **Van Eijk, H. J., Kroos, M. J., Hoogendoorn, G. A., and Wallenberg, H. C. S.,** Serum ferritin and iron stores during pregnancy, *Clin. Chim. Acta*, 83, 81, 1978.

107. **Kaneshige, E.,** Serum ferritin as an assessment of iron stores and other hematologic parameters during pregnancy, *Obstet. Gyn.*, 57, 238, 1981.

108. **Saarinen, U. M. and Siimes, M. A.,** Serum ferritin in assessment of iron nutrition in healthy infants, *Acta Paediatr. Scand.*, 67, 741, 1978.

109. **Siimes, M. A., Addiego, J. E., and Dallman, P. R.,** Ferritin in serum: diagnosis of iron deficiency and iron overload in infants and children, *Blood,* 43, 581, 1974.

110. **Milman, N. and Ibsen, K.,** Serum ferritin in Danish children and adolescents, *Scand. J. Haematol.,* 33, 260, 1984.

111. **Casale, G., Bonora, C., Migliavacca, A., Zurita, I. E., and de Nicola, P.,** Serum ferritin and ageing, *Age Ageing,* 10, 119, 1981.

112. **Seamonds, B., Anderson, K., and Whitaker, B.,** Reference intervals for ferritin: age dependence, *Clin. Chem.,* 10, 1515, 1980.

113. **Loria, A., Hershko, C., and Konijn, A. M.,** Serum ferritin in an elderly population, *J. Gerontol.,* 34, 521, 1979.

114. **Touitou, Y., Proust, J., Carayon, A., Klinger, E., Nakache, J.-P., Huard, D., and Sachet, A.,** Plasma ferritin in old age: influence of biological and pathological factors in a large elderly population, *Clin. Chim. Acta,* 149, 37, 1985.

115. **Milman, N., Anderson, H. C., and Pedersen, N. S.,** Serum ferritin and iron status in "healthy" elderly individuals, *Scand. J. Clin. Lab. Invest.,* 46, 19, 1986.

116. **Charlton, R. W., Hawkins, O. M., Mavor, W. O., and Bothwell, T. H.,** Hepatic storage iron concentration in different population groups, *Am. J. Clin. Nutr.,* 23, 358, 1970.

117. **Celada, A., Herreros, V., and de Castro, S.,** Liver iron storage in a Spanish aging population, *Am. J. Clin. Nutr.,* 2662, 1980.

118. **Bentley, D. P. and Williams, P.,** Serum ferritin concentration as an index of storage iron in rheumatoid arthritis, *J. Clin. Path.,* 27, 786, 1974.

119. **Birgegard, G., Hallgren, R., Killander, A., Stromberg, A., Venge, P., and Wide, L.,** Serum ferritin during infection: a longitudinal study, *Scand. J. Haematol.,* 21, 333, 1978.

120. **Prieto, J., Barry, M., and Sherlock, S.,** Serum ferritin in patients with iron overload and acute and chronic liver diseases, *Gastroenterology,* 68, 525, 1975.

121. **Valberg, L. S., Ghent, C. N., Lloyd, D. A., Frei, J. V., and Chamberlain, M. J.,** Diagnostic efficacy of tests for the detection of iron overload in chronic liver disease, *Can. Med. Assoc. J.,* 119, 229, 1978.

122. **Kew, M. C., Torrance, J. D., Derman, D., Simon, M., MacNab, G. M., Charlton, R. W., and Bothwell, T. H.,** Serum and tumor ferritins in primary liver cell cancer, *Gut,* 19, 294, 1978.

123. **Hann, H. L., Levy, L., and Evans, A. E.,** Serum ferritin as a guide to therapy in neuroblastoma, *Cancer Res.,* 40, 1411, 1980.

124. **Campanini, S., Arosio, P., Levi, S., Ceriotti, F., Murone, M., and Marconi, C.,** Analysis of the iron status of professional cyclists during a 3 week road race, *Haematologica,* 73, 111, 1988.

125. **Kristensen, H., Fex, G., and Treel, E.,** Serum ferritin, gamma glutamyl-transferase and alcohol consumption in healthy, middle-aged men, *Drug Alcohol Depend.,* 8, 43, 1981.

126. **Lundin, L., Hallgren, R., Birgegard, G., and Wide, L.,** Serum ferritin in alcoholics and the relation to liver damage, iron state and erythropoietic activity, *Acta Med. Scand.,* 209, 327, 1981.

127. **Meyer, T. E., Kassianides, C., Bothwell, T. H., and Green, A.,** Effects of heavy alcohol consumption on serum ferritin concentrations, *S. Afr. Med. J.,* 66, 573, 1984.

128. **Irving, M. G., Halliday, J. W., and Powell, L. W.,** Association between alcoholism and increased hepatic iron stores, *Alcoholism (N.Y.),* 12, 7, 1988.

129. Food Consumption Statistics 1976-1985, *OECD (Paris),* 1988.

130. The Surgeon General's Report on Nutrition and Health DHHS (PHS) Publ. No. 88-50210, US Department of Health and Human Services, Washington, D.C., 1988.

131. **Cade, J. E., Barker, D. J. P., Margetts, B. M., and Morris, J. A.,** Diet and inequalities of health in three English towns, *Br. Med. J.,* 296, 1359, 1988.

130

132. **Dadone, M. M., Kushner, J. P., Edwards, C. Q., Bishop, D. T., and Skolnick, M. H.,** Hereditary hemochromatosis: analysis of laboratory expression of the disease by genotyping 18 pedigrees, *Am. J. Clin. Pathol.,* 78, 196, 1982.

133. **Leggett, B. A., Halliday, J. W., Brown, N. N., Bryant, S., and Powell, L. W.,** Prevalence of haemochromatosis amongst asymptomatic Australians, *Br. J. Haematol.,* 74, 525, 1990.

134. **Niederau, C., Fischer, R., Sonnenberg, A., Stremmel, W., Trampisch, H. J., and Strohmeyer, G.,** Survival and causes of death in cirrhotic and noncirrhotic patients with primary hemochromatosis, *N. Engl. J. Med.,* 313, 1256, 1985.

135. **Beaumont, C., Simon, M., Fauchet, R., Hespel, J.-P., Brissot, P., Genetet, B., and Bourel, M.,** Serum ferritin as a possible marker of the hemochromatosis allele, *N. Engl. J. Med.,* 301, 169, 1979.

136. **Basset, M. L., Doran, T. J., Halliday, J. W., Bashir, H. V., and Powell, L. W.,** Idiopathic haemochromatosis: demonstration of homozygous-heterozygous mating by HLA typing of families, *Hum. Genet.,* 60, 353, 1982.

137. **Borwein, S. T., Ghent, C. N., Flanagan, P. R., Chamberlain, M. J., and Valberg, L. S.,** Genetic and phenotypic expression of hemochromatosis in Canadians, *Clin. Invest. Med.,* 6, 171, 1983.

138. **Edwards, C. Q., Griffen, L. M., Goldgar, D., Drummond, C., Skolnick, M. H., Kushner, J. P.,** Prevalence of hemochromatosis among 11,065 presumably health blood donors, *N. Engl. J. Med.,* 318, 1355, 1988.

139. **Tanner, A. R., Desai, S., Lu, W., and Wright, R.,** Screening for haemochromatosis in the U.K.: preliminary results, *Gut,* 26, A1139, 1985.

140. **Elliott, R., Tait, A., Lin, B. P. C., Smith, C. I., and Dent, O. F.,** Prevalence of haemochromatosis in a random sample of asymptomatic men, *Aust. N.Z. J. Med.,* 16, 491, 1986.

141. **Meyer, T. E., Baynes, R., Bothwell, T. H., Jenkins, T., Jooste, P. L., du Toit, E. D., Martell, R., and Jacobs, P.,** Phenotypic expression of the HLA linked iron-loading gene in males over the age of 40 years: a population study using serial serum ferritin estimations, *J. Intern. Med.,* 227, 397, 1990.

142. **Olsson, K. S., Ritter, B., Rosen, U., Heedman, P. A., Staugard, F.,** Prevalence of iron overload in central Sweden, *Acta Med. Scand.,* 213, 145, 1983.

143. **Lindmark, B. and Eriksson, S.,** Regional differences in the idiopathic haemochromatosis gene frequency in Sweden, *Acta Med. Scand.,* 218, 299, 1985.

144. **Hallberg, L., Bjorn-Rasmussen, E., and Junger, I.,** Prevalence of hereditary haemochromatosis in two Swedish urban areas, *J. Int. Med.,* 225, 249, 1989.

145. **Karlsson, M., Ikkala, E., Reunanen, A., Takkunen, H., Vuori, E., and Makinen, J.,** Prevalence of haemochromatosis in Findland, *Acta Med. Scand.,* 224, 385, 1988.

146. **Motulsky, A. G.,** Genetics of hemochromatosis, *N. Engl. J. Med.,* 301, 1291, 1979.

147. **Rotter, J. I. and Diamond, J. M.,** What maintains the frequencies of human genetic diseases?, *Nature,* 329, 289, 1987.

148. **Bhargava, M., Kumar, N., Iyer, P., Bhargava, S. K., and Kumar, R.,** Serum ferritin levels in normal Indian subjects, *Indian J. Med. Res.,* 86, 65, 1987.

4. Hemochromatosis and Other Diseases Associated with Iron Overload

JUNE W. HALLIDAY and LAWRIE W. POWELL

The Liver Unit, Queensland Institute of Medical Research,
The Bancroft Centre, Herston, Brisbane, Australia

I. INTRODUCTION

The body of a healthy adult male normally contains about 90 mmol (5 g) of iron and a female somewhat less. Of this iron, approximately 80% is present in compounds such as hemoglobin, myoglobin, and tissue enzymes, while the remainder (about 1 g) represents a store which is located largely in the reticuloendothelial (RE) system. Approximately one third of these iron stores are in the liver. Storage iron exists in two forms: first, in the large iron-storage protein, ferritin, and second, as hemosiderin, a poorly defined molecule which consists of aggregates derived from ferrtin. The concentration of hemosiderin relative to that of ferritin rises with increasing iron concentration in the tissues.

There is no physiological mechanism for the excretion of excess iron. Losses from the skin, gastrointestinal tract and genitourinary tract amount to only about 1 mg/day in the adult male and approximately double this in premenopausal women. Normal iron balance is maintained through regulation of iron absorption by the duodenum and proximal intestine, but the actual mechanism is unknown. The most important factor in the physiological regulation of mucosal iron absorption, however, is the total body iron content. The available data suggest that the ultimate control of iron uptake and transport by the intestine lies primarily within the intestinal cell itself and that this is influenced by other factors such as the degree of erythropoiesis, but the presence of circulating "messengers" cannot be discounted.[1]

The lack of a major excretory pathway for iron in man means that any increase in iron intake, either by a prolonged increase in iron absorption or as a consequence of the administration of parenteral iron, must produce an increase in iron stores in the body unless there is a concomitant pathological increase in iron losses, e.g., by blood loss.

II. NORMAL IRON METABOLISM

In order to understand abnormal iron metabolism it is necessary to establish a background of the present state of knowledge of normal iron metabolism.

A. IRON ABSORPTION

Iron absorption is regulated via poorly understood mechanisms to maintain body iron stores at optimal levels. In the normal subject, absorption is greater than normal when the stores are depleted and diminished when stores are increased. Iron is absorbed both as heme and non-heme iron. In an average Western diet, non-heme iron accounts for over 90% of total iron. Highly refined foods commonly used in Western countries contain approximately 90 μmol (5 mg) iron per 1000 calories. Normal males consuming 3000 calories per day would, therefore, obtain no more than 270 μmol (15 mg) iron per day of which 9 to 27 μmol (0.5 to 1.5 mg) would be absorbed. It is thus apparent that the possible range of absorption from the normal diet is quite small, extending from less than 9 μmol (0.5 mg) daily in the iron-replete subject to approximately 72 μmol (4 mg) in the iron-deficient subject.[2]

The availability of dietary iron may be modified by other factors including dietary fiber, tannins (e.g., in tea) and drugs such as cholestyramine and tetracyclines, all of which result in decreased iron absorption.[2] (See also Chapters 3 and 19).

Much interest has been focused on the possible role of membrane receptors for the iron-binding proteins transferrin and ferritin in iron absorption. However, recent evidence points to the fact that the transferrin receptor does not play a direct role in the absorption of iron,[3] and there are no data on the possible role of a ferritin receptor.

The recent discovery of an iron responsive element (IRE) in the untranslated regions of the mRNAs for both the transferrin receptor and ferritin[4-8] suggested the possibility that a protein binding to this sequence might be involved in iron storage and perhaps also in the control of iron absorption. When the cytoplasmic iron concentration is low, a 90 kDa cytoplasmic protein binds RNA sequences corresponding to the IREs from both ferritin and transferrin receptor transcripts, simultaneously decreasing ferritin translation while protecting the transferrin receptor mRNA from endonuclease activity. This results in reduced ferritin synthesis and increased expression of the transferrin receptor.[9] The reverse applies in cellular iron overload. An IRE-binding protein gene has been mapped to the human chromosome 9. It appears to contain an iron-sulfur cluster and has a 40% homology with the enzyme aconitase.[10] (See also Chapters 1 and 2).

Interest has recently been revived in the reexamination of intestinal iron-binding proteins. Several newly identified iron-binding proteins in the intestine have been described. Peters et al.[11-13] have identified a basolateral membrane-binding site for recently absorbed iron which shows increased binding *in vivo* following chronic hypoxia, a state which is known to be associated with increased iron absorption. They have suggested that this binding site may be involved in an iron-transfer step in intestinal absorption of iron. Conrad et al.[14] have reported a further iron-binding compound of molecular size approximately 56 kDa. They also suggest that this newly identified protein, which is immunologically distinct from transferrin and ferritin, may be important in the regulation of iron absorption in the small intestinal mucosa. Teichman and Stremmel[15] have found evidence for a facilitated transport mechanism mediated by a 54 kDa iron-binding protein located in the microvillous membranes. Further genetic and biochemical investigation of each of these proteins will be necessary to establish their role in normal and abnormal iron absorption.

B. IRON DELIVERY TO TISSUES

The interaction between transferrin and the erythroid cell involves three main steps: the binding of the iron-transferrin complex to specific cell receptors and the internalization of the protein-receptor complex through the cell membrane, followed by the release of iron within the cell. Within the reticulocyte, transferrin concentrates in endosomes where a low intravesicular acid pH facilitates the removal of iron from transferrin. This receptor-mediated endocytosis releases iron to safe storage. In other cells, such as hepatocytes, this mechanism of iron delivery is only one of several and others may predominate at the concentration of transferrin in serum.

C. IRON EXCRETION

Daily iron losses amount to approximately 18 μmol (1 mg) in adult males.[2] Approximately two thirds of this are lost via the gut, and most of the remainder is lost in the urine and skin. These losses are reduced by about half in iron deficiency and may rise to three times normal in iron overload. In the female, additional losses are incurred. The mean normal menstrual losses, when expressed in terms of daily iron balance, are approximately 9 μmol (0.5 mg), although there is much variation. It has been calculated that approximately 18 mmol (1 g) of iron is needed for each pregnancy. This is equivalent to an average daily requirement of between 90 and 110 μmol (5 and 6 mg) throughout the last two trimesters. Urinary losses of iron are about 1.8 μmol (0.1 mg) per day. The wide variation in iron intake, iron losses, and iron requirements among various groups in a community and between different populations causes considerable difficulty in planning programs for dietary iron fortification in order to eliminate iron deficiency without exacerbating iron overload in those with the inherited disorder.

D. IRON TOXICITY

The development of fibrosis and collagen deposition in areas associated with dense parenchymal cell iron deposits and the impressive clinical, biochemical, and histological improvement which follows iron removal has led to the suggestion that iron is a causative agent of fibrosis. Many recent studies have shown conclusively that excess iron is accompanied by increased lipid peroxidation,[16-19] and there is now convincing evidence that the presence of iron in parenchymal cells over many years is an important etiological factor in determining tissue damage, although a causal relation between iron-induced lipid peroxidation and fibrosis has not been firmly established. However, other undefined factors may also be important for individual cases in determining the extent of hepatic damage and which particular organs are affected, as, for example, in relation to the development of diabetes mellitus and particularly in the arthropathy (chondrocalcinosis), which is encountered in about 25% of patients (see later) but which appears to bear no relation to the iron overload.

E. MECHANISMS OF PRODUCTION OF IRON OVERLOAD

Iron overload may be produced by several mechanisms:

An inappropriate increase in the absorption of iron from the gut mucosa. This occurs in genetic hemochromatosis when an accumulation of 15 to 40 g of iron may be observed over a period of 20 or more years. With increasing body iron stores, absorption decreases toward the level found in the normal individual. However, the level of iron absorption remains inappropriate for the level of iron stores. When iron is removed by phlebotomy, absorption returns to its former high level. The cause of the abnormal iron absorption in hemochromatosis has not been identified. Disorders of erythropoiesis are also associated with increased iron absorption. However, gross iron overload is usually restricted to those conditions with ineffective erythropoiesis, e.g., thalassemia major and hereditary sideroblastic anemia (see below).

Parenteral administration of iron. This can occur via blood transfusions (e.g., in aplastic anemias or thalassemia) or by therapeutic injections of iron preparations (e.g., in some patients on renal dialysis). Parenterally administered iron undergoes RE processing before it becomes available to other body tissues and this usually results in predominantly RE iron-loading. Cellular dysfunction and tissue injury appear to be related more closely to parenchymal than to RE iron loading.

Increased oral intake (e.g., of iron medications) over a prolonged period. If such intake is massive and sufficient to overcome the mucosal regulation mechanisms, iron overload will result. The iron overload previously seen in South African blacks was attributable to large amounts of "dietary" iron consumed with ethanol resulting from the brewing of "Kaffir beer" in large iron pots. Iron is present in this beer (fermented from maize and sorghum) and the absorption of iron from these fermented beverages has been shown to be comparable to that from a solution of inorganic ferric salts. Several reports have concluded that the syndrome of hemochromatosis has occurred in Caucasian subjects following medicinal iron intake totaling more than 18 mol (1000 g) over many years. It is possible that such reported cases may also have carried the gene for hemochromatosis. Elucidation of this problem must await the identification of the gene responsible for hemochromatosis.

The association of liver disease (especially cirrhosis and porta systemic shunting) with various degrees of iron overload. This connection has been recognized for over a century and has resulted in much controversy as to the distinction from hemochromatosis. The precise pathogenesis of the increased iron storage is still uncertain. However, excess iron storage associated with liver disease is usually complicated by factors such as ineffective erythropoiesis, folate deficiency, or hemolytic anemia. It is also important to emphasize that subjects with alcoholic liver disease associated with *gross* iron overload are usually homozygous for the HLA-linked iron-loading (hemochromatosis) gene.[20,21]

TABLE 1
Clinical Causes of Iron Overload

1. Genetic hemochromatosis.
2. Iron overload associated with chronic anemia:
   A. Increased absorption (ineffective erythropoeisis with bone marrow hyperplasia)
   B. Multiple blood transfusions (hypoplastic bone marrow)
   C. Combination of increased absorption and blood transfusions
3. Iron overload associated with excessive oral intake over a prolonged period
4. Iron overload associated with cirrhosis

In some conditions more than one of the above mechanisms may apply. Thus, in patients with ineffective erythropoiesis (e.g., thalassemia), increased iron absorption can be demonstrated, but the patients also require transfusion. This combination often results in massive iron overload with clinical and pathological features that are similar but not identical to those of the genetic disease.

The clinical conditions associated with iron overload are summarized in Table 1. The term hemochromatosis is now usually reserved for the genetic disease. The designation of "iron overload secondary to or associated with" other primary conditions avoids the need for the use of the confusing term "hemosiderosis".

III. IRON OVERLOAD: DEFINITIONS AND CLASSIFICATION

Hemochromatosis is an iron-storage disease in which an inappropriate increase in intestinal iron absorption results in deposition of iron with eventual tissue damage and functional impairment of the organs involved, especially the liver, pancreas, heart, and pituitary. Hemochromatosis implies progressive iron overload leading to fibrosis and organ failure. The essential feature is an increase in total body iron with predominantly parenchymal cell deposition. The inappropriate iron absorption may result from a genetically determined error of iron metabolism (primarily genetic or hereditary hemochromatosis) in which the basic metabolic defect leading to the increased iron absorption is unknown or from ineffective erythropoiesis (secondary iron overload). Excessive body iron stores have also been described in association with a high dietary intake of iron and also with some forms of liver disease, e.g., after porta-systemic shunting. Although there is debate about the definitions, the following terminology is now commonly used: (i) genetic or hereditary hemochromatosis — the inherited disease associated with an abnormal gene tightly linked to the A locus of the HLA complex; (ii) acquired iron overload arising as a result of another disease, usually an iron-loading anemia such as thalassemia or sideroblastic anemia in which increased erythropoiesis is present.

IV. GENETIC (HEREDITARY) HEMOCHROMATOSIS

A. DEFINITION AND PREVALENCE

By definition, the term "genetic or hereditary hemochromatosis" should be used for those patients in whom there is evidence of familial, HLA-linked parenchymal iron loading. In practice the diagnosis is a presumptive one if no definite family history is available, since there is no genetic or phenotypic marker for the disease other than iron loading.

It is now established that hemochromatosis is inherited as an autosomal recessive trait (see later) and that the susceptibility locus is tightly linked to the HLA-A locus of the histocompatibility antigen complex on chromosome 6.[22-24] Numerous recent genetic studies have allowed estimates of the prevalence of the disease to be revised. The gene frequency has been calculated to be approximately 1 in 20 and the calculated homozygote frequency to be about 1 in 300.[25,26] Thus, contrary to earlier beliefs, it is clear that hemochromatosis is among the most common genetic disorders in Western countries, with a gene carrier rate of 1 in 10, i.e., higher than that of cystic fibrosis and phenylketonuria.[26]

However, expression of the disease is modified by several factors, especially blood loss (e.g., associated with menstruation and pregnancy in women). The *clinical expression* of disease is observed five to ten times more frequently in males than in females. The disease is rarely clinically evident below age 20, although with family screening, asymptomatic subjects with iron overload can be identified, even in young menstruating women. Approximately 70% of patients become symptomatic in the fifth and sixth decade.[27]

Hemochromatosis is quite rare among other population groups, e.g., in Asia, where the HLA-A3 locus is relatively uncommon. Because of a similarity in geographical distribution of case reports and the current settlements of Celtic peoples, Simon et al.[23,24] have proposed that hemochromatosis is basically a disease of Celtic peoples, arising from a new mutation in ancestral Celtic groups. The disease locus lies close to the HLA-A locus on chromosome 6 and the disease may have risen to high frequencies because of a selective effect on the MHC region, because of advantageous interaction with specific HLA alleles, or because of a selective advantage to the disease gene itself.

B. GENETIC ASPECTS

Sheldon[28] proposed in 1935 that hemochromatosis resulted from an inherited error of iron metabolism which led to progressive body iron loading. An increased frequency of the HLA alleles, A3, B14 and A3, B7, was initially reported[29,30] and demonstrated a strong linkage between the disease locus and the HLA-A locus on chromosome 6. These findings have since been confirmed and extended by numerous other groups, particularly in England, Salt Lake City,[31] and Australia.[32,33] In the latter studies there was a stronger association of hemochromatosis with HLA-A3, B7 than with A3, B14. The increase in

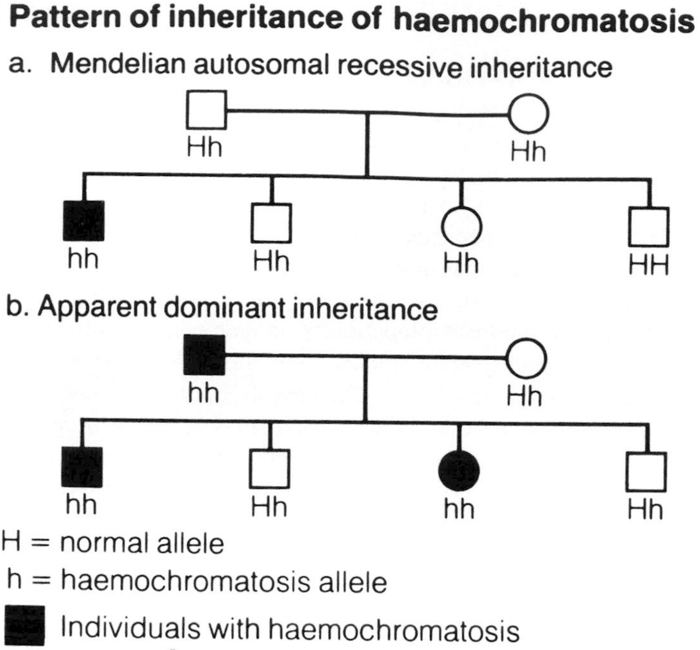

Pattern of inheritance of haemochromatosis

a. Mendelian autosomal recessive inheritance

b. Apparent dominant inheritance

H = normal allele
h = haemochromatosis allele
■ Individuals with haemochromatosis

FIGURE 1. Pattern of inheritance of hemochromatosis. (From Halliday, J. W. and Powell, L. W., Haemochromatosis, in *Medicine Internal 1990*, The Medicine Group, U.K., 3496. With permission.)

HLA-B7 probably reflects the linkage disequilibrium between HLA-B7 and A3 in these populations, since there is no association with B7 when the effect of A3 is removed.

HLA typing of first-degree relatives of the proband allows the pattern of inheritance within a family to be determined. Affected siblings of the proband usually have two HLA haplotypes identical to those of the proband and are presumed to be homozygous for the iron-loading gene. Unaffected siblings have either one HLA haplotype identical to the proband (i.e., heterozygous) or neither haplotype identical (homozygous normal). Such studies have confirmed the inheritance as an autosomal recessive trait[23,24,34,35] (Figure 1). Furthermore, the distribution of haplotypes identical to those of the proband among affected siblings fits the criterion proposed by Thomson and Bodmer[36] for a recessively inherited disease coded by an HLA-linked susceptibility gene with a frequency of at least 0.05. In Australia, the majority of relatives predicted by HLA typing to be homozygous exhibit full clinical and biochemical expression of the disease, although this depends on iron intake and physiological blood loss. In a recent study by Powell et al.[37] 47 of 50 homozygous relatives as determined by HLA studies expressed the disease either at first assessment or during a follow-up period of up to 8 years. In contrast, heterozygotes may demonstrate minor biochemical abnormalities of iron status but rarely, if ever, develop a progressive increase in body iron stores of the order seen in homozygotes.[24,37] In rare "heterozygotes" who appear to develop progressive iron overload, a chromosomal recombination resulting in misclassification of homozygotes as heterozygotes is likely.[22,24,38] In addition, the high carrier frequency means that putative heterozygous offspring of an affected individual may be homozygous due to homozygous-heterozygous mating.

The calculated gene frequency and homozygote and heterozygote frequencies for the disease are approximately 5, 0.3, and 10%, respectively, in populations of European origin.[25] *Hemochromatosis is thus probably the most common disease inherited as an autosomal recessive trait.*

C. PATHOGENESIS

The various hypotheses that have been advanced for the underlying metabolic defect in this disease have included (a) an abnormal avidity of liver and other tissues for iron, (b) abnormal kinetics of the iron-transferrin complex or of the transferrin receptor,[39] (c) aberrant reticuloendothelial function, (d) abnormal luminal factors, including abnormalities in pancreatic and gastric secretions,[2,40] and (e) abnormal mucosal cell function.[41] However, despite extensive studies, no consistent defects in luminal secretions, the intestinal mucosal cell, the RE system, or in the transferrin molecule or in its ability to bind iron have been demonstrated.[3]

D. THE BASIC BIOCHEMICAL DEFECT IN HEMOCHROMATOSIS

Despite some recent advances, the present questions still relate to two major areas: (a) what is the site of the primary defect?, and (b) what is the nature of the primary defect?

Concerning the site of the primary defect, candidates at this time include the intestinal mucosa, the liver, the RE system, or a universal abnormality. Most recent work has focused on the gut, although some recent work relating to liver transplantation is also relevant.

The intestinal mucosa — If there is one indisputable fact in hemochromatosis it is that iron absorption is increased above the expected level in "steady-state" patients with the disease, i.e., in the absence of phlebotomy. Even in the presence of an iron load in such patients, iron absorption remains high. An obvious implication of this is that "normal" regulation of iron absorption is not occurring. Other causes of an increased iron absorption immediately called to mind include increased erythropoiesis, hypoxia, pregnancy, and, of course, iron deficiency. Perhaps because the early investigators were often hematologists and concerned with the major health problem of iron deficiency, examination of the mechanisms of cellular iron uptake was frequently undertaken using the reticulocyte. This led to attempts to relate intestinal uptake and transfer to the function of transferrin and transferrin receptor as it had been demonstrated in these cells.

Transferrin and the transferrin receptor in the gut — There is little evidence that transferrin as it occurs in serum is synthesized in intestinal cells, and recently Pietrangelo and colleagues failed to demonstrate transferrin mRNA in mucosal cells.[43] It has also been hypothesized that the transferrin receptor is involved in iron absorption. Recent work, however, supports the hypothesis that the transferrin receptor is concerned more with the transport of iron *from* the plasma to the mucosal cell, presumably for use within the cell, which may imply that the endosomal pathway of iron entry is necessary to deliver the iron to the appropriate intracellular cell destination.

It has been suggested that hemochromatosis relates to a failure to "switch" from neonatal to adult control of iron absorption. Anderson[44] and Srai et al.[45,48] have studied these changes. Anderson[44] showed that the intestine of the pre-term rat demonstrated a high level of duodenal transferrin receptor (TfR) along the full length of the crypt-villous axis, but soon after birth a gradation in staining intensity was seen, reducing toward the villous tip. The crypt receptor density remained high at all ages. There was no correlation between iron absorption and transferrin receptor expression in either neonates or adult animals. Furthermore, the changes in both villous transferrin receptor concentration and iron absorption which occur around weaning were *inversely* related. The transferrin receptor concentration increased on weaning at which time iron absorption decreased. Banerjee and colleagues[47] showed no increase in gut transferrin receptors in hemochromatosis. Most evidence now, therefore, would not favor the involvement of transferrin and the transferrin receptor pathway directly in iron absorption. The presence of the gene for each of these proteins on chromosome 3 is also consistent with their noninvolvement in hemochromatosis.[4]

The role of ferritin in iron absorption — Several groups of investigators have examined ferritin protein and, more recently, ferritin mRNAs in both the liver and the gut, first in animals with iron overload and more recently in human subjects with hemochromatosis. For some years now it has been recognized that the level of ferritin in the gut in chronic iron overload is less than might be expected. In the 1970s Britten and Raval[48,49] showed that ferritin synthesis in the gut could be stimulated by small doses of iron in both iron-replete and iron-deficient rats. Other studies[50] showed that the ferritin concentration in the gut of hemochromatosis subjects was proportional to the serum ferritin concentration, but the levels in the gut were lower than expected from those of normal subjects. Nevertheless, a small dose of oral iron given to a hemochromatotic subject resulted in a highly significant increase in the concentration of ferritin in the gut in that subject, implying that their gut could still respond to an increased iron load. In addition, there was no change in the isoferritin profile of gut ferritin between hemochromatosis and normal subjects. In 1989, using enterocytes from human duodenal biopsies, Whittaker et al.[41] studied 17 normal and 7 patients with untreated hemochromatosis.

With monoclonal antibodies specific for each of the two subunits, H and L ferritin, they measured the amounts of each protein (ng/mg protein) and showed that both H and L ferritin concentrations were reduced by approximately 75% in three iron-depleted subjects. In hemochromatosis the concentrations of both H and L ferritin were lower than predicted by the associated serum ferritin concentration and were comparable with the concentrations found in normal, iron-replete subjects. They showed no change in the ratio of H and L ferritin as indeed was predicted by earlier studies of isoferritin profiles.[50] In 1989 Fracanzani et al.[42] studied H and L ferritin in the gut by immunohistochemical means. They studied 24 patients with genetic hemochromatosis, two of whom were treated. They reported an absence of ferritin granules in duodenal epithelial cells of the apical villi in 87% of patients with hemochromatosis. There was no difference in ferritin in antral mucosa or duodenal lamina propria, including macrophages, the amount varying only with body iron loading whether of primary or secondary cause. There did not appear to be any difference between H and L ferritins. More recently, Pietrangelo et al.[43] have studied the regulation of ferritin and other gene expression in the duodenum of normal, anemic, and siderotic subjects. The iron-overloaded subjects included four with genetic hemochromatosis, all of whom were iron-loaded. Of interest is the fact that no mRNA for transferrin was detectable in the gut biopsies. However, they detected a higher level of TfR mRNA in the hemochromatotic subjects consistent with earlier observations of Banerjee et al.[47] At the same time, both H- and L-ferritin mRNA was significantly lower in the genetic hemochromatosis subjects, and an abnormally low level of ferritin transcripts was seen in the genetic hemochromatosis patients. An increase in ferritin mRNA was seen in patients with secondary iron overload. Histone H_3 mRNA was unchanged in all samples, which seemed to indicate no changes in the proliferative state of the cells. Thus, both TfR mRNA and ferritin mRNA are still regulated in concert in hemochromatosis. This appears to make it unlikely that the IRE-binding protein which so elegantly up- and down-regulates these two proteins, is functioning abnormally.[6,8,51,52] In addition, the gene for this protein is located on chromosome 9 and not 6.[53] Recent mapping and linkage studies[54] would also place at least one of the H-ferritin pseudogenes on chromosome 6 centromeric to the hemochromatosis locus which makes this unlikely to be a candidate gene for the disease.

The role of nonprotein carriers in the gut — The experiments of Peters et al.[11-13,55] investigating the linkage of increased iron absorption with increased erythropoiesis indicated a dissociation between these two processes. In mice with experimentally altered erythropoietic activity, they showed enhanced iron uptake *in vitro* in response to hypoxia, comparable to that seen in normal mice. *In vivo,* the transfer of iron to the carcass was markedly reduced in animals with obliterated bone marrows; nevertheless, such animals did respond to an induced reticulocytosis. They also found no response of iron absorption to erythropoietin, as is also seen in nephrectomized patients given this drug. Elegant studies supported the much earlier work implying regulation both at the point of uptake and the point of transfer to the body. Their studies also suggested that the search for iron-carrier molecules should include those other than proteins, e.g., fatty acids such as oleic acid. However, the mechanism by which increased erythropoiesis results in a rapid increase in iron absorption was not elucidated by these experiments.

New intestinal iron-binding proteins — What role do they play in iron absorption? Are they altered in hemochromatosis? Is the change primary or secondary? Recently, two new membrane iron-binding proteins have been described, one by Teichmann and Stremmel[15] and one by Conrad et al.[14] Following isolation of an iron(Fe)-binding protein from rat mucosa cells, Teichman and Stremmel[15] isolated a 160-kDa iron-binding protein — (a trimer of 54 kDa monomers) from solubilized *human* microvillous membrane proteins. It was localized to brushborder plasma membranes and was present in human intestinal mucosa and liver but not in the esophagus. An antibody against this protein inhibited Fe^{3+} uptake by more than 50%. Preliminary calculations revealed that this protein has the capacity to provide for the calculated daily iron uptake in a normal adult (personal communication). Recently reported studies from this group have indicated that the protein is upregulated in hemochromatosis and remains so after phlebotomy therapy. A postulated regulatory function may be relevant. Conrad et al. reported a 56-kDa iron-binding protein in rat duodenal mucosa in the apical cytoplasm of cells of the small intestine.[14] The relation of these two proteins is unclear, and both appear to be concerned with iron uptake rather than transport out of the cell, although this remains to be elucidated.

The role of low-molecular-weight iron in mucosal cells in hemochromatosis — Changes in both ferritin and TfR concentration response to "iron" concentration. All these changes could still be secondary to an abnormally low iron concentration in the mucosal cell, which implies that the iron transport system of out of these cells to the plasma is bypassing the normal pathways by which it can stimulate ferritin synthesis. This could also explain the decreased iron observed in RE cells in hemochromatosis. Either a molecule which is essential to iron removal from cells is upregulated or an abnormal pathway through the cell is preventing the iron from acting on IRE-binding proteins.

The liver: does the hemochromatosis defect lie in the liver? — It would seem that modern transplantation technologies might be able to answer this question as they have done for other metabolic diseases, e.g., Wilson's disease. Rat transplantation experiments[56] have been used in attempts to provide some answers. A summary of early results seemed to indicate that there was some evidence for a "message" being transported from the liver in relation to its iron stores, which caused increases and decreases in iron absorption in appropriate circumstances. Human liver transplantation has now provided some details on the fate both of those hemochromatotics who have been transplanted and those "normal" subjects who have inadvertently been given a liver from a previously undiagnosed hemochromatotic. Preliminary data could be consistent with either a primary defect in the liver or a more generalized defect, e.g., in membrane transport in the parenchymal cells of many organs. So far there has been no convincing envidence for or against a primary liver defect which is correctable by transplanatation, but only time will provide the data.

The RE system — A very early observation in hemochromatosis in contrast to secondary iron overload was the relative paucity of iron and ferritin to be seen in macrophages in the gut and elsewhere. A whole series of past investigations have failed to reveal any defect in the ferritin synthetic capabilities of these cells or in their ability to take up iron. The possibility of an increased transport of iron out of these cells has also been examined.[57,58] Enhanced ferritin release has been observed in mononuclear cells of patients with hemochromatosis whether treated or not.[57,58] Fillet et al.[58] showed that the early release phase of iron from RE cells was considerably enhanced in patients with hemochromatosis. The mechanism by which this enhanced release occurs has not been elucidated but may be related to the basic defect in hemochromatosis.

A universal cellular defect? — The implications so far still favor a defect (i.e., an increase) in iron release from cells of the gut and possibly from the RE cells. However, if one examines the liver in patients with hemochromatosis in whom there has been some damage or hepatic process in addition to iron overload, e.g., grossly excessive alcohol consumption, iron is stored in the Kupffer cells, indicating some capability for RE iron storage. Hence, one might conclude that the apparent absence of iron and ferritin from these cells is merely a secondary reflection of the route by which the iron enters the cells. Evidence for any universal cellular defect so far remains unconfirmed. Reverse genetics proceeding from chromosomal localization of the gene is likely to provide us soon with the relevant gene which will open up an enormous vista of future studies of iron metabolism. The elucidation of the basic metabolic defect must presumably await the cloning and sequencing of the HLA-A-linked gene on the short arm of chromosome 6. The fact that the only iron-loading gene so far documented is tightly linked to the HLA loci and displays linkage disequilibrium with HLA-A alleles suggests that abnormalities of a key protein coded at a single locus result in overt hemochromatosis. However, a clear understanding of the function of the disease gene is hampered by the observation that the expression of the disease phenotype and the age of symptomatic onset can be highly variable even within the one family. This suggests that not only may some individuals carry a mutation causing a more severe form of the disease, but also that the interaction of the hemochromatosis gene with other genes may be variable. A number of genes have been considered potential candidates for the HC gene on the basis of their function. Modern genetic techniques such as genetic linkage analysis, *in situ* hybridization, and somatic cell hybrid deletion mapping panel analysis have demonstrated that most of them can be excluded on the basis of incorrect chromosomal location.

E. PATHOLOGY

In the fully established disease, the total iron content of the body is usually between 360 and 720 mmol (20 and 40 g).[11] Iron deposits are heaviest in the liver and pancreas, in which the iron concentration is 50 to 100 times normal. The iron content of other organs is also elevated from 5 to 24 times normal, particularly in the endocrine glands, cardiac muscle, and skin. A notable exception is the testis, the iron content of which is relatively low despite the fact that impaired gonadal function is a characteristic and early feature of the disease. The gonadal atrophy is due to iron deposition in the pituitary.

The detailed pathological findings in the disease have been described elsewhere.[28] The most characteristic and diagnostically the most important findings are seen in the liver. This is usually greatly enlarged, weighing over 2000 g. The cut surface has a striking reddish-brown color and is firm in consistency. Histologically, the two outstanding features are extensive pigmentation and fibrosis. The appearances are best appreciated in autopsy or wedge-biopsy specimens. They show a characteristic pattern of fibrosis and iron deposition with dense fibrous septa forming a network surrounding groups of lobules (''holly-leaf'' pattern) somewhat analogous to that seen in chronic biliary disease. A fully established cirrhosis with nodularity develops comparatively late in the disease. Hemosiderin deposits characteristically appear first in the periportal parenchyma, being found within lysosomes in the pericanalicular cytoplasm of the hepatocytes. Later, they are distributed widely throughout the lobules as well as in biliary duct epithelium, Kupffer cells, and connective tissue. There is recent evidence that the structure of the iron cores in hemosiderin differs in different types of iron overload, e.g., in thalassemia and hemochromatosis. The significance of this is unknown. Cell necrosis and inflammation are usually absent and the parenchymal cells otherwise appear normal. It is now known that alcoholic liver disease itself does not lead to iron overload of the degree seen in hemochromatosis, and the distinction can be made readily by measuring the hepatic iron concentration.[59,60] However, in alcoholic subjects the features of alcoholic liver disease may be superimposed on the above appearances.

In patients with hemochromatosis secondary to erythropoietic disorders such as thalassemia, hemosiderin deposits are much more prominent in Kupffer and other endothelial cells, but in other respects the appearance of the liver closely resembles that of the genetic form of the disease.

Microscopic examination of the pancreas usually shows heavy deposits of hemosiderin in the acinar cells. Hemosiderin is also found in the heart muscle fibers in nearly all cases of well-established hemochromatosis, but fibrosis is rare. Hemosiderin is also deposited in the conducting fibers of the atrioventricular node and is presumably responsible for the cardiac arrhythmias which occur in this disease. The pituitary, adrenal, thyroid, and parathyroid glands frequently contain extensive hemosiderin deposits, although evidence of functional impairment is usually confined to the pituitary. The epidermis of the skin is atropic with increased melanin in the cells of the basal layer. The characteristic metallic gray hue results from increased melanin (with or without iron) in the dermis. Increased iron deposition in the skin is variable and tends to occur around the sweat glands.

F. CLINICAL FEATURES

In patients with advanced disease, common symptoms include lethargy, loss of weight, loss of libido, abdominal pain, joint pain, or symptoms related to diabetes. The most prominent physical signs are hepatomegaly (in 95% of symptomatic patients), skin pigmentation (a characteristic metallic gray), testicular atrophy, loss of body hair, arthropathy, and heart failure. Cardiac failure may be the earliest manifestation in young adults (it is the presenting complaint in 5 to 15% of patients), and rapid clinical deterioration may occur in such subjects and may lead to death.[61] It characteristically takes the form of arrhythmias or progressively severe heart failure. Cardiac failure has been shown to occur in thalassemia in association with the administration of ascorbic acid during chelation therapy,[62] and the potential hazards of ingestion of excess ascorbic acid in subjects with iron overload must be stressed, especially as ascorbic acid also facilitates iron absorption. Symptoms of congestive heart failure may develop quite rapidly with progression to death if untreated.[63] The heart is diffusely enlarged, and such cases may be misdiagnosed as idiopathic cardiomyopathy if other overt manifestations are absent. However, with the widespread use of phlebotomy therapy, these complications appear to be much less common.

A comparatively recent description and characteristic feature in some 25 to 50% of cases is the presence of an arthropathy characterized by the deposition of calcium pyrophosphate and iron in the synovium — *chondrocalcinosis*. Both small and large joints are involved, predominantly the first and second metacarpophalangeal and knee joints, with pain, swelling, and limitation of movement. There is a correlation between the degree of chondrocalcinosis and the severity of joint disease, but the exact relationship of the iron deposition to the arthritis is unclear. Symptoms and progress of the arthropathy are not related to the degree of iron loading, and the course of the disease is not influenced by phlebotomy therapy.

Primary liver cell cancer is increased as a complication of hemochromatosis, and this is presumably related to the increase in life span as a result of more effective therapy of the disease. Hepatic cirrhosis appears to be an important prerequisite for the development of malignant hepatoma. The relative risk is 200-fold in cirrhotic subjects with hemochromatosis,[64,65] but this complication is very rare in precirrhotic cases that are adequately treated. *Thus, the early diagnosis of the disease is most important.*

G. PRECIRRHOTIC (EARLY OF PRESYMPTOMATIC) HEMOCHROMATOSIS

Screening for iron overload in the families of probands now allows the diagnosis to be made in young relatives. These subjects are usually asymptomatic and physical findings may be absent or restricted to mild hepatomegaly.

There is increasing evidence that early detection and treatment of the disease prolongs life and may delay or prevent irreversible complications.[2] It is, therefore, of prime importance to ensure that all blood relatives of the proband are screened for the disease. There is now good evidence that iron deposition precedes fibrosis and other evidence of tissue injury.[2,18,59] Experimental observations in the rat using the carbonyl iron model are also consistent with this sequence of events.[16-19] Cirrhosis does not develop if adequate venesection therapy is instituted in the pre-cirrhotic stage of the disease.[2,66,67] Early cases are now often diagnosed after finding an elevated serum iron on routine biochemical analysis. This should be followed by measurement of transferrin saturation and serum ferritin levels. The high prevalence of the gene for this disease in populations of European origin and the easy prevention of complications may justify inclusion of measurement of the serum iron concentration and transferrin saturation in standard health checks.[26]

H. DIAGNOSIS AND DIFFERENTIAL DIAGNOSIS

The diagnosis of symptomatic hemochromatosis is usually made on the basis of the above clinical features, with or without a positive family history, together with laboratory investigations indicative of excessive iron stores and tissue damage. These include serum iron level > 30 μmol/1 (> 170 μg/100 ml) associated with an elevation of percentage transferrin saturation (greater than 50%) and an elevated serum ferritin concentration.[68,69] Hepatic biopsy is very important in defining the the extent of tissue damage as well as in allowing both histochemical assessment of tissue iron and measurement of hepatic iron concentration.[59,60] In the absence of causes of secondary iron overload the ultimate diagnosis rests on the demonstration of increased body iron stores. Chemical analysis of iron in tissue obtained by biopsy or at necropsy is very reliable, while calculation of the amount of iron removed by "quantitative" phlebotomy gives a good retrospective estimate of iron stores.[2,59,60] Presymptomatic homozygotes usually have values for hepatic

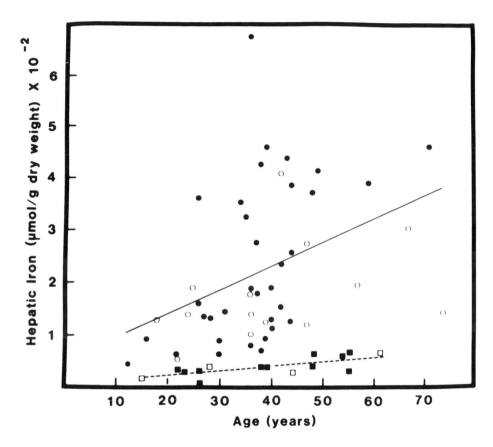

FIGURE 2. Age-related rise in hepatic iron concentration in subjects with hemochromatosis. Hepatic iron concentration vs. age in hemochromatosis homozygotes (circles) and heterozygotes (squares). Solid line (homozygotes) and broken line (heterozygotes) indicate the linear regression curves. Solid symbols = men; open symbols = women. (From Summers, K. M., Halliday, J. W., and Powell, L. W., *Hepatology,* 12, 20, 1990. With permission.)

iron concentration more than twice the upper limit of normal (i.e., > 80 μmol/g dry weight (Figure 2) and the hepatic iron index is usually greater than 2 in homozygotes (Figure 3).[59] Tests involving the upper limits of measurement of urinary iron excretion after injection of chelating agents are cumbersome and have now largely been replaced by the above. Computed tomography (CT), squid biomagnetometry, and magnetic resonance imaging of hepatic iron[70,71] have been investigated as noninvasive tests for the detection of iron overload. CT shows increased density of the liver due to iron deposition, but dual-energy scanning is necessary and the lower limits for accurate assessment of liver iron are debatable. In addition, measurements may be complicated by the presence of fat in a biopsy. Magnetic resonance can also detect increase tissue iron but it is costly, and the relatively poor sensitivity

148

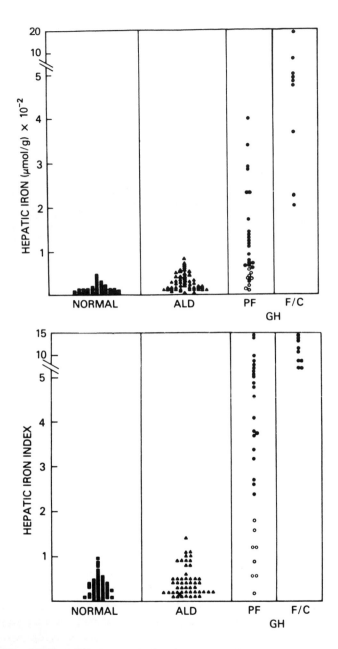

FIGURE 3. (A) Hepatic iron concentrations in normal subjects (NORMAL), patients with ALD, and GH subjects. PF = prefibrotic; F/C = fibrotic or cirrhotic. GH heterozygotes are shown by open circles; homozygotes are shown by closed circles. (B) Hepatic iron index (ratio of iron concentration to age) in normal subjects. (NORMAL), ALD subjects, and GH subjects. PF = prefibrotic, F/C = fibrotic or cirrhotic. GH heterozygotes are shown by open circles; homozygotes are shown by closed circles. (From Bassett, M. L., Halliday, J. W., and Powell, L. W., *Hepatology,* 1, 120, 1981. With permission.)

at lower iron concentrations limits its value. If the techniques are simplified and become widely available, they could be useful non-invasive screening tests, particularly in the follow-up of patients or in those in whom biopsy cannot be performed without excessive risk. Liver biopsy will remain the gold standard for the determination of the morphology and the degree of hepatic injury. The most satisfactory noninvasive screening tests for *precirrhotic hemochromatosis* at present are the transferrin saturation and the serum ferritin concentration. Since each has limitations, both are usually performed. In the presence of parenchymal iron overload the transferrin saturation is usually greater than 50% and the serum ferritin rises above the normal range when the hepatic iron stores are about twice normal. Repeated fasting serum transferrin saturations greater than 62% suggest homozygosity for hemochromatosis.[72] However, two points should be noted. First, the serum ferritin level may be elevated out of proportion to body iron stores when there is hepatocellular necrosis, especially in alcoholic liver disease. Second, some rare families have been reported in which the serum ferritin concentration has been normal in relatives despite unequivocal increase in body iron stores. The reason for this is uncertain and appears to be an exceptional situation. The serum ferritin concentration usually rises in proportion to total body iron stores until it reaches levels of 1000 ng/ml or more.[35] A recent population survey has indicated that, at least in some populations, levels up to 250 µg/ml in females and 400 µg/ml in males may be present with normal iron stores.[26] Representative values for serum ferritin, transferrin saturation, hepatic iron, and hepatic iron index in probands and relatives are given in Figure 4.

Since the HC locus is tightly linked to the HLA-A locus on chromosome 6, HLA-typing in families is helpful in determining the probability of a sibling being a homozygote or heterozygote.[37,68,73] Thus, siblings sharing two HLA haplotypes with a patient (putative homozygotes) are at high risk of developing iron overload and should be checked on a regular basis for the disease (Figure 5).

For practical purposes, all first-degree relatives of patients with symptomatic hemochromatosis should be screened for the disease by physical examination and by measurement of transferrin saturation and serum ferritin level. These tests should also be performed if an elevated serum iron level is detected unexpectedly on biochemical analysis. If both these indices are normal, the probability of the subject having increased iron stores is very low.[69] If either test is abnormal on more than one occasion, liver biopsy should be performed for quantitative assessment of tissue iron concentration and determination of the presence of fibrosis or cirrhosis (Figure 6).

I. TREATMENT AND PROGNOSIS

There is strong circumstantial evidence that venesection therapy prolongs life and that tissue damage is at least partially reversible.[67] The excess iron

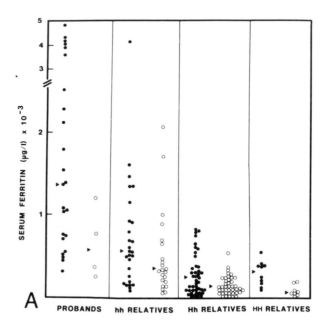

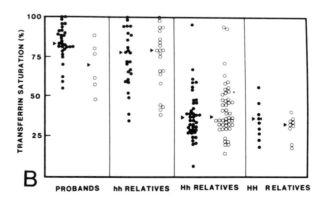

FIGURE 4. Iron indices in probands and relatives. Indicators of iron status of probands and relatives at diagnosis of hemochromatosis (if affected) or at most recent assessment (if not affected); hh relatives, putative homozygous affected relatives; Hh relatives, putative heterozygous relatives; HH relatives, putative homozygous normal relatives. Males are shown by closed circles; females are shown by open circles; median values are shown by closed arrows. (A) Serum ferritin concentration; (B) serum transferrin concentration; (C) hepatic iron concentration (HIC); (D) hepatic iron index (HIC divided by age). (From Powell, L. W., Summers, K., Board, P. G., Axelsen, E., Webb, S., and Halliday, J. W., *Gastroenterology,* 98, 1625, 1990. With permission.)

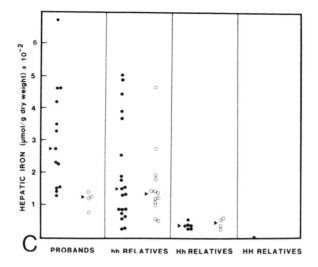

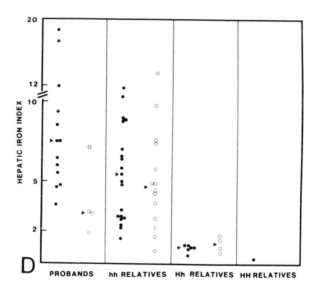

FIGURE 4 continued.

should be removed as rapidly as possible to minimize the risk of complications, especially primary liver cell cancer. Weekly phlebotomies, each of 500 ml, are usually well tolerated. Since the average patient with hemochromatosis has 360 to 720 mmol (20 to 40 g) of stored iron, this phlebotomy schedule may have to be continued for up to 2 to 3 years. During this period the plasma

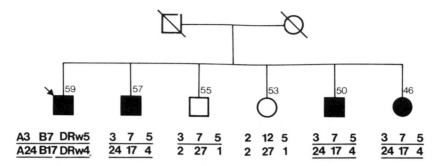

FIGURE 5. HLA typing of a family with hemochromatosis demonstrating identical HLA haplotypes in affected siblings and nonidentical haplotypes in unaffected siblings. Homozygotes are shown by closed squares and circles; underlining represents an HC allele. (From Bassett, M. L., Halliday, J. W., and Powell, L. W., *Semin. Liver Dis.*, 4, 217, 1984. With permission.)

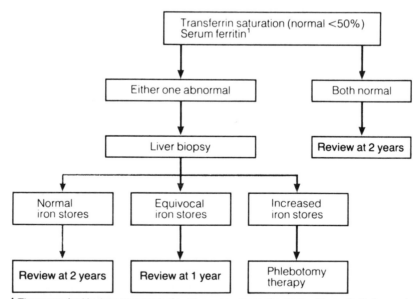

[1] The serum ferritin rises progressively with age in untreated patients. (Upper limit of normal is 150 ng/ml for women, 200 ng/ml for men.)

FIGURE 6. Screening for genetic hemochromatosis in families. The serum ferritin rises progressively with age in untreated patients. (Upper limit of normal is 150 ng/ml for women and 200 ng/ml for men.) (From Halliday, J. W. and Powell, L. W., Haemochromatosis, in *Medicine Internal 1990*, The Medicine Group, U.K., 3496. With permission.)

iron concentration and iron transferrin saturation remain high and fall only when available iron stores are depleted. In contrast, plasma ferritin levels fall progressively, reflecting body iron stores. Venesection should therefore be continued as required to keep the plasma transferrin saturation within normal limits and the ferritin levels in the low normal range.

Many complications of the disease improve or disappear after adequate venesection therapy. The exceptions are diabetes, testicular atrophy, and articular chondrocalcinosis. However, insulin requirements in diabetic patients frequently decrease after venesection therapy and replacement therapy with testosterone may be helpful. Therapy with desferrioxamine is not usually practicable in hemochromatosis because the amount of iron excreted, 270 to 360 μmol/day (15 to 20 mg/day), does not compare with that removed by venesections. However, when venesection therapy is not feasible, for example, in cardiac failure or hemochromatosis secondary to chronic anemia, therapy with iron-chelating agents should be used. Desferrioxamine can be given intravenously in glucose-saline following each transfusion (e.g., 1 g every 8 h) and up to 18 μmol (1 g) of iron may be excreted over 2 to 3 days during such therapy. Long-term therapy can be instituted with subcutaneous infusions overnight twice or thrice weekly and can be very successful.

The mean survival after diagnosis in 1935 was 4.4 years[74] when treatment was limited to supportive measures for diabetes, liver disease, and cardiac failure. At that time, 14% of patients developed primary liver cell cancer. In contrast, of patients treated by phlebotomy at the present time, 89% have a 5-year survival rate from the time of diagnosis,[75] although the incidence of primary hepatocellular cancer has increased to 25 to 30% with longer survival.[64,65] Most complications are preventable in individuals whose tissues are overloaded with iron but not yet damaged, as long as the excess iron is removed and future accumulation of iron is prevented.[34,69] Malignant hepatoma develops only very rarely if the disease is treated in the precirrhotic phase,[76] and two large studies have shown no increase in other forms of internal malignancy in the disease.[64,65] The prognosis for survival in treated precirrhotic subjects does not differ from the general population.[65] In patients and their relatives with early disease, the complications of iron overload are preventable.

V. SECONDARY (ACQUIRED) IRON OVERLOAD

A. HEMOCHROMATOSIS ASSOCIATED WITH CHRONIC ANEMIAS

Increased erythropoeisis results in increased iron absorption either in humans or experimentally induced animals. In the human, such increased iron absorption occurs primarily in those forms of hemolytic anemia associated with ineffective erythropoeisis, as in thalassemia major and hereditary side-roblastic anemia. Hemochromatosis has been described in association with other disorders, such as chronic refractory anemias and congenital sphero-cytosis, but it is likely that such patients carried the gene for hemochromatosis. Diseases associated with ineffective erythropoeisis and increased iron absorption lead to predominantly parenchymal iron loading, whereas when the iron load has been acquired primarily parenterally, i.e., by transfusion, there is predominantly RE cell involvement at least in the initial stages of loading. Fibrosis and functional impairment of the affected organs are seen more often in the former group. The full clinicopathological syndrome of hemochromatosis, including cardiac failure, diabetes mellitus, and hypopituitarism, has been described in patients with iron-loading anemias.

Cautious phlebotomy and chelating agents are used for iron removal. Intensive regular chelation therapy with desferrioxamine has been shown in a controlled trial to be effective in reducing the iron load and delaying the onset of hepatic fibrosis. The development of more effective oral chelating agents is eagerly awaited for this group of patients. At present, desferrioxamine remains the most effective form of chelation therapy, but new oral chelating agents are currently undergoing therapeutic trials. Desferrioxamine should be given by slow subcutaneous or intravenous infusion and the subject should be ascorbic-acid replete. However, excess ascorbate should be avoided since this may aggravate iron toxicity (see above).

B. CIRRHOSIS WITH SUBSEQUENT SECONDARY IRON OVERLOAD

As discussed above, it has long been recognized that patients with hepatic cirrhosis may secondarily develop increased stainable hepatic iron.[77] However, the increase in body iron stores is usually small (2 to 3 g). The problem has now been greatly clarified by the recognition of the HLA-related genetic disease (discussed previously) and may be summarized as follows:

1. A proporption of patients with hepatic cirrhosis accumulate iron but rarely do the body iron stores or hepatic iron concentrations reach levels comparable with those seen in patients with hemochromatosis.[64,78,79] When gross iron overload is encountered in association with cirrhosis, the genetic disease is usually responsible.
2. The factors that have been suggested as contributing to increased iron absorption and iron accumulation in patients with cirrhosis of the liver are

    a. Increased oral iron intake in alcoholic beverages or iron tablets
    b. Stimulation of absorption of inorganic iron by alcohol
    c. Pancreatic insufficiency

d. Folic acid deficiency

e. Portacaval shunt surgery

These factors and the relevant literature have been discussed in detail elsewhere.[2,32]

3. There is an increased incidence of alcoholism in patients with idiopathic hemochromatosis, varying from between 25 and 50% of patients. The reason for this is still unclear. However, systematic comparisons of alcoholic and non-alcoholic subjects with hemochromatosis as defined above have shown no significant different between the two groups with respect to the clinical and pathological features or to the degree of iron overload, except for the presence of active hepatocellular disease in some alcoholic patients. A detailed study of the pathology of the liver in hemochromatosis revealed that the hepatic findings were the same in alcoholic and non-alcoholic patients, except that in about 25% of the alcoholic patients there were changes of alcoholic liver disease super-imposed on the underlying hemochromatosis.[77] This is an incidence of alcoholic liver disease very similar to that reported among heavy drinkers in the general population.

Thus, the available data suggest that the majority of alcoholic subject with excessive iron overload possess the basic genetic defect of hemochromatosis and that the iron accumulation and liver injury have been accelerated by alcoholism.

4. Persons who are heterozygous for the hemochromatosis allele rarely, if ever, develop a progressive increase in body iron stores even with alcoholism or prolonged intake of dietary iron (Figure 1).[34,69]

5. While phlebotomy therapy is indicated in patients with primary idio-pathic hemochromatosis, whether alcoholic or non-alcoholic, it has not been demonstrated to have a therapeutic role in the alcoholic cirrhotic with increased iron stores.[74]

C. DIETARY IRON OVERLOAD

Gross iron overload resulting from excess absorption of orally ingested iron is very rare in all populations that have been studied with the single exception of the blacks of South Africa, among whom it was previously common (so-called "Bantu-type hemochromatosis"). The disease in that population has been extensively reviewed and will not be discussed further.

The prolonged ingestion of pharmacological doses of iron may lead to excessive iron accumulation. However, the data of Powell[77] suggest that less than massive doses of oral iron do not lead to increased iron stores. An association with the gene for hemochromatosis cannot be excluded until a gene probe becomes available for use in such patients.

ACKNOWLEDGMENTS

The authors acknowledge the support of the National Health and Medical Research Council of Australia and the Mayne Bequest Fund of the University of Queensland.

REFERENCES

1. **Bothwell, T. H.,** The control of iron absorption, *Br. J. Haematol.,* 14, 453, 1968.
2. **Bothwell, T. H., Charlton, R. W., Cook, J. D., and Finch, C. A.,** *Iron Metabolism in Man,* Blackwell Scientific, Oxford, 1979.
3. **Anderson, G. J., Powell, L. W., and Halliday, J. W.,** Transferrin receptor distribution and regulation in the rat small intestine: effect of iron stores and erythropoeisis, *Gastroenterology,* 98, 576, 1990.
4. **Casey, J. L., Di Jeso, B., Rao, K., Klausner, R. D., and Harford, J. B.,** Two genetiloci participate in the regulation by iron of the gene for the human transferrin receptor, *Proc. Natl. Acad. Sci. U.S.A.,* 85, 1787, 1988b.
5. **Casey, J. L., Di Jeso, B., Rao, K., Rouault, T. A., Klausner, R. D., and Harford, J. B.,** Deletional analysis of the promoter region of the human transferrin receptor gene, *Nucleic Acid Res.,* 16, 629, 1988a.
6. **Casey, J. L., Hentze, M. W., Koeller, D. M., Caughman, S. W., Roualt, T. A., Klausner, R. D., and Harford, J. B.,** Iron-responsive elements: regulatory DNA sequences that control mRNA levels and translation, *Science,* 240, 924, 1988.
7. **Caughman, S. W., Hentze, M. W., Rouault, T. A., Harford, J. B., and Klausner, R. D.,** The iron-responsive element is the single element responsible for iron-dependent translational regulation of ferritin biosynthesis, *J. Biol. Chem.,* 263, 19048, 1988.
8. **Leibold, F. A. and Munro, H. N.,** Cytoplasmic protein binds *in vitro* to a highly conserved sequence in the 51 untranslated region of ferritin heavy and light subunit mRNAs, *Proc. Natl. Acad. Sci. U.S.A.,* 85, 2171, 1988.
9. **Hentze, M. W., Caughman, S. W., Casey, J. W., Koeller, D. M., Rouault, T. A., Harford, J. B., and Klausner, R. D.,** A model for the structure and functions of iron-responsive elements, *Gene,* 72, 201, 1988.
10. **Rouault, T. A., Stout, C. D., Kaptain, S., Harford, J. B., and Klausner, R. D.,** Structural relationship between an iron-regulated RNA-binding protein (IRE-BP) and aconitase: functional implications, *Cell,* 64, 881, 1991.
11. **Peters, T. J.,** Mechanisms of cellular iron uptake and release, *Proc. Second Int. Haemochromatosis Conf.,* Gold Coast, Australia, 1989, 35.
12. **Raja, K. B., Simpson, R. J., Pippard, M. J., and Peters, T. J.,** *In vivo* studies on the relationship between intestinal iron (Fe^{3+}) absorption, hypoxia and erythropoeisis in the mouse, *Br. J. Haematol.,* 68, 373, 1988.
13. **Simpson, R. J., Moore, R., and Peters, T. J.,** Significance of non-esterified fatty acids in iron uptake by intestinal brush-border membrane vesicles, *Biochim. Biophys. Acta,* 941, 39, 1988.

14. **Conrad, M. E., Umbreit, J. N., Moore, E. G., Peterson, D. A., and Jones, B. M.,** A newly identified iron binding protein in duodenal mucosa of rats, *J. Biol. Chem.,* 265, 5273, 1990.
15. **Teichman, R. and Stremmel, W.,** Iron uptake by human upper small intestine microvillous membrane vesicles: indication for a facilitated transport mechanism medicated by a membrane iron-binding protein, *J. Clin. Invest.,* 86, 2145, 1990.
16. **Bacon, B. R., Tavill, A. S., Brittenham, G. M., Park, C. H., and Recknagel, R. O.,** Hepatic lipid peroxidation *in vivo* in rats with chronic iron overload, *J. Clin. Invest.,* 71, 429, 1983.
17. **Fletcher, L. M., Roberts, F. D., Irving, M. G., Powell, L. W., and Halliday, J. W.,** Effects of iron loading on free radical scavening enzymes and lipid peroxidation in rat liver, *Gastroenterology,* 97, 1011, 1989.
18. **Bacon, B. R. and Britton, R. S.,** The pathology of hepatic iron overload: A free radical-mediated process?, *Hepatology,* 11, 127, 1990.
19. **Britton, R. S., O'Neill, R., and Bacon, B. R.,** Hepatic mitochondrial malondialdehyde metabolism in rats with chronic iron overload, *Hepatology,* 11, 93, 1990.
20. **Powell, L. W.,** Iron storage in relatives of patients with haemochromatosis and in relatives of patients with alcoholic cirrhosis and haemosiderosis: a comparative study of 27 families, *Q. J. Med.,* 34, 427, 1965.
21. **Powell, L. W.,** The role of alcoholism in hepatic iron storage disease, *Ann. N.Y. Acad. Sci.,* 252, 124, 1975.
22. **Simon, M., Alexandre, J. L., Bourel, M., et al.,** Heredity of idiopathic hemochromatosis: a study of 106 families, *Clin. Genet.,* 11, 327, 1977.
23. **Simon, M., Alexandre, J.-L., Fauchet, R., et al.,** The genetics of hemochromatosis, *Prog. Med. Genet.,* 4, 135, 1980.
24. **Simon, M. and Brissot, P.,** The genetics of hemochromatosis, *Hepatology,* 6, 116, 1988.
25. **Edwards, C. Q., Griffin, L. M., Goldgar, D., Drummond, C., Skolnick, M. H., and Kushner, J. P.,** Prevalence of hemochromatosis among 11,065 presumably healthy blood donors, *N. Engl. J. Med.,* 318, 1355, 1988.
26. **Leggett, B. A., Brown, N. N., Bryant, S., Duplock, L., Powell, L. W., and Halliday, J. W.,** Factors affecting the concentration of ferritin in serum in a healthy Australian population, *Clin. Chem.,* 36, 1350, 1990.
27. **Williams, R., Scheuer, P. J., and Sherlock, S.,** The inheritance of idiopathic hemochromatosis: a clinical and liver biopsy study of 16 families, *Q. J. Med.,* 31, 249, 1962.
28. **Sheldon, J. H.,** Hemochromatosis, *London Oxford University Press,* 1935.
29. **Fauchet, R., Simon, M., Genetet, B., Kerbaol, M., Bansard, J. Y., Genetet, N., and Bourel, M.,** HLA-A, B, C, D and lymphocytes B antigens typing in idiopathic hemochromatosis with the study of 5 families, *Tissue Antigens,* 10, 206, 1977.
30. **Fauchet, R., Genetet, N., Genetet, B., Simon, M., and Bourel, M.,** HLA determinants in idiopathic hemochromatosis, *Tissue Antigens,* 14, 10, 1979.
31. **Cartwright, G. E., Edwards, C. Q., and Skolnick, M.,** Letter to editors: genetics of hemochromatosis, *N. Engl. J. Med.,* 301, 1291, 1979.
32. **Bassett, M. L., Halliday, J. W., and Powell, L. W.,** Genetic hemochromatosis, *Semin. Liver Dis.,* 4, 217, 1984.
33. **Summers, K. M., Tam, K. S., Halliday, J. W., and Powell, L. W.,** HLA determinants in an Australian population of hemochromatosis patients and their families, *Am. J. Hum. Genet.,* 45, 41, 1989.
34. **Bassett, M. L., Halliday, J. W., and Powell, L. W.,** HLA typing in idiopathic hemochromatosis: distinction between homozygotes and heterozygotes with biochemical expression, *Hepatology,* 1, 120, 1981.
35. **Edwards, C. Q., Carroll, M., Bray, P., and Cartwright, G. E.,** Hereditary hemochromatosis, *N. Engl. J. Med.,* 297, 7, 1977.

158

36. **Thomson, G. and Bodmer, W.,** The genetic analysis of HLA and disease associations, in *HLA and Disease,* Dausset, J. and Svejgaard, A., Eds., Williams & Wilkins, Baltimore, 1977, 84.

37. **Powell, L. W., Summers, K., Board, P. G., Axelsen, E., Webb, S., and Halliday, J. W.,** Expression of hemochromatosis in homozygous subjects: implications for early diagnosis and prevention, *Gastroenterology,* 98, 1625, 1990.

38. **Powell, L. W., Ferluga, J., Halliday, J. W., Bassett, M. L., Kohonen-Corish, M. K., and Serjeantson, S.,** Genetic hemochromatosis and HLA linkage, *Hum. Genet.,* 77, 55, 1987.

39. **Sciot, R., Paterson, A. C., Van Den Oord, J. J., and Desmet, V. J.,** Lack of hepatic transferrin receptor expression in hemochromatosis, *Hepatology,* 7, 831, 1987.

40. **Powell, L. W., Campbell, C. B., and Wilson, E.,** Intestinal mucosal uptake of iron and iron retention in idiopathic hemochromatosis as evidence of a mucosal abnormality, *Gut,* 11, 727, 1970.

41. **Whittaker, P., Skikne, B. S., Covell, A. M., Flowers, C., Cooke, A., and Lynch, S. L.,** Duodenal iron proteins in idiopathic hemochromatosis, *J. Clin. Invest.,* 83, 261, 1989.

42. **Francanzani, A. L., Fargion, S., Romeno, R., Piperno, A., Arosio, P., and Fiorelli, G.,** Immunohistochemical evidence for a lack of ferritin in duodenal absorptive epithelial cells in idiopathic hemochromatosis, *Gastroenterology,* 96, 1071, 1989.

43. **Pietrangelo, A., Rocchi, E., Rigo, G., Ferrari, A. L., Perini, M., Ventura, E., and Cario, G.,** Regulation of transferrin, transferrin receptor and ferritin gene expression in the duodenum of normal anemic and siderotic subjects, *Gastroenterology,* in press.

44. **Anderson, G. J., Walsh, M. D., Powell, L. W., and Halliday, J. W.,** Intestinal transferrin receptors and iron absorption in the neonatal rat, *Br. J. Haematol.,* 77, 229, 1991.

45. **Srai, S. K. S., Epstein, O., Denham, E. S., and McIntyre, N.,** The ontogeny of iron absorption and its possible relationship to pathogenesis of haemochromatosis, *Hepatology,* 4, 1033, 1984.

46. **Srai, S. K. S., Denham, E., and Epstein, O.,** Development changes in the villous uptake of iron and enterocyte iron binding proteins in the guinea pig duodenum, *Gut,* 28, A1333, 1987.

47. **Banerjee, D., Flanagan, P. R., Cluett, J., and Valberg, L. S.,** Transferrin receptors in the human gastrointestinal tract, *Gastroenterology,* 91, 861, 1986.

48. **Brittin, G. M. and Ravel, D.,** Duodenal ferritin synthesis during iron absorption in the iron-deficient rat, *J. Lab. Clin. Med.,* 75, 811, 1970.

49. **Brittin, G. M. and Raval, D.,** Duodenal ferritin synthesis in iron-replete and iron-deficient rats: response to small doses of iron, *J. Lab. Clin. Med.,* 77, 54, 1971.

50. **Halliday, J. W., Mack, U., and Powell, L. W.,** Duodenal ferritin content and structure: relationship with body iron stores in man, *Arch. Intern. Med.,* 138, 1109, 1978.

51. **Theil, E. C.,** Regulation of ferritin and transferrin receptor mRNAs, *J. Biol. Chem.,* 265, 4771, 1990.

52. **Klausner, R. D.,** From receptors to genes — insights from molecular iron metabolism, *Clin. Res.,* 36, 494, 1988.

53. **Hentze, M. W., Seuanez, H. N., O'Brien, S. J., Harford, J. B., and Klausner, R. D.,** Chromosomal localization of nucleic acid-binding proteins by affinity mapping: assignment of the IRE-binding protein gene to human chromosome 9, *Nucleic Acids Res.,* 6103, 1989.

54. **Summers, K. M., Tam, K. S., Bartley, P. B., Drysdale, J., Zoghbi, H. Y., Halliday, J. W., and Powell, L. W.,** Fine mapping of a chromosome 6 ferritin heavy chain gene: relevance to haemochromatosis, *Hum. Genet.,* 88, 175, 1991.

55. **Osterloh, K. R. S., Simpson, R. J., Snape, S., and Peters, T. J.,** Intestinal iron absorption and mucosal transferrin in rats subjected to hypoxia, *Blut,* 55, 421, 1987.

56. **Adams, P. C., Reece, A. S., Powell, L. W., and Halliday, J. W.,** Hepatic iron in the control of iron absorption in a rat liver transplantation model, *Transplantation,* 48, 19, 1989.

57. **Flanagan, P. R., Lam, D., Banerjee, D., and Valberg, L. S.,** Ferritin release by mononuclear cells in hereditary hemochromatosis, *J. Lab. Clin. Med.,* 113, 145, 1989.

58. **Fillet, G., Beguin, Y., and Baldelli, L.,** Model of reticuloendothelial iron metabolism in humans: abnormal behaviour in idiopathic hemochromatosis and in inflammation, *Blood,* 74, 844, 1989.

59. **Bassett, M. L., Halliday, J. W., and Powell, L. W.,** Value of hepatic iron measurements in early hemochromatosis and determination of the critical iron level associated with fibrosis, *Hepatology,* 6, 24, 1986.

60. **Summers, K. M., Halliday, J. W., and Powell, L. W.,** Identification of homozygous hemochromatosis subjects by measurements of hepatic iron index, *Hepatology,* 12, 20, 1990.

61. **Leon, M. B., Borer, J. S., Bacharach, S. L., Green, M. V., Benz, E. J., Griffith, P., and Nienhuis, A. W.,** Detection of early cardiac dysfunction in patients with severe β-thalassemia and chronic iron overload, *N. Engl. J. Med.,* 301, 1143, 1979.

62. **Nienhuis, A. W.,** Vitamin C and iron, *N. Engl. J. Med.,* 304, 170, 1981.

63. **McLaren, C., Bett, J. H. N., Nye, J. A., and Halliday, J. W.,** Congestive cardiomyopathy and haemochromatosis — rapid progression possibly accelerated by excessive ingestion of ascorbic acid, *Aust. N.Z. J. Med.,* 12, 187, 1982.

64. **Bradbear, R. A., Bain, C., Siskind, V., et al.,** Cohort study of internal malignancy in genetic hemochromatosis and other nonalcoholic liver diseases, *J.N.C.I.,* 74, 81, 1985.

65. **Niederau, C., Fisher, R., Sonnenberg, A., Stremmel, W., Trammpisch, H. J., and Strohmeyer, G.,** Survival and causes of death in cirrhotic and non-cirrhotic patients with primary hemochromatosis, *N. Engl. J. Med.,* 313, 1256, 1985.

66. **Grace, N. D. and Greenberg, M. S.,** Phlebotomy in the treatment of iron overload: a controlled trial (preliminary report), *Gastroenterology,* 60, 744, 1971.

67. **Williams, R., Smith, P. M., Spicer, E. J. F., et al.,** Venesection therapy in idiopathic hemochromatosis, *Q. J. Med.,* 38, 1, 1969.

68. **Bassett, M. L., Halliday, J. W., and Powell, L. W.,** Early detection of idiopathic hemochromatosis, relative value of serum-ferritin and HLA typing, *Lancet,* 2, 4, 1979.

69. **Bassett, M. L., Halliday, J. W., Ferris, R. A., and Powell, L. W.,** Diagnosis of hemochromatosis in young subjects: predictive accuracy of serum iron, transferrin saturation and serum ferritin, *Gastroenterology,* 87, 628, 1984.

70. **Chapman, R. W. G., Williams, G., Bydder, G., et al.,** Computed tomography for determining liver iron content in primary haemochromatosis, *Br. Med. J.,* 1, 440, 1980.

71. **Howard, J. M., Ghent, C. N., Carey, L. S., et al.,** Diagnostic efficacy of hepatic computed tomography in the detection of body iron overload, *Gastroenterology,* 84, 209, 1983.

72. **Dadone, M. M., Kushner, J. P., Edwards, C. Q., Bishop, D. T., and Skolnick, M. H.,** Hereditary hemochromatosis: analysis of laboratory expression of the disease by genotype in 18 pedigrees, *Am. J. Clin. Pathol.,* 78, 196, 1982.

73. **Bassett, M. L., Doran, T. J., Halliday, J. W., et al.,** Idiopathic hemochromatosis: demonstration of homozygous-heterozygous mating by HLA typing of families, *Hum. Genet.,* 60, 352, 1982.

74. **Grace, N. D. and Powell, L. W.,** Iron storage disorders of the liver, *Gastroenterology,* 64, 1257, 1974.

75. **Finch, S. C. and Finch, C. A.,** Idiopathic hemochromatosis, an iron storage disease. 1. Iron metabolism in hemochromatosis, *Medicine,* 34, 381, 1955.

76. **Powell, L. W. and Kerr, J. F. R.,** The pathology of the liver in hemochromatosis, in *Pathobiology Annual,* Joacim, H., Ed., Appleton-Century-Crofts, New York, 1975, 317.

77. **Powell, L. W.,** Iron storage in relatives of patients with hemochromatosis and in relatives of patients with alcoholic cirrhosis and hemosiderosis: a comparative study of 27 families, *Q. J. Med.,* 34, 427, 1965.
78. **Simon, M., Bourel, M., Genetet, B., et al.,** Idiopathic hemochromatosis and iron overload in alcoholic liver disease: differentiation by HLA phenotype, *Gastroenterology,* 73, 655, 1977.
79. **Zimmerman, H. J., Chomet, B., Kulesch, M. H., and McWhorter, C. A.,** Hepatic hemosiderin deposits: incidence in 558 biopsies from patients with and without intrinsic hepatic disease, *Arch. Intern. Med.,* 197, 494, 1961.

5. Iron and the Immune System

JEREMY H. BROCK

*University Department of Immunology, Western Infirmary,
Glasgow, Scotland, U.K.*

I. INTRODUCTION

The immune system consists of a complex series of cellular and molecular interactions, the activation of which is designed to recognize and then destroy foreign or altered molecules and organisms. As advances have been made in molecular and cellular biology, so the mystery surrounding much of the phenomenology of the immune system has been stripped away to reveal in detail the intricate recognition and metabolic events involved. This has led to a realization that mechanisms previously thought to have little or nothing to do with the immune system are crucial if the system is to function normally. One such area that has received increasing attention in recent years is the interaction between the immune system and iron metabolism, and it is this interface which forms the basis of this chapter.

Immunity is frequently divided into specific and nonspecific (or innate) immunity. Into the latter category fall a number of mechanisms, which include the ability of iron-binding proteins such as transferrin and lactoferrin to retard microbial growth. This topic is dealt with in the following chapter and will not be considered here, so this chapter will therefore concentrate on the specific immune response. It will discuss experimental and clinical evidence for the role played by iron in the immune system and consider how these observations may be explained by the way in which iron and iron-binding proteins interact with the cells and molecules of the immune system. The whole area has been reviewed in detail fairly recently,[1] and so this chapter will concentrate as far as possible on the most recent findings.

Evidence for the role of iron in the immune system in man inevitably comes mainly from clinical studies of patients with abnormal iron metabolism. There have been numerous studies of patients suffering from various degrees of iron deficiency and a rather smaller number of studies of patients with iron overload due either to inherited abnormalities in iron regulation (hereditary hemochromatosis) or to transfusional iron overload, mainly in patients with β-thalassemia. Such studies are prone to various difficulties, such as ensuring the absence of other deficiencies in patients with iron deficiency, obtaining genuinely normal controls in studies carried out in developing countries, and differentiating between epiphenomena and genuine effects of iron when dealing with iron overload. For this reason, researchers have sought to overcome these problems by using animal models, in which other variables are more readily controlled. The present state of knowledge, drawing on both clinical and experimental studies, is summarized in Table 1.

II. IRON DEFICIENCY

A large number of clinical studies of the effects of iron deficiency on the immune system have been carried out. The results have been rather variable, as discussed in a number of reviews,[2-7] but some defects have been reported fairly consistently.

TABLE 1
Effect of Iron Deficiency and Iron Overload on Immune Function

Function	Iron deficiency	Iron overload
Total lymphocyte number	NORMAL	NORMAL
Proportion of T cells	DECREASED	normal
Number/proportion of B-cells	normal?	normal
CD4:CD8 ratio	normal	DECREASED
CD2 expression	—	increased[1]
Skin test response	DECREASED	decreased
Response to mitogens	decreased	DECREASED
Immunoglobulin levels/synthesis	normal?[2]	?
Lymphocyte cytotoxicity	normal	normal?
Macrophage/monocyte phagocytosis	decreased	?
Macrophage/monocyte cyto-toxicity/intracellular killing	decreased?	decreased
Neutrophil phagocytosis	NORMAL	decreased[3]
Neutrophil intracellular killing	DECREASED	decreased[3]
Myeloperoxidase activity	DECREASED	—
Superoxide production	normal?	—

Note: **CAPITALS** = consistent finding — several reports, all or almost all in agreement; **lower case** = quite good evidence — most reports in accordance, but some contrary findings, or evidence based on only a small number of reports; **lower case** plus ? = not certain, but balance of evidence favors conclusion shown; **?** = contradictory findings — impossible to draw conclusions; — = no data.

[1] Normal in clinical studies, decreased in animal studies.
[2] Only in hereditary hemochromatosis.
[3] Only in transfused thalassemia patients.

A. T-LYMPHOCYTE FUNCTION

Total lymphocyte numbers are usually unchanged in iron deficiency,[8,9] although the proportion of T cells is often reduced.[8-12] However, a more recent study of subjects in which iron deficiency was due to blood loss rather than to inadequate iron nutrition showed the reverse, i.e., a decrease in total lymphocyte numbers but a normal proportion of T cells.[13] This study also reported a normal CD4:CD8 ratio.

Several clinical studies have assessed T-cell function in iron deficiency. *In vivo* studies using skin tests have invariably found depressed responses,[8,12,14-17] but more variable results were obtained when T-cell function was measured *in vitro* by the proliferative response to mitogens. This controversial area has been discussed by Farthing,[4] who concluded that in adults the responses were normal in iron-deficient pregnant females[9] but depressed in men or non-pregnant females.[14,17-20] A more recent study using T-cell colony formation rather than thymidine incorporation to assay T-cell proliferation also reported depressed responses in adults.[21] However, no explanation could be found for the conflicting results of studies in children, where reports showing depressed responses[8,10,15,16,22] are balanced by those showing no effect.[12,23-25] Animal studies have tended to support the findings of reduced T-lymphocyte proliferation in iron deficiency,[26-29] and more recently it has been found that in iron-deficient mice the thymus was depleted of thymocytes, though there was no evidence of impaired thymic endocrine function.[30] In animal studies, the degree of iron deficiency induced is usually more severe than that seen in human subjects, although a recent study reported decreased T-cell responses to mitogens in both moderate and severe iron deficiency.[31] One might speculate that in situations where iron deficiency is a quasi-physiological condition, i.e., in pregnancy or young children, the immune system compensates for any potential defects in T-cell function, but cannot or does not do so when the deficiency is severe or occurs in otherwise normal adults. In this connection it is noteworthy that mitochondrial abnormalities have been found in electron microscope studies of lymphocytes from iron-deficient adults[32,33] in whom the condition had probably been present for some time.

B. B-LYMPHOCYTE FUNCTION AND ANTIBODY PRODUCTION

There are fewer clinical reports on the effect of iron deficiency on B-cell function and less evidence of abnormalities than in T cells. B-cell numbers and proportions are reported as normal in two studies,[11,12] and depressed in a third,[13] while various studies on serum immunoglobulin or specific antibody levels have failed to reveal any consistent effect of iron deficiency.[8,9,11,13,16,34] Vaccination of iron-deficient children with tetanus toxoid resulted in normal antibody titers,[8] and a reported failure of iron-deficient children to mount a normal antibody response to diphtheria toxoid[35] did not contain adequate documentation of the subjects to eliminate other nutritional abnormalities.

However, these results tend to differ from those obtained in animal studies. Iron-deficient rats or mice showed decreased antibody production,[28,36-38] and proliferative responses to the B-cell mitogen lipopolysaccharide were impaired.[31] Numbers of IgA- and IgM-bearing B cells in the jejunal mucosa of iron-deficient weanling rats were reduced, suggesting that mucosal immunity might also be adversely affected.[39] However, in one recent study an impaired response to influenza virus in severely iron-deficient rats was thought to be due to the associated reduction in food intake, as a similar impairment occurred in the pair-fed group.[40] Thus, the ability of iron deficiency to impair B-cell function remains less convincing than its effect on T cells. Possible reasons for this are discussed later.

C. LYMPHOCYTE CYTOTOXICITY

There is little evidence that iron deficiency adversely affects lymphocyte cytotoxic activity. A recent study reported decreased antibody-dependent cytotoxic activity (ADCC) in lymphocytes from iron-deficient adults,[13] although correction of iron deficiency failed to normalize cytotoxic activity, suggesting that some other defect might have been responsible. There appear to be no clinical reports on the effect of iron deficiency on NK cell activity, so one suspects that such activity is probably normal. Iron-deficient rat pups were found to have decreased NK cell activity,[41] but it is not clear whether this reflected impaired NK activity or a decrease in the proportion of NK cells in the spleen cell population. Decreased α-interferon production by macrophages may be partly responsible.[42]

D. IRON REQUIREMENTS OF LYMPHOCYTES

What are the mechanisms behind the defects in lymphocyte function associated with iron deficiency? It is now well established that lymphocyte activation is accompanied by increased uptake of iron via the transferrin-transferrin receptor system[43] and that in the absence of transferrin-bound iron, lymphocyte proliferation is usually impaired. Blockade of transferrin-iron uptake, either by monoclonal antibodies to the transferrin receptor[44-48] or by apotransferrin,[45] prevents T-cell proliferation. However, the effect of monoclonal antibodies is complex, and an ability to cross-link receptors is more important than merely blocking transferrin binding,[49] perhaps because cross-linking prevents normal recycling of the receptors. The impaired T-cell function seen in iron-deficiency can therefore by explained, at least in part, by an inadequate supply of transferrin-bound iron to transferrin-receptor-bearing activated T-cells, and indeed the decreased mitogen responses of lymphocytes from iron-deficient mice were found to be due to the low saturation of serum transferrin.[28] The requirement for iron in T-cell proliferation is usually dependent on the induction of transferrin receptor expression via the interaction of interleukin-2 (IL-2) with its receptor.[50,51] However, stimulation with phorbol ester plus calcium ionophore can induce expression of transferrin receptors without a requirement for IL-2,[52] and in the presence of submitogenic levels of phorbol ester a monoclonal antibody to the transferrin receptor was found to stimulate rather than inhibit proliferation.[53] Studies in which cells are stimulated with specific antigens rather than mitogens would be helpful in resolving these differences.

It has been reported that cloned human TH1 helper cells are much more strongly inhibited by iron deprivation than TH2 clones.[54] This difference was due, at least in part, to the presence of larger iron storage pools in the TH2 cells. Since the TH1 subset is important in delayed-type hypersensitivity responses this observation may help explain the frequent reports of depressed skin-test responses in iron-deficient patients. This recent evidence for differences in iron requirements between T-cell subpopulations is important and further studies of this type may help explain some of the inconsistencies in the results of clinical studies.

For B lymphocytes, delivery of transferrin-bound iron is also important for proliferation,[55] but the role of transferrin may be more complex than in

T-cell activation. In B-cells stimulated with staphylococcal protein A it was found that immunoglobulin synthesis could precede transferrin receptor expression,[56] suggesting that antibody production might not have a rigorous requirement for iron. This might explain why iron deficiency tends to have a greater effect on cell-mediated immunity than on antibody production. However, when B-cells were stimulated with LPS or anti-μ-chain antibodies *in vitro*[57,58] or anti-δ-chain antibodies *in vivo*,[59] transferrin receptors could be detected at only 3 to 4 h after activation, reminiscent of the early expression on T-cells activated with phorbol ester plus a calcium ionophore.

Furthermore, transferrin enhances *in vitro* production of IgM and, in particular, IgE by blood mononuclear cells,[60] thought it it not clear whether transferrin stimulates the B-cells directly or acts indirectly by enhancing T-helper cell activation.

E. MACROPHAGE FUNCTION

Relatively little attention has been paid to the effect of iron deficiency on macrophage function. In a recent clinical study,[61] macrophages from iron-deficient children showed normal cytotoxic activity and IL-1 release. However, in animal studies iron deficiency reduced *in vivo* clearance of poly-vinylpyrollidone and α-interferon synthesis in rats[62] and *in vitro* synthesis of IL-1 in mice.[63] The *in vitro* tumoricidal activity of splenic macrophages from iron-deficient mice was also impaired.[64] A possible explanation comes from findings showing that macrophages depleted of iron *in vitro* showed reduced hydrogen peroxide release,[65] and that iron may be important in the production of nitric oxide,[66] both of which may contribute to monocyte/macrophage cytotoxic and antimicrobial activity.

F. NEUTROPHIL FUNCTION

The effect of iron deficiency on neutrophil function has been more extensively investigated. The majority of clinical studies concluded that phagocytic activity was unaffected,[8,16,67-69] but that bactericidal activity was impaired.[8,10,16,22,69,70] However, two groups failed to find any defect in bactericidal activity,[23,71] and in a more recent study claiming defective bactericidal activity[72] it is not clear whether the authors were measuring phagocytosis or intracellular killing. Since the generation of reactive oxygen derivatives and the activity of the myeloperoxidase-halide system are important in microbicidal activity, some workers have studied the effect of iron deficiency on these parameters. As with bactericidal activity, a majority have reported impairment,[8,68,72-74] but some have reported no effect.[16,70,71]

Animal studies of the effect of iron deficiency on neutrophil function are relatively few but tend to confirm the existence of defects in oxygen metabolism[75-79] and bactericidal activity,[77] though not in phagocytic uptake.[77] It is perhaps noteworthy that two of the more recent experimental studies reported that while myeloperoxidase activity was decreased, superoxide production was normal.[78,79] Impaired functioning of the myeloperoxidase halide system may therefore be the key to the reduced bactericidal activity.

There is little information about other neutrophil activities. Chemotaxis measured *in vitro* was found to be normal,[16,71] although in iron-deficient rats recruitment of neutrophils to the lung and peritoneum following an inflammatory stimulus was reduced.[78] Lysozyme production appears to be normal.[76]

G. COMPLEMENT

There are few studies of the effect of iron deficiency on other aspects of the immune system. Levels of complement components C3,[8,34] C4,[34] and total hemolytic activity[8] were unchanged in iron-deficient children.[34]

III. IRON OVERLOAD

The effect of iron overload on the immune system has received less attention than iron deficiency, and there are fewer clinical studies. Most such studies deal with transfusional iron overload, either in β-thalassemia or in renal failure patients, although some have been carried out in patients with hereditary hemochromatosis. The subject has recently been reviewed by De Sousa.[80,81]

A. T-LYMPHOCYTES

Evidence for a defect in responses to T-cell mitogens in iron overload is scarce. In thalassemia patients, depressed T-lymphocyte responses to PHA[82-84] and in the mixed lymphocyte reaction[82] have been reported, and skin-test responses to *Candida albicans* were impaired.[82] The situation in hemochromatosis is confused, since a report of normal lymphocyte responses to Con-A[85] was contradicted in a later publication by the same group[86] when depressed responses were reported. There appears to be no information on lymphocyte proliferation in animal studies of iron overload, although IL-2 production following Con-A stimulation was found to be impaired in iron-overloaded mice.[87]

In contrast to the paucity of data on mitogen responses of lymphocytes in iron overload, there have been quite a number of studies on T-cell subsets and marker expression. The most consistent finding is a reduced CD4:CD8 ratio. In thalassemia, this is due mainly to a reduction in the number of CD4 cells,[82,88-90] although increased numbers of CD8 cells have also been reported.[82,89] It is possible that this is not a result of iron loading, but arises from chronic alloantigen stimulation due to repeated blood transfusions.[89,91] Nevertheless, elevated CD8 levels have also been reported in hereditary hemochromatosis,[86] although as with responses to PHA, this group had reported contrary findings in an earlier study.[85]

Other T-cell markers may be affected by iron overload. In both their studies Bryan and co-workers[85,86] found that the proportion of cells expressing the CD2 epitope responsible for formation of thermostable E-rosettes was increased in hemochromatosis patients. There appears to be no evidence of abnormal CD2 expression in iron-overloaded thalassemia patients, although an abnormally high proportion of cells expressing CD1 have been reported in thalassemia intermedia.[88] This was reversed by incubation of the cells with a crude thymic extract for 48 h, suggesting that an abnormality in maturation may have been responsible. Further studies will be required to determine whether this abnormality is directly related to iron overload.

B. B-LYMPHOCYTES

Evidence for abnormal B-cell function in iron overload is contradictory. In hereditary hemochromatosis, Bryan and co-workers[86] found that the *in vitro* proliferative response to pokeweed mitogen was impaired, but the situation is again confused by a report of normal responses in this group's earlier publication.[85] There was no consistent effect on PWM-stimulated immuno-globulin synthesis,[86] and patients' immunoglobulin levels were normal.[85] In thalassemia, both B-cell numbers and immunoglobulin levels were elevated,[82] but *in vitro* production of plaque-forming cells in response to PWM was reduced.[92] However, as with T-cell abnormalities it is not certain whether these findings are necessarily related to iron overload. Elevated spontaneous immunoglobulin production by B-cells was found in both hemochromatosis[85] and thalassemia patients.[92]

C. EFFECT OF IRON ON LYMPHOCYTES *IN VITRO*

Evidence for abnormal lymphocyte numbers and/or function in iron overload is supported by *in vitro* studies showing that nontransferrin-bound iron can affect various functions. Although transferrin-bound iron enhances lymphocyte proliferation, iron in the form of hydrophilic chelates (citrate or nitrolotriacetate) or ferric salts is often inhibitory.[55,93-96] This may be due to hydrolysis followed by polymerization and binding to the cell membrane.[97,98] Such binding might especially affect the CD2 molecule, as recognition of this marker by sheep red cells[99] or monoclonal antibodies[100] is reduced by exposure of lymphocytes to ferric citrate. Since CD2 is important in lymphocyte activation, this might help explain the inhibitory effect of Fe-citrate on *in vitro* lymphocyte proliferation and the impaired immune responsiveness found in some clinical studies of iron overload. However, this depressed CD2 reactivity is in direct contrast to the previously mentioned increased number of CD2+ cells found in patients with hereditary hemochromatosis. Further studies which can differentiate between total cell levels of CD2 and the availability of surface CD2 molecules to sheep erythrocytes or antibodies may help resolve this discrepancy.

Nearly all studies on the effect of excess iron on T-cells *in vitro* have examined the total T-cell populations. However, Good and co-workers[101] found that the inhibitory effect of excess iron on T-cell cloning efficiency was more pronounced on murine CD4+ memory cells and CD8+ cytotoxic cells than on CD8− helper cells, due in part to an increase in T-suppressor function. Generation of human CD4+ clones was also inhibited by Fe-citrate,[102] and Fe-nitrilotriacetate selectivity inhibited proliferation of human CD4+ cells.[103]

In iron overload, serum ferritin levels are elevated and this may contribute to immunosuppression, as lymphocytes can bind ferritin, particularly the H-subunit,[104-107] which inhibits mitogen-stimulated T-cell proliferation.[108,109] Ferritin can depress DTH responses when injected into mice,[110] and clinical evidence also suggests that ferritin may have an immunosuppressive effect.[111]

D. NK CELLS AND CYTOTOXIC T-CELLS

NK cell activity is reduced in β-thalassemia,[91,112,113] and since incubation of NK cells *in vitro* with the iron chelator desferrioxamine partially reversed the defect,[114] it was suggested that iron overload was responsible.[113,114] However, administration of desferrioxamine to patients failed to alter NK activity,[112] and NK function was found to be normal in hereditary hemochromatosis.[115] It therefore seems likely that the depressed NK activity in thalassemia is due to mechanisms unrelated to iron overload.

Decreased cytotoxic T-cell activity was found in spleen cells from iron-overloaded mice.[87] This was due to impaired production of IL-2, rather than to a decrease in the number of precursor cells in the spleen. Cytotoxic T-cell function in human iron overload appears not to have been investigated.

E. MACROPHAGE/MONOCYTE FUNCTION

The role of the macrophage as a phagocytic defense mechanism against infection does not seem to be greatly impaired in iron overload. In hemochromatosis this might not seem surprising given that macrophage is largely spared from iron overload (see Chapter 4), although defective *in vitro* phagocytosis of *Staphylococcus aureus* has been reported in some patients,[116,117] and in one case an improvement was noted after phlebotomy.[116] Defective intracellular killing by monocytes from thalassemia patients[118] and from patients with other transfusion-related iron overload[117] has been reported, but ingestion was not affected. In the case of the thalassemia patients the defect was not found in patients <10 years old and was inversely related to serum ferritin levels, suggesting that iron overload was the causative factor. However, the defect was not related to the number of blood transfusions and did not disappear when the patients were treated with desferrioxamine.

The role of iron in the microbicidal activity of monocytes is complex. On the one hand iron may enhance activity, as killing of trypanosomes by macrophages was increased if the cells were exposed to Fe-lactoferrin, but not apolactoferrin,[119] and iron-loaded bacteria were more susceptible than iron-poor organisms to killing by hydrogen peroxide[120,121] and by monocytes.[121] On the other hand reducing macrophage intracellular iron levels by incubation with desferrioxamine or γ-interferon enhanced their ability to kill intracellular pathogens,[122,123] probably by preventing intracellular multiplication. This suggests that levels of iron within macrophages need to be carefully regulated to provide optimal microbicidal activity, and, indeed, it has been shown that killing of *Listeria* by macrophages was related to the iron content of the cells at low iron levels, but killing by thioglycolate-elicited macrophages was only effective when high initial intracellular iron levels were reduced by incubation of the cells with apotransferrin.[124] Although these findings go some way to explaining the defects in monocyte/macrophage function observed in transfusional iron overload, they seem unlikely to account for the impaired bactericidal activity of monocytes from hemochromatosis patients, as these cells are largely spared from iron overloading. Possibly, inhibition results from interaction with non-transferrin-bound iron in the serum of these patients.

F. NEUTROPHIL FUNCTION

Several studies have reported impaired neutrophil function associated with transfusional iron overload. In renal-failure patients undergoing hemodialysis, both ingestion and intracellular killing mechanisms were impaired.[125,126] Decreased phagocytosis seems to be due to an intrinsic defect in neutrophil function, whereas impairment of intracellular killing was related to a factor present in the patient's serum. Similar defects have been noted in β-thalassemia patients with transfusional iron overload,[127-129] and, moreover, it seems likely that the serum factor responsible for decreased bactericidal activity was non-transferrin-bound iron, as the defect could be abolished by adding desferrioxamine to the patient serum.[128]

There is little information on neutrophil function in primary iron overload, but the limited data available suggest that this has less effect on neutrophil function, which was normal in patients with hereditary hemochromatosis,[116,117] even though monocyte phagocytosis was impaired.

The inhibitory effect of iron overload on neutrophil function may be due to interaction of non-transferrin-bound iron with the neutrophil membrane, as iron citrate or ascorbate were found to bind to neutrophils and catalyze the production of toxic oxygen intermediates from neutrophil-derived superoxide.[130-132] On the other hand neutrophils, unlike macrophages, do not kill iron-loaded microorganisms better than those with normal iron levels.[120,121] This is probably because the myeloperoxidase-halide system does not require catalytic iron, unlike killing by hydroxyl radicals, which is a relatively more important mechanism in monocytes and macrophages.

G. OTHER INTERACTIONS BETWEEN IRON AND THE IMMUNE SYSTEM

Two recent observations that do not readily fit into any of the previous sections and for which the mechanisms involved are unclear deserve comment.

First, a protein produced by suppressor T-cells which inhibits antibody production and delayed hypersensitivity responses appears to require iron for its activity.[133] Iron (and to a lesser extent other metal ions) appears to act by inducing the oxidation of the protein from an inactive to an active form. The relationship of this protein to other molecules with immunoregulatory properties such as cytokines is unclear, and the nature of the metal-binding site has not yet been determined.

It has also been reported that iron-saturated bovine transferrin, human lactoferrin, and chicken ovotransferrin facilitate bone-marrow grafting in mice. Apotransferrin was ineffective.[134] It is difficult to envisage what the underlying mechanism might be, given the diversity of the proteins involved and the fact that the recipients' own (murine) transferrin must presumably be inactive. The quantities used (100 μg per mouse per day) were too small to have any generalized effect on iron status.

IV. CONCLUSIONS

It is evident that the interrelationship between iron metabolism and the immune system is complex. In general, this relationship reflects the fact that iron is on the one hand an essential requirement for many metabolic processes, while on the other it may become toxic if metabolism is abnormal. Thus, the role of iron in immune function must be seen in the wider context of its role in the biology and biochemistry of the whole organism, rather than as some kind of special relationship between the two systems. Discussion of the role of iron in the immune system is therefore to some extent an artificial exercise unless it is viewed within the context of other biological activities of iron. Fortunately, many of these are discussed elsewhere in this book.

The immune system seems to be relatively robust, insofar as it only becomes malfunctional in the face of fairly major derangements of iron metabolism. Transferrin is probably the key factor in maintaining normal immune function over an iron status that varies fairly widely. One may speculate that iron deficiency only impairs normal immunological function when the degree of iron saturation of transferrin is so low that iron delivery to critical cells and tissues is diminished. On the other hand, iron overload will only cause damage when transferrin becomes fully saturated and non-transferrin-bound iron is present in the circulation. This may bind to cells of the immune system and impair their function through the generation of toxic oxygen radicals and, perhaps, by other mechanisms. Nevertheless, it is possible that as the functions of cell subsets, particularly lymphocytes, become better known, subtle differences in their iron requirements may appear, which in turn could lead to iron acting as a "fine tuner" for the immune system. Hopefully, future work will test the validity of this proposal.

172

REFERENCES

1. **De Sousa, M. and Brock, J. H.**, *Iron in Immunity, Cancer and Inflammation*, Wiley, Chichester, 1989.
2. **Brock, J. H. and Mainou-Fowler, T.**, Iron and immunity, *Proc. Nutr. Soc.*, 305, 1986.
3. **Dallman, P. R.**, Iron deficiency and the immune response, *Am. J. Clin. Nutr.*, 46, 329, 1987.
4. **Farthing, M. J. G.**, Iron and immunity, *Acta Paediatr. Scand.*, Suppl. 361, 44, 1989.
5. **Hershko, C., Peto, T. E. A., and Weatherall, D. J.**, Iron and infection, *Br. Med. J.*, 296, 600, 1988.
6. **Dhur, A., Galán, P., and Hercberg, S.**, Iron status, immune capacity and resistance to infections, *Comp. Biochem. Physiol.*, 94A, 11, 1989.
7. **Kuvibidila, S.**, Iron deficiency, cell mediated immunity and resistance against infections: present knowledge and controversies, *Nutr. Res.*, 7, 989, 1987.
8. **Chandra, R. K.**, Impaired immunocompetence associated with iron deficiency, *J. Pediatr.*, 86, 899, 1975.
9. **Prema, K., Ramalakshmi, B. A., Madhava Peddi, R., and Babu, S.**, Immune status of anaemic pregnant women, *Br. J. Obstet. Gynaecol.*, 89, 222, 1982.
10. **Srikantia, S. G., Prasad, J. S., Bhaskaram, C., and Krishnamachari, K. A. V. R.**, Anaemia and the immune response, *Lancet*, 1, 1307, 1976.
11. **Bagchi, K., Mohanram, M., and Reddy, V.**, Humoral immune response in children with iron deficiency, *Br. Med. J.*, 208, 1249, 1980.
12. **Krantman, H. J., Young, S. R., Ank, B. J., O'Donnell, C. M., Rachelefsky, G. S., and Stiehm, E. R.**, Immune function in pure iron deficiency, *Am. J. Dis. Child.*, 136, 840, 1982.
13. **Santos, P. C. and Falcão, R. P.**, Decreased lymphocyte subsets and K-cell activity in iron deficiency anemia, *Acta Haematol.*, 84, 118, 1990.
14. **Joynson, D. H. M., Jacobs, A., Walker, D. M., and Dolby, A. F.**, Defect in cell mediated immunity in patients with iron-deficiency anaemia, *Lancet*, 2, 1058, 1972.
15. **Bhaskaram, C. and Reddy, V.**, Cell-mediated immunity in iron- and vitamin-deficient children, *Br. Med. J.*, 3, 522, 1975.
16. **Macdougall, L. G., Anderson, R., McNab, G. M., and Katz, J.**, The immune response in iron-deficient children: impaired cellular defense mechanisms with altered humoral components, *J. Pediatr.*, 86, 833, 1975.
17. **Swarup-Mitra, S. and Sinha, A. K.**, Cell-mediated immunity in nutritional anaemia, *Ind. J. Med. Res.*, 79, 354, 1984.
18. **Fletcher, J., Mather, J., Lewis, M. J., and Whiting, G.**, Mouth lesions in iron-deficient anemia: relationship to *Candida albicans* in saliva and to impairment of lymphocyte transformation, *J. Infect. Dis.*, 131, 44, 1975.
19. **Sawitsky, B., Kanter, R., and Sawitsky, A.**, Lymphocyte response to phytomitogens in iron deficiency, *Am. J. Med. Sci.*, 272, 153, 1976.
20. **Moraes-de-Souza, H., Kerbauy, J., Yamamoto, M., da-Silva, M. P., and dos-Santos, M. R. M.**, Depressed cell-mediated immunity in iron-deficiency anemia due to chronic loss of blood, *Braz. J. Med. Biol. Res.*, 17, 143, 1984.
21. **Wakabayashi, Y., Sugimoto, M., Ishiyama, T., and Hirose, S.**, Effect of iron on T-cell colony formation in patients with iron deficiency anemia, *Acta Haematol. Jpn.*, 51, 691, 1988.
22. **Rao, B. S. N.**, Studies on iron-deficiency anemia, *Ind. J. Med. Res.*, 68, 58, 1978.
23. **Kulapongs, P., Vithayasai, V., Suskind, R., and Olsen, R. E.**, Cell mediated immunity and phagocytosis and killing function in children with severe iron-deficiency anaemia, *Lancet*, 2, 689, 1974.
24. **Gupta, K. K., Dhatt, P. S., and Singh, H.**, Cell-mediated immunity in children with iron-deficiency anaemia, *Ind. J. Pediat.*, 49, 507, 1982.

25. **Grosch-Wörner, I., Grosse-Wilde, H., Bender-Götze, C., and Schüfer, K. H.,** Lymphozytenfunktionen bei kindern mit eisenmangel, *Klin. Wochenschr.,* 62, 1091, 1984.
26. **Kuvibidila, S. R., Baliga, B. S., and Suskind, R. M.,** Effects of iron deficiency anemia on delayed cutaneous hypersensitivity in mice, *Am. J. Clin. Nutr.,* 34, 2635, 1981.
27. **Kuvibidila, S., Nauss, K. M., Baliga, B. S., and Suskind, R. M.,** Impairment of blastogenic response of splenic lymphocytes from iron-deficient mice: *in vivo* repletion, *Am. J. Clin. Nutr.,* 37, 15, 1983.
28. **Mainou-Fowler, T. and Brock, J. H.,** Effect of iron deficiency on the response of mouse lymphocytes to concanavalin A: the importance of transferrin-bound iron, *Immunology,* 54, 325, 1985.
29. **Soyano, A., Candellet, D., and Layrisse, M.,** Effect of iron-deficiency on the mitogen-induced proliferative response of rat lymphocytes, *Int. Arch. Allergy. Appl. Immunol.,* 69, 353, 1982.
30. **Kuvibidila, S., Dardenne, M., Savino, W., and Lepault, F.,** Influence of iron-deficiency anemia on selected thymus functions in mice: thymulin biological activity, T-cell subsets, and thymocyte proliferation, *Am. J. Clin. Nutr.,* 51, 228, 1990.
31. **Kuvibidila, S. and Sarpong, D.,** Mitogenic response of lymph nodes and spleen lymphocytes from mice with moderate and severe iron deficiency anemia, *Nutr. Res.,* 10, 195, 1990.
32. **Jarvis, J. H. and Jacobs, A.,** Morphological abnormalities in lymphocyte mitochondria associated with iron-deficiency anaemia, *J. Clin. Pathol.,* 27, 973, 1974.
33. **Jiménez, A., Sánchez, A., Vázquez, A., and Olmos, J. M.,** Alteraciones mitochondriales en los linfocitos de pacientes con anemia ferropénica, *Morfol. Norm. Patol.,* 6B, 279, 1982.
34. **Galán, P., Davila, M., Mekki, N., and Hercberg, S.,** Iron deficiency, inflammatory processes and humoral immunity in children, *Int. J. Vit. Nutr. Res.,* 58, 225, 1988.
35. **MacDougall, L. G. and Jacobs, M. R.,** The immune response in iron-deficient children. Isohemagglutinin titres and antibody response to imunisation, *South Afr. Med. J.,* 53, 405, 1978.
36. **Nalder, B. N., Mahoney, A. W., Ramakrishnan, R., and Hendricks, D. G.,** Sensitivity of the immunological response to the nutritional status of rats, *J. Nutr.,* 102, 535, 1972.
37. **Kochanowski, B. A. and Sherman, A. R.,** Decreased antibody formation in iron-deficient rat pups — effect of iron repletion, *Am. J. Clin. Nutr.,* 41, 278, 1985.
38. **Kuvibidila, S. R., Baliga, B. S., and Suskind, R. M.,** Generation of plaque forming cells in iron-deficient anemic mice, *Nutr. Rep. Int.,* 26, 871, 1982.
39. **Perkkiö, M. V., Jansson, L. T., Dallman, P. R., Siimes, M. A., and Savilahti, E.,** sIGA- and IgM-containing cells in the intestinal mucosa of iron-deficient rats, *Am. J. Clin. Nutr.,* 46, 341, 1987.
40. **Dhur, A., Galán, P., Hannoun, C., Huot, K., and Hercberg, S.,** Effects of iron deficiency upon the antibody response to influenza virus in rats, *J. Nutr. Biochem.,* 1, 629, 1990.
41. **Sherman, A. R. and Lockwood, J. F.,** Impaired natural killer cell activity in iron-deficient rat pups, *J. Nutr.,* 117, 567, 1987.
42. **Hallquist, N. A. and Sherman, A. R.,** Effect of iron deficiency on the stimulation of natural killer cells by macrophage-produced interferon, *Nutr. Res.,* 9, 283, 1989.
43. **Brock, J. H. and Mainou-Fowler, T.,** The role of iron and transferrin in lymphocyte transformation, *Immunol. Today,* 4, 347, 1983.
44. **Kemp, J. D., Thorson, J. A., McAlmont, T. H., Horowitz, M., Cowdery, J. S., and Ballas, Z. K.,** Role of transferrin receptor in lymphocyte growth: a rat IgG monoclonal antibody against the murine transferrin receptor produces highly selective inhibition of T and B cell activation protocols, *J. Immunol.,* 138, 2422, 1987.

45. **Brock, J. H., Mainou-Fowler, T., and Webster, L. M.,** Evidence that transferrin may function exclusively as an iron donor in promoting lymphocyte proliferation, *Immunology,* 57, 105, 1986.

46. **Rammensee, H., Lesley, J., Trowbridge, I., and Bevan, M.,** Antibodies against the transferrin receptor block the induction of cytotoxic T lymphocytes. A new method for antigen-specific negative selection *in vitro, Eur. J. Immunol.,* 15, 687, 1985.

47. **Kemp, J. D., Thorson, J. A., Gómez, F., Smith, K. M., Cowdery, J. S., and Ballas, Z. K.,** Inhibition of lymphocyte activation with anti-transferrin receptor Mabs: a comparison of three reagents and further studies of their range of effects and mechanism of action, *Cell. Immunol.,* 122, 218, 1989.

48. **Suciu-Foca, N., Rosochacki, S. J., Cai, J., Reed, E., Rubinstein, P., and King, D. W.,** Immunological and biochemical characterization of an epitope of the transferrin receptor involved in the production of interferon-γ and B-cell growth factor, *Cell. Immunol.,* 110, 265, 1987.

49. **Trowbridge, I. S.,** Potential clinical uses of anti-transferrin receptor monoclonal antibodies, in *Iron in Immunity, Cancer and Inflammation,* de Sousa, M. and Brock, J. H., Eds., Wiley, Chichester, 1989, 341.

50. **Hamilton, T. A.,** Regulation of transferrin receptor expression in concanavalin A stimulated and Gross virus transformed rat lymphoblasts, *J. Cell. Physiol.,* 113, 40, 1982.

51. **Neckers, L. M. and Cossman, J.,** Transferrin receptor induction in mitogen-stimulated human T lymphocytes is required for DNA synthesis and is regulated by interleukin 2, *Proc. Natl. Acad. Sci. U.S.A.,* 89, 3494, 1983.

52. **Kumagai, N., Benedict, S. H., Mills, G. B., and Gelfand, E. W.,** Comparison of phorbol ester/calcium ionophore and phytohemagglutinin-induced signaling in human T lymphocytes. Demonstration of interleukin 2-independent transferrin receptor gene expression, *J. Immunol.,* 140, 37, 1988.

53. **Cano, E., Pizarro, A., Redondo, J. M., Sánchez-Madrid, F., Bernabeu, C., and Fresno, M.,** Induction of T cell activation by monoclonal antibodies specific for the transferrin receptor, *Eur. J. Immunol.,* 20, 765, 1990.

54. **Thorson, J. A., Smith, K. M., Gómez, F., Naumann, P. W., and Kemp, J. D.,** Role of iron in T cell activation: TH1 clones differ from TH2 clones in their sensitivity to inhibition of DNA synthesis caused by IGG Mabs against the transferrin receptor and the iron chelator desferrioxamine, *Cell. Immunol.,* 134, 126, 1991.

55. **Brock, J. H.,** The effect of iron and transferrin on the response of serum-free cultures of mouse lymphocytes to concanavalin A and lipopolysaccharide, *Immunology,* 43, 387, 1981.

56. **Neckers, L. M., Yenokida, G., and James, S. P.,** The role of the transferrin receptor in human B-lymphocyte activation, *J. Immunol.,* 133, 2437, 1984.

57. **Ashman, R. F.,** B lymphocyte activation: the transferrin receptor as a prototype intermediate activation molecule, *J. Lab. Clin. Med.,* 116, 759, 1990.

58. **Futran, J., Kemp, J. D., Field, E. H., Vora, A., and Ashman, R. F.,** Transferrin receptor synthesis is an early event in B cell activation, *J. Immunol.,* 143, 787, 1989.

59. **Weber, R. J. and Finkelman, F. D.,** Increased expression of B lymphocyte receptor for transferrin by *in vivo* crosslinking of cell surface IgD, *Cell. Immunol.,* 104, 400, 1987.

60. **Van der Pouw-Kraan, T., van Kooten, C., van Oers, R., and Aarden, L. A.,** Human transferrin allows efficient IgE production by anti-CD3-stimulated human lymphocytes at low cell densities, *Eur. J. Immunol.,* 21, 385, 1991.

61. **Bhaskaram, P., Sharada, K., Sivakumar, B., Rao, K. V., and Nair, M.,** Effect of iron and vitamin A deficiencies on macrophage function in children, *Nutr. Res.,* 9, 35, 1989.

62. **Kuvibidila, S. R. and Wade, S.,** Macrophage function as studied by the clearance of ^{125}I-labeled polyvinylpyrollidone in iron-deficient and iron replete mice, *J. Nutr.,* 117, 170, 1987.

63. **Helyar, L. and Sherman, A. R.,** Iron deficiency and interleukin 1 production by rat leukocytes, *Am. J. Clin. Nutr.,* 46, 346, 1987.
64. **Kuvibidila, S. R., Baliga, B. S., and Suskind, R. M.,** The effect of iron-deficiency anemia on cytolytic activity of mice spleen and peritoneal cells against allogenic tumor cells, *Am. J. Clin. Nutr.,* 38, 238, 1983.
65. **Thompson, H. L., Stevenson, J., and Brock, J. H.,** The effect of iron and agar on production of hydrogen peroxide by stimulated and activated mouse peritoneal macrophages, *FEBS Lett.,* 200, 283, 1986.
66. **Vanin, A. F., Kubrina, L. N., Kurbanov, I. S., Mordvintsev, P. I., Khrapova, N. V., Galagan, M. E., and Matkhanov, É. I.,** Iron as an inducer of the formation of nitric oxide in animal organisms, *Biochemistry (USSR),* 54, 1609, 1989.
67. **Arbeter, A., Echeverri, L., Franco, D., Munson, D., Vélez, H., and Vitale, J. J.,** Nutrition and infection, *Fed. Proc.,* 30, 1421, 1971.
68. **Chandra, R. K.,** Reduced bactericidal capacity of polymorphs in iron deficiency, *Arch. Dis. Child.,* 48, 864, 1973.
69. **Walter, T., Arredondo, S., Arévalo, M., and Stekel, A.,** Effect of iron therapy on phagocytosis and bactericidal activity in neutrophils of iron deficient infants, *Am. J. Clin. Nutr.,* 44, 877, 1986.
70. **Yetgin, S., Altay, C., Ciliv, G., and Laleli, Y.,** Myeloperoxidase activity and bactericidal function of PMN in iron deficiency, *Acta Haematol.,* 61, 10, 1979.
71. **Van Heerden, C., Oosthuizen, R., Van Wyk, H., Prinsloo, P., and Anderson, R.,** Evaluation of neutrophil and lymphocyte function in subjects with iron deficiency, *South Afri. Med. J.,* 24, 111, 1983.
72. **Hasan, S. M., Aziz, M., Ahmad, P., and Aggarwal, M.,** Phagocyte metabolic functions in iron deficiency anaemia of Indian children, *J. Trop. Pediatr.,* 35, 6, 1989.
73. **Turgeon-O'Brien, H., Amiot, J., Lemieux, L., and Dillon, J.-C.,** Myeloperoxidase activity of polymorphonuclear leukocytes in iron deficiency anemia and the anemia of chronic disorders, *Acta Haematol.,* 74, 151, 1985.
74. **Prasad, J. S.,** Leukocyte function in iron-deficiency anemia, *Am. J. Clin. Nutr.,* 32, 550, 1979.
75. **Mackler, B., Person, R., Ochs, H., and Finch, C. A.,** Iron deficiency in the rat: effects on neutrophil activation and metabolism, *Pediatr. Res.,* 18, 549, 1984.
76. **Celada, A., Herreros, V., Pugin, P., and Rudolf, M.,** Reduced leucocyte alkaline phosphatase activity and decreased NBT reduction test in induced iron deficiency, *Br. J. Haematol.,* 43, 457, 1979.
77. **Moore, L. L. and Humbert, J. R.,** Neutrophil bactericidal dysfunction towards oxidant radical-sensitive microorganisms during experimental iron deficiency, *Pediatr. Res.,* 18, 684, 1984.
78. **Sullivan, J. R., Till, G. O., Ward, P. A., and Newton, R. B.,** Nutritional iron restriction diminishes acute complement-dependent lung injury, *Nutr. Res.,* 9, 625, 1989.
79. **Murakawa, H., Bland, C. E., Willis, W. T., and Dallman, P. R.,** Iron deficiency and neutrophil function: different rates of correction of the depressions in oxidative burst and myeloperoxidase activity after iron treatment, *Blood,* 69, 1464, 1987.
80. **de Sousa, M.,** The immunology of iron overload, in *Iron in Immunity, Cancer and Inflammation,* de Sousa, M. and Brock, J. H., Eds., Wiley, Chichester, 1989, 247.
81. **de Sousa, M.,** Immune cell functions in iron overload, *Clin. Exp. Immunol.,* 75, 1, 1989.
82. **Dwyer, J., Wood, C., McNamara, J., Williams, A., Andiman, W., Rink, L., O'Connor, T., and Pearson, H.,** Abnormalities in the immune system of children with beta-thalassemia major, *Clin. Exp. Immunol.,* 68, 621, 1987.
83. **Munn, C. G., Markenson, A. L., Kapadia, A., and de Sousa, M.,** Impaired T cell mitogen responses in some patients with thalassemia intermedia, *Thymus,* 3, 119, 1981.

84. **Pattanapanyasat, K.,** Expression of cell surface transferrin receptor following *in vitro* stimulation of peripheral blood lymphocytes in patients with β-thalassemia and iron-deficiency anaemia, *Eur. J. Haematol.,* 44, 190, 1990.

85. **Bryan, C. F., Leech, S. H., Ducos, R., Edwards, C. Q., Kushner, J. P., Skolnick, M. H., Bozelka, B., Linn, J. C., and Gaumer, R.,** Thermostable erythrocyte rosette-forming lymphocytes in hereditary hemochromatosis. I. Identification in peripheral blood, *J. Clin. Immunol.,* 4, 134, 1984.

86. **Bryan, C. F., Leech, S. H., Kumar, P., Gaumer, R., Bozelka, B., and Morgan, J.,** The immune system in hereditary hemochromatosis: a quantitative and functional assessment of the cellular arm, *Am. J. Med. Sci.,* 301, 55, 1991.

87. **Good, M. F., Chapman, D. E., Powell, L. W., and Halliday, J. W.,** The effect of experimental iron-overload on splenic T- cell function: analysis using cloning techniques, *Clin. Exp. Immunol.,* 68, 375, 1987.

88. **Guglielmo, P., Cunsolo, F., Lombardo, T., Sortino G., Giustolisi, R., Cacciola, E., and Cacciola, E.,** T-subset abnormalities in thalassemia intermedia: possible evidence for a thymus functional deficiency, *Acta Haematol.,* 72, 361, 1984.

89. **Grady, R. W., Akbar, A., Giardina, P. J., Hilgartner, M. W., and de Sousa, M.,** Disproportionate lymphoid cell subsets in thalassemia major: the relative contributions of transfusion and splenectomy, *Br. J. Haematol.,* 72, 361, 1985.

90. **Pardalos, G., Kannakoudi-Tsaklidis, F., Malaka-Zafirin, M., Tsantali, H., and Papaevangelou, G.,** Iron-related disturbances of cell-mediated immunity in multitransfused children with thalassemia major, *Clin. Exp. Immunol.,* 68, 138, 1987.

91. **Kaplan, J., Sarnaik, S., Gitlin, J., and Lusher, J.,** Diminished helper/suppressor lymphocyte ratios and natural killer activity in recipients of repeated blood transfusions, *Blood,* 64, 308, 1984.

92. **Nualart, P., Estevez, M. E., Ballart, I. J., de Miani, S. A., Peñalver, J., and Sen, L.,** Effect of alpha interferon on the altered T-B-cell immunoregulation in patients with thalassemia major, *Am. J. Hematol.,* 24, 151, 1987.

93. **Djeha, A. and Brock, J. H.,** Uptake and intracellular handling of iron from transferrin and iron chelators by mitogen-stimulated mouse lymphocytes, *Biochim. Biophys. Acta,* in press.

94. **Bryan, C. F., Nishiya, K., Pollack, M. S., Dupont, B., and de Sousa, M.,** Differential inhibition of the MLR by iron: association with HLA phenotype, *Immunogenetics,* 12, 129, 1981.

95. **Taylor, P. G., Soyano, A., Romano, E., and Layrisse, M.,** Physiological and non-physiological forms of iron affect differently proliferation and ferritin synthesis in human mononuclear cells *in vitro, Tohoku J. Exp. Med.,* 153, 285, 1987.

96. **Keown, P. and Descamps-Latscha, B.,** *In vitro* suppression of cell-mediated immunity by ferroproteins and ferric salts, *Cell. Immunol.,* 80, 257, 1983.

97. **Nishiya, K., de Sousa, M., Tsoi, E., Bognacki, J., and de Harven, E.,** Regulation of expression of a human lymphoid cell surface marker by iron, *Cell. Immunol.,* 53, 71, 1980.

98. **Soyano, A., Fernández, E., and Romano, E.,** Suppressive effects of iron on *in vitro* lymphocyte function: formation of iron polymers as a possible explanation, *Int. Arch. Allergy Appl. Immunol.,* 76, 376, 1985.

99. **de Sousa, M. and Nishiya, K.,** Inhibition of E-rosette formation by two iron salts, *Cell. Immunol.,* 38, 203, 1978.

100. **Carvalho, G. S. and de Sousa, M.,** Iron exerts a specific inhibitory effect on CD2 expression of human PBL, *Immunol. Lett.,* 19, 163, 1988.

101. **Good, M. F., Powell, L. W., and Halliday, J. W.,** The effect of non-transferrin-bound iron on murine T lymphocyte subsets: analysis by clonal techniques, *Clin. Exp. Immunol.,* 70, 164, 1987.

102. **Good, M. F., Chapman, D. E., Powell, L. W., and Halliday, J. W.**, The effect of iron (Fe^{3+}) on the cloning efficiency of human memory T4$^+$ lymphocytes, *Clin. Exp. Immunol.*, 66, 340, 1986.

103. **Djeha, A. and Brock, J. H.**, Effect of transferrin, lactoferrin and chelated iron on human T-lymphocytes, *Br. J. Haematol.*, in press.

104. **Cragg, S. J., Hoy, T. G., and Jacobs, A.**, The expression of cell surface ferritin by peripheral blood lymphocytes and monocytes, *Br. J. Haematol.*, 57, 679, 1984.

105. **Pattanapanyasat, K., Hoy, T. G., and Jacobs, A.**, The response of intracellular and surface ferritin after T-cell stimulation *in vitro*, *Clin. Sci.*, 73, 605, 1987.

106. **Anderson, G. J., Faulk, W. P., Arosio, P., Moss, D., Powell, L. W., and Halliday, J. W.**, Identification of H- and L-ferritin subunit binding sites in human T and B lymphoid cells, *Br. J. Haematol.*, 73, 260, 1989.

107. **Konijn, A. M., Meyron-Holtz, E. G., Levy, R., Ben-Bassat, H., and Matzner, Y.**, Specific binding of placental acidic isoferritin to cells of the T-cell line HD-MDR, *FEBS Lett.*, 263, 229, 1990.

108. **Matzner, Y., Hershko, C., Polliack, A., Konijn, A., and Izak, G.**, Suppressive effect of ferritin on *in vitro* lymphocyte function, *Br. J. Haematol.*, 42, 345, 1979.

109. **Matzner, Y., Konijn, A. M., Shlomai, Z., and Ben-Bassat, H.**, Differential effect of isolated placental isoferritins on *in vitro* T-lymphocyte function, *Br. J. Haematol.*, 59, 443, 1985.

110. **Harada, T., Baba, M., Torii, I., and Morikawa, S.**, Ferritin selectively suppresses delayed-type hypersensitivity responses at induction or effector phase, *Cell. Immunol.*, 109, 75, 1987.

111. **Moroz, C., Giler, S. H., Kupfer, B., and Urca, C.**, Lymphocytes bearing surface ferritin in patients with Hodgkin's disease and breast cancer, *N. Engl. J. Med.*, 296, 1173, 1977.

112. **Gascon, P., Zoumbos, N. C., and Young, N. S.**, Immunological abnormalities in patients receiving multiple blood transfusions, *Ann. Intern. Med.*, 100, 173, 1984.

113. **Akbar, A. N., Fitzgerald-Bocarsly, P. A., de Sousa, M., Giardina, P. J., Hilgartner, M. W., and Grady, R. W.**, Decreased natural killer activity in thalassemia major: a possible consequence of iron overload, *J. Immunol.*, 136, 1635, 1986.

114. **Akbar, A. N., Fitzgerald-Bocarsly, P. A., Giardina, P. J., Hilgartner, M. W., and Grady, R. W.**, Modulation of the defective natural killer activity seen in thalassaemia major with desferrioxamine and α-interferon, *Clin. Exp. Immunol.*, 70, 345, 1987.

115. **Chapman, D. E., Good, M. F., Powell, L. W., and Halliday, J. W.**, The effect of iron, iron-binding proteins and iron-overload on human natural killer cell activity, *J. Gastroenterol. Hepatol.*, 3, 9, 1988.

116. **Van Asbeck, B. S., Verbrugh, H. A., van Oost, B. A., Marx, J. J. M., Imhof, H., and Verhoef, J.**, *Listeria monocytogenes* meningitis and decreased phagocytosis associated with iron overload, *Br. Med. J.*, 284, 542, 1982.

117. **Van Asbeck, B. S., Marx, J. J. M., Struyvenberg, J., and Verhoef, J.**, Functional defects in phagocytic cells from patients with iron overload, *J. Infect.*, 8, 232, 1984.

118. **Ballart, I. J., Estevez, M. E., Sen, L., Diez, R. A., Giuntoli, R. A., de Miani, S. A., and Peñalver, J.**, Progessive dysfunction of monocytes associated with iron overload and age in patients with thalassemia major, *Blood*, 67, 105, 1986.

119. **Lima, M. F. and Kierszenbaum, F.**, Lactoferrin effects on phagocytic cell function. II. The presence of iron is required for the lactoferrin molecule to stimulate intracellular killing by macrophages but not to enhance the uptake of particles and microorganisms, *J. Immunol.*, 139, 1647, 1987.

120. **Hoepelman, I. M., Bezemer, W. A., Vandenbroucke-Grauls, C. M. J. E., Marx, J. J. M., and Verhoef, J.**, Bacterial iron enhances oxygen radical-mediated killing of *Staphylococcus aureus* by phagocytes, *Infect. Immun.*, 58, 26, 1990.

121. **Sambri, V., Cevenini, R., and la Paca, M.**, Susceptibility of iron-loaded *Borrelia burgdorferi* to killing by hydrogen peroxide and human polymorphonuclear leucocytes, *FEMS Microbiol. Lett.*, 81, 67, 1991.

122. **Lane, T. E., Wu-Hsieh, B. A., and Howard, D. H.,** Iron limitation and the gamma interferon-mediated antihistoplasma state of murine macrophages, *Infect. Immun.*, 59, 2274, 1991.

123. **Byrd, T. F. and Horwitz, M. A.,** Interferon gamma-activated human monocytes down-regulate transferrin receptors and inhibit the intracellular multiplication of *Legionella pneomophila* by limiting the availability of iron, *J. Clin. Invest.*, 83, 1457, 1989.

124. **Alford, C. E., King, T. E., and Campbell, P. A.,** Role of transferrin, transferrin receptors, and iron in macrophage listericidal activity, *J. Exp. Med.*, 174, 459, 1991.

125. **Waterlot, Y., Cantinieaux, B., Hariga-Muller, H., de Maertelaere-Laurent, E., Vanherweghem, J. L., and Fondu, P.,** Impaired phagocytic activity of neutrophils in patients receiving haemodialysis: the critical role of iron overload, *Br. Med. J.*, 291, 501, 1985.

126. **Flament, J., Goldman, M., Waterlot, Y., Dupont, E., Wybran, J., and Vanherweghem, J.-L.,** Impairment of phagocytic oxidative metabolism in hemodialyzed patients with iron overload, *Clin. Nephrol.*, 25, 227, 1986.

127. **Cantinieaux, B., Hariga, C., Ferster, A., de Maertelaere, E., Toppet, M., and Fondu, P.,** Neutrophil dysfunctions in thalassemia major: the role of cell iron overload, *Eur. J. Haematol.*, 39, 28, 1987.

128. **Cantinieaux, B., Hariga, C., Ferster, A., Toppet, M., and Fondu, P.,** Desferrioxamine improves neutrophil phagocytosis in thalassemia major, *Am. J. Haematol.*, 35, 13, 1990.

129. **Martino, M., Rossi, M. E., Resti, M., Vullo, C., and Vierucci, A.,** Changes in superoxide anion production in neutrophils from multitransfused β-thalassemia patients: correlation with ferritin levels and liver damage, *Acta Haematol.*, 71, 289, 1984.

130. **Hoepelman, I. M., Jaarsma, E. Y., Verhoef, J., and Marx, J. J. M.,** Polynuclear iron complexes impair the function of polymorphonuclear granulocytes, *Br. J. Haematol.*, 68, 385, 1988.

131. **Hoepelman, I. M., Jaarsma, E. Y., Verhoef, J., and Marx, J. J. M.,** Effect of iron on polymorphonuclear granulocyte phagocytic capacity: role of oxidation state and effect of ascorbic acid, *Br. J. Haematol.*, 70, 495, 1988.

132. **Hoepelman, I. M., Bezmer, W. A., van Doornmalen, E., Verhoef, J., and Marx, J. J. M.,** Lipid peroxidation of human granulocytes (PMN) and monocytes by iron complexes, *Br. J. Haematol.*, 72, 584, 1989.

133. **Schnaper, H. W.,** Divalent metal requirement for soluble immune response suppressor (SIRS) activity, *Cell. Immunol.*, 118, 157, 1989.

134. **Pierpaoli, W., Dall'ara, A., Yi, C., Neri, P., Santucci, A., and Choay, J.,** Iron carrier proteins facilitate engraftment of allogeneic bone marrow and enduring hemopoeitic chimerism in the lethally irradiated host, *Cell. Immunol.*, 134, 225, 1991.

6. Cellular Acquisition of Iron and the Iron-Withholding Defense Against Microbial and Neoplastic Invasion*

EUGENE D. WEINBERG

Department of Biology and Program in Medical Sciences, Indiana University, Bloomington, Indiana

* Dedicated to Professor J. B. (Joe) Neilands in honor of his distinguished career as architect, developer, and dean of the science of microbial cell acquisition of iron.

I. INTRODUCTION

The scientific study of the components of immune defense against infection and neoplasia began near the close of the 19th century. At that time, it also was recognized that, in addition to the immune defense system, potential hosts must possess natural (i.e., nonspecific) resistance against threatening invaders. Were natural resistance not to exist, nonimmune individuals would fail to survive initial exposure to microbial pathogens or to cancer cells.

Early in the 20th century, various natural physical and a few chemical barriers were identified in specific tissues. Examples include the flushing action of tears and urine, the ciliary sweeping of the bronchii, the gastric acidity, and the presence of lysozyme in various body fluids and in leukocytic defense cells. In the 1960s, a natural defense component with broad spectrum activity, the alternative pathway for activation of complement, was discovered.

The elements of still another natural defense system that functions in nearly all host tissues and fluids and that has very broad spectrum activity began to be identified 60 years ago. In 1931, a clinical pathologist in Chicago asked a straightforward question: do ill persons alter their concentration of plasma iron? He found, indeed, that patients who have infection, neoplasia, or other causes of inflammatory stress have a profound depression of plasma iron.[1] Numerous subsequent studies have shown that the depression begins quite early in the incubation stage of the disease, that the reduction can be as great as 70%, and that normal levels of plasma iron rapidly reappear as the patients recover.[2] Additional features of the iron-withholding defense system have been discovered and will be described in Section III.

Notwithstanding the remarkable efficacy of our iron-witholding defense system, hosts do at times develop fungal, bacterial, or protozoan infections or malignant neoplasms. Two principal reasons account for such development. First, highly virulent microbial or neoplastic cell strains have evolved strategies to obtain growth-essential iron from normal tissues, despite vigorous attempts by the host to maintain inaccessibility of the metal. Second, numerous cultural practices of humans tend to elevate levels of iron in various tissues which results in neutralization of the iron-withholding defense system.

The strategies of iron acquisition practiced by virulent invaders will be described in Section II, and the conditions that compromise iron withholding will be reviewed in Section IV. Methods for strengthening iron withholding will be discussed in Section V.

II. MICROBIAL AND NEOPLASTIC CELL ACQUISITION OF IRON

A. FUNGI, BACTERIA, PROTOZOA

In 1911, a British veterinary microbiologist, F. W. Twort, observed that a mycobacterial species that causes severe enteritis in calves would grow in pure culture only if provided with a chemical synthesized by other myco-bacteria.[3] This compound, the very first bacterial growth factor to be dis-covered, was shown 30 years later to be mycobactin, an hydroxamate sid-erophore.[4] During the past four decades, many additional microbial (and some higher plant) siderophores have been discovered. Chemical species of micro-bial siderophores include at least 21 kinds of fungal and 11 kinds of bacterial hydroxamates as well as about 11 types of bacterial catechols.[5] Hydroxamates contain oxidized peptide moieties; catechols possess units of 2,3-dihydroxy-benzoic acid. Other classes of microbial molecules with siderophoric activity also have been described.[6]

To contain the six strong binding sites for the ferric iron, the size of siderophoric molecules ranges between 500 and 1000 Da.[7] Thus, the ferrated molecules cannot simply diffuse into cells but must be bound to specific-receptor proteins and then actively transported into and/or through the cell membrane. Intracellular release of the iron atom occurs by reduction to the ferrous state or by modification of the ligand.[8] The deferrated siderophore then may either be stored, degraded, or excreted. Formation of the sidero-phores, their precursors, and their receptor-binding proteins is coordinately inhibited by the concentration of 10 to 60 μM iron commonly present as a contaminant in the various kinds of complex media employed by microbiol-ogists. Derepression of synthesis of the iron acquisition systems occurs in low iron culture media (0.1 to 1.0 μM iron) as well as in host tissue envi-ronments.

As may be noted in Table 1, microbial cells can acquire iron by a variety of mechanisms in addition to use of siderophores. Some strains, in fact, can engage in alternative strategies depending on the particular environmental niche. An important potential source of iron for many bacterial, protozoan, and neoplastic cells is heme. The ability of invading pathogens to lyse eryth-rocytes and digest hemoglobin to release the iron-containing porphyrin has long been known to be an important feature of virulence. Not surprisingly, the synthesis of erythrocyte lysins (hemolysins) generally is derepressed in low iron media and in host tissue environments.[6]

A variety of bacterial pathogens obtain iron directly from transferrin. Often, the ferrated protein can bind to specific protein receptors on the cell surface, and the metal can be removed in the presence of a reducing agent such as L-cysteine.[9] Alternatively, as catabolic acids from defense cells and pathogens accumulate in the infected site, the decline in pH value causes transferrin to release its atoms of iron.

A recent survey of 48 published reports on 27 strains of bacterial species noted a mean of five iron-repressed outer membrane or outer envelope proteins per strain (Table 2). Some of these proteins bind either ferrated siderophores, heme, ferrated transferrins, or ferrated lactoferrins. Not all of the iron-re-pressed proteins are involved in iron acquisition. The functions of many

TABLE 1
Strategies for Microbial Cell Acquisition of Iron

Strategy	Selected examples		
	Fungi	Bacteria	Protozoa
Acquire ferric ions by use of siderophores	Many groups	Many groups	—
Acquire iron by assimilation of heme	—	Many groups	Entamoeba, Naegleria
Acquire ferric ions directly from transferrin	—	Aeromonas, Bacteroides,[9] Bordetella,[10] Hemophilus, Neisseria, Pasteurella, Treponema[11]	Plasmodium
Acquire ferric ions directly from lactoferrin	—	Aeromonas, Hemophilus, Mycoplasma,[12] Neisseria, Treponema[11]	Trichomonas
Reduce ferric ions at cell membrane and assimilate ferrous ions	Saccharomyces	Bifidobacterium, Listeria, Streptococcus	—
Occupy host intracellular niche (oxidation state of iron unknown)	Histoplasma	Legionella, Listeria, Salmonella, Yersinia	Trypanasoma
Occupy acidic, anaerobic niches that favor ferrous ions	—	Clostridium	Naegleria
Abstain from use of iron	—	Lactobacillus	—

Note: Unless otherwise designated, references are contained in Reference 6.

TABLE 2
Examples of Iron-Regulated Synthesis of Outer Membrane Proteins

Bacterial species	Proteins produced in	
	Low-iron medium	High-iron medium
Azotobacter vinelandii	77[a],81,85,93	NR[b]
Bacteroides fragilis[9]	44 (Haem),23,49,89	NR
Campylobacter jejuni	74,76,82	NR
Erwinia chrysanthemi	78,82,88	NR
Escherichia coli	25,74 (Aerobactin); 78 (ferrichrome); 90 (inner membrane); 81 (enterobactin), 83	90 (inner membrane)
E. coli-Shigella flexneri	76 (aerobactin)	NR
Hemophilus influenzae[13]	43,58 (hTf),92,94,98 (hTf),105-106 (hLf)	24,65
Hem. parainfluenzae[14]	80-82 (enterobactin)	NR
Klebsiella aerogenes	69,70,73,75,78	18.5
K. pneumoniae	69,70,73,75,78,83	22,48
Mycobacterium smegmatis (outer envelope)	25,29 (exochelin),84,180	NR
Neisseria gonorrhoeae[15]	19,37 (Fe),70,76,84,86,97,100 (hTf),105 (hLf)	33
N. meningitidis	31,37 (Fe),69,70,71 (hTf),84,94,95-100 (hTf),105 (hLf)	43
Paracoccus denitrificans	76-84 (Four proteins)	23
Pasteurella haemolytica[16]	71,77,100 (bTf)	NR
Pseudomonas aeruginosa	14 (Pyochelin),66,75,80,86	17,22
P. chloraphis	82	22,32,75
P. sp. B10	85 (Pseudobactin)	NR
P. species	76,88,89,92	45,46,93
P. syringae	47,74-80 (Eight proteins)	NR
Salmonella typhi	78,81	NR

TABLE 2 (continued)
Examples of Iron-Regulated Synthesis of Outer Membrane Proteins

Bacterial species	Proteins produced in	
	Low-iron medium	High-iron medium
S. typhimurium	77,79,82	NR
Shigella flexneri	74 (aerobactin),81,83 (enterobactin)	High 80s (two)
Vibrio anguillarum	79,86	45,68
V. cholerae	62,73,75,76,77,220	NR
V. vulnificus	74,81,85	NR
Yersinia enterocolitica	79,81	NR

Note: hTf = human transferrin, bTf = bovine transferrin, hLf = human lactoferrin. Unless otherwise designated, references are contained in Reference 6.

a   kDa.
b   None recognized.

remain unknown. Nearly half of the strains studied synthesized other outer membrane proteins in high iron media. These iron-derepressed proteins might either function in low affinity iron uptake systems, be related to bacterioferritins, or be involved in prevention of excessive intake of the metal.

Within each microbial group, the level of virulence generally is strongly correlated with ability to acquire iron in the particular host. For example, Gram-negative bacterial strains have been divided into four classes on the basis of the strains' observed virulence when iron availability is varied.[17] Strains of class I, usually capable of causing disseminated septicemias, can extract the metal from host defense proteins of normal or even of lowered iron saturation. Virulence of class II, in contrast, is related to the amount of iron saturation of transferrin. Pathogenicity of this class is lowered by the defenses of iron withholding and elevated by iron excess. Class III strains normally are nonvirulent but can cause lesions in hosts stressed with excess iron. Strains of class IV remain nonvirulent even with added iron. They apparently lack other attributes required for survival and growth in host tissues.

Often an initial distinction between the ability or lack of ability to overcome defenses of iron withholding can be made on well-established taxonomic bases. For instance, in a study of strains of *Hemophilus influenzae* type *b*, *H. parainfluenzae*, and *H. paraphropilus*, each could acquire iron from free hemoglobin but only the major pathogen (*H. influenzae* type *b*) was capable of utilizing iron from hemoglobin bound to haptoglobin.[14] In the genus *Neisseria*, strains of the pathogen *N. meningitidis* obtained iron from transferrin; strains of the commensals, *N. flava* and *N. sicca*, could not.[18] In a different study of 29 strains of *N. gonorrhoeae*, 21 strains of *N. meningitidis*, and 45 strains of commensal *Neisseria* — 100% of the two pathogenic species but only 22% of the nonpathogens could obtain iron from transferrin saturated 25% with the metal.[19] In the genus *Staphylococcus*, 16 strains of the major pathogen, *S. aureus*, could grow in the presence of transferrin whereas 19 strains of the commensal, *S. epidermidis*, could not.[20]

Legionella pneumophila requires an iron reductase to obtain iron.[21] Virulent strains show maximum activity of the reductase with NADH which remains constant in the intracellular macrophage environment in which the bacteria reside. In contrast, avirulent strains require NADPH which decreases markedly during phagocytosis.

Plasmodium vivax, a protozoan agent of human malaria, grows well in reticulocytes but not in mature human erythrocytes. Unlike erythrocytes, the reticulocytes have transferrin receptors to acquire iron. In contrast, *P. falciparum* survives and reproduces quite well in mature erythrocytes. Consequently, it produces a much greater parasitemia and dangerous illness. *Plasmodium falciparum* apparently stimulates its host erythrocytes to acquire transferrin iron. Possibly the pathogen synthesizes transferrin receptors and inserts them into the host cell surface membranes.[6]

As is true for *Plasmodium,* pathogenic bacteria that produce transferrin-binding proteins and thus obtain iron directly from transferrin (e.g., *Bordetella, Hemophilus, Neisseria, Pasteurella*) generally are restricted to particular host species. For instance, *Neisseria menigitidis,* a pathogen in humans but not in cattle, can secure iron by binding human transferrin or human lactoferrin but cannot bind bovine transferrin or bovine lactoferrin.[22] Thus, the growth-essential metal is much more readily withheld from the pathogen by cattle than by humans. *Hemophilus somnus,* an important pathogen of cattle but not of humans, can obtain iron from bovine but not from human, porcine, or avian transferrin.[23] Strains of *Pasteurella hemolytica* type 1 (pathogenic for cattle) are capable of using bovine but not human, porcine, equine, or avian transferrin.[16] In contrast, pathogenic bacteria that acquire iron via siderophores generally can cause disease in multiple host species.

Components of systems designed to exclude excess iron from microbial cells are beginning to be identified. The term siderophrax (Greek for [Gr.]: iron excluder) has been designated for molecules that protect cells from iron toxicity.[6] Possible examples include some of the iron derepressed outer membrane proteins (Table 2) and, in *Azotobacter,* a catechol melanin.[24] Moreover, in coliform bacteria, an excess of ferrous ions combines with a histidine-rich, 17-kDa protein termed Fur to suppress transcription of genes that code for constituents of iron acquisition systems.[25]

B. NEOPLASTIC AND TRANSFORMED CELLS

In 1972, Holley proposed that "the crucial change in a malignant cell is an alteration in the cell surface membrane that results in increased internal concentrations of nutrients that regulate cell growth".[26] Numerous studies in the subsequent 20 years have found that one of the nutrients relevant to the Holley hypothesis is iron.[27] Although normal and neoplastic cells have a similar qualitative need for the metal, the continuous proliferation of the tumor cells would be expected to necessitate their requirement for an enhanced and perhaps diversified supply of iron. For example, leukemic cell lines have been described in which, unlike normal cells, DNA synthesis can be catalyzed by iron acquired from ferric citrate in the absence of transferrin.[28] Small-cell lung cancer cells can synthesize their own transferrin, a finding that may explain why this neoplasm, despite little vascularization, has an extremely short doubling time.[29] Human melanoma cells produce an iron-binding 97-kDa glycoprotein that is associated with the cell membrane and is structurally and functionally related to transferrin.[30] Only trace amounts of the protein are found in normal tissues.

In normal nonmultiplying B lymphocytes, expression of transferrin receptors (TfRs) is a multistep, tightly regulated process that requires antigen or mitogen stimulation, interleukin growth factors, and acquisition of interleukin receptors. In contrast, proliferating malignant B lymphocytes express

TfRs constitutively.[31] Most clonogenic leukemia cells express TfRs whereas most pluripotent hematopoietic progenitor cells do not.[32] Cultured virus-transformed myogenic cells expressed more than twice as many TfRs as did normal cells that were multiplying at the same rate.[33]

In a study of expressed TfRs in human surgical specimens, the distribution in normal tissues was observed in a limited number of sites.[34] In contrast, of 87 malignant samples, TfRs were found in 70. The positive specimens included the majority of carcinomas, all of the sarcomas and Hodgkin's lymphomas, and two thirds of other lymphomas. Some of the 17 negative specimens had high mitotic rates and presumably were acquiring iron via nontransferrin carriers. Similarly, in two series of breast carcinomas,[35,36] greater amounts of TfRs were detected in malignant samples than in the corresponding normal tissues. Aggressive lymphomas have been found to display an epitope of TfR that is not seen in indolent lymphomas or in normal cells.[37]

In summary of this section, pathogenic fungi, bacteria, and protozoa as well as neoplastic cells can acquire iron from their hosts via a diversity of strategies. The virulence of specific strains, and their host and tissue ranges, often are determined by the efficiency of the available strategies.

III. HOSTS ATTEMPT TO WITHHOLD AND WITHDRAW IRON FROM INVADERS

A. CONSTITUTIVE DEFENSES IN PLACE PRIOR TO INVASION

The various features of the iron-withinholding/withdrawal defense system in vertebrate hosts are summarized in Table 3. The constitutive components, transferrin (Tf) and lactoferrin (Lf), constantly are present in every body fluid except urine. Presumably the kidney has not been able to evolve a mechanism for selective excretion of Tf or Lf. Thus, it is not surprising that urinary tract infections predominate in the array of infectious disease episodes that require clinical assistance.

Note that nearly all of the body fluids that contain Lf are contaminated with normal flora. Were Lf not to be present, qualitative and quantitative changes in these flora, with consequent development of infectious processes, would be expected. For instance, Lf in saliva apparently prevents excessive replication of *Actinobacillus actinomycetemcomitans,* a potential periodontopathogen.[39] In human colostrum and milk, the quantity of 200 μM Lf favors the establishment of nonpathogenic flora in the nursling intestine.[40] In contrast, the low concentration of 2 μM Lf in bovine milk permits a useful flora to develop in the digestive tract of calves. Unfortunately, in human infants fed bovine rather than human milk, the lack of adequate Lf permits establishment of bacterial flora that predispose to enteritis.

TABLE 3
Features of the Iron-Witholding Defense System

Constitutive components
    Transferrin in plasma and perspiration
    Lactoferrin in tears, nasal exudate, saliva, bronchial mucus, gastrointestinal fluid, hepatic
      bile, cervical mucus, seminal fluid, milk, and secondary granules of neutrophils
    Ovotransferrin in egg white

Processes induced at time of microbial or neoplastic cell invasion

[a] Suppression of assimilation of ≤80% of dietary iron

[a] Suppression of iron efflux from macrophages that have digested effete erythrocytes to result
      in ≤70% reduction in plasma iron

[a] Release of neutrophils from bone marrow into peripheral circulation and then into site of
      invasion of extracellular bacteria followed by discharge of secondary granules
    Release of apolactoferrin from secondary granules followed by binding of iron in septic sites
      even if pH is as low as 4
    Macrophage scavenging of lactoferrin-iron in septic areas and in sites surrounding clusters
      of tumor cells

[a] Increased synthesis of ferritin by macrophages to accommodate iron from phagocytosed
      lactoferrin iron. Increased conversion of iron-rich ferritin to hemosiderin within macro-
      phages
    Synthesis of nitric oxide (from L-arginine) by macrophages activated by interferon-γ to effect
      efflux of nonheme iron from neoplastic and microbial cells and from macrophages them-
      selves
    Suppression of growth of bacteria in phagosomes of macrophages by interferon-γ activation
      that results in downshift of expression of transferrin receptors
    Induction in B lymphocytes of synthesis of immunoglobulins to iron-repressed outer mem-
      brane proteins of Gram-negative bacterial pathogens

[a]   Activated by interleukin-1 or tumor necrosis factor-α.

From Weinberg, E. D., *Drug Metab. Rev.*, 22, 531, 1990. With permission.

Lactoferrin is present in a highly unsaturated form to permit maximum iron-scavenging activity. Transferrin, however, has a dual function. It must not only withold iron from pathogenic microorganisms but also transport the metal to host cells. Fortunately in humans, the normal level of transferrin iron saturation of 20 to 30% permits the protein to be microbiostatic toward many potential invaders. The level of iron saturation has prognostic value. For example, in a series of 33 patients with pneumococcal pneumonia, 10 had abnormally high saturation.[41] Of these, six died and three had complications. Of the 23 persons with normal transferrin iron saturation, only three died and the remaining 20 patients recovered with no complications.

B. INDUCED DEFENSES MOUNTED AT TIMES OF INVASION

A very early response to microbial or neoplastic cell invasion is a lowering of the transferrin-bound plasma iron value often by as much as 70%.[2] This consistent physiological response to insult occurs also in inflammatory conditions caused by collagen diseases, cardiovascular accidents, surgery, obstetric complications, or other traumatic injuries. In patients stressed concurrently by two kinds of insult, e.g., surgery plus infection, reductions in plasma iron as great as 90 to 93% have been recorded.[42] Even in 1-year-old children inoculated with live measles virus vaccine (surely, a "benign" insult), plasma iron was lowered from a normal mean value of 10 μM down to 5.5 μM.[43] Transferrin iron saturation was lowered from a mean value of 17.2% down to 8.0%. Although the reduction in iron values cannot prevent replication of viruses, the hypoferremic response of the children would protect them from secondary streptococcal infection, a common and dangerous sequel of clinical measles. Ironically, had the iron values of the children been monitored during the hypoferremic episode by uninformed persons, the children would have been mislabeled "iron deficient". Thus, they might then have been fed or injected with excessive, detrimental amounts of iron.

A recent review of 29 patients "diagnosed" as having iron deficiency anemia by practitioners in a teaching hospital revealed that only 11 were correctly identified.[44] Most of the 18 misdiagnosed patients had the hypoferremic response to inflammatory stress. The hematologists who conducted the review believe that this problem of misdiagnosis is not unique to hospital-based specialists but also applies more widely.

The importance of the hypoferremic response to insult has been emphasized by the observation that, unlike the febrile defense response, it can be mobilized at birth. When endotoxin was injected into neonatal guinea pigs at the time of birth, plasma iron was lowered by 40% during the first day of life and by 50% during the second day.[45] In contrast, fever could not be evoked by i.p. injection of endotoxin until the animals had achieved an age of 8 d.

In a study of airborne legionellosis in adult guinea pigs, the development of the hypoferremic response was observed to occur very early in the infection.[46] Within 24 h of exposure to the inoculum, the animals had achieved a reduction in plasma iron of 33% and, by 48 h, of 87%. Temperature, on the other hand, was not elevated until the second day, and migration of leukocytes into the affected alveoli did not occur until the fourth day.

During each of the first 4 d after exposure of humans to the bacterial agent of tularemia, their mean plasma iron level decreased, respectively, by 20, 30, 50, and 55%.[47] In contrast, the febrile defense response was absent on the first two days. It developed partially on the third day and fully on the fourth day.

Plasma iron turns over about ten times daily, and hypoferremia quickly can be achieved by suppression of the release of the metal from splenic and hepatic macrophages that have processed decaying erythrocytes. In healthy persons, the quantity of plasma iron is only 0.3% of the amount of storage iron. Accordingly, withholding of $\leq 70\%$ of the plasma iron by macrophages during the inflammatory response should present no logistical problem. Of course, synthesis of additional ferritin as well as hemosiderin is required. The amino acids most likely are derived from catabolized muscle protein.

When human monocytes differentiate into macrophages, their intracellular ferritin increases from 10 ng/10^6 cells to approximately 1000 ng/10^6 cells.[48] In mature macrophages of noninflammed hosts, the ratio of hemosiderin iron to ferritin is 0:03:1 whereas in similar cells exposed to inflammatory agents, the ratio was observed to increase to 0.28:1.[49]

The majority of studies on stress hypoferremia have been performed with endothermic vertebrates. However, the defense is practiced also by ectotherms. For example, lizards inoculated with *Aeromonas hydrophila*[50] and rainbow trout injected i.p. with endotoxin[51] lowered their concentrations of plasma iron. In the latter study, the transferrin iron saturation value was lowered from 20 to 38% down to 8 to 18% within 24 h of injection of endotoxin.

The normal recycling of iron from macrophages can be blocked by a considerable variety of inducers of inflammation; e.g., microbial and neoplastic cell invaders, endotoxin, thioglycollate, or turpentine.[52,53] The inducers stimulate mononuclear leukocytes to form a 15 to 17-kDa peptide hormone, originally called leukocyte endogenous mediator (LEM) and, more recently, interleukin-1 (IL-1). This cytokine is formed by induced alveolar, peritoneal, and Kupffer macrophages; by peripheral blood monocytes; and by macrophage-derived cell culture lines. Following induction, several hours are required to obtain synthesis and secretion of mature IL-1.[54] Additional hours are needed for cytokine function. In an early study, partially purified rabbit LEM injected i.p. in rats caused a 67% reduction in plasma iron within 8 h and provided protection against a lethal dose of *Salmonella typhimurium*.[55] In a recent report, human recombinant IL-1 injected i.m. in rats caused an 87% reduction in plasma iron within 6 h.[56]

Iron has been found to potentiate the biological effects of radiation.[57] Accordingly, inducers of iron withholding such as IL-1 could be predicted to have radioprotective activity. Evidence for such activity has been described.[58]

In addition to stimulating apoferritin synthesis in macrophages, IL-1 performs more than 60 other activities that involve at least 21 types of target cells.[59] Among these manifold functions are several that assist further in the iron-withholding defense. IL-1 stimulates the release of mature neutrophils from the bone marrow as well as their mobilization to and activation at the site of invasion. Activation involves degranulation in which secondary specific granules of the neutrophils release apolactoferrin (Lf). Unlike Tf, Lf can bind iron at pH values as low as 4. When the molecules of apo-Lf have scavenged sufficient iron to become about 40% saturated, they are assimilated by macrophages that have been attracted to the site of invasion.

Interleukin-1 shares many of its multiple systemic activities with tumor necrosis factor-α (TNF). Like IL-1, TNF also is produced by monocytes and can mediate a wide range of immunologic and metabolic activities.[60] Another cytokine whose functions overlap those of IL-1 and TNF is IL-6. Like IL-1 and TNF, IL-6 has good hypoferremic activity.[61]

Activated macrophages participate in iron scavenging not only in infected areas but also in site threatened by tumor cell invasion. A variety of solid tumors have been observed to be surrounded by macrophages that contain large amounts of iron and ferritin.[27] Examples include sarcomas, lymphomas, and neuroblastomas.

In addition to their important defense roles as retainers and scavengers of iron, macrophages — when activated by interferon-γ (IFN-γ) and provided with L-arginine — can induce a withdrawal of nonheme iron from fungal, bacterial, protozoan, and neoplastic cells. The targeted cells in some cases remain viable but are unable to synthesize DNA or maintain oxidative metabolism. The iron withdrawal factors formed by activated macrophages consist of unstable products of L-arginine catabolism termed reactive nitrogen intermediates (RNI) and exemplified by nitric oxide, nitrite, and nitrate. Authentic nitric oxide possesses iron withdrawal activity.[62] The RNI are derived from the guanido atom(s) of L-arginine when about 30% of the amino acid is converted to L-citrulline. In contrast, mammalian nonactivated macrophages catabolize L-arginine entirely to L-ornithine and urea.

Murine lung vascular endothelial cells also can produce RNI when activated by IFN-γ or TNF-α provided that L-arginine is available as the substrate. Nitric oxide produced by these cells has been shown to lyse reticulum cell sarcoma cells.[63] Even tumor cells themselves can be induced to lose nonheme iron when activated by IFN-γ and provided with L-arginine for conversion to nitric oxide.[64]

Still another method of iron deprivation of invaders involves limiting the uptake of the metal into macrophages that are harboring intracellular pathogens. Human blood monocytes fail to support the intracellular growth of *Legionella pneumophila* when in contact with 15 μM deferoxamine or when activated by IFN-γ.[65] Monocytes exposed to the cytokine showed a 73% reduction in expressed TfRs as compared with infected cells in the absence of IFN-γ. Similarly, mouse peritoneal macrophages, activated by IFN-γ, failed to support growth of *Histoplasma capsulatum*.[66] For this activity of the cytokine, L-arginine is not required.

As mentioned in Section II, many pathogenic microorganisms and neoplastic cells can utilize heme as an alternative source of iron. Hosts attempt to render heme unavailable, at least to bacteria, by complexing it with haptoglobin, hemopexin, or albumen. Some strains of coliform bacteria are unable to use heme that is complexed to haptoglobin.[67] However, some strains of streptococci,[68] staphylococci,[68] *Vibrio*,[69] and *Aeromonas*[70] can acquire iron from the complex. Strains of *Hemophilus*[71] but not *Neisseria*[72] could obtain iron from heme bound to hemopexin or albumen.

Yet another method of iron deprivation practiced by vertebrate hosts is the development of antibodies to the protein components of iron acquisition systems of extracellular bacterial pathogens. Examples in humans have been reported in patients recovering from meningococcal meningitis[73] and Gram-negative bacterial urinary tract infections,[74] as well as in advanced cystic fibrosis patients who have lung infections caused by *Pseudomonas aeruginosa*.[75] Accordingly, it is easily to predict that vaccine efficacy would be much improved by using antigens from bacteria that had been grown in low iron medium, and such a prediction has been confirmed.[76]

To summarize this section, hosts attempt to withhold and to withdraw iron from microbial and neoplastic cells in a variety of ways. Powerful iron-binding proteins are stationed in all body fluids except urine. Early in an invasion, cytokines such as interleukin-1 and tumor necrosis factor-α stimulate ferrtin synthesis in macrophages which permits enhanced intracellular iron retention to result in hypoferremia. The cytokines also induce an outpouring of neutrophils to the site of extracellular bacterial invasion with discharge of apo-Lf. The protein binds iron and is then scavenged by macrophages that have migrated to the site. Macrophages also scavenge iron in areas of tumor cell growth. Furthermore, macrophages activated by interferon-γ produce reactive nitrogen intermediates (RNI) from L-arginine. The RNI, exemplified by nitric oxide, cause microbial and neoplastic cells to lose nonheme iron, with consequent cessation of their DNA synthesis. Infected macrophages activated by IFN-γ also can starve their intracellular pathogens by downshifting expression of TfRs. Finally, hosts recovering from extracellular bacterial infections develop humoral immunity that blocks the function of protein components of the pathogen's iron acquisition systems.

IV. CONDITIONS THAT COMPROMISE THE IRON-WITHHOLDING DEFENSE SYSTEM

Manifold ways whereby the iron-withholding defense system can be compromised are contained in Table 4. The conditions listed are associated with increased susceptibility to fungal, bacterial, protozoan and neoplastic cell invasion as well as to increased incidence of cardiomyopathy, arthropathy, and endocrine deficits.[38] Microbial genera that contain strains in which growth in body fluids, cells, tissues, and/or intact vertebrate hosts is stimulated by excess iron are listed in Table 5. The association of excess iron with neoplastic cell growth is summarized in Table 6.

Excessive iron not only serves as a growth-essential nutrient for microbial and neoplastic cell invaders but also suppresses chemotaxis, phagocytosis, and microbicidal action of mononuclear and polymorphonuclear leukocytes.[77,78] Furthermore, iron overload reduces (1) migration of B and T lymphocytes into the lymphatic system,[79] (2) the number of IL-2 secreting cells and of T helper cells,[80,81] (3) the activity of natural killer cells,[82,83] and (4) the tumoricidal activity of macrophages.[84]

A few examples of the clinical association of iron overload with infection are presented as follows. (The clinical association of cancer and iron is discussed in Chapter 13 of this volume.) The danger of excessive dietary iron is well illustrated in a recent study of mice infected with *Mycobacterium paratuberculosis*.[85] The animals were fed either a low amount of iron (similar to that in natural diets) or a high amount (similar to that in laboratory chow). Increased iron intake resulted in increased frequency of residual and progressive mycobacterial infection. Similarly, hamsters infected with the protozoan *Entamoeba histolytica* had twice the number of infective lesions when fed excess iron.[86a] Human infants fed high-iron formula had a threefold greater risk of developing salmonellosis than those fed low-iron formula.[86b] In an autopsy series on captive rock hyraxes that had hemochromatosis, the large majority were found to have died of infection.[87]

Likewise in human hemochromatosis, the common (though often unrecognized) terminal event is septicemia.[88] Such Gram-negative bacteria as *Yersinia enterocolitica*[89,90] and *Vibrio vulnificus*[91] especially are troublesome. Indeed, *V. vulnificus* cannot multiply in normal human sera but grows rapidly in hemochromatotic human sera.[92] The growth was found to be due solely to the presence of extra iron.

TABLE 4
Cultural and Clinical Conditions that Compromise the Iron-Withholding Defense System

Excessive intake of iron via intestinal absorption
  Excessive consumption of red meats or of blood (heme iron)
  Adulteration of processed foods with inorganic iron
  Use of iron cookware
  Excessive consumption of ethanol
  Possible cell receptor defect in hereditary hemochromatosis
  Accidental ingestion of, or over-medication with, iron tablets
  Excessive consumption of ascorbic acid with inorganic iron
  Pancreatic deficiency of bicarbonate ions
  Erythropoietic defects due to:
    Folic acid deficiency
    Porphyria cutanea tarda
    Various hemoglobinopathies
    Various anemias
  Asplenia

Parenteral iron
  Intravenous multiple transfusions of whole blood or erythrocytes
  Intramuscular iron dextran

Inhaled iron
  Mining iron ore, welding or grinding steel
  Painting with iron oxide powder
  Exposure to amosite, crocidolite, or tremolite (but not chrysotile) asbestos
  Cigarette smoking

Shifting iron from body compartments into plasma
  Release of stored iron from hepatocytes injured by hepatitis
  Release of erythrocyte iron during hemolytic disease episodes
  Suppression of cellular iron assimilation from plasma by such antitumor drugs as cisplatinum and *Vinca* alkaloids

Reduction of normal menstrual excretion of iron in premenopausal women
  Hysterectomy
  Ingestion of high dose oral contraceptive agents

Lack of transferrin or lactoferrin
  Congenital defect in synthesis
  Lack of dietary amino acids for synthesis
    Kwashiorkor
    Jejunoileal bypass

From Weinberg, E. D., *Drug Metab. Rev.*, 22, 531, 1990. With permission.

TABLE 5
Microbial Genera with Strains Whose Growth in Body Fluids, Cells, Tissues, and/or Intact Vertebrate Hosts Is Stimulated by Excess Iron

Fungi and Protozoa	Gram-positive and acid-fast bacteria	Gram-negative bacteria
Candida	Bacillus	Acinetobacter
Cryptococcus	Clostridium	Aeromonas
Entamoeba	Corynebacterium	Alcaligenes
Histoplasma	Erysipelothrix	Campylobacter
Naegleria	Listeria	Enterobacter
Plasmodium	Mycobacterium	Escherichia
Pneumocystis	Staphylococcus	Klebsiella
Pythium	Streptococcus	Legionella
Rhizopus		Moraxella
Torulopsis		Neisseria
Trichophyton		Pasteurella
Trichosporon		Proteus
Trypanasoma		Pseudomonas
		Salmonella
		Shigella
		Vibrio
		Yersinia

From Weinberg, E. D., *Physiol. Rev.*, 64, 65, 1984. With permission.

TABLE 6
Association of Excess Iron with Enhanced Neoplastic Cell Growth

Route of entry of excess iron	Hosts	Types of neoplasms
Ingested	Rodents	Adenocarcinomas, colorectal tumors, hepatomas, mammary gland tumors, plasmacytomas
	Humans	Hepatocellular carcinomas, lung cancers
Injected	Rodents	Hepatocellular carcinomas, leukemias, sarcomas
	Humans	Sarcomas
Inhaled	Humans	Lung cancers, mesotheliomas
Unknown	Humans	Hepatocellular carcinomas, leukemias, lung cancers, lymphomas, neuroblastomas

From Weinberg, E. D., *Biol. Trace Elem. Res.*, in press. With permission.

In addition to hemochromatosis, other causes of iron overload predispose to yersiniosis. These include oral overdoses of inorganic iron tablets,[93] use of iron cookware,[94] and alcoholism,[95] as well as injected iron combined with dextran[96] or injected hemoglobin in multiple blood transfusions.[97,98] Similarly, children with hypotransferrinemia due to kwashiorkor[99] are at increased risk of yersiniosis.[97] Sicklemia patients, during episodes of hyperferremia, likewise have increased risk of yersiniosis.[100] Patients who release stored iron from hepatocytes (in episodes of hepatitis) or hemoglobin iron from erythrocytes (in episodes of malaria and other hemolytic diseases) develop an hyperferremia that frequently results in appearance of such Gram-negative bacterial infections as systemic salmonellosis.[101]

A potentially dangerous practice is the contemplated addition of animal hemoglobin to human food. For instance, cured beef sausage, containing $0.002\ \mu M$ nitrite, was inoculated with 400 spores per gram of *Clostridium botulinum*.[102] The control samples contained detectable toxin within 4 weeks. In contrast, samples adulterated with 5% bovine hemoglobin had toxin within 1 week. On the other hand, samples supplemented with 5% bovine plasma that contained unsaturated transferrin had no detectable toxin after 10 weeks.

Persons who received multiple blood transfusions at the time of surgery were found to develop 3.5 times as many bacterial infections as nontransfused persons in the same surgical unit.[103] Moreover, the leading drug employed to remove iron by chelation, i.e., deferoxamine, can function as a siderophore for various fungal and bacterial pathogens. Thus, patients treated with the drug have, at times, developed such conditions as yersiniosis,[104,105] vibriosis,[106] or fungal infections.[107,108] Children, deficient in neutrophilic lactoferrin, are at increased risk for Gram-positive and Gram-negative bacterial infections as well as for fungal infections.[109]

In normal full-term infants, the risk of Gram-negative bacterial septicemias,[110] respiratory infections,[111] and malaria[112] was increased by injected iron dextran. Supplementation of infant milk formulas with iron has been associated with increased severity of infant botulism[113] and with an increased incidence of sudden infant death syndrome.[114]

To summarize this section, the iron-withholding defense system can be compromised either by excessive amounts of iron in various body comparments or a deficiency in iron-withholding proteins. Numerous reports of increased fungal, bacterial, and protozoan infections as well as increased neoplastic cell growth are associated with a compromised iron-withholding defense.

TABLE 7
Methods for Lowering the Exposure of Humans to Iron

Reduction of amount of ingested iron
    Items that should be reduced
        Iron adulteration of processed foods; intake of red meats, ethanol, ascorbic acid, iron med-
           ications (unless person has a correctly diagnosed iron deficiency); and use of iron cookware
    Items that should be increased
        Ingestion of tea and unrefined grains that contain phytic acid

Reduction of amount of injected iron
    Substitute human recombinant erythropoietin for blood transfusions whenever possible
    Eliminate injected iron medications (unless person has a correctly diagnosed iron
      deficiency)

Reduction of amount of inhaled iron
    Enhanced worker protection equipment in ferrous metals industries
    Convert asbestos industry to focus on use of chrysotile and to abandon use of crocidolite,
      amosite, and tremolite
    Avoid inhalation of cigarette tars

Removal of appropriate quantities of blood and iron
    Avoid use of high dose oral contraceptive agents, as well as premenopausal hysterectomies,
      to permit normal menstrual iron excretion
    Establish appropriate schedules of phlebotomy in persons who have hereditary hemochro-
      matosis or other iron-overload disease
    Continue development of orally effective iron-chelating drugs for use in iron-overloaded
      persons who cannot be phlebotomized (e.g., thalassemics)

V. METHODS FOR STRENGTHENING THE IRON-WITHHOLDING DEFENSE SYSTEM

A. LOWERING THE EXPOSURE OF HOSTS TO IRON

Examples of procedures for lowering the exposure of hosts to iron are contained in Table 7. (See also Chapter 19). To ensure success of these procedures, a healthy iron-withholding defense system must be sustained. For instance, good protein nutrition is required to supply amino acids for construction of adequate levels of transferrin and lactoferrin.[2] In addition to nutritional control, appropriate hormonal balance should be maintained. An example of hormonal modulation of iron withholding is observed in users of oral contraceptive agents.[115] In these persons, the 13-fold increase in vaginal mucous lactoferrin that normally would develop just after menses fails to occur.

B. SUPPRESSION OF IRON ASSIMILATION IN INVADING CELLS

Convalescent sera of animals and humans recovering from Gram-negative bacterial infections contain immunoglobulins to iron-repressed outer membrane proteins.[2] Thus, to ensure expression of iron-repressed epitopes, vaccines are being developed that are derived from bacteria grown in low-iron media. For instance, such a vaccine gave 99% protection to lambs challenged with *Pasteurella hemolytica* whereas a vaccine prepared from bacteria grown in high-iron medium gave only 47% protection.[76] However, iron-regulated proteins can be subject to antigenic variation. Accordingly, it will be important to employ bacterial strains that express highly conserved epitopes.[15,116,117]

A variety of methods to prevent neoplastic cells from acquiring iron presently are in clinical or experimental use.[27] Such drugs as cisplatinum and the *Vinca rosea* alkaloids, and possibly hydroxyurea, interfere with endocytosis of Tf-Fe. Deferoxamine (DFO) has antitumor activity in animals and humans. The action of DFO is synergistic with hydroxyurea as well as with monoclonal antibodies to TfR. Transferrin gallium binds to TfR and is endocytosed but the gallium ion is incapable of catalyzing the iron-dependent M2 subunit of ribonucleotide reductase. Synergistic inhibition of tumor cells occurs with gallium and hydroxyurea as well as with sequential use of DF and gallium.[118]

Normal biological modifiers that effect iron withholding such as interleukin-1 and tumor necrosis factor-α or that induce iron withdrawal such as nitric oxide are appropriate candidates for research and development of novel chemotherapeutic modalities. However, the two cytokines have multiple functions, and nitric oxide causes vascular smooth muscle relaxation and inhibition of platelet aggregation. Thus, the chemicals may need to be introduced directly into the tumor site rather than to be administered systemically.

To summarize this section, practices recommended to lower ingested, injected, and inhaled quantities of iron are beginning to show associations with reduced incidence of infection and neoplasia. Immunological and pharmacological methods for prevention of iron assimilation by microbial and neoplastic cells are being developed in experimental and clinical protocols.

VI. CONCLUSIONS

An important component of virulence of strains of fungal, bacterial, protozoan, and neoplastic cells is their ability to acquire iron from their vertebrate hosts. The latter attempt to withhold the growth-essential metal from the invading cells in a variety of ways. These include (1) continuous stationing of powerful iron-binding proteins at most sites of invasions, (2) lowering iron in body fluids and in diseased sites during invasions, (3) withdrawal of nonheme iron from microbial and neoplastic cells, and (4) synthesis of immunoglobulins to protein components of microbial iron acquisition systems.

The iron-withholding defense system can be compromised either by excessive amounts of iron in various body compartments or a deficiency of iron-withholding proteins. Compromised persons are at high risk for development of infection and neoplasia. The iron-withholding defense system can be strengthened by (1) lowering the exposure of hosts to ingested, injected, and inhaled quantities of iron; and (2) suppressing by immunological and pharmacological methods the ability of invaders to assimilate iron.

REFERENCES

1. **Locke, A., Main, E. R., and Rosbach, D. O.,** The copper and non-hemoglobinous iron contents of the blood serum in disease, *J. Clin. Invest.,* 11, 527, 1932.
2. **Weinberg, E. D.,** Iron withholding: a defense against infection and neoplasia, *Physiol. Rev.,* 64, 65, 1984.
3. **Twort, F. W. and Ingram, G. L. Y.,** A method for isolating and cultivating the *Mycobacterium enteriditis* chromicae pseudotuberculosis bovis, Johne, and some experiments on the preparation of a diagnostic vaccine for pseudotuberculosis enteritis of bovines, *Proc. R. Soc. London, Ser. B,* 84, 517, 1912.
4. **Snow, G. A.,** Mycobactins: iron-chelating growth factors from mycobacteria, *Microbiol. Rev.,* 34, 99, 1970.
5. **Neilands, J. B.,** Siderophore systems of bacteria and fungi, in *Metal Ions and Bacteria,* Beveridge, T. J. and Doyle, R. J., Eds., John Wiley & Sons, New York, 1989, 141.
6. **Weinberg, E. D.,** Cellular regulation of iron assimilation, *Q. Rev. Biol.,* 64, 261, 1989.
7. **Neilands, J. B.,** Methodology of siderophores, *Struct. Bonding (Berlin),* 58, 1, 1984.
8. **Byers, B. R.,** Pathogenic iron acquisition, *Life Chem. Rep.,* 4, 143, 1987.
9. **Otto, B. R., Sparrius, M., Verwey-van Vught, A. M. J. J., and MacLaren, D. M.,** Iron-regulated outer membrane protein of *Bacteroides fragilis* involved in heme uptake, *Infect. Immun.,* 58, 3954, 1990.
10. **Redhead, K. and Hill, T.,** Acquisition of iron from transferrin by *Bordetella pertussis, FEMS Microbiol. Lett.,* 77, 303, 1991.
11. **Alderete, J. F., Peterson, K. M., and Baseman, J.,** Affinities of *Treponema pallidum* for human lactoferrin and transferrin, *Genitourin. Med.,* 64, 359, 1988.
12. **Tryon, V. V. and Baseman, J.,** The acquisition of human lactoferrin by *Mycoplasma pneumoniae, Microb. Pathogenesis,* 3, 437, 1987.
13. **Schryvers, A. B.,** Identification of the transferrin- and lactoferrin-binding proteins in *Haemophilus influenzae, J. Med. Microbiol.,* 29, 121, 1989.
14. **Williams, P., Morton, D. J., Tower, K. J., Stevenson, P., and Griffiths, E.,** Utilization of enterobactin and other exogenous iron sources by *Haemophilus influenzae, H. parainfluenzae* and *H. paraphrophilus, J. Gen. Microbiol.,* 136, 2343, 1990.
15. **van Putten, J. P. M.,** Iron acquisition and the pathogenesis of meningococcal and gonococcal disease, *Med. Microbiol. Immunol.,* 179, 289, 1990.

200

16. **Ogunnawariwo, J. A. and Schryvers, A. B.,** Iron acquisition in *Pasteurella haemolytica:* expression and identification of a bovine-specific transferrin receptor, *Infect. Immun.,* 58, 2091, 1990.

17. **Payne, S. M. and Finkelstein, R. A.,** The critical role of iron in host-bacterial infections, *J. Clin. Invest.,* 61, 1428, 1978.

18. **Simonson, C., Brener, D., and De Voe, I. W.,** Expression of a high affinity mechanism for acquisition of transferrin iron by *Neisseria meningitidis, Infect. Immun.,* 36, 107, 1982.

19. **Mickelson, P. A. and Sparling, P. F.,** Ability of *Neisseria gonorrhoeae, Neisseria meningitidis,* and commensal *Neisseria* species to obtain iron from transferrin and iron compounds, *Infect. Immun.,* 33, 555, 1981.

20. **McFarlane, H., Reddy, S., Adcock, K. J., Adeshina, H., Cooke, A. R., and Akene, J.,** Immunity, transferrin, and survival in kwashiorkor, *Br. Med. J.,* 4, 268, 1970.

21. **Johnson, W., Varner, L., and Poch, M.,** Acquisition of iron by *Legionella pneumophila:* role of iron reductase, *Infect. Immun.,* 59, 2376, 1991.

22. **Schryvers, A. B. and Gonzalez, G. C.,** Comparison of the abilities of differences sources in iron to enhance *Neisseria meningitidis* infection in mice, *Infect. Immun.,* 57, 2425, 1989.

23. **Ogunnariwo, J. A., Cheng, C., Ford, J., and Schryvers, A. B.,** Response of *Haemophilus somnus* to iron limitation: expression and identification of a bovine-specific transferrin receptor, *Microb. Pathogenesis,* 9, 397, 1990.

24. **Shivprasad, S. and Page, W. J.,** Catechol formation and melanization by Na + -dependent *Azobacter chroococcum:* a protective mechanism for aeroadaptation?, *Appl. Environ. Microbiol.,* 55, 1811, 1989.

25. **Bagg, A. and Neilands, J. B.,** Molecular mechanism of regulation of siderophore mediated iron assimilation, *Microbiol. Rev.,* 51, 509, 1987.

26. **Holley, R. W.,** A unifying hypothesis concerning the nature of malignant growth, *Proc. Natl. Acad. Sci. U.S.A.,* 69, 2840, 1972.

27. **Weinberg, E. D.,** Roles of iron in neoplasia: promotion, prevention, and therapy, *Biol. Trace Elem. Res.,* in press.

28. **Basset, P., Quesneau, Y., and Zwiller, J.,** Iron-induced L1210 cell growth: evidence of a transferrin independent iron transport, *Cancer Res.,* 46, 1644, 1986.

29. **Vostrejs, M., Moran, P. L., and Seligman, P. A.,** Transferrin synthesis by small cell lung cancer cells acts as an autocrine regulator of cellular proliferation, *J. Clin. Invest.,* 82, 231, 1988.

30. **Brown, J. P., Hewick, R. W., and Hellstrom, I.,** Human melanoma associated antigen p97 is structurally and functionally related to transferrin, *Nature (London),* 296, 171, 1982.

31. **Neckers, L. M.,** Transferrin receptors regulate proliferation of normal and malignant B cells, *Curr. Top. Microbiol. Immunol.,* 113, 62, 1984.

32. **Cazzola, M., Bergamaschi, G., Dezza, L., and Arosio, P.,** Manipulations of cellular iron metabolism for modulating normal and malignant cell proliferation: achievements and prospects, *Blood,* 75, 1903, 1990.

33. **Sorokin, L. M., Morgan, E. H., and Yeoh, G. C. T.,** Transformation-induced changes in transferrin and iron metabolism in myogenic cells, *Cancer Res.,* 49, 1941, 1989.

34. **Gatter, K. C., Brown, G., and Trowbridge, I. S.,** Transferrin receptors in human tissues: their distribution and possible clinical relevance, *J. Clin. Pathol.,* 36, 539, 1983.

35. **Faulk, W. P., Hsi, B. L., and Stevens, P. L.,** Transferrin and transferrin receptors in carcinoma of breast, *Lancet,* 2, 390, 1980.

36. **Shindelman, J. E., Ortmeyer, A. E., and Sussman, H.,** Demonstration of the transferrin receptor in human breast cancer tissue, *Int. J. Cancer,* 27, 329, 1981.

37. **Esserman, L., Takahashi, S., and Rojas, V.,** An epitope of the transferrin receptor is exposed on the cell surface of high-grade but not low-grade human lymphomas, *Blood,* 74, 2718, 1989.
38. **Weinberg, E. D.,** Cellular iron metabolism in health and disease, *Drug Metab. Rev.,* 22, 531, 1990.
39. **Kalmar, J. R. and Arnold, R. R.,** Killing of *Actinobacillus actinomycetem comitans* by human lactoferrin, *Infect. Immun.,* 56, 2552, 1988.
40. **Reiter, B.,** The biological significance of lactoferrin, *Int. J. Tissue React.,* 5, 87, 1983.
41. **Lambert, C. C. and Hunter, R. L.,** Low levels of unsaturated transferrin as a predictor of survival in pneumococcal pneumonia, *Ann. Clin. Lab. Sci.,* 20, 140, 1990.
42. **Fitzsimons, E. J. and Levine, S. R.,** Rapid drop in serum iron concentration associated with stress, *Am. J. Med. Sci.,* 285, 12, 1973.
43. **Olivares, M., Walter, T., Osorio, H., Chadud, P., and Schlesinger, L.,** Anemia of a mild viral infection: the measles vaccine as a model, *Pediatrics,* 84, 851, 1989.
44. **Arthur, C. K. and Isbister, J. P.,** Iron deficiency: misunderstood, misdiagnosed and mistreated, *Drugs,* 33, 171, 1987.
45. **Blatteis, C. M., Mashburn, T. A., Jr., and Ahokas, R. A.,** Fever and trace metal changes in endotoxin-challenged neonates, *Pfluegers Arch.,* 389, 177, 1981.
46. **Hambleton, P., Bailey, N. E., Fitzgeorge, R. B., and Baskerville, A.,** Clinical chemical responses to experimental airborne legionellosis in the guinea pig, *Br. J. Exp. Pathol.,* 66, 173, 1985.
47. **Pekarek, R. S., Bostian, K. A., Bartelloni, P. J., Calia, F. M., and Beisel, W. R.,** The effects of *Francisella tularensis* infection on iron metabolism in man, *Am. J. Med. Sci.,* 258, 14, 1969.
48. **Andreesen, R., Osterholz, J., and Bodemann, H.,** Expression of transferrin receptors and intracellular ferritin during terminal differentiation of human monocytes, *Blut,* 49, 195, 1984.
49. **Alvarez-Hernandez, X., Felstein, M. V., and Brock, J. H.,** The relationship between iron release, ferritin synthesis and intracellular iron distribution in mouse peritoneal macrophages, *Biochim. Biophys. Acta,* 886, 214, 1986.
50. **Grieger, T. A. and Kluger, M. J.,** Effects of bacteria and temperature on free serum iron levels in the lizard *Dipsosaurus dorsalis, Physiologist,* 20, 37, 1977.
51. **Congleton, J. L. and Wagner, E. J.,** Acute-phase hypoferremic response to lipopolysaccharide in rainbow trout *(Onchorhynchus mykiss), Comp. Biochem. Physiol.,* 98A, 195, 1991.
52. **Konin, A. M. and Hershko, C.,** The anaemia of inflammation and chronic disease, in *Iron in Immunity, Cancer and Inflammation,* M. de Sousa and J. H. Brock, Eds., John Wiley & Sons, Chichester, 1989, 111.
53. **Mitsuyama, M., Igaraski, K.-I., and Kawamura, I.,** Difference in the induction of macrophage interleukin-1 production between viable and killed cells of *Listeria monocytogenes, Infect. Immun.,* 58, 1254, 1990.
54. **Lee, G. R.,** The anemia of chronic disease, *Semin. Hematol.,* 20, 61, 1983.
55. **Kampschmidt, R. F. and Pulliam, L. A.,** Stimulation of antimicrobial activity in the rat with leukocytic endogenous mediator, *J. Retic. Soc.,* 17, 162, 1975.
56. **Uchida, T., Yamagiwa, A., and Nakamura, K.,** The effect of interleukin-1 on iron metabolism in rats, *Eur. J. Haematol.,* 46, 1, 1991.
57. **Stevens, R. G. and Kalkworf, D. R.,** Iron, radiation and cancer, *Environ. Health Perspect.,* 87, 291, 1990.
58. **Neta, R., Douches, S., and Oppenheim, J. J.,** Interleukin-1 is a radioprotector, *J. Immunol.,* 136, 2483, 1986.

202

59. **Malkovsky, M., Sondel, P. M., and Strober, W.,** The interleukins in acquired disease, *Clin. Exp. Immunol.,* 74, 151, 1988.

60. **Alvarez-Hernandez, X., Liceaga, J., McKay, I. C., and Brock, J. H.,** Induction of hypoferremia and modulation of macrophage iron metabolism by tumor necrosis factor, *Lab. Invest.,* 61, 319, 1989.

61. **Sakata, Y., Morimoto, A., Long, N. C., and Murakami, N.,** Fever and acute phase response induced in rabbits by intravenous and intracerebroventricular injection of interleukin-6, *Cytokine,* 3, 199, 1991.

62. **Hibbs, J. B., Jr., Taintor, R. R., Vavrin, Z., and Rachlin, E. M.,** Nitric oxide: a cytotoxic activated macrophage effector molecule, *Biochem. Biophys. Res. Commun.,* 157, 87, 1988.

63. **Li, L., Kilbourn, R. G., Adams, J., and Fidler, I. J.,** Role of nitric oxide in lysis of tumor cells by cytokine-activated endothelial cells, *Cancer Res.,* 51, 2531, 1991.

64. **Amber, I. J., Hibbs, J. B., Jr., and Parker, C. J.,** Activated macrophage conditioned medium: identification of the soluble factors inducing cytotoxicity and the L-arginine dependent effector mechanism, *J. Leuk. Biol.,* 49, 610, 1991.

65. **Byrd, T. F. and Horwitz, M. A.,** Interferon gamma-activated human monocytes down regulate transferrin receptors and inhibit the intracellular multiplication of *Legionella pneumophila* by limiting the availability of iron, *J. Clin. Invest.,* 83, 1457, 1989.

66. **Lane, T. E., Wu-Hsieh, B. A., and Howard, D. H.,** Iron limitation and the gamma interferon-mediated antihistoplasma state of murine macrophages, *Infect. Immun.,* 59, 2274, 1991.

67. **Eaton, J. W., Brandt, P., Mahoney, J. R., and Lee, J. T.,** Haptoglobin: a natural bacteriostat, *Science,* 215, 691, 1982.

68. **Francis, R. T., Jr., Booth, J. W., and Becker, R. R.,** Uptake of iron from hemoglobin and the haptoglobin-hemoglobin complex by hemolytic bacteria, *Int. J. Biochem.,* 17, 767, 1985.

69. **Zakaria-Meehan, Z., Massad, G., Simpson, L. M., Travis, J. C., and Oliver, J. D.,** Ability of *Vibrio vulnificus* to obtain iron from hemoglobin-haptoglobin complexes, *Infect. Immun.,* 56, 275, 1988.

70. **Massad, G., Arceneaux, J. E. L., and Byers, B. R.,** Acquisition of iron from host sources by mesophilic *Aeromonas* species, *J. Gen. Microbiol.,* 137, 237, 1991.

71. **Stull, T. L.,** Protein sources of heme for *Haemophilus influenzae, Infect. Immun.,* 55, 148, 1987.

72. **Dyer, D. W., West, E. P., and Sparling, P. F.,** Effects of serum carrier proteins on the growth of pathogenic *Neisseriae* with heme-bound iron, *Infect. Immun.,* 55, 2171, 1987.

73. **Black, J. R., Dyer, D. W., Thompson, M. K., and Sparling, P. F.,** Human immune response to iron-repressible outer membrane proteins of *Neisseria meningitidis, Infect. Immun.,* 54, 710, 1986.

74. **Shand, G. H., Anwar, H., Kadurugamuwa, J., Brown, M. R. W., Silverman, S. H., and Melling, J.,** *In vivo* evidence that bacteria in urinary tract infection grow under iron-restricted conditions, *Infect. Immun.,* 48, 35, 1985.

75. **Shand, G. H., Pedersen, S. S., Brown, M. R. W., and Hoiby, N.,** Serum antibodies to *Pseudomonas aeruginosa* outer-membrane proteins and iron-regulated membrane proteins at different stages of chronic cystic fibrosis lung infection, *J. Med. Microbiol.,* 34, 203, 1991.

76. **Gilmour, N. J. L., Donachie, W., Sutherland, A. D., Gilmour, J. S., Jones, G. E., and Quirie, M.,** Vaccine containing iron-regulated proteins of *Pasteurella haemolytica* A2 enhances protection against experimental pasteurellosis in lambs, *Vaccine,* 9, 137, 1991.

77. **Waterlot, Y., Cantinieaux, B., and Hariga-Muller, C.,** Impaired phagocytic activity of neutrophils in patients receiving haemodialysis: the critical role of iron overload, *Br. Med. J.,* 291, 503, 1985.

78. **Cantinieaux, B., Hariga, C., and Ferster, A.,** Neutrophil dysfunctions in thalassemia major: the role of cell iron overload, *Eur. J. Haematol.,* 39, 28, 1987.

79. **de Sousa, M.,** Lymphoid cell positioning: a new proposal for the mechanism of control of lymphoid cell migration, *Symp. Soc. Exp. Biol.,* 32, 393, 1978.

80. **Pardalos, G., Kanakoudi-Tsakalidis, F., and Malaka-Zafiriu, M.,** Iron-related disturbances of cell-mediated immunity in multitransfused children with thalassemia major, *Clin. Exp. Immunol.,* 68, 138, 1987.

81. **Good, M. F., Chapman, D. E., Powell, L. W., and Halliday, J. W.,** The effect of experimental iron-overload on splenic T cell function: analysis using clonal techniques, *Clin. Exp. Immunol.,* 68, 375, 1987.

82. **Akbar, A. N., Fitzgerald-Bocarsley, P. A., and de Sousa, M.,** Decreased natural killer activity in thalassemia major: a possible consequence of iron overload, *J. Immunol.,* 136, 1635, 1986.

83. **Kaplan, J., Sarnaik, S., Gitlin, J., and Lusher, J.,** Diminished helper/suppressor lymphocyte ratios and natural killer activity in recipients of repeated blood transfusions, *Blood,* 64, 308, 1984.

84. **Green, R., Esperaza, I., and Schreiber, R.,** Iron inhibits the nonspecific tumorcidal activity of macrophages, *Ann. N.Y. Acad. Sci.,* 526, 301, 1988.

85. **Lepper, A. W. D., Jarrett, R. G., and Lewis, V. M.,** The effect of different levels of iron intake on the multiplication of *Mycobacterium paratuberculosis* in C57 and C3H mice, *Vet. Microbiol.,* 16, 369, 1988.

86. **Diamond, L. S., Harlow, D. R., Phillips, B. P., and Keister, D. B.,** *Entamoeba histolyica:* iron and nutritional immunity, *Arch. Invest. Med.,* 9 (Suppl. 1), 329, 1978.

86a. **Haddock, R. L., Cousens, S. N., and Cruzman, C. C.,** Infant diet and salmonellosis, *Am. J. Publ. Health,* 81, 977, 1991.

87. **Rahg, J. E., Burek, J. D., Strindberg, J. D., and Monteli, R. J.,** Hemochromatosis in the rock hyrax, in *The Comparative Pathology of Zoo Animals,* Monteli, R. J. and Migaki, G., Eds., Smithsonian Institute Press, Washington, D.C., 1980, 113.

88. **Fairbanks, V. F., Fahey, J. L., and Beutler, E.,** *Clinical Disorders of Iron Metabolism,* 2nd ed., Grune & Stratton, New York, 1971, 437.

89. **Chiesa, C., Pacifico, L., and Renzuli, E.,** *Yersinia* hepatic abscesses and iron overload, *J. Am. Med. Assoc.,* 257, 3230, 1987.

90. **Adams, P. C. and Gregor, J.,** Hemochromatosis and yersiniosis, *Can. J. Gastroenterol.,* 4, 160, 1990.

91. **Blake, P. A., Merson, M. H., and Weaver, R. E.,** Disease caused by a marine vibrio, *N. Engl. J. Med.,* 300, 1, 1979.

92. **Chart, H. and Griffiths, E.,** The availability of iron and the growth of *Vibrio vulnificus* in sera from patients with haemochromatosis, *FEMS Microbiol. Lett.,* 26, 227, 1985.

93. **Melby, K., Slordahl, S., Gutteberg, T. J., and Nordbro, S. A.,** Septicaemia due to *Yersinia enterolcolitica* after oral overdoses of iron, *Br. Med. J.,* 285, 467, 1982.

94. **Robins-Browne, R. M., Rabson, A. R., and Koornhof, H. J.,** Generalized infection with *Yersinia enterocolitica* and the role of iron, *Contrib. Microbiol. Immunol.,* 5, 277, 1979.

95. **Capron, J.-P., Capron-Chivrac, D., and Tossou, H.,** Spontaneous *Yersinia enterocolitica* peritonitis in idiopathic hemochromatosis, *Gastroenterology,* 87, 1372, 1984.

96. **Leighton, P. M. and MacSween, H. M.,** *Yersinia* hepatic abscesses subsequent to long-term iron therapy, *JAMA,* 257, 964, 1987.

97. **Butzler, J. P., Alexander, M., and Segers, A.,** Enteritis, abscess and septicemia due to *Yersinia enterocolitica* in a child with thalassemia, *J. Pediatr.,* 93, 619, 1978.

98. **Boelaert, J. R., Van Landuyt, H. W., and Valcke, Y. J.,** The role of iron overload in *Yersinia enterocolitica* and *Yersinia pseudotuberculosis* bacteremia in hemodialysis patients, *J. Infect. Dis.,* 156, 384, 1987.

99. **McFarlane, H., Reddy, S., and Cooke, A.,** Immunoglobulins, transfferin, caeruloplasmin and heterophile antibodies in kwashiorkor, *Trop. Geogr. Med.,* 22, 61, 1970.

100. **Bradley, J. M. and Skinner, J. I.,** Isolation of *Yersinia pseudotuberculosis* serotype V from the blood of a patient with sickle-cell anemia, *J. Med. Microbiol.,* 7, 383, 1974.

101. **Weinberg, E. D.,** Iron and infection, *Microbiol. Rev.,* 42, 45, 1978.

102. **Miller, A. J. and Menichillo, D. A.,** Blood fraction effects on the antibotulinal efficacy of nitrite in model beef sausage, *J. Food Sci.,* 56, 1158, 1991.

103. **Tartter, P. I., Quintero, S., and Barron, D. M.,** Perioperative blood transfusion associated with infectious complications after colorectal cancer operations, *Am. J. Surg.,* 152, 479, 1986.

104. **Boyce, N., Thomson, N. M., and Wood, C.,** Life-threatening sepsis complicating heavy metal chelation therapy with desferrioxamine, *Aust. N.Z. J. Med.,* 15, 654, 1985.

105. **Gallant, T., Freedman, M. H., Vellend, H., and Francomb, W. H.,** *Yersinia* sepsis in patients with iron overload treated with deferoxamine, *N. Engl. J. Med.,* 314, 1643, 1986.

106. **Mehtar, S.,** Adult epiglottitis due to *Vibrio vulnificus, Br. Med. J.,* 296, 827, 1988.

107. **Sane, A., Manzi, S., and Perfect, J.,** Deferoxamine treatment as a risk factor for zygomycete infection, *J. Infect. Dis.,* 159, 151, 1989.

108. **Sathapatayavongs, B., Leelachaikul, P., and Prachaktam, P.,** Human pythiosis associated with thalassemia hemoglobinopathy syndrome, *J. Infect. Dis.,* 159, 274, 1989.

109. **Breton-Gorius, J., Mason, D. Y., and Buriot, D.,** Lactoferrin deficiency as a consequence of a lack of specific granules in neutrophils from a patient with recurrent infections, *Am. J. Pathol.,* 99, 413, 1980.

110. **Barry, D. M. J. and Reeve, A. W.,** Iron and infection, *Br. Med. J.,* 296, 1736, 1988.

111. **Oppenheimer, S. J. MacFarlane, S. B. J., and Moody, J. B.,** Effect of iron prophylaxis on morbidity due to infectious disease: report on clinical studies in Papua New Guinea, *Trans. R. Soc. Trop. Med. Hyg.,* 80, 596, 1986.

112. **Oppenheimer, S. J., Gibson, F. D., and Macfarlane, S. B.,** Iron supplementation increases prevalence and effects of malaria: report on clinical studies in Papua New Guinea, *Trans. R. Soc. Trop. Med. Hyg.,* 80, 603, 1986.

113. **Arnon, S. S.,** Infant botulism, *Annu. Rev. Med.,* 31, 541, 1980.

114. **Moore, A. and Worwood, M.,** Iron and the sudden infant death syndrome, *Br. Med. J.,* 298, 1642, 1989.

115. **Cohen, M. S., Britigan, B. E., French, M., and Bean, K.,** Preliminary observations on the lactoferrin secretion in human vaginal mucus: variation during the menstrual cycle, evidence of hormonal regulation, and implications for infection with *Neisseria gonorrhoeae, Am. J. Obstet. Gynecol.,* 157, 1122, 1987.

116. **Banerjee-Bhatnagar, N. and Frasch, C. E.,** Expression of *Neisseria meningitidis* iron-regulated outer membrane proteins, including a 70-kilodalton transferrin receptor, and their potential for use as vaccines, *Infect. Immun.,* 58, 2875, 1990.

117. **Pettersson, A., Kuipers, B., Pelzer, M., Verhagen, E., Tiesjema, R. H., Tommassen, J., and Poolman, J. T.,** Monoclonal antibodies against the 70-kilodalton iron-regulated protein of *Neisseria meningitidis* are bactericidal and strain specific, *Infect. Immun.,* 58, 3036, 1990.

118. **Chitambar, C. R. and Naresimhan, J.,** Targeting iron-dependent DNA synthesis with gallium and transferrin-gallium, *Pathobiology,* 59, 3, 1991.

Part III
Iron and Oxidative Stress

7. Iron and Damage to Biomolecules

BARRY HALLIWELL

Division of Pulmonary-Critical Care Medicine, UC Davis Medical Center, Sacramento, California

I. INTRODUCTION

It is now well established that reactive oxygen species are continuously produced *in vivo*. In consequence, organisms have evolved not only antioxidant defense systems to protect against them, but also repair systems that prevent the accumulation of oxidatively damaged molecules.[1-3] The term reactive oxygen species (ROS) is a collective one that includes oxygen radicals (species containing one or more unpaired electrons, such as superoxide [O_2^-] and hydroxyl [$OH^.$]) and certain nonradical derivatives of oxygen, such as hydrogen peroxide (H_2O_2), singlet oxygen $^1\Delta g$, hypochlorous acid (HOCl), and ozone (O_3). Hydroxyl radical is produced in living organisms by at least two mechanisms: reaction of transition metal ions with H_2O_2 (see Section II) and homolytic fission of water due to background exposure to ionizing radiation.[4] Hydroxyl radical is a fearsomely reactive species that can attack all biological molecules, usually setting off free-radical chain reactions.[1,4]

Superoxide radical (O_2^-) is much less reactive than $OH^.$, but there are a number of biological targets that can be attacked by it. Thus, O_2^- reacts with nitric oxide ($NO^.$), a free radical produced by phagocytes and vascular endothelial cells, to give peroxynitrite.[5] Nitric oxide, or a derivative of it, acts upon smooth muscle cells in vessel walls to produce relaxation. By opposing its action, therefore, O_2^- can act as a vasoconstrictor, and this may have deleterious effects in some clinical situations.[6] There is considerable debate in the literature as to whether this interaction of O_2^- and $NO^.$ might be damaging to cells[7] or even whether it might occur physiologically as a means of regulating vascular muscle tone.[8] Thus, one possibility is that peroxynitrite could decompose to form $OH^.$.[5,7,9] Superoxide may also attack enzymes containing an iron-sulfur cluster, such as bacterial dihydroxyacid dehydratase, aconitase, or 6-phosphogluconate dehydrogenase.[10,11] It may also inactivate the NADH dehydrogenase complex of the mitochondrial electron transport chain.[12] Some of the O_2^- production that occurs *in vivo* appears to be a chemical accident, due to autoxidation reactions and the leakage of electrons from electron transport chains.[3,10] Sometimes O_2^- is made deliberately, e.g., by activated phagocytes[13] and, to a lesser extent, by other cell types such as fibroblasts and lymphocytes.[14-16] Removal of excess O_2^- by superoxide dismutase (SOD) enzymes is an important physiological antioxidant defense mechanism in aerobic organisms.[3,10,17,18]

SOD enzymes convert O_2^- into O_2 and H_2O_2, which might also have metabolic functions.[19-21] H_2O_2 crosses cell membranes easily and it can attack, apparently directly, a few cellular targets. For example, high levels of H_2O_2 can inactivate the glycolytic enzyme glyceraldehyde-3-phosphate dehydrogenase in mammalian cells[22] and the enzymes fructose bisphosphatase in chloroplasts,[23] and aconitase in plant mitochondria.[24]

On the whole, however, O_2^- and H_2O_2 have limited chemical reactivity. For example, increased generation of O_2^- and H_2O_2 within cells often leads to DNA damage, but neither of these species reacts directly with DNA.[25]

Interest has, therefore, focused on their ability to generate more reactive species, such as OH·, *in vivo*. Most,[1,25,26] but not all,[9] of these proposed reactions involve transition metal ions.

II. TRANSITION METALS AND FREE-RADICAL REACTIONS

An important feature of the chemistry of transition metals is their variable oxidation number. Thus, titanium has oxidation numbers of III and IV; copper, I and II; and nickel, II and III. Possession of oxidation numbers differing by one allows transition metal salts to participate in single-electron transfer reactions, for example:

$$Cu(II) + e^- \rightleftarrows Cu(I) \tag{1}$$

$$Fe(II) \rightleftarrows Fe(III) + e^- \tag{2}$$

$$Ti(III) \rightleftarrows Ti(IV) + e^- \tag{3}$$

Thus, several transition metal ions can reduce H_2O_2 in a one-electron reaction to generate OH·, by the overall reaction:

$$M^{n+} + H_2O_2 \rightarrow M^{(n+1)+} + OH^· + OH^- \tag{4}$$

where M^{n+} can be Ti(III), Cu(I), Fe(II), Co(II), or Ni(II). Indeed, chemists have frequently used mixtures of Ti(III) and H_2O_2 as a source of OH· in the laboratory, because the reaction is fairly simple:[27,28]

$$Ti(III) + H_2O_2 \rightarrow Ti(IV) + OH^· + OH^- \tag{5}$$

By contrast, the reactions of iron and copper compounds with H_2O_2 are by no means simple. For a long time, it was debated as to whether any OH· is formed at all when copper ions react with H_2O_2 (reviewed in References 26 and 29). Only recently has the production of OH· been confirmed by examining the pattern of damage to the purine and pyrimidine bases of DNA exposed to copper ions and H_2O_2, and by showing that this pattern is characteristic of attack by OH·.[30]

The most stable oxidation number of iron is Fe(III) (ferric). Thus, Fe^{2+} ions in aqueous solution oxidize to form Fe(III) at a rate depending on the pH, the buffer present, and on O_2 tension. Hence, a simple aerobic aqueous solution of a Fe(II) salt is a source of free radicals. Concentrated Fe(II) solutions have been shown to damage many biological molecules, such as hyaluronic acid[31] and DNA,[32] in the presence of oxygen.

$$Fe(II) + O_2 \rightarrow Fe(III) + O_2^{\cdot-} \tag{6}$$

$$2O_2^{\cdot-} + 2H^+ \rightarrow H_2O_2 + O_2 \tag{7}$$
nonenzymic dismutation of superoxide

$$Fe(II) + H_2O_2 \rightarrow Fe(III) + OH^{\cdot} + OH^- \tag{8}$$

$$OH^{\cdot} + biomolecule \rightarrow damage \tag{9}$$

Iron can also exist in ferryl (Fe[IV], $Fe=O^{2+}$) and perferryl (Fe[V], $Fe=O^{3+}$) states.[33,34] Ferryl species are important oxidizing agents at the active sites of several enzymes, including cytochromes P-450 and horseradish peroxidase: they can be powerful oxidizing and hydroxylating agents, depending on the precise chemistry taking place at the enzyme active site.[33] By contrast perferryl species appear to be less reactive,[1,26] e.g., they are present at the active site of horseradish peroxidase compound III (oxyperoxidase), a poorly active form of the enzyme that can be generated[35] by reaction of the "resting" (ferric) enzyme with $O_2^{\cdot}$:

$$Peroxidase\text{-}heme\ Fe(III) + O_2^{\cdot-} \rightarrow Peroxidase\text{-}heme\text{--}Fe^{2+}\text{--}O_2 \tag{10}$$

A. THE FENTON REACTION

Several transition metal salts react with H_2O_2 to form $OH^{\cdot}$; however, in terms of the possibility of $OH^{\cdot}$ generation *in vivo,* most attention has been paid to iron,[26,36] although interest in copper is increasing.[26,29,30] Fe^{2+} ions react with H_2O_2 to form $OH^{\cdot}$ by the so-called Fenton reaction, which is usually written as:

$$Fe(II) + H_2O_2 \rightarrow Fe(III) + OH^{\cdot} + OH^- \tag{11}$$

In fact, Fenton chemistry is far more complex. Thus, the initial product of reaction (11) may be an oxo-iron complex, possibly ferryl, that then decomposes to form $OH^{\cdot}$ (reviewed in Reference 26):

$$Fe(II) + H_2O_2 \rightarrow FeOH^{3+}\ (or\ FeO^{2+}) \rightarrow OH^{\cdot} + Fe(III) \tag{12}$$

Different ligands to the iron(II) may stabilize this intermediate, so that little $OH^{\cdot}$ is formed, whereas others destabilize it. Thus, iron-ethylenediaminetetraacetic acid (EDTA) chelates are good sources of $OH^{\cdot}$ in the presence of H_2O_2, (and have been used as sources of $OH^{\cdot}$ to measure rate constants for reactions of this radical[38]) whereas heme rings appear to stabilize ferryl species.[26,33] The fact that multiple reactive species are generated when iron chelates are mixed with H_2O_2 goes a long way toward explaining the long-lived controversy as to whether $OH^{\cdot}$ is the damaging species generated in Fenton reactions.[26,36] This depends on the precise molecular form of the iron, especially the chelating agent to which it is bound.[26,37,39] Iron ions bind to most biological molecules and laboratory reagents, such as buffers, and the resulting chelates have very different chemical properties.[37,39] The same is true for copper.[26,40]

Reactions 11 and 12 generate Fe(III). Most ferric complexes react more slowly (if at all) with H_2O_2 than do Fe(II) complexes, so that reducing agents stimulate Fenton reactions. This can occur with ascorbate,[26,36] e.g.:

$$Fe(III) + ascorbate \rightarrow Fe(II) + semidehydroascorbate \qquad (13)$$

Hence, iron salt/ascorbate/H_2O_2 mixtures are good sources of $OH^{\cdot}$ radical[26,36] and have been used to generate $OH^{\cdot}$ for determination of reaction rate constants.[38]

Superoxide can reduce certain ferric chelates. Thus, reaction of Fe(III) with $O_2^{\cdot-}$ appears to proceed via a perferryl intermediate:

$$Fe(III) + O_2^{\cdot-} \rightleftarrows [Fe^{3+} - O_2^{-} \leftrightarrow Fe^{2+} - O_2] \rightleftarrows Fe^{3+} + O_2 \qquad (14)$$

The sum of Reactions 11 and 14, ignoring the oxo-iron intermediates, is

$$O_2^{\cdot-} + H_2O_2 \xrightarrow{\text{Fe}} OH^{\cdot} + OH^{-} + O_2 \qquad (15)$$

This reaction is often called the iron-catalyzed Haber-Weiss reaction, or sometimes the superoxide-driven Fenton reaction. This reaction appears to account for a significant part of the damage that is caused to living cells by excess generation of ROS (reviewed in References 1, 25, 26, 41-43). It has been argued that[1,26,43] just as oxidative stress is known to cause rises in intracellular free Ca^{2+} ions by interfering with normal Ca^{2+}-sequestering mechanisms,[44] oxidative stress also increases the iron ion concentration available within cells to catalyze free-radical reactions.[43] For example, Ferrali et al.[45] showed that iron ion release plays an important part in mediating the toxic effects of allyl alcohol in mice. Reaction 15 can be inhibited by a number of iron-chelating agents, such as desferrioxamine,[46] which has been shown to offer protection against oxidative damage in a large number of biological systems, some of which are listed in Table 1. Desferrioxamine has been widely and effectively used to clear excess body iron stores from thalassemic patients.

Since desferrioxamine does not penetrate cells rapidly,[47] it cannot be given orally, and many thalassemic patients do not comply with subcutaneous infusion regimes. The search for cheap orally active alternatives to desferriox-

TABLE 1
Action of Desferrioxamine on Animal Models of Tissue Injury by Disease or Toxins

System studied	Action of desferrioxamine
Adjuvant arthritis in rats	Decreased incidence and severity of joint inflammation
Urate or carrageenan-induced footpad swelling in rats	Low doses increase urate-induced swelling; high doses anti-inflammatory in both systems
Glynn-Dumonde synovitis in guinea pigs	Stimulates acute inflammatory induction phase: repeated administration depresses chronic phase
Allergic air pouch inflammation in rats	Aggravates acute inflammation but suppresses the chronic phase
Acute lung injury in rats after complement activation	Highly protective
Immune-complex-induced vasculitis in rats	Highly protective
Alloxan-induced reduction in parasitemia in mice infected with *Plasmodium vinckei*	Protects the parasites: however, DFX itself can inhibit the intra-erythrocytic development of parasites by depriving them of essential iron
Hemorrhagic shock in dogs	High protective
Ischemia/reperfusion in *ex vivo* cat ileum	Highly protective
Ischemia/reperfusion in isolated hearts and open-chest animals (rats, dogs, rabbits)	Highly protective against free-radical induced stunning and arrhythmias; not clear if infarct size decreased
Rejection of islet allografts in mice	Decreases rejection
Ischemia/reperfusion of skin flaps	Highly protective
Allergic encephalomyelitis in rats	Constant subcutaneous infusion is protective
Antibody-dependent glomerular injury in rabbits	Highly protective
Paraquat toxicity (rats, mice)	Variable reports; most show protection, but some report exacerbation of toxicity; high DFX levels might also affect paraquat uptake by type II cells (Van der Wal et al., *Biochem. Pharmacol.*, 39, 665, 1990)
Post-transplantation lung function in dogs after transplant of stored lungs	Improvements in lung preservation and early post-transplantation function (Conte et al., *J. Thorac. Cardiovasc. Surg.*, 101, 1024, 1991)
Pathological effects of copper deficiency in rats	Ameliorated by DFX apparently by preventing tissue iron overload (Fields et al., *Metabolism*, 40, 105, 1991)
Retinal injury by high light exposure in albino rats	Less injury observed (Li et al., *Current Eye Res.*, 10, 133, 1991)

Note: References supporting the statements may be found in Reference 49 unless specifically cited in the table.

amine has led to the development of a range of hydroxypyridone iron chelators. Before using chelating agents in this way, it would seem essential to ensure that they do not promote free-radical reactions, such as OH˙ generation.[48,49] Preliminary clinical evaluation of hydroxypyridones suggests that at least some of them are more toxic than desferrioxamine.[48] Hydroxypyridones can apparently remove iron ions from transferrin and lactoferrin,[50,51] which are "safe" forms of iron unable to catalyze free-radical reactions (Section III). Hydroxypyridones form 3:1 complexes with iron ions, which do not appear to catalyze generation of free OH˙ radicals.[52] However, 2:1 and 1:1 hydroxypyridone:iron ion chelates may be able to catalyze OH˙ formation.[52] Hence, one can envisage a scenario in which the hydroxypyridones remove iron ions from safe forms and create iron complexes active in catalyzing free-radical reactions. This could contribute to the increased toxicity reported for these chelating agents.

B. FERRIC-DEPENDENT FORMATION OF HYDROXYL RADICALS

Although chelates of Fe(II) generally react much faster with H_2O_2 than do Fe(III) chelates, the latter reaction cannot always be ignored. Gutteridge[53,54] was the first to demonstrate experimentally, using the deoxyribose assay (Section IV.A) for OH˙, that certain ferric chelates react with H_2O_2 to form OH˙, in a process involving O_2^{-} and almost completely inhibitable by SOD. Ferric-EDTA and ferric-nitrilotriacetic acid (NTA) were especially effective.[53,54] However, some scientists have been skeptical. Aruoma et al.,[55] therefore, studied the mechanism of damage to isolated DNA by various ferric chelates in the presence of H_2O_2. The pattern of damage to the DNA bases confirmed the production of OH˙. Ferric-NTA produced the most DNA base damage in the presence of H_2O_2, and SOD had a marked inhibitory effect.[55] It is disturbing to note that NTA, previously a common constituent of detergents, is now widely distributed in the environment.[56]

III. SOURCES OF IRON FOR FENTON CHEMISTRY *IN VIVO*

The importance of iron ions in mediating oxidative damage (e.g., Table 1) naturally leads to the question as to what forms of iron might be available to catalyze radical reactions *in vivo*.

It must not be forgotten that iron is a remarkably useful metal in nature; we depend on it to transport (hemoglobin), store (myoglobin), and utilize (cytochromes, cytochrome oxidase) oxygen for respiration. Iron is also an essential component in the active sites of many enzymes (e.g., aconitase, proline hydroxylase), including enzymes that protect against reactive oxygen species (iron-containing SOD enzymes in bacteria and some higher plants, catalase in most aerobic organisms). In mammals, iron is absorbed from the gut and enters the plasma attached to the protein transferrin, which binds 2 mol of Fe(III) per mole of protein with very high affinity at pH 7.4. In plasma from healthy human adults, the average iron loading of transferrin is 20 to 30% of maximum. Hence, there is an excess of iron-binding capacity, which means that the content of "free" ionic iron in plasma should be effectively nil, a result confirmed by experiments using the bleomycin assay (Section III.D). A protein similar to transferrin, known as lactoferrin, is found in several body fluids and in milk and is produced by phagocytic cells. Lactoferrin also binds 2 mol of Fe(III) per mole of protein.

Transferrin enters cells by endocytosis, and the pH of the vacuole containing it is then lowered. This causes release of iron from the protein. The unloaded transferrin (apotransferrin) is ejected from the cell, and the iron ions released from it are used in the synthesis of intracellular iron-containing proteins.[57] Excess iron is stored in the protein ferritin. At present, the chemical nature and subcellular distribution of the "iron transit pool" within cells are completely unknown, except that the pool seems to be kept very small.[57] Fuller details of mammalian iron metabolism may be found in Chapters 1 through 6.

We thus have several forms of iron *in vivo* that could potentially act as catalysts of Fenton chemistry.

A. LACTOFERRIN AND TRANSFERRIN

Early reports that iron-loaded lactoferrin (2 mol of Fe(III) per mole of protein) is an efficient catalyst of OH˙ radical formation from O_2^- and H_2O_2 have now been disproved, as have similar claims for transferrin (reviewed in References 26 and 58). Indeed, from simple chemical considerations, it would be expected that little or none of any OH˙ formed by iron ions attached to a protein could escape from the protein and be measurable outside it: the OH˙ would attack the protein instead, in view of the very high reactivity of this radical. In some earlier studies claiming that lactoferrin and transferrin are catalysts of OH˙ production, it is likely that iron ions became detached from the protein during the assay, and these released iron ions were the real catalysts of the observed OH˙ production.[26,58]

Further evidence that lactoferrin does not participate in OH˙ generation is provided by the observation that activated human neutrophils do not produce OH˙ (as detected by spin trapping, aromatic hydroxylation, or deoxyribose degradation) unless iron ions are added to the reaction mixture, even though activated neutrophils release O_2^-, H_2O_2, and lactoferrin extracellularly.[59,60] Indeed, it has been argued that one function of the secretion of lactoferrin by activated neutrophils is to minimize OH˙ production in the surrounding environment, by chelating "catalytic" iron ions.[59,61] Lactoferrin and transferrin are similar in many respects, but a major difference in their properties is that iron can be released from transferrin at pH values of 5.6 and below, whereas lactoferrin holds on to its iron down to pH values of 4.0 or less. The author has argued[61] that the low pH that can be produced in the microenvironment of activated phagocytic cells adhering to a surface could lead to release of iron from transferrin, and that one biological role of lactoferrin could be to bind some of this iron at low pH values as a protective mechanism. The ability of lactoferrin to resist damage by oxidants generated at sites of inflammation[62] is consistent with such a role.

B. FERRITIN AND HEMOSIDERIN

Ferritin is often regarded as a safe storage form of iron, yet ferritin has been shown to stimulate the formation of $OH^{\cdot}$ radicals from $O_2^{\cdot -}$ and H_2O_2. This is not due to a reaction with the intact protein: superoxide mobilizes iron ions from ferritin, leading to iron-catalyzed production of $OH^{\cdot}$ radicals.[63] A rate constant of $2 \times 10^6 \ M^{-1} \ s^{-1}$ has been calculated for reaction of $O_2^{\cdot -}$ with horse spleen ferritin.[64] Hence, generation of $O_2^{\cdot -}$ and H_2O_2 adjacent to ferritin deposits could cause cell damage.[63] However, the amount of iron that can be released from ferritin by $O_2^{\cdot -}$ is only a very small percentage of the total iron stored in the protein,[65] i.e., ferritin-bound iron is much safer than an equivalent amount of "free" iron.

O'Connell et al.[66] have shown that hemosiderin iron can also participate in $OH^{\cdot}$ generation, although hemosiderin is usually less active than ferritin because it is more difficult to mobilize iron from it. Perhaps conversion of stored ferritin to hemosiderin (as happens in human liver during iron overload disease) is biologically advantageous.[66] The precise "availability" of iron in hemosiderin depends on the type of iron core present.[67]

Since transferrin will not stimulate free-radical reactions and most iron in human blood plasma is bound to this protein, it follows that in plasma from healthy humans no iron is available to stimulate free-radical reactions.[21,26,68] Indeed, plasma does not stimulate lipid peroxidation or $OH^{\cdot}$ formation: it can inhibit them by binding any necessary irons.[21,26,68] This lack of free iron also prevents the growth of most types of bacteria.[69] Unlike cells, human plasma and other human body fluids contain only very low levels of antioxidant defense enzymes, such as catalase, SOD, or glutathione peroxidase.[68] Gutteridge and I have argued[21,26,68] that some of the $O_2^{\cdot -}$ and H_2O_2 generated in extracellular compartments (e.g., by phagocytes, endothelial cells, or lymphocytes[13-16]) may be employed for useful purposes, such as cellular signaling and regulation of vascular tone (Section II). Use of $O_2^{\cdot -}$ and H_2O_2 in this way would not necessarily be dangerous because, in the absence of catalytic metal ions, they cannot lead to formation of $OH^{\cdot}$ and other highly oxidizing species. Copper ions are similarly unavailable in human plasma;[70] most or all of plasma copper is attached to the protein ceruloplasmin, which has antioxidant properties (reviewed in Reference 71). Thus, a major form of antioxidant defense in human plasma is the prevention of transition metal ions from participating in the generation of reactive oxygen species.[21,68] For example, ascorbic acid has been claimed to be "the most important antioxidant" in plasma.[72] However, ascorbate can only exert its antioxidant actions[72,73] in the absence of transition metal ions. Ascorbate/iron ion or ascorbate/copper ion mixtures are cytotoxic.[26,73]

C. HEMOGLOBIN AND MYOGLOBIN

Hemoglobin is transported in erythrocytes, which are rich in the antioxidant defense enzymes, catalase, SOD, and glutathione peroxidase. However, isolated hemoglobin[74,75] (and myoglobin[76]) are degraded on exposure to excess H_2O_2 to release catalytic iron ions from the heme ring. In addition, both proteins react with H_2O_2 to form an oxidizing species capable of stimulating lipid peroxidation (reviewed in Reference 77). In the case of hemoglobin, the chemical nature of this oxidizing species is not yet known. Reaction of H_2O_2 with the protein probably generates a heme ferryl species plus an amino acid radical. In the case of myoglobin, it has been suggested that a tyrosine peroxyl radical, capable of abstracting hydrogen and initiating lipid peroxidation, is formed upon exposure of the myoglobin to H_2O_2.[78,79]

Thus, as Figure 1 emphasizes, hemoglobin outside the erythrocyte is potentially a dangerous protein.[75,80,81] For example, spasm of cerebral arteries can be a significant late complication of hemorrhagic stroke, and it has been proposed that release of hemoglobin from erythrocytes in the clot and subsequent free-radical reactions are involved.[80] Similarly, the reaction of myoglobin with H_2O_2 has been suggested to be one mechanism contributing to myocardial reperfusion injury.[82] Prolonged exercise, or severe trauma to muscles (as in "crush injury"),[83] can cause release of myoglobin into the circulation, where it would be capable of stimulating free-radical reactions if H_2O_2 were available. By contrast with its stimulatory effect upon reactions dependent upon free metal ions, ascorbate usually inhibits peroxidation stimulated by heme protein/H_2O_2 mixtures, because it acts as an alternative substrate for oxidation.[77,84]

D. 'SIMPLE' IRON CHELATES

As explained at the beginning of this section, a small transit pool of iron, probably in a low molecular mass form, is present within mammalian cells. The exact chemical nature of this pool is not clear, but it may represent iron ions attached to phosphate esters (such as ATP, ADP, or GTP), to organic acids (such as citrate) and perhaps to the polar head groups of membrane lipids, or to DNA. All these iron complexes are capable[25,26,29,85,86] of decomposing H_2O_2 to form OH·. For example, at least some of the DNA damage caused by exposing mammalian cells to oxidative stress may involve OH· generation by metal ions bound upon, or very close to, the DNA.[25,42]

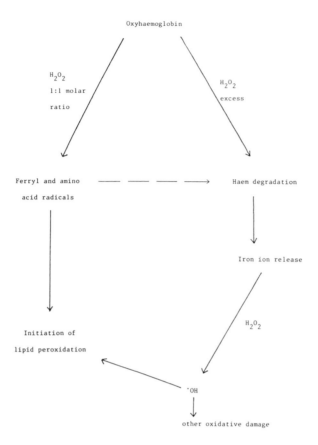

FIGURE 1. Hemoglobin — a dangerous protein. Hemoglobin is normally transported inside erythrocytes, cells rich in antioxidant defense enzymes. Free hemoglobin is very sensitive to attack by H_2O_2, potentially resulting in an exacerbation of oxidative damage.

E. THE BLEOMYCIN ASSAY

Gutteridge et al. (reviewed in Reference 87) developed the bleomycin assay as a first attempt to measure the availability of iron, in a form catalytic for free-radical reactions, in human body fluids. The assay is based on the ability of the glycopeptide antitumor antibiotic bleomycin to degrade DNA in the presence of an iron salt, O_2, and a suitable reducing agent. During this reaction, base-propenals are released and rapidly break down to yield malondialdehyde. Binding of the bleomycin-iron-O_2 complex to DNA makes the reaction site specific, and antioxidants rarely interfere. The bleomycin assay, therefore, can be applied directly to biological fluids, where it detects iron available to the bleomycin molecule.[87] The assay requires stringent removal of adventitious iron associated with laboratory water, buffers, other reagents, and the bleomycin molecule itself. This can be done by using Chelex resin or, more efficiently, by employing the iron-binding properties of transferrins.[88] Iron detected in the assay is then a measure of iron available from the biological sample to bleomycin, and can be measured at concentrations as low as 0.5 μM. Application of the bleomycin assay shows that blood serum or plasma prepared from healthy human subjects does not contain iron available to bleomycin.[87,89] This agrees with observations that the bleomycin assay, as usually carried out, does not measure iron bound to the transferrin, lactoferrin, or ferritin proteins in plasma or serum.[87]

When the bleomycin assay is applied to plasma or serum from patients with iron overload, resulting from the disease idiopathic hemochromatosis, bleomycin-detectable iron is present,[87,89-91] and its concentration is highly correlated to that of serum ferritin.[91] As the iron overload is brought under control by phlebotomy therapy, concentrations of bleomycin-detectable iron decline.[91] Studies by high-performance liquid chromatography (HPLC) and proton Hahn spin-echo nuclear magnetic resonance (NMR) suggest that at least some, and perhaps all, of the bleomycin-detectable iron in the plasma of these patients is in a low molecular mass form, existing as complexes with citrate, and possible as ternary iron-citrate-acetate complexes.[90] Whereas plasma from healthy humans inhibits iron-dependent free-radical reactions, largely because of the iron-binding capacity present, plasma from iron-overloaded hemochromatosis patients stimulates such reactions.[89] Thus, at least in the case of iron overload, the forms of iron measured by the bleomycin assay do seem capable of stimulating free-radical reactions.

Bleomycin-detectable iron has also been measured in human sweat,[87] in some cerebrospinal fluid (CSF) samples,[87,92] in synovial fluid from human knee joints,[87,93] and in extracts of several bacterial strains.[87] About 40% of synovial fluid samples withdrawn from the knee joints of patients with active rheumatoid arthritis contain bleomycin-detectable iron; the fluids in which iron is measurable have lower total antioxidant activity than the synovial fluids which register negative in the bleomycin assay.[93] Further work is needed to determine the precise molecular nature of bleomycin-detectable iron in human sweat, CSF, and synovial fluid, since the assay measures only iron that can be chelated by the bleomycin molecule under the assay conditions employed.

F. SUMMARY: WHAT IS THE SOURCE OF CATALYTIC IRON *IN VIVO?*

When the ideas that the toxicity of O_2^- and H_2O_2 involves OH· were first being formulated, there was much debate about the availability of catalytic metal ions *in vivo,* with several investigators being dubious about their existence (reviewed in References 21, 26, and 29). The picture emerging is now much clearer. Organisms take great care in the handling of iron,[69] using transport proteins such as transferrin and storage proteins such as ferritin and minimizing the size of the intracellular iron pool.[57] Indeed this sequestration of transition metals may be regarded as an important contribution to antioxidant defenses.[21,26,68] However, oxidative stress can itself provide the iron necessary for Fenton chemistry (Section III.B and C), for example, by mobilizing iron from ferritin (via O_2^-) or by degrading heme proteins to release iron (via H_2O_2).

The availability of iron to stimulate free-radical reactions *in vivo* is very limited. For example, concentrations of bleomycin-detectable iron in samples of human body fluids are often 0 and rarely greater than 3 μM, except in iron-overloaded patients.[87,89] Gutteridge and I have thus argued that formation of OH· and of other damaging radicals *in vivo* may be limited by the supply of transition metals.[1,21,26,43,66,68,87] Thus, if no catalytic metal ions are available, then O_2^- and H_2O_2 will have limited, if any, damaging effects. This principle underlines the importance of examining the availability and distribution of catalytic metal ions in explaining oxidative damage to cells. In general, iron and copper ions act to convert poorly reactive species (O_2^-, H_2O_2, thiols, lipid hydroperoxides) into more reactive, cytotoxic ones (OH·, ferryl, aldehydes, etc.) as summarized in Table 2.

G. TISSUE INJURY AND IRON-DEPENDENT FREE-RADICAL REACTIONS

Tissue injury, by any mechanism, has the potential to stimulate free-radical reactions, one reason being that cell destruction liberates intracellular transition metal ions into the extracellular environment. This increased "decompartmentalization" of iron ions has been demonstrated after chemotherapy in patients with acute myeloid leukemia,[94] in dogs subjected to hemorrhagic shock,[95] and in patients with fulminant hepatic failure.[96] Some areas of the human brain (e.g., the globus pallidus and the substantia nigra) are low in iron, yet cerebrospinal fluid has no significant iron-binding capacity because its content of transferrin is very low.[92,97] Most brain iron is protein bound, but little is known of its molecular nature.[97] Iron seems to play essential roles in learning and memory, perhaps because iron ions are required for the correct binding of certain neurotransmitters to their receptors.[97]

Although a high content of iron may be essential for brain function,[97] its presence means that any injury to brain cells can result in release of iron ions that stimulate free-radical reactions. Homogenates of the brain peroxidize very rapidly *in vitro:* indeed, peroxidation of ox brain homogenates has been used for many years as an assay to measure antioxidant activity, and the peroxidation is largely inhibited by several iron-chelating agents.[98] Ischemic or traumatic injury might be thought of as essentially causing a partial disruption of brain tissue (partial homogenization) that stimulates free-radical reactions.[99]

In addition, there is a high concentration of ascorbic acid in the gray and white matter of the CNS. The choroid plexus has a specific active transport system that raises ascorbate concentrations in the cerebrospinal fluid to greater than the plasma level, and neural cells have a second transport system that

TABLE 2
Role of Metal Ions in Converting Less Reactive to More Reactive Species

$\left.\begin{array}{l} O_2^- \\ H_2O_2 \end{array}\right\}$ $\xrightarrow{\text{Fe/Cu}^a}$ OH·

Lipid peroxides (ROOH) $\xrightarrow{\text{Fe/Cu}^b}$ RO· (alkoxyl), RO₂· (peroxyl), cytotoxic aldehyde

Thiols (RSH) $\xrightarrow{\text{Fe/Cu plus } O_2^c}$ O_2^-, H_2O_2, thiyl (RS·), OH·

NAD(P)H $\xrightarrow{\text{Fe/Cu plus } O_2^c}$ NAD(P)·, O_2^-, H_2O_2, OH·

Ascorbic acid $\xrightarrow{\text{Cu/Fe}^d}$ Semidehydroascorbate radicals, OH·, H_2O_2, degradation products of ascorbate

Catecholamines, related autoxidizable molecules $\xrightarrow{\text{Fe/Cu/Mn plus } O_2^c}$ O_2^-, H_2O_2, OH·, semiquinones (or other radicals derived from the oxidizing compounds)

[a] The iron or copper catalyzed Haber-Weiss reaction.

[b] Lipid peroxide decomposition is metal ion-dependent, and eventually produces highly cytotoxic products such as 4-hydroxy-2,3-*trans*-nonenal, and less toxic ones such as malondialdehyde.

[c] Most so-called autoxidations are stimulated by traces of transition metal ions, and proceed by free-radical mechanisms.

[d] Copper ions are especially effective in decomposing ascorbic acid, and ascorbate/copper or ascorbate/iron mixtures are cytotoxic.

concentrates intracellular ascorbate even more.[100] Ascorbic acid in the absence of transition metal ions has antioxidant properties, but if catalytic iron were released in the CNS as a result of injury,[99] ascorbic acid might then stimulate free-radical reactions within the brain and CSF.[101-104] Thus, there is considerable current interest in the possibility that antioxidants and iron-chelating agents might be clinically useful in diminishing tissue injury resulting from ischemia or trauma of the CNS.[99,104] (See Chapter 12.)

It is also possible that iron-dependent free-radical reactions contribute to damage of the substantia nigra observed in patients suffering from Parkinson's disease. Thus, Dexter et al.[105] have reported increased nigral iron and decreased brain ferritin levels in Parkinsonian patients, and they speculate that increased iron-dependent lipid peroxidation could contribute to cell destruction. Riederer et al.[106,107] reported increased nigral iron and increased ferritin in Parkinsonian brains, as well as decreased reduced glutathione (GSH). Of course, it must be remembered that nigral cell injury (by any mechanism) could lead to iron release and more free-radical reactions, even if the cause of the injury had nothing to do with free radicals. The question that remains to be answered is "does any such secondary radical generation contribute significantly to the disease pathology?" (See also Chapters 14 and 15.)

IV. SITE SPECIFICITY AND FENTON CHEMISTRY

High energy irradiation of aqueous solutions produces a substantial yield of hydroxyl radicals, which can be removed by added hydroxyl radical scavengers at rates that depend only on their concentrations and on the second-order rate constants of these scavengers for reaction with $OH^{\cdot}$. Indeed, competition kinetics are employed in this way to determine rate constants for reaction of scavengers with $OH^{\cdot}$, using the technique of pulse radiolysis. Using this approach, the kinetics are usually simple since the $OH^{\cdot}$ radicals are produced in free solution and can react directly and competitively with any added scavenger. However, when these same scavengers, with their known rate constants, are added to Fenton chemistry reactions involving biological molecules, they do not always inhibit $OH^{\cdot}$ radical damage to a detector molecule (a chemical added to the reaction that will be damaged by $OH^{\cdot}$ radicals in some easily measurable way) to the extent predicted from those rate constants. This important anomaly can often be explained by the concept of site specificity. Since iron ions cannot exist free in aqueous solution, they must either bind to a biological molecule, a buffer, or some other constituent of the reaction mixture, or else they will eventually precipitate out of solution as polymerized ferric hydroxides and oxyhydroxides. The damage due to $OH^{\cdot}$ will thus be "directed onto" the site of iron binding.

The biological implications of site specificity of $OH^{\cdot}$ formation are profound. I have already explained that a major determinant of the actual toxicity of O_2^- and H_2O_2 to cells may well be the availability and location of metal

TABLE 3
Some Problems in the Use of Hydroxyl Radical Scavengers in Biological Systems

An inhibition by a single scavenger proves nothing, especially if that scavenger is thiourea, which reacts with O_2^-, H_2O_2, HOCl, and alkoxyl radicals, weakly inhibits xanthine oxidase, and may also chelate metal ions necessary for OH· production. Ethanol also reacts with alkoxyl radicals, although mannitol and formate do not. A range of scavengers should be used and the inhibition they exert correlated with the published rate constants for reaction of the scavengers with OH·.

The scavenger and the molecule being used to detect OH· should show competition kinetics, i.e., they should be competing for the same species.

Reaction of OH· radical with a scavenger produces a secondary radical that might itself do damage in certain systems. For example, formate and ethanol radicals can attack serum albumin and azide radical attacks tryptophan and tyrosine. This may sometimes account for failure to protect by one scavenger.

If buffers such as Tris or "Goods buffers" are present, they can be attacked by OH· to give buffer-derived radicals whose properties must be considered.

OH· radical is often formed in biological systems by reaction of H_2O_2 with metal ions bound at specific sites. The OH· then reacts with the binding molecule and is not accessible to added scavengers of OH·. For example, H_2O_2-dependent damage to the DNA of mammalian cells may be due to reaction of H_2O_2 with metal ions bound to the DNA.

Note: Based on discussions in References 1 and 26.

ion catalysts of OH· radical formation. If, for example, catalytic iron salts are bound to DNA or to membrane lipids, introduction of H_2O_2 and O_2^- will, in the first case, fragment the DNA and in the other could initiate lipid peroxidation (Section IV). Indeed, the use of OH· scavengers in biological systems is fraught with problems, some of which are listed in Table 3.

The type of biological damage produced by site specific OH· radical generation will often not resemble that produced by attack of free OH· (e.g., generated by ionizing radiation) upon the biomolecule. This has been demonstrated for carbohydrates,[108] nucleic acids,[25,30] and proteins.[109,110]

A. THE DEOXYRIBOSE ASSAY

The difference between damage to molecules by OH· generated in free solution and by OH· generated by metal ions bound to a target can be illustrated by studies using deoxyribose, introduced in 1981 as a simple detector molecule for OH· generated in biological systems.[111] The pentose sugar 2-deoxy-D-ribose is attacked by OH· radicals to yield a mixture of products. On heating with thiobarbituric acid at low pH, some or all of these products react to form a pink chromogen that can be measured by its absorbance at 532 nm; this chromogen is indistinguishable from a thiobarbituric acid-malondialdehyde (TBA-MDA) adduct.[111,112] Generation of the pink TBA-MDA adduct can be used as a simple assay for OH· generation in biological systems, provided that suitable control experiments are performed.[73,111]

If deoxyribose is incubated with H_2O_2 and a ferrous-EDTA complex (or a ferric-EDTA complex in the presence of a reducing agent, such as ascorbate or O_2^-), the resulting deoxyribose degradation to TBA-reactive material is inhibited by any added scavenger of $OH^{\cdot}$ to an extent that depends only on the concentration of scavenger relative to deoxyribose and on the scavenger's second-order rate constant for reaction with $OH^{\cdot}$.[26,73,112] It seems that, when $OH^{\cdot}$ is generated by reaction of ferrous EDTA with H_2O_2, any $OH^{\cdot}$ that escapes scavenging by the EDTA enters free solution and is equally accessible to deoxyribose and to any added scavenger.[73,112] Indeed, the deoxyribose assay in the presence of ferric-EDTA, H_2O_2, and a reducing agent provides a simple method for determining rate constants for the reaction of substrates with $OH^{\cdot}$, which has been used in several studies.[73,113]

If deoxyribose is incubated with H_2O_2 and Fe^{2+} (or Fe[III] plus a reductant) in the absence of EDTA, it is still degraded into products that can react to form a TBA-MDA chromogen. However, some $OH^{\cdot}$ scavengers (such as ethanol, formate, dimethylsulfoxide, and 2-hydroxyethylpiperazine-N'-2-ethanesulfonic acid [HEPES]) no longer inhibit the deoxyribose degradation whereas others (such as mannitol, thiourea, and hydroxychloroquine) still do. Two possible explanations of this observation have been advanced. One is that the deoxyribose-degrading species is not $OH^{\cdot}$ but some other oxidant, such as ferryl.[29] It is known that oxidants other than $OH^{\cdot}$ can degrade deoxyribose to a TBA-reactive material. For example, such a deoxyribose-degrading oxidant is produced by reaction of human oxyhemoglobin with equimolar H_2O_2.[75] An alternative explanation, which the author prefers, is that unchelated iron ions added to deoxyribose-containing reaction mixtures become bound to deoxyribose. When the bound iron ions react with H_2O_2, some or all of the $OH^{\cdot}$ formed immediately attack the deoxyribose, and scavengers cannot easily prevent this site-specific attack.[73,112]

Consistent with such an explanation, evidence for a weak binding of both ferrous and ferric iron to deoxyribose at physiological pH has been obtained (reviewed in Reference 73). Further, the metal-binding ability of a compound has been shown to be a major determinant of its ability to inhibit deoxyribose degradation in the presence of H_2O_2 and Fe^{2+} (or ferric salts plus a reducing agent). For example, citrate (which chelates iron) is a poor scavenger of $OH^{\cdot}$ relative to most other molecules (rate constant about $10^7 \ M^{-1} \ s^{-1}$) but citrate is a good inhibitor of deoxyribose degradation in the presence of H_2O_2, $FeCl_3$, and ascorbate.[113] Indeed, the deoxyribose assay has been used to test the ability of several substances to interfere with site-specific iron-dependent generation of $OH^{\cdot}$ radicals.[73,113]

V. IRON AND LIPID PEROXIDATION

Imposition of oxidative stress upon mammalian cells leads to several metabolic dysfunctions, including DNA damage, depletion of adenosine 5'-triphosphate (ATP), GSH oxidation, rises in intracellular free Ca^{2+}, enzyme inactivation, and lipid peroxidation.[23,25,26,44,114] Transition metal ions are intimately associated with many of these events, but they play an especially important role in the process of lipid peroxidation.[26,115,116]

There is considerable confusion in the literature about the role played by iron in stimulating lipid peroxidation, but the basics are simple. Iron ions react with H_2O_2 to form OH·, which is known to be capable of initiating peroxidation, by abstracting hydrogen atoms from fatty acid side chains of lipids, as demonstrated using OH· generated by radiolysis of water.[1,4,26] However, most scientists[1,26,115-117] find that addition of catalase or scavengers of OH· to isolated cellular membrane fractions (e.g., plasma membrane fractions, microsomes) or to liposomes undergoing peroxidation in the presence of ferrous salts or of ferric salts plus reducing agents (such as ascorbate) does not inhibit the peroxidation. This lack of effect is despite the fact that OH· radicals can usually be detected in the reaction mixtures by such techniques as aromatic hydroxylation, spin trapping, or the deoxyribose method, and detection of these OH· radicals is inhibited by catalase or scavengers. It follows that OH· is being generated in the reaction mixtures, but is not required for peroxidation to proceed.[117] How can this be explained?

It is unlikely that the lack of action of OH· scavengers means that the required OH· formation is site specific, involving iron ions bound to the membrane, so that any OH· formed reacts immediately with the membrane components and is not available for scavenging. Membrane-bound iron certainly does participate in lipid peroxidation.[115,118] However, a source of H_2O_2 would still be required, and thus catalase should still inhibit. The fact that it does not has led several scientists to suggest that first-chain initiation of lipid peroxidation in membrane systems incubated with iron salts in the presence of O_2 is achieved by reactive species other than OH·.[115,116] Ferryl is one possibility. However, ferryl formation by reaction of iron salts with H_2O_2 would still require a source of H_2O_2, and inhibition by peroxide-removing enzymes such as catalase would be expected. Perferryl could conceivably be involved. However, what is known of the chemistry of perferryl complexes suggests that they would be insufficiently reactive to abstract H or to insert oxygen directly into fatty acid side chains, although their participation cannot be ruled out.[119]

Studies on the kinetics of microsomal or liposomal lipid peroxidation in the presence of ferrous and/or ferric salts led Minotti and Aust[116] to propose that initiation of peroxidation requires an iron(II)-iron(III)-oxygen complex, or at least a specific critical 1:1 ratio of Fe^{2+} to Fe(III). This proposal was based on observations that Fe^{2+}-dependent peroxidation in membrane systems proceeds most rapidly in the presence of Fe(III). Indeed, comparable experimental results have been obtained by several other groups (discussed in Reference 120). Attempts to isolate the Fe(II)-Fe(III) complex have not been successful, however, and it has been observed that Pb^{2+} and Al(III) can replace Fe(III) in stimulating Fe^{2+}-dependent peroxidation in liposomes and microsomes.[120] If other metal ions can replace Fe(III), then a specific Fe(II)-Fe(III) complex cannot be required for the initiation of peroxidation. The ability of Al(III) and Pb^{2+} ions to stimulate iron-dependent lipid peroxidation might be relevant to the neurotoxicity of these two metals.[121] (See Chapter 15.)

It has long been known (e.g., Reference 122) that iron plays a second important role in lipid peroxidation. Pure lipid hydroperoxides are fairly stable at physiological temperatures, but, in the presence of transition metal complexes, especially iron salts, their decomposition is greatly accelerated. Thus, ferrous iron can react with lipid peroxides in a way similar to its reaction with H_2O_2: it causes fission of O—O bonds to form alkoxyl (often shortened to alkoxy) radicals by the overall reaction:

$$R\text{—OOH} + Fe^{2+}\text{—complex} \rightarrow Fe^{3+}\text{—complex} + R\text{—O}^{\cdot} + OH^- \quad (16)$$

lipid   alkoxyl

hydroperoxide   radical

Iron(III) can form both peroxyl and alkoxyl radicals.[123] The overall equation below probably represents the sum of several stages:

$$R\text{—OOH} + Fe^{3+}\text{—complex} \rightarrow RO_2^{\cdot} + Fe^{2+}\text{—complex} + H^+ \quad (17)$$

peroxyl

radical

The resulting Fe^{2+} complex can then react with R—OOH to give alkoxyl radicals.

The reactions of ferrous ions with lipid hydroperoxides may be faster than their reactions with H_2O_2, depending on the ligand to which the iron is bound.[26,85] Predictably, reactions of Fe(III) with hydroperoxides seem much slower than those of Fe(II), but precise rate constants have not yet been determined.[117] Thus, in general, iron(II) and its complexes stimulate membrane peroxidation more than iron(III) does. This may be explained by the greater solubility of Fe^{2+} salts in solution, the faster rate at which lipid peroxides are decomposed by Fe^{2+}, and the higher reactivity of the alkoxyl radicals thus produced. Hence, the rate of peroxidation of purified membrane lipids or microsomal fractions in the presence of Fe(III) complexes is usually increased by the addition of reducing agents. Effective reductants include ascorbic acid, certain thiols, O_2^-, and, in the case of microsomes, reduced nicotinamide adenine dinucleotide phosphate (NADPH) to provide a source of electrons for NADPH-cytochrome P-450 reductase.[115] The variable effects of certain chelating agents (e.g., EDTA, DTPA) on lipid peroxidation can, at least in part, be explained by their ability to influence these different reactions. For example, EDTA can often stimulate the reaction of iron ions with H_2O_2, while slowing their reaction with lipid peroxides.[124]

Commercially available lipids are all contaminated with lipid peroxides (e.g., Reference 125), so that liposomes or micelles made from them will already contain traces of such peroxides (the purchase of high-purity [99.9%] fatty acids is no safeguard, since purity refers to contamination with other fatty acids, not to peroxide content). When cells are injured, lipid peroxidation is favored and traces of lipid peroxides are formed enzymatically in tissues by cyclooxygenase and lipoxygenase enzymes. Thus, membrane fractions isolated from disrupted cells should also contain some lipid peroxide.

When iron salts are added to isolated membrane fractions, the lipid peroxides present will be decomposed by Reactions 16 and 17 to generate peroxyl and alkoxyl radicals. Both radicals can abstract H$^\cdot$ and propagate lipid peroxidation. Thus, there is no need for OH$^\cdot$ formation and first-chain initiation; the added metal ions are doing no more than stimulating further lipid peroxidation by breaking down lipid peroxides. It is not impossible that the putative abilities of ferryl, perferryl, and Fe(II)-Fe(III)-O_2 complexes to initiate lipid peroxidation are explicable by the abilities of these complexes to degrade traces of lipid peroxides in the membrane systems that were being studied. Experiments on peroxide-free lipid systems (which are very difficult to obtain[125a]) are urgently required to establish firmly whether various iron-oxygen complexes are really capable of abstracting hydrogen. The author feels that more such chemical studies, and fewer repetitive biochemical experiments on isolated membrane and lipid fractions will lead to more progress in this field.

We saw in Section II that low-molecular-mass iron complexes can react with H_2O_2 to form OH$^\cdot$, but that reaction of most iron proteins with H_2O_2 and/or O_2^- does not result in formation of OH$^\cdot$ detectable outside the protein, unless iron is released from the protein under the reaction conditions being used. The range of iron complexes that can stimulate lipid peroxidation is wider. Thus, not only are Fe^{2+} salts and simple complexes (e.g., Fe^{2+}-adenosine 5′-diphosphate [ADP]) effective, but also (under certain circumstances) free heme, met- and oxyhemoglobin, metmyoglobin, cytochromes (including cytochromes c and P-450), horseradish peroxidase, and lactoperoxidase (reviewed in References 1, 26, 74, 115, 126-128). Ferritin stimulates lipid peroxidation to an extent proportional to the amount of iron it contains,[129] whereas hemosiderin usually stimulates much less strongly (on a unit iron basis),[126] although this might depend on the exact type of iron core present in the hemosiderin studied.

Sometimes the stimulation of lipid peroxidation by iron proteins is due to a release of iron from the protein under the conditions of the experiment. For example, stimulation of lipid peroxidation in liposomes by ferritin or hemosiderin is almost completely inhibitable by desferrioxamine, suggesting that it is mediated by released iron ions.[126,129] Stimulation of peroxidation by myoglobin and hemoglobin can involve both iron release from the protein by peroxides[74-76] and reactions brought about by the intact protein itself, such as initiation by tyrosine peroxyl radicals[78,79] (see Section III.C). Even catalase (a heme-containing protein) is weakly effective in stimulating peroxide decomposition under certain circumstances, an action that has sometimes caused problems in attempts to use catalase as a probe for the role of H_2O_2 in peroxidizing lipid systems.[130]

By contrast, iron correctly bound to the two specific iron-binding sites of transferrin or lactoferrin does not promote decomposition of either H_2O_2 or of lipid hydroperoxides, i.e., iron bound to these two proteins is safe in terms of inability to catalyze free-radical reactions (Section III.A).

VI. CONCLUSION

Transition metal ions are important promoters of free-radical reactions: they convert less-reactive to more-reactive species (summarized in Table 2). Hence, organisms have evolved to handle them carefully, and thus the availability of metal ions catalytic for free-radical reactions is very limited *in vivo* in healthy subjects. Their location and concentration control, to a considerable extent, the damage that can be done by oxidative stress. An inspection of the pathology suffered by patients with prolonged iron overload disease (Table 4) illustrates how important this metal ion sequestration is for health. In tissue injury and human disease, however, metal ions may become more available. Hence, antioxidants of several types, including metal ion chelators (Table 1), may have therapeutic benefit.[49,131]

TABLE 4
Some Consequences of
Prolonged Iron Overload in
Hemochromatosis

(In Descending Order of Frequency)
Hepatomegaly
Skin pigmentation
Joint inflammation
Diabetes mellitus
Cardiac abnormalities
Testicular atrophy
Peripheral neuritis
Hepatoma

Note: In newly diagnosed iron-overloaded hemochromatosis patients
serum nonheme iron is elevated,
transferrin saturation is at or close
to 100%, and bleomycin-detectable iron is often present. Heart
and pancreatic β cells are highly
sensitive to free-radical damage,[1]
and iron is intimately involved in
the pathology of chronic joint inflammation.[1,31,61]

Data abstracted from McLaren et al., *CRC
Crit. Rev. Clin. Lab. Sci.*, 19, 205, 1985.

REFERENCES

1. **Halliwell, B. and Gutteridge, J. M. C.,** *Free Radicals in Biology and Medicine,* 2nd ed., Clarendon Press, Oxford, 1989.
2. **Sies, H.,** *Oxidative Stress: Oxidants and Antioxidants,* Academic Press, New York, 1991.
3. **Fridovich, I.,** Superoxide dismutase: an adaptation to a paramagnetic gas, *J. Biol. Chem.,* 264, 7761, 1989.
4. **Von Sonntag, C.,** *The Chemical Basis of Radiation Biology,* Taylor & Francis, London, 1987.
5. **Saran, M., Michel, C., and Bors, W.,** Reactions of NO with O_2^-. Implications for the action of endothelium-derived relaxing factor, *Free Radical Res. Commun.,* 10, 221, 1990.
6. **Laurindo, F. R. M., da Luz, P. L., Uint, L., Rocha, T. F., and Jaeger, R. G.,** Evidence for superoxide radical-dependent coronary vasospasm after angioplasty in intact dogs, *Circulation,* 83, 1705, 1991.
7. **Radi, R., Beckman, J. S., Bush, K. M., and Freeman, B. A.,** Peroxynitrite oxidation of sulfhydryls. The cytotoxic potential of superoxide and nitric oxide, *J. Biol. Chem.,* 266, 4244, 1990.

8. **Halliwell, B.**, Superoxide, iron, vascular endothelium and reperfusion injury, *Free Radical Res. Commun.*, 5, 315, 1989.

9. **Beckman, J. S., Beckman, T. W., Chen, J., Marshall, P. A., and Freeman, B. A.**, Apparent hydroxy radical production by peroxynitrite: implications for endothelial injury from nitric oxide and superoxide, *Proc. Natl. Acad. Sci. U.S.A.*, 87, 1620, 1990.

10. **Imlay, J. A. and Fridovich, I.**, Assays of metabolic superoxide production in *Escherichia coli*, *J. Biol. Chem.*, 266, 6957, 1991.

11. **Gardner, P. R. and Fridovich, I.**, Superoxide sensitivity of the *Escherichia coli* 6-phosphogluconate dehydratase, *J. Biol. Chem.*, 266, 1478, 1991.

12. **Zhang, Y., Marcillat, O., Giulivi, C., Ernster, L., and Davies, K. J. A.**, The oxidative inactivation of mitochondrial electron transport chain components and ATPase, *J. Biol. Chem.*, 265, 16330, 1990.

13. **Babior, B. M. and Woodman, R. C.**, Chronic granulomatous disease, *Semin. Hematol.*, 27, 247, 1990.

14. **Murrell, G. A. C., Francis, M. J. O., and Bromley, L.**, Modulation of fibroblast proliferation by oxygen free radicals, *Biochem. J.*, 265, 659, 1990.

15. **Maly, F. E.**, The B-lymphocyte: a newly-recognized source of reactive oxygen species with immunoregulatory potential, *Free Radical Res. Commun.*, 8, 143, 1990.

16. **Meier, B., Radeke, H., Selle, S., Raspe, H. H., Sies, H., Resch, K., and Habermehl, G. G.**, Human fibroblasts release reactive oxygen species in response to treatment with synovial fluids from patients suffering from arthritis, *Free Radical Res. Commun.*, 8, 149, 1990.

17. **Touati, D.**, The molecular genetics of superoxide dismutase in *E. coli*. An approach to understanding the biological role and regulation of SODs in relation to other elements of the defence system against oxygen toxicity, *Free Radical Res. Commun.*, 8, 1, 1989.

18. **Chang, E. C., Crawford, B. F., Hong, Z., Bilinski, T., and Kosman, D. J.**, Genetic and biochemical characterization of Cu, Zn superoxide dismutase mutants in *Saccharomyces cerevisiae*, *J. Biol. Chem.*, 266, 4417, 1991.

19. **Dupuy, C., Virion, A., Ohayon, R., Kamiewski, J., Deme, D., and Pommier, J.**, Mechanism of hydrogen peroxide formation catalyzed by NADPH oxidase in thyroid plasma membrane, *J. Biol. Chem.*, 266, 3739, 1991.

20. **Shapiro, B. M.**, The control of oxidative stress at fertilization, *Science*, 252, 533, 1991.

21. **Halliwell, B. and Gutteridge, J. M. C.**, Oxygen free radicals and iron in relation to biology and medicine. Some problems and concepts, *Arch. Biochem. Biophys.*, 246, 501, 1986.

22. **Hyslop, P. A., Hinshaw, D. B., Halsey, W. A., Jr., Schraufstatter, I. U., Sauerheber, R. D., Spragg, R. G., Jackson, J. H., and Cochrane, C. G.**, Mechanisms of oxidant-mediated cell injury. The glycolytic and mitochondrial pathways of ADP phosphorylation are major intracellular targets inactivated by hydrogen peroxide, *J. Biol. Chem.*, 263, 1665, 1988.

23. **Charles, S. A. and Halliwell, B.**, Light-activation of fructose bisphosphatase in isolated spinach chloroplasts and deactivation by hydrogen peroxide. A physiological role for the thioredoxin system, *Planta*, 151, 242, 1981.

24. **Verniquet, F., Gaillard, J., Neuberger, M., and Douce, R.**, Rapid inactivation of aconitase by hydrogen peroxide, *Biochem. J.*, 276, 648, 1991.

25. **Halliwell, B. and Aruoma, O. I.**, DNA damage by oxygen-derived species. Its mechanism and measurement in mammalian systems, *FEBS Lett.*, 281, 9, 1991.

26. **Halliwell, B. and Gutteridge, J. M. C.**, Role of free radicals and catalytic metal ions in human disease: an overview, *Methods Enzymol.*, 186, 1, 1990.

27. **Dixon, W. T. and Norman, R. O. C.**, Free radicals formed during the oxidation and reduction of peroxides, *Nature (London)*, 196, 891, 1962.

28. **Jefcoate, C. R. E. and Norman, R. O. C.**, Electron spin resonance studies, Part XIV, Hydroxylation, Part IV. Reactions of anisole, acetanilide, fluorobenzene and some phenols with the titanium(III)-hydrogen peroxide system, *J. Chem. Soc.*, B, 48, 1968.

29. **Sutton, H. C. and Winterbourn, C. C.,** On the participation of higher oxidation states of iron and copper in Fenton reactions, *Free Radical Biol. Med.,* 6, 53, 1989.

30. **Aruoma, O. I., Halliwell, B., Gajewski, E., and Dizdaroglu, M.,** Copper ion-dependent damage to the bases in DNA in the presence of hydrogen peroxide, *Biochem. J.,* 273, 601, 1991.

31. **Wong, S. F., Halliwell, B., Richmond, R., and Skowroneck, W. R.,** The role of superoxide and hydroxyl radicals in the degradation of hyaluronic acid induced by metal ions and by ascorbic acid, *J. Inorg. Biochem.,* 14, 127, 1981.

32. **Loeb, L. A., James, E. A., Waltersdorph, A. M., and Klebanoff, S. J.,** Mutagenesis by the autoxidation of iron with isolated DNA, *Proc. Natl. Acad. Sci. U.S.A.,* 8, 3918, 1988.

33. **Ortiz de Montellano, P. R.,** Free radical modification of prosthetic heme groups, *Pharmacol. Ther.,* 48, 95, 1990.

34. **Bielski, B. H. J.,** Studies of hypervalent iron, *Free Radical Res. Commun.,* 12, 469, 1991.

35. **Metodiewa, D. and Dunford, H. B.,** The reactions of horseradish peroxidase, lactoperoxidase and myeloperoxidase with enzymatically generated superoxide, *Arch. Biochem. Biophys.,* 272, 245, 1989.

36. **Walling, C.,** The nature of the primary oxidants in oxidations mediated by metal ions, in *Proc. 3rd Int. Symp. Oxidases Related Redox Systems,* King, T. E., Mason, H. S., and Morrison, M., Eds., Pergamon Press, Oxford, 1982, 85.

37. **Gutteridge, J. M. C., Mait, L., and Poyer, L.,** Superoxide dismutase and Fenton chemistry, *Biochem. J.,* 269, 169, 1990.

38. **Halliwell, B., Gutteridge, J. M. C., and Aruoma, O. I.,** The deoxyribose method: a simple test-tube assay for determination of rate constants for reactions of hydroxyl radicals, *Anal. Biochem.,* 165, 215, 1987.

39. **Burkitt, M. J. and Gilbert, B. C.,** The autoxidation of iron(II) in aqueous systems: the effect of iron chelation by physiological, nonphysiological and therapeutic chelators on the generation of reactive oxygen species and the inducement of biomolecular damage, *Free Radical Res. Commun.,* 14, 107, 1991.

40. **Simpson, J. A., Cheeseman, K. H., Smith, S. E., and Dean, R. T.,** Free radical generation by copper ions and hydrogen peroxide, *Biochem. J.,* 254, 519, 1988.

41. **Kyle, M. E., Nakae, D., Sakaida, I., Miccadei, S., and Farber, J. L.,** Endocytosis of superoxide dismutase is required in order for the enzyme to protect hepatocytes from the cytotoxicity of hydrogen peroxide, *J. Biol. Chem.,* 263, 3784, 1988.

42. **Imlay, J. A. and Linn, S.,** DNA damage and oxygen radical toxicity, *Science,* 240, 1302, 1988.

43. **Halliwell, B.,** Oxidants and human disease: some new concepts, *FASEB J.,* 1, 358, 1987.

44. **Orrenius, S., McConkey, D. J., Bellomo, G., and Nicotera, P.,** Role of Ca^{2+} in toxic cell killing, *Trends Pharmacol. Sci.,* 10, 281, 1989.

45. **Ferrali, M., Ciccoli, L., Signorini, C., and Comporti, M.,** Iron release and erythrocyte damage in allyl alcohol intoxication in mice, *Biochem. Pharmacol.,* 40, 1485, 1990.

46. **Gutteridge, J. M. C., Richmond, R., and Halliwell, B.,** Inhibition of the iron-catalyzed formation of hydroxyl radicals from superoxide and of lipid peroxidation by desferrioxamine, *Biochem. J.,* 184, 469, 1979.

47. **Lloyd, J. B., Cable, H., and Rice-Evans, C.,** Evidence that desferrioxamine cannot enter cells by passive diffusion, *Biochem. Pharmacol.,* 41, 1361, 1991.

48. Editorial, Oral iron chelators, *Lancet,* 2, 1016, 1989.

49. **Halliwell, B.,** Protection against tissue damage *in vivo* by desferrioxamine. What is its mechanism of action?, *Free Rad. Biol. Med.,* 7, 645, 1989.

50. **Kontoghiorghes, G. J.,** The study of iron mobilization from transferrin using α-ketohydroxy heteroaromatic chelators, *Biochim. Biophys. Acta,* 869, 141, 1986.

51. **Kontoghiorghes, G. J.,** Iron mobilization from lactoferrin by chelators at physiological pH, *Biochim. Biophys. Acta,* 882, 267, 1986.

52. **Kontoghiorghes, G. J., Jackson, M. J., and Lunec, J.,** *In vitro* screening of iron chelators using models of free radical damage, *Free Radical Res. Commun.,* 2, 115, 1986.

53. **Gutteridge, J. M. C.,** Superoxide dismutase inhibits the superoxide-driven Fenton reaction at two different levels: implications for a wider protective role, *FEBS Lett.,* 185, 19, 1985.

54. **Gutteridge, J. M. C.,** Superoxide-dependent formation of hydroxyl radicals from ferric complexes and hydrogen peroxide — an evaluation of 14 iron chelators, *Free Radical Res. Commun.,* 9, 19, 1991.

55. **Aruoma, O. I., Halliwell, B., Gajewski, E., and Dizdaroglu, M.,** Damage to the bases in DNA induced by hydrogen peroxide and ferric ion chelates, *J. Biol. Chem.,* 264, 20509, 1989.

56. **Aruoma, O. I. and Halliwell, B.,** DNA damage and free radicals, *Chem. Br.,* 149, 1991.

57. **Crichton, R. R. and Charloteaux-Wauters, M.,** Iron transport and storage, *Eur. J. Biochem.,* 164, 485, 1987.

58. **Aruoma, O. I. and Halliwell, B.,** Superoxide-dependent and ascorbate-dependent formation of hydroxyl radicals from hydrogen peroxide in the presence of iron. Are lactoferrin and transferrin promoters of hydroxyl radical generation?, *Biochem. J.,* 241, 273, 1987.

59. **Britigan, B. E., Rosen, G. M., Thompson, B. Y., Chai, Y., and Cohen, M. S.,** Stimulated neutrophils limit iron-catalyzed hydroxyl radical formation as detected by spin-trapping, *J. Biol. Chem.,* 261, 1706, 1986.

60. **Kaur, H., Fagerheim, I., Grootveld, M., Puppo, A., and Halliwell, B.,** Aromatic hydroxylation of phenylalanine as an assay for hydroxyl radicals. Application to activated human neutrophils and to the heme protein leghemoglobin, *Anal. Biochem.,* 172, 360, 1988.

61. **Halliwell, B., Gutteridge, J. M. C., and Blake, D. R.,** Metal ions and oxygen radical reactions in human inflammatory joint disease, *Philos. Trans. R. Soc. London, Ser B,* 311, 659, 1985.

62. **Halliwell, B., Aruoma, O. I., Wasil, M., and Gutteridge, J. M. C.,** The resistance of transferrin, lactoferrin, and ceruloplasmin to oxidative damage, *Biochem. J.,* 256, 311, 1988.

63. **Biemond, P., Van Eijk, H. G., Swaak, A. J. G., and Koster, J. F.,** Iron mobilization from ferritin by superoxide derived from stimulated polymorphonuclear leukocytes. Possible mechanism in inflammation diseases, *J. Clin. Invest.,* 73, 1576, 1984.

64. **Buettner, G. R., Saran, M., and Bors, W.,** The kinetics of the reaction of ferritin with superoxide, *Free Radical Res. Commun.,* 2, 369, 1987.

65. **Bolann, B. J. and Ulvik, R. J.,** On the limited ability of superoxide to release iron from ferritin, *Eur. J. Biochem.,* 193, 899, 1990.

66. **O'Connell, M. J., Halliwell, B., Moorhouse, C. P., Aruoma, O. I., Baum, H., and Peters, T. J.,** Formation of hydroxyl radicals in the presence of ferritin and haemosiderin, *Biochem. J.,* 234, 724, 1986.

67. **Mann, S., Wade, V. J., Dickson, D. P. E., Reid, N. M. K., Ward, R. J., O'Connell, M., and Peters, T. J.,** Structural specificity of haemosiderin iron cores in iron-overload diseases, *FEBS Lett.,* 234, 69, 1988.

68. **Halliwell, B. and Gutteridge, J. M. C.,** The antioxidants of human extracellular fluids, *Arch. Biochem. Biophys.,* 280, 1, 1990.

69. **Weinberg, A. B.,** Cellular iron metabolism in health and disease, *Drug Metab. Rev.,* 22, 531, 1990.

70. **Evans, P. J., Bomford, A., and Halliwell, B.,** Non-caeruloplasmin copper and ferroxidase activity in mammalian serum, *Free Radical Res. Commun.,* 7, 55, 1989.

71. **Gutteridge, J. M. C. and Stocks, J.,** Caeruloplasmin: physiological and pathological perspectives, *CRC Crit. Rev. Clin. Lab. Sci.,* 14, 257, 1981.

72. **Frei, B., England, L., and Ames, B. N.,** Ascorbate is an outstanding antioxidant in human blood plasma, *Proc. Natl. Acad. Sci. U.S.A.,* 86, 6377, 1989.

73. **Halliwell, B.,** How to characterize a biological antioxidant, *Free Radical Red. Commun.,* 9, 1, 1990.

74. **Gutteridge, J. M. C.,** Iron promoters of the Fenton reaction and lipid peroxidation can be released from haemoglobin by peroxides, *FEBS Lett.,* 201, 291, 1986.

75. **Puppo, A. and Halliwell, B.,** Formation of hydroxyl radicals from hydrogen peroxide in the presence of iron. Is haemoglobin a biological Fenton catalyst?, *Biochem. J.,* 249, 185, 1988.

76. **Puppo, A. and Halliwell, B.,** Formation of hydroxyl radicals in biological systems. Does myoglobin stimulate hydroxyl radical production from hydrogen peroxide?, *Free Radical Res. Commun.,* 4, 415, 1988.

77. **Kanner, J., German, J. B., and Kinsella, J. E.,** Initiation of lipid peroxidation in biological systems, *CRC Crit. Rev. Food Sci. Nutr.,* 25, 317, 1987.

78. **Davies, M. J.,** Detection of myoglobin-derived radicals on reaction of metmyoglobin with hydrogen peroxide and other peroxidic compounds, *Free Radical Res. Commun.,* 10, 361, 1990.

79. **Davies, M. J.,** Identification of a globin free radical in equine myoglobin treated with peroxides, *Biochim. Biophys. Acta,* 1077, 86, 1991.

80. **Steele, J. A., Stockbridge, N., Maljkovic, G., and Weir, B.,** Free radicals mediate actions of oxyhemoglobin on cerebrovascular smooth muscle cells, *Circulation,* 68, 416, 1991.

81. **Seibert, A. F., Taylor, A. E., Bass, J. B., and Haynes, J., Jr.,** Hemoglobin potentiates oxidant injury in isolated rat lungs, *Am. J. Physiol.,* 200, H1980, 1991.

82. **Arduini, A., Eddy, L., and Hochstein, P.,** Detection of ferryl myoglobin in the isolated ischemic rat heart, *Free Radical Biol. Med.,* 9, 511, 1990.

83. **Odeh, M.,** The role of reperfusion-induced injury in the pathogenesis of the crush syndrome, *N. Engl. J. Med.,* 324, 1417, 1991.

84. **Rice-Evans, C., Okunade, G., and Khan, R.,** The suppression of iron release from activated myoglobin by physiological electron donors and by desferrioxamine, *Free Radical Res. Commun.,* 7, 45, 1989.

85. **Rush, J. D., Maskos, Z., and Koppenol, W. H.,** Reactions of iron(II) nucleotide complexes with hydrogen peroxide, *FEBS Lett.,* 261, 121, 1990.

86. **Gutteridge, J. M. C., Nagy, I. Z., Maidt, L., and Floyd, R. A.,** ADP-iron as a Fenton reagent: radical reactions detected by spin trapping, hydrogen abstraction, and aromatic hydroxylation, *Arch. Biochem. Biophys.,* 277, 422, 1990.

87. **Gutteridge, J. M. C. and Halliwell, B.,** Radical-promoting loosely-bound iron in biological fluids and the bleomycin assay, *Life Chem. Rep.,* 4, 113, 1987.

88. **Gutteridge, J. M. C.,** A method for removal of trace iron contamination from biological buffers, *FEBS Lett.,* 214, 362, 1987.

89. **Gutteridge, J. M. C., Rowley, D. A., Griffiths, E., and Halliwell, B.,** Low-molecular-weight iron complexes and oxygen radical reactions in idiopathic haemochromatosis, *Clin. Sci.,* 68, 463, 1985.

90. **Grootveld, M., Bell, J. D., Halliwell, B., Aruoma, O. I., Bomford, A., and Sadler, P. J.,** Non-transferrin-bound iron in plasma or serum from patients with idiopathic hemochromatosis. Characterization by high-performance liquid chromatography and nuclear magnetic resonance spectroscopy, *J. Biol. Chem.,* 264, 4417, 1989.

91. **Aruoma, O. I., Bomford, A., Polson, R. J., and Halliwell, B.,** Non-transferrin-bound iron in plasma from hemochromatosis patients. Effect of phlebotomy therapy, *Blood,* 72, 1416, 1988.

92. **Heiskala, H., Gutteridge, J. M. C., Westermarck, T., Alanen, T., and Santavuori, P.**, Bleomycin-detectable iron and phenanthroline-detectable copper in the cerebrospinal fluid of patients with neuronal ceroid-lipofuscinoses, *Am. J. Med. Genet.*, Suppl., 5, 193, 1988.

93. **Gutteridge, J. M. C.**, Bleomycin-detectable iron in knee-joint synovial fluid from arthritic patients and its relationship to the extracellular antioxidant activities of caeruloplasmin, transferrin, and lactoferrin, *Biochem. J.*, 245, 415, 1987.

94. **Halliwell, B., Aruoma, O. I., Mufti, G., and Bomford, A.**, Bleomycin-detectable iron in serum from leukaemic patients before and after chemotherapy, *FEBS Lett.*, 241, 202, 1988.

95. **Sanan, S., Sharma, G., Malholtra, R., Sanan, D. P., Jain, P., and Vadhera, P.**, Protection by desferrioxamine against histopathological changes in the liver in the post-oligaemic phase of clinical haemorrhagic shock in dogs. Correlation with improved survival rate and recovery, *Free Radical Res. Commun.*, 6, 29, 1989.

96. **Halliwell, B.**, Free radicals, tissue injury and human disease. Some lessons from fulminant hepatic failure, ischaemia-reperfusion, rheumatoid arthritis and adult respiratory distress syndrome, in *Proc. SCAARF Meet.*, in press.

97. **Youdim, M. B. H.**, *Brain Iron. Neurochemical and Behavioural Aspects*, Taylor & Francis, New York, 1988.

98. **Stocks, J., Gutteridge, J. M. C., Sharp, R. F., and Dormandy, T. L.**, The inhibition of lipid autoxidation by human serum and its relationship to serum proteins and alpha tocopherol, *Clin. Sci.*, 47, 223, 1974.

99. **Halliwell, B. and Gutteridge, J. M. C.**, Oxygen radicals and the nervous system, *Trends Neurosci.*, 8, 22, 1985.

100. **Spector, R. and Eells, J.**, Deoxynucleoside and vitamin transport into the central nervous system, *Fed. Proc.*, 43, 196, 1984.

101. **Rosen, A. D. and Frumin, N. V.**, Focal epileptogenesis following intracortical haemoglobin injection, *Exp. Neurol.*, 66, 277, 1979.

102. **Willmore, L. J., Triggs, W. J., and Gray, J. D.**, The role of iron-induced hippocampal peroxidation in acute epileptogenesis, *Brain Res.*, 382, 422, 1986.

103. **Willmore, L. J., Ballinger, W. E., Boggs, W., Sypert, G. W., and Rubin, J. J.**, Dendritic alterations in rat isocortex within an iron-induced chronic epileptic focus, *Neurosurgery*, 7, 142, 1980.

104. **Hall, E. D. and Braughler, J. M.**, Central nervous system trauma and stroke. Physiological and pharmacological evidence for involvement of oxygen radicals and lipid peroxidation, *Free Radical Biol. Med.*, 6, 303, 1989.

105. **Dexter, D. T., Wells, F. R., Lees, A. J., Agid, F., Agid, Y., Jenner, P., and Marsen, C. D.**, Increased nigral iron content and alterations in other metal ions occurring in brain in Parkinson's disease, *J. Neurochem.*, 52, 1830, 1989.

106. **Riederer, P., Sofic, E., Rausche, W. D., Schmidt, B., Reynolds, G. P., Jallinger, K., and Youdim, M. B. H.**, Transition metals, ferritin, glutathione and ascorbic acid in Parkinsonian brains, *J. Neurochem.*, 52, 515, 1989.

107. **Sofic, E., Paulus, W., Jellinger, K., Riederer, P., and Youdim, M. B. H.**, Selective increase of iron in substantia nigra zona compacta of Parkinsonian brains, *J. Neurochem.*, 56, 978, 1991.

108. **Creeth, J. M.**, Oxidation products of ovarian cyst mucins. Characterization by density-gradient analysis, *Carbohydrate Res.*, 178, 314, 1988.

109. **Stadtman, E. R. and Oliver, C. N.**, Metal-catalyzed oxidation of proteins. Physiological consequences, *J. Biol. Chem.*, 266, 2005, 1991.

110. **Marx, G. and Chevion, M.**, Site-specific modification of albumin by free radicals. Reaction with copper(II) and ascorbate, *Biochem. J.*, 236, 397, 1986.

111. **Halliwell, B. and Gutteridge, J. M. C.**, Formation of a thiobarbituric-acid-reactive substance from deoxyribose in the presence of iron salts, *FEBS Lett.*, 128, 347, 1981.

112. **Gutteridge, J. M. C.,** Reactivity of hydroxyl and hydroxyl-like radical discriminated by release of thiobarbituric-acid-reactive material from deoxyribose, nucleosides, and benzoate, *Biochem. J.,* 224, 761, 1984.

113. **Aruoma, O. I. and Halliwell, B.,** The iron-binding and hydroxyl radical scavenging action of anti-inflammatory drugs, *Xenobiotica,* 18, 459, 1988.

114. **Cochrane, C. J., Schraufstatter, I. U., Hyslop, P., and Jackson, J.,** Cellular and biochemical events in oxidant injury, in Halliwell, B., *Oxygen Radicals and Tissue Injury,* Halliwell, B., Ed., FASEB, 1988, 49.

115. **Aust, S. D., Morehouse, L. A., and Thomas, C. E.,** Role of metals in oxygen radical reactions, *J. Free Radical Biol. Med.,* 1, 3, 1985.

116. **Minotti, G. and Aust, S. D.,** The role of iron in the initiation of lipid peroxidation, *Chem. Phys. Lipids,* 44, 191, 1987.

117. **Halliwell, B. and Gutteridge, J. M. C.,** Oxygen toxicity, oxygen radicals, transition metals, and disease, *Biochem. J.,* 219, 1, 1984.

118. **Borg, D. C. and Schaich, K. M.,** Iron and iron-derived radicals, in *Oxygen Radicals and Tissue Injury,* Halliwell, B., Ed., FASEB, 1988, 27.

119. **Ursini, F., Maiorino, M., Hochstein, P., and Ernster, L.,** Microsomal lipid peroxidation: mechanisms of initiation. The role of iron and iron chelators, *Free Radical Biol. Med.,* 6, 31, 1989.

120. **Aruoma, O. I., Halliwell, B., Laughton, M. J., Quinlan, G. J., and Gutteridge, J. M. C.,** The mechanism of initiation of lipid peroxidation. Evidence against a requirement for an iron(II)-iron(III) complex, *Biochem. J.,* 258, 617, 1988.

121. **Quinlan, G. J., Halliwell, B., Moorhouse, C. P., and Gutteridge, J. M. C.,** Action of lead(II) and aluminium(III) ions on iron-stimulated lipid peroxidation in liposomes, erythrocytes, and rat liver microsomal fractions, *Biochim. Biophys. Acta,* 962, 196, 1988.

122. **O'Brien, P. J.,** Intracellular mechanisms for the decomposition of a lipid peroxide. I. Decomposition of a lipid peroxide by metal ions, heme compounds and nucleophiles, *Can. J. Biochem.,* 47, 485, 1969.

123. **Davies, M. J. and Slater, T. F.,** Studies on the metal-ion and lipoxygenase-catalysed breakdown of hydroperoxides using electron-spin-resonance spectroscopy, *Biochem. J.,* 245, 167, 1987.

124. **Gutteridge, J. M. C.,** Iron-EDTA stimulated phospholipid peroxidation: a reaction changing from alkoxyl to hydroxyl radical dependent initiation, *Biochem. J.,* 224, 697, 1984.

125. **Gutteridge, J. M. C. and Kerry, P. J.,** Detection by fluorescence of peroxides and carbonyls in samples of arachidonic acid, *Br. J. Pharmacol.,* 76, 459, 1982.

125a. **Bielski, B.,** personal communication.

126. **O'Connell, M. J., Ward, R. J., Baum, H., and Peters, T. J.,** The role of iron in ferritin and haemosiderin-mediated lipid peroxidation in liposomes, *Biochem. J.,* 229, 135, 1985.

127. **Radi, R., Turrens, J. F., and Freeman, B. A.,** Cytochrome c-catalyzed membrane lipid peroxidation by hydrogen peroxide, *Arch. Biochem. Biophys.,* 288, 118, 1991.

128. **Kim, E. H. and Sevanian, A.,** Hematin — and peroxide-catalyzed peroxidation of phospholipid liposomes, *Arch. Biochem. Biophys.,* 288, 324, 1991.

129. **Gutteridge, J. M. C., Halliwell, B., Treffry, A., Harrison, P. M., and Blake, D. R.,** Effect of ferritin-containing fractions with different iron loading on lipid peroxidation, *Biochem. J.,* 209, 557, 1983.

130. **Gutteridge, J. M. C., Beard, A. P. C., and Quinlan, G. J.,** Superoxide-dependent lipid peroxidation. Problems with the use of catalase as a specific probe for Fenton-derived hydroxyl radicals, *Biochem. Biophys. Res. Commun.,* 117, 901, 1983.

131. **Halliwell, B.,** Drug antioxidant effects, a basis for drug selection?, *Drugs,* 42, 569, 1991.

8. Lipofuscin, Lysosomes, and Iron

Ulf T. Brunk, Massoud R. Marzabadi, and Charles B. Jones

Department of Pathology II, University of Linköping, Linköping, Sweden

I. INTRODUCTION

Lipofuscin, or age pigment, accumulates with age in the lysosomal vacuome of a variety of postmitotic cell types in animals belonging to widely divergent phylogenetic groups.[1-4] Indeed, it is the only age-associated intracellular alteration which has been considered to be almost universal. Although these cellular deposits have been widely regarded by the classical cytologists as an index of aging, their significance and relationship to aging processes have remained somewhat ambiguous because the chemical composition of the pigment is heterogeneous and its identification cannot be based on any single or distinct compound. However, lipofuscin invariably contains polymerized residues of peroxidized lipids and proteins and seems to be incorporated into the secondary lysosomes by autophagocytosis of cellular constituents undergoing peroxidation events within this vacuome.[5,6]

Ever since its discovery more than a century ago, lipofuscin has retained the interest of gerontologists in the hope that this marker of cellular aging may provide clues to the underlying mechanism of aging. Accordingly, a variety of experimental and comparative studies have been conducted to identify the factors that influence lipofuscinogenesis and may link it to the aging process. Although we are still in the midst of this quest, a considerable amount of knowledge has been gained to lead to the postulation of two hypotheses regarding the causes of lipofuscin accumulation and its role in the aging process. One hypothesis proposes oxidative stress, i.e., the ratio of prooxidants to antioxidants as the main factor,[2,6-8] while the other hypothesis regards a decline in the degradative ability of cells to be primarily responsible for lipofuscin formation.[9-12] The two hypotheses are not necessarily mutually incompatible as it is possible that oxidative reactions involving lipid and protein peroxidation, among others, may induce both a decline in the activity of lytic enzymes as well as an increase in the production of modified molecules that are precursors of lipofuscin. Nevertheless, the key difference between the two hypotheses is which of the two processes plays the most dominant role in lipofuscinogenesis. It is fair to say, in general, the first hypothesis is more popular among gerontologists while the second is favored by pathologists and some experimentalists dealing with the accumulation of "ceroid", a related pigmented substance which appears to be an early, immature, variety of lipofuscin.

The rationale for understanding the nature and mechanism of lipofuscinogenesis remains compelling, namely, that processes associated with its formation, or cellular effects, may be directly or indirectly related to the mechanisms of cellular aging.

II. CHARACTERISTICS OF LIPOFUSCIN

Lipofuscin is a yellowish-brown pigment which is sequestered within cytoplasmic granules. The pigment is absent from postmitotic cells of young animals, but can occupy up to 20% of the cytoplasmic volume in old animals.[13] In histological sections, the lipofuscin-containing granules appear rounded or oblong 1 to 5 μm in diameter and increase in both size and number with age. When examined with the aid of a transmission electron microscope, lipofuscin-containing granules exhibit a single-limiting membrane enclosing variable amounts of materials with vacuolar, granular, or lamellar organization.[14]

Lipofuscin has been histochemically characterized as a heterogeneous compound with some unifying characteristics as follows: basophilic due to the presence of acidic groups, with a pKa of about 3 to 4; periodic acid-Schiff positive, probably due to the presence of carbonyl lipids or carbon chains with adjacent aldehyde groups; stainable by lipid stains such as Sudan black B and by reagents specific for proteins; and exhibiting positive localization of lysosomal enzymes.[4,15] There is, however, considerable variation in the staining response of lipofuscin in different tissues at different ages and under different physiological conditions. It is generally believed that this variability is partially related to its stage of oxidation and cross-linking. As these processes progress, the substances undergo characteristic changes which are reflected in their reactions to different stains, e.g., loss of sudanophilia.[16] One of the main characteristics of lipofuscin granules, which has been widely used for their identification and recently also for quantification, is the emittance of intense yellowish autofluorescence when excited with ultraviolet and blue light. The excitation maximum of the *in situ* and isolated lipofuscin granules has been reported to range from 340 to 480 nm, whereas the emission maximum ranges between 530 and 560 nm.[9]

Chemical analyses of isolated lipofuscin have indicated the presence of three major components: 19 to 51% lipids, 30 to 50% proteins, and 9 to 30% acid hydrolysis-resistant residues. Extracts of isolated lipofuscin in chloroform contain a complex mixture of fluorescent substances.[17,18] Contamination with flavins and peroxidation during the extraction process may create artifactual increased values if not compensated.[19]

III. MECHANISMS OF LIPOFUSCIN FORMATION

Lysosomes are known to participate in the intracellular digestion of compounds taken up by way of endocytosis in heterophagosomes, as well as of intracellular material sequestrated during autophagy in autophagosomes. During these events hydrolytic enzymes are mixed with the enclosed materials through fusion between lysosomes and phagosomes. Primary as well as secondary lysosomes are believed to contribute their lytic enzymes to the degradative process.[20] The lysosomal membrane-bound system of hydrolytic enzymes controls a major part of intracellular catablism of macromolecules and encloses some 40 enzymes, such as proteases, nucleases, glycosidases, lipases, phospholipases, phosphatases, and sulfatases. These enzymes, being acid hydrolases, function in the pH 5 acidity maintained within the lysosomal system by the ATP-dependent H^+ pump of the lysosomal membrane.[21]

Residual bodies, including the morphologically distinctive subgroup named lipofuscin granules, are special types of secondary lysosomes with characteristic ultrastructure and special cytochemical features.[4] Their origin is debated, but evidence has accumulated to indicate that they may form as a result of incomplete degradation of material taken up during endocytosis and/or incomplete decomposition following autophagocytosis. Residual bodies accumulate as a result of continuous autophagocytosis in combination with inability of the cells to rid themselves of the residues of digestion to a sufficient degree.[22] Residual bodies are mainly found in nondividing (postmitotic cells) which are unable to prevent the accumulation of these bodies by way of cell division.

Studies on cultured human glial cells with electron-dense marker particles added to the culture medium have shown residual bodies (lipofuscin granules) to form part of a vacuome system which by fusion and fission allows material within membrane-limited vacuoles to spread throughout the system, although at any one moment it is discontinuous.[23] Residual bodies thus form an integral part of the lysosomal vacuome system and regularly receive lytic enzymes by fusion with other types of lysosomes. These findings are consistent with de Duve's exoplasmic vacuome concept.[24]

A major difficulty in elucidating the mechanism of lipofuscin formation is the inability to define chemically what actually constitutes lipofuscin. To confound matters, pathological conditions such as storage diseases, due to inadequacy of degradative enzymes or to unknown causes, have also been used as models to study lipofuscin composition and lipofuscinogenesis.[10,18] The results obtained from such studies are difficult to interpret because the material present may not be identical to lipofuscin that is formed during the normal course of aging, and data from such studies should be interpreted in view of these complicating factors.

Investigations on the mechanism of lipofuscin formation have proceeded along two different lines, the morphological and the biochemical. At the morphological level, the preponderance of evidence suggests that lipofuscin-containing granules are secondary lysosomes of the residual body variety arising from autophagocytosis of cytoplasmic constituents.[6] The lipids within lipofuscin granules seem to undergo progressive oxidation as reflected by the characteristic changes in their staining reactions, e.g., the gradual loss of sudanophilia and increased stainability with Nile blue sulfate.[16]

Biochemical studies on the origin of lipofuscin have given rise to two different schools of thought. According to one view, lipofuscin accumulation represents a storage phenomenon occurring due to the inability of cells to degrade normal cellular constituents such as retinoyl complexes, polyisoprenols of the dolichol class, and intracellular membranes.[10,11,18] This view is primarily based on chemical analysis of pigment accumulating under pathological or experimental conditions. The reasoning seems to be that if the cells had adequate degradative ability, these substances would not accumulate with time. However, it has not been proven that such a deficiency exists in normal tissues during aging or whether reduction in degradative ability is a cause of lipofuscinogenesis. Moreover, lipofuscin accumulation seems to be a process starting early in life and not restricted to old age.[25]

The other school of thought regards lipofuscin to be an end product of molecular damage to cell organelles by oxygen free radicals.[5,7,26] Studies supporting this view have attempted to identify molecular events which could inflict oxidative damage to cell organelles, leading to their autophagocytosis and subsequent partial degradation or, alternatively, to intralysosomal peroxidation occurring after cellular material becomes sequestered within the lysosomal vacuome during normal autophagocytosis.[27] Following peroxidation of degradation fragments, polymerization of these fragments would result in products resistent to normal enzymatic degradation. Most experimental studies have focused on peroxidation of lipids, the subsequent reactions of the lipid breakdown products, and the reactions resulting in the production of the characteristic fluorophores within lipofuscin.[7] The biochemical concept of fluorophore formation, developed mainly by Tappel and co-workers,[7] considers lipid autooxidative reactions to play a crucial role. Figure 1 illustrates the formation of fluorescent products during lipid peroxidation events. Following the free-radical initiation and propagation steps, lipid hydroperoxides, cyclic peroxides, and cyclic endoperoxides are formed, which further decompose to carbonyl compounds, among them malondialdehyde. The reaction of carbonyl compounds with side-chain amino groups present in proteins, free amino acids, amino phospholipids, and nucleic acids produces conjugated Schiff's bases that have strong optical absorptions as well as fluorescence features, the chromophoric system responsible for fluorescence being $-N=C-C=C-N-$. Malondialdehyde, possessing two carbonyl groups, can cross-link two amino-containing compounds to produce fluorescent products of the general structure $R_1-N=CH-CH=CH-NH-R_2$, termed aminoiminopropene Schiff's bases. The fluorescence wavelength seems to depend on the type of side chains (R_1 and R_2) in the amino group-containing molecule. An alternative route leading to fluorescent product formation during lipid peroxidation is the polymerization of aldehydes.

We have experimentally investigated the relationship between oxidative stress and lipofuscinogenesis in cultured human glial cells[28] and rat cardiac myocytes.[26,29] Effects of various ambient oxygen concentrations (5, 20, and 40%) on the lipofuscin concentration were examined at different ages of the culture. Lipofuscin was quantified by microspectrofluorometry of individual cells (see below). The yellow autofluorescence due to lipofuscin increased in direct relationship to ambient oxygen concentration with culture age (Figures 2 and 3). Light and transmission electron microscopic examination of the cells at different ages indicated a progressive time- and oxygen-dependent increase in the frequency and size of lipofuscin-containing organelles. Further support for the involvement of oxidative stress in lipofuscinogenesis was

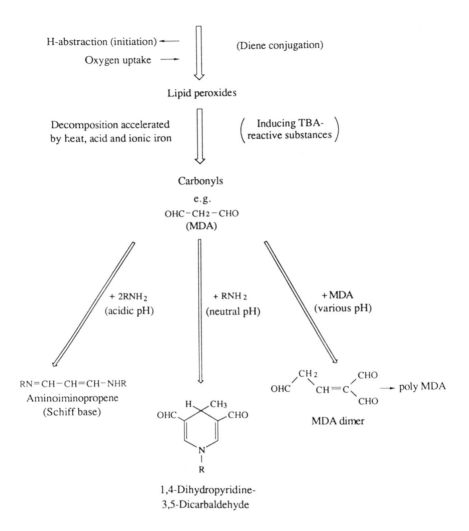

FIGURE 1. Fluorescent materials produced from iron-catalyzed peroxidation of membrane lipids. (Modified from Halliwell and Gutteridge, Eds., *Free Radicals in Biology and Medicine*, Clarendon Press, Oxford, 1989.)

provided by the effects of iron and the iron chelator desferrioxamine on lipofuscin concentration in rat cardiac myocytes in culture. Augmentation of iron in the culture medium markedly increased the level of lipofuscin accumulation, whereas desferrioxamine had the opposite effect. Both iron and desferrioxamine are endocytosed and will end up in the lysosomal vacuome after fusion between endosomes and primary or secondary lysosomes where

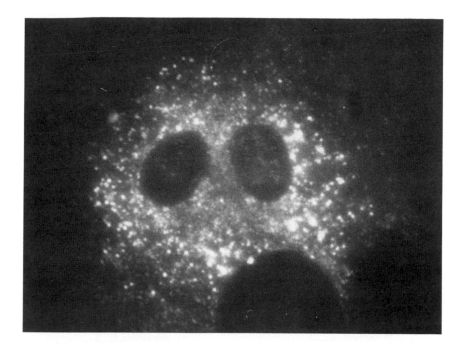

FIGURE 2. Photomicrograph of cardiac myocytes from a culture kept in 40% oxygen, 55% nitrogen, and 5% carbon dioxide for 12 d. Cells show numerous autofluorescent yellow granules in the perinuclear area when excited with blue light. (From Sohal, R. S., Marzabadi, M. R., Galaris, D., and Brunk, U. T., *Free-Radical Biol. Med.*, 6, 23, 1989. With permission.)

they influence the intralysosomal mileu and the conditions for lipofuscinogenesis. These findings can be understood in terms of iron potentiation of oxidative stress, probably by means of a superoxide ($O_2^{\cdot -}$) or another reducing agent such as glutathione, ascorbic acid, or cysteine-driven Fenton reaction[30] (Reactions 1 and 2).

$$X\text{–}Fe^{3+} + O_2^{\cdot -} \rightarrow X\text{–}Fe^{2+} + O_2 \qquad (1)$$

$$X\text{–}Fe^{2+} + H_2O_2 \rightarrow X\text{–}Fe^{3+} + OH^- + OH^{\cdot} \qquad (2)$$

Hydroxyl radicals ($OH^{\cdot}$) are very potent radicals abstracting hydrogen from all available molecules and initiating peroxidation (Figure 1). It is believed that lipofuscinogenesis is mainly an intralysosomal process and that iron added to the culture medium enters the lysosomal vacuome following endocytotic uptake. The effects of 30 μM ferric iron added to the culture medium on lipofuscin levels were mainly examined on neonatal cardiac myocytes kept under 20 and 40% oxygen.[29] At both 6 and 12 d of culture age, the amount of lipofuscin found in myocytes exposed to 30 μM ferric iron

244

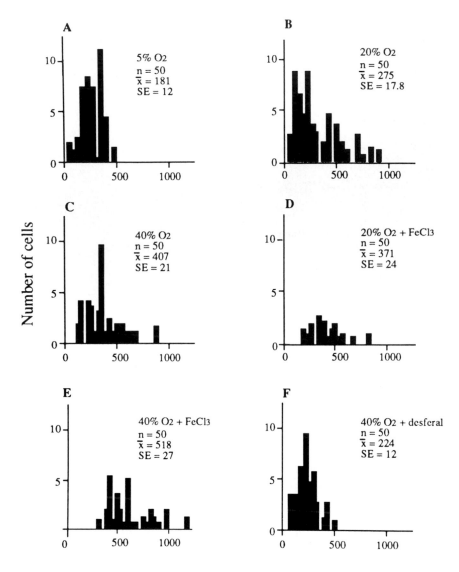

FIGURE 3. Computer-generated histograms of autofluorescence exhibited by cardiac myocytes kept in 5, 20, or 40% oxygen for 12 d. The additional effect of $FeCl_3$ and desferrioxamine is also shown. Abscissa: autofluorescence/cell (arbitrary units); ordinate: number of cells. A total of 50 cells were examined in each group.

was markedly greater than in the controls. Again, the effects were more pronounced under 40% than under 20% oxygen. In a separate experiment, effects of various concentrations of desferrioxamine, which binds iron, on lipofuscin content were examined.[29] The amount of lipofuscin was found to be inversely related to the concentration of desferrioxamine. Interestingly,

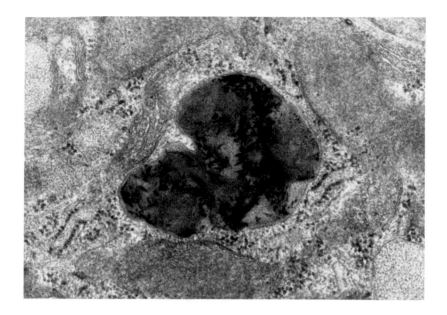

FIGURE 4. Electron micrograph of a lipofuscin-containing organelle in a myocyte cultured for 8 d in a medium containing 30 μM FeCl$_3$ showing dense needle-shaped material (arrow) shown to be iron when analyzed with energy dispersive X-ray analysis. (From Thaw, H. H., Brunk, U. T., and Collin, V. P., *Mech. Ageing Dev.*, 24, 211, 1984. With permission.)

the protective effects of desferrioxamine against lipofuscin accumulation were more pronounced in cells kept under 40% oxygen as compared to those kept under 20% oxygen. Thus, oxygen and iron seem to act synergistically to accelerate lipofuscin accumulation as would be expected if oxygen free radicals are a causal factor in lipofuscinogenesis.

Electron microscopic examination and energy dispersive X-ray microanalysis of cells exposed to ferric iron[29] indicated that iron is sequestered in the lipofuscin-containing organelles (Figure 4).

The accumulation of lipofuscin pigment is a phenomenon which occurs under physiological conditions and appears to be inevitable with age. It is now well established that the material constituting lipofuscin is located in the lysosomal vacuome,[6,22] though the presence of these age pigments therein has been a matter of dispute as to whether it has any effects on cell function.[22] Regardless of its possible influence on the lysosomal function and stability, it could be assumed that the accumulation velocity for age pigment will be influenced by some functional properties of lysosomes: (1) the rate at which autophagocytosis or endocytosis presents material rich in phospholipids and proteins to the lysosomal system, (2) the efficiency of the lysosomal enzymes in degrading this material, (3) the degree of peroxidation inside the lysosomal vacuome, and (4) the cellular capacity to exocytose undegradable residues. Peroxidation will also be influenced by cytosolic formation and degradation

of O_2^- and H_2O_2 as well as the amount of reactive iron outside and inside
.the lysosomal vacuome. Peroxidation initiated in the cytosol may influence
factors leading to autophagocytosis. Age pigment, being located in lysosomes
and therefore mixed with lytic enzymes which are capable of degrading almost
all types of organic material, are essentially a nondegradable end product.
Under normal conditions the intralysosomal localization of lipofuscin could
provide secondary antioxidant defense[31] because this complex polymerized
compound does not appear to interfere with cell functions, at least not until
loading is very substantial.[22] Eventually, however, this nondigestible lipofuscin may cause cellular impairment by forcing the cell to supply large
amounts of the multiple degradative enzymes to a system containing material
which cannot be lysed. Also, lipofuscin-overloaded lysosomes might be unable to further handle peroxidized material formed during oxidative stress,
which would increase intracellular concentration of products of lipid peroxidation, such as malondialdehyde (MDA), impairing several critical cellular
targets.

IV. QUANTIFICATION OF LIPOFUSCIN

Understanding the mechanism of lipofuscinogenesis has been hampered
by a confusion in terminology, the purported chemical nature, as well as the
methods employed for the quantification of lipofuscin (see References 8 and
32 for detailed discussions). Most of the confusion can be traced to the lack
of knowledge of the chemical nature of lipofuscin as well as the absence of
any specific compound of known chemical compositions that can specifically
label lipofuscin. Classically, the term lipofuscin has been used to refer to the
material emitting greenish to yellowish-orange autofluorescence when excited
with blue light and studied in cells and tissues using fluorescence light microscopy. This material is present in membrane-bound organelles that can be
identified as secondary lysosomes. Presently, lipofuscin is being identified
and measured by four different methods:

1.   The most reliable method measures the autofluorescence of lipofuscin
     granules and employs microspectrofluorometry of cells *in situ.*
2.   Another method uses cytochemical staining and morphometry of sec-
     tioned material and can only provide semiquantitative measurements.
     The drawback of this method is that it cannot determine if all the granules
     under study exhibit fluorescence; and if they do, of what intensity.
3.   Another morphological method employs electron microscopy and mor-
     phometry of sectioned material. It suffers from the handicap that it
     cannot specifically identify the relative fluorescent content of the sec-
     ondary lysosomes.
4.   One method that has been frequently used in recent studies and the one
     which has contributed to the current confusion in terminology is based
     on the measurement of blue-emitting fluorescence in the organic solvent

extracts of tissues.[28] Studies using this method have generated much controversy because the results are often at odds with those obtained by microspectrofluorometry.

We therefore suggest that the term "lipofuscin" be used only for the material that specifically exhibits *in situ* the characteristics of lipofuscin, namely, greenish-yellowish autofluorescence emanating from the lysosomal vacuome. In our opinion, microspectrofluorometry of the *in situ* granules is currently the most reliable method for the quantification of lipofuscin. The discrepancies between emission values for fluorometric and microfluorometric measurements on tissue extracts and intact cells, respectively, may be due to the large differences in concentration of at least 1:1000 between lipofuscin containing lysosomes of intact cells and in extracts of cells and tissues. Materials believed to constitute lipofuscin have been shown to have metachromatic properties showing red shifting of fluorescence emission by increased concentration.[33] This simple fact may well explain these quoted discrepancies.

V. THE LYSOSOMAL VACUOME, IRON, AND OTHER HEAVY METALS IN HEALTH AND DISEASE

Iron is an essential element in many important metalloorganic compounds including most of the electron transfer systems involved in a variety of redox processes. A normal human male contains about 4.5 g of iron and has a daily absorption of about 1 mg from the diet with about the same daily amount of the metal lost from the body. About two thirds of total body iron is a part of hemoglobin while the rest is in myoglobin ($\pm 15\%$), various redox active enzymes, or stored as ferritin and hemosiderin ($\pm 15\%$). Iron is handled with extreme care by the body and is almost always kept bound within stable metalloorganic compounds. The reason for this is iron in free form can catalyze a variety of processes involved in oxidative alterations and degradation of many organic molecules including lipids, proteins, and nucleic acids. (See also Chapters 1 and 7.) A small amount of iron (0.2%) is bound to the iron-transport protein transferrin with a total plasma iron turnover of about 35 mg/d. Some iron is bound to lactoferrin in white blood cells, in mucosal cells, and in the milk of lactation. Transferrin transports iron to all cells and interacts with plasma membrane-bound transferrin receptors, inducing a receptor-mediated endocytotic uptake. The resulting endosomes are acidified which leads to a cleavage of iron from the apotransferrin molecule with the latter being returned to the plasma membrane for a repeat cycle. The released iron chelates to various cellular chelators — including ATP, GTP, phosphate esters, and citrate — although probably many important normal iron chelators are still to be discovered. This process creates a small pool of "non-protein-bound iron" which can be utilized in the synthesis of various iron-containing metalloproteins. Some iron is stored as intracellular ferritin which can be autophagocytosed and degraded within the lysosomal vacuome resulting in release of the iron into the nonprotein iron pool mentioned earlier. Moreover, iron is released from cellular organelles such as mitochondria and endoplasmic reticulum following autophagocytosis and degradation within the lysosomal vacuome. Thus, within endosomes and lysosomes for a short period of time iron is in a loosely bound state. This fact might render these organelles especially vulnerable to oxidative stress as will be discussed further.

Although lysosomal organelles have been investigated intensively since their recognition by de Duve, relatively little is known about their nonenzymatic contents. The lysosomes are known to contain proteins other than enzymes and small amounts of phospholipids, probably as part of membranes, glycolipids, and mucopolysaccharides. Nondigestive materials are known to accumulate in old lysosomes, also known as residual bodies, such as the lipofuscin pigment granules often seen in liver cells, heart muscle cells, and nerve cells.[4] Recently heavy metals have been found in lysosomes in pathological conditions[34,35] and normally[36-39] in certain types of cells. The intracellular distribution of normally occurring heavy metals is not known in detail. Histochemical studies, both electron microscopic[36,38,40] and light microscopic,[37,39] indicate that zinc occurs in high concentrations in the specific granules of mast cells, pancreatic islet cells, mossy fibers of the hippocampus, Paneth's cells, and eosinophilic leukocytes.

In mammary epithelial cells of mice, especially after the age of 20 weeks, lysosomes are rich in ferritin-like particles.[41] Such particles are also demonstrated in lysosomal fractions of liver homogenate. Furthermore, iron has been found to be associated with lipofuscin in lysosomes in several organs including the liver.[42]

When abnormally large amounts of heavy metals occur in tissues, the lysosomes appear to be involved. In Wilson's disease the lysosomes of hepatic cells contain a considerably increased amount of copper. This has been shown through combined biochemical, histochemical, and electron probe microanalysis.[35]

In experimental lead and mercury intoxication the cytochemical sulfide-silver method, or Timm technique for demonstration of heavy metals, shows an accumulation of mercury within granules which, judging from their size and arrangement, conform well with lysosomes in the kidney, liver, and brain.[43,44]

The reason for the presence of heavy metals in lysosomes is not obvious. Small amounts of heavy metals are normal cellular constituents. Manganese, iron, cobalt, and zinc are especially essential to metabolism, and enzyme activity is often dependent on their presence. In true metalloenzymes the metal is firmly bound as a constituent of the molecule. Other enzymes are activated by metal ions,[45] and metals may also be part of nonenzyme proteins or act as linking agents between different molecules.

Lysosomes are known to contain a large spectrum of hydrolytic enzymes, and some of the normally occurring heavy metals may be involved in their activities. According to the lysosomal concept, these organelles are involved in endocytosis and autophagocytosis during degradation of exogenous and endogenous materials.[46] Metals are taken up during endocytotic activity or brought into lysosomes during degradation of endogenous structures such as mitochondria containing many metal-dependent oxidative enzyme systems. Metals could accumulate in residual bodies together with the nondigestible materials, and different types of lysosomes may vary in the content of heavy metals. With the light microscope it is not possible to determine which type or types of lysosomes contain the heavy metals, and this requires electron microscopic methods. Presently available modifications of the sulfide-silver method for electron microscopy[36,38,40] are capable of showing large amounts of zinc in the mossy fibers of the hippocampus and in the granules of eosinophilic leukocytes and mast cells.

In hemochromatosis there is lysosomal overload of iron in hepatic parenchymal cells.[47] (See Chapter 4.) The iron-binding capacity of transferrin in the serum is exceeded in the iron-overloaded patients resulting in nontransferrin-bound iron to be present. This iron may bind to albumin, citrate, or other chelating agents and be taken up by liver cells resulting in lysosomal storage of increased amounts of iron. Iron overload may also result from repeated transfusions for anemia as in thalassemia major. Lysosomal overload of iron could result in Fenton reactions (see following), peroxidation of lysosomal membranes, and leakage of lytic enzymes to the cell sap with ensuing cell damage. This hypothesis has not been proven but could explain the cell degeneration and fibrosis in the liver, heart, and pancreatic β-cells in states of abnormal iron accumulation within the lysosomes of these cells.

VI. LYSOSOMES, IRON, AND OXIDATIVE STRESS

Hydrogen peroxide (H_2O_2) is a product of numerous oxidases in the cytosol, mitochondrial matrix and outer membrane, and plasma membrane; it is a ubiquitous compound in all cells. This slightly oxidative species also may be a result of many nonenzymatic autooxidative processes,[48] and, probably above all, as a result of electron leakage from the electron transportation complexes of the inner mitochondrial membrane to surrounding oxygen (Reaction 3). In mammalian cells, between 3 and 5% of all consumed oxygen is believed to result in the production of H_2O_2, usually through the intermediate formation of superoxide anion radicals ($O_2^{\cdot-}$) with ensuing spontaneous or enzymatic (SOD) dismutation (Reaction 4).

$$O_2 + e^- \rightarrow O_2^{\cdot-} \tag{3}$$

$$O_2^{\cdot-} + O_2^{\cdot-} + 2H^+ \rightarrow H_2O_2 + O_2 \tag{4}$$

Since H_2O_2 is a component of the Fenton reaction, leading to formation of the very reactive hydroxyl radical ($OH^{\cdot}$; see Reaction 2), the cellular location of H_2O_2 and iron is of great interest in oxidative-induced cellular pathology.

Under normal conditions the combined effects of catalase and glutathione peroxidase seem adequate to handle the H_2O_2 formed without upsetting the normal GSH/GSSG ratio, which in turn is dependent on the activity of glutatione reductase and the NADPH/NADP$^+$ ratio.[49,50] Little is known about the consequences of a cytosolic increase in H_2O_2 concentration as might occur suddenly during reperfusion conditions following ischemia,[49,50] during metabolism of several xenobiotics,[50] or more slowly during aging and inflammation.[49,50]

It is well known that H_2O_2 is cytotoxic to a variety of cells and organisms ranging from bacteria to vertebrate.[50] Being a weak oxidant, H_2O_2 can inactivate a few enzymes directly by oxidation of their essential thiol ($-SH$) groups,[50] although derangement of the GSH/GSSG and NADPH/NADP$^+$ ratios probably would have greater impact on cell metabolism. Whether these or some other metabolic alterations account for the acute cell death as can be produced with several types of mammalian cells in culture by the addition to the media of H_2O_2 in the μM range, however, seems uncertain or even improbable.

An alternative explanation would be OH$^{\cdot}$-inflicted damage following Fenton type reactions (Reaction 2). Essentially the hydroxyl radical reacts with a large variety of molecules immediately at the site where it is formed (site specificity). The chemistry of these reactions is complicated, but has been worked out to some extent for a number of organic compounds.[50] Among those most studied are the peroxidative chain reactions that take place with polyunsaturated fatty acids of membrane phospholipids in the presence of oxygen (Reactions 5 to 7).

$$LH + OH^{\cdot} \rightarrow L^{\cdot} + H_2O \tag{5}$$

$$L^{\cdot} + O_2 \rightarrow LOO^{\cdot} \tag{6}$$

$$LOO^{\cdot} + LH \rightarrow LOOH + L^{\cdot} \tag{7}$$

Cellular hydroperoxides formed are unstable and degrade easily, particularly in the presence of transition metal complexes including iron and copper salts, to carbonyls and other products, several of which are toxic or even themselves radicals such as alkoxyl and peroxyl radicals (Reactions 8 and 9).

$$ROOH + Fe^{2+}-complex \rightarrow Fe^{3+}-complex + RO^{\cdot} + OH^- \tag{8}$$

$$ROOH + Fe^{3+}-complex \rightarrow Fe^{2+}-complex + ROO^{\cdot} + H^+ \tag{9}$$

The decomposition of H_2O_2 with formation of OH$^{\cdot}$ requires catalysis by transition metals, usually iron as indicated in Reaction 2. The cellular occurrence of Fe^{2+}, in reactive form, would thus constitute a great threat to cellular integrity. Organisms utilize and store iron with great care and almost always keep it a chelated form in the non-protein-bound pool or in stable metalloorganic compounds. Probably only during the passage through the lysosomal vacuome does iron exist in a loosely bound form and then only for short periods of time.[49] This occurs as iron is released from its apoprotein moiety of transferrin in acidified endosomes, and in secondary lysosomes following autophagocytosis of iron-containing compounds and structures, such as ferritin, mitochondria, or endoplasmic reticulum. In cells such as Kuppfer cells and macrophages the lysosomal vacuome may be enriched in iron during phagocytosis of red blood cells or of cellular debris. Moreover, the acidic pH of the lysosomal or prelysosomal vesicles (pH 4.5 to 5.5) governs both dissociation of iron from metalloorganic compounds and the reduction of Fe^{3+} to Fe^{2+}. Secondary lysosomes might constitute *loci minora resistentia* as possible sites for the formation of OH˙ by Fenton reactions, with ensuing damage to the surrounding membranes. Severe damage would jeopardize cell integrity by leakage of powerful hydrolytic enzymes to the cell sap, followed by autolysis.

Acridine orange (AO) is a weak base belonging to the group of lysosomo-tropic agents that accumulate and are trapped in the lysosomal vacuome of living cells due to the acid conditions within the vacuome.[51-53] Reflecting its lipid solubility, AO passes cellular membranes passively, as long as it is still an uncharged molecule. Due to its capacity to accept protons in acid pH ranges it is converted to a positively charged compound within the lysosomal vacuome and becomes retained since the molecule in its charged form does not freely pass membranes.[51] Living cells exposed to a low concentration of AO in their ordinary medium for about 10 min and then transferred to medium without AO show bright red lysosomes when studied in the fluorescence microscope using blue-activating light. When cells are affected by a fixative, membrane permeability changes occur; the red, granular (lysosomal) fluo-rescence does not show; and the ordinary staining of DNA (green) and RNA (red) of fixed cells appears[53] (DNA-RNA staining by AO, however, requires much higher AO concentration than lysosomal staining of living cells). The retention of a granular red fluorescence in living cells can be regarded as an indication of lysosomal integrity with membranes capable of retaining a pH gradiant and the internal acid milieu. When this acidity disappears, the AO is converted back to a weak uncharged base that diffuses out to the cell sap resulting in change from granular red to diffuse green fluorescence.

When cells from the established macrophage-like cell line J-774 were exposed to 30 μ*M* $FeCl_3$ for 6 to 12 h in culture, the lysosomal vacuomes of these cells were enriched in iron. This could be demonstrated with the Timm or silver enhancement technique, which is a sensitive way of dem-onstrating heavy metals in cells and tissue.[39] When such cells were exposed to hydrogen peroxide in the range of 100 to 500 μ*M* following acridine orange

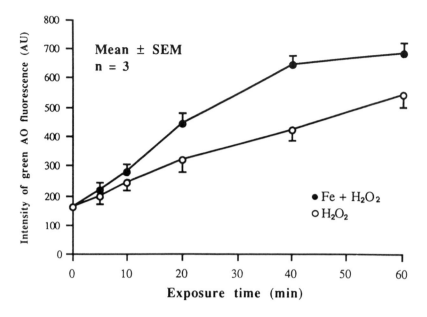

FIGURE 5. Cells were grown with and without 30 μM $FeCl_3$ in the medium, rinsed and exposed to 500 μM H_2O_2 in PBS for different periods of time. The increase in green fluorescence (indicating leakage of AO from lysosomes to the cytosole) differed between the two groups of cells indicating iron-induced lysosomal membrane lability.

staining, the increasing green fluorescence was much more rapid in iron-exposed cells than in control ones[54] as shown in Figure 5.

This indicates that Fenton reactions might have occurred intralysosomally resulting in hydroxyl radical production and initiation of peroxidative processes with ensuing membrane damage and loss of the proton gradient across the membrane.[54] The results point to the possibility that oxidative stress and postischemic reperfusion resulting in increased cellular levels of hydrogen peroxide might constitute a threat to lysosomal integrity if these organelles contain enhanced amounts of iron in reactive form.

AO, apart from being a weak base, is also a potent photosensitizer during photolysis in many systems.[52,55] When blue light is trapped by AO, the molecules become excited and in the presence of molecular oxygen produce singlet oxygen (O_2') and superoxide ($O_2^{\cdot-}$). Although the details are still incompletely known, the production of these reactive agents appears responsible for the membrane change found in the photolytic reactions.[55] When living cells are exposed to short wave blue light, the lysosomes previously filled with AO can be seen in the fluorescence microscope to gradually lose the red fluorescence, and after some time almost no granular red fluorescence remains. The velocity of this process should give an indication of capacity of the membranes of the lysosomal vacuome to withstand the attack of the radicals formed and resultant lipid peroxidation of the lysosomal membranes.

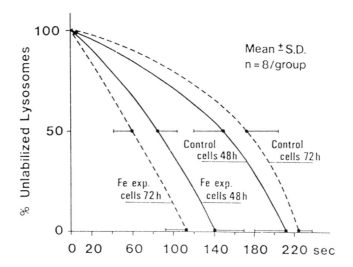

FIGURE 6. Rate of disappearance of granular red fluorescence from AO exposed MPMs during continuous exposure to blue light (in a Leitz fluorescence microscope equipped with an HPO lamp and a BG 12 filter utilizing transmitted light) in control cells and cells exposed to 60 μM Fe^{3+} in culture medium for 48 and 72 h. The controls as well as Fe^{3+} exposed MPMs were subjected continuously to blue light and observed for a period of 5 min in the fluorescence microscope.

Retention periods of lysosomal AO under illumination with blue light were found to be much shorter for iron-loaded lysosomes than for normal ones,[56] as shown in Figure 6.

The measurements of size of the iron-loaded lysosomes indicate that these lysosomes were not significantly larger (thus not more fragile due to expansion) than lysosomes of control cells.[56] The evidence would, therefore, favor an iron-dependent change or damage in the lysosomal membrane resulting in equilibration of the pH between lysosomal contents and the rest of the cell. Nevertheless, it should be kept in mind that the membrane change resulting in lost ability of the lysosomes to retain protons may not necessarily be associated with increased fragility of the lysosomal membrane or leakiness to large molecules such as hydrolytic enzymes.

The effect of lysosomal damage by photolysis was demonstrated by keeping the AO treated, blue light-exposed cells in culture medium for an additional 1 h at either 0 or 37°C. The cells kept at 37°C under ordinary culture conditions rapidly started to bleb, soon rounded up and detached from the plastic bottom of the dishes, while the cells that were kept at 0°C remained almost unaltered.[55] The cells exposed to AO and blue light and then kept for 1 h at 0°C were morphologically intact but observed to have a weak, diffuse, nongranular reaction product when a Gomori-type reaction for acid phosphatase was performed.[55] These findings indicate that lysosomal enzymes may diffuse out into the cell sap as a result of photooxidative damage. At 37°C this will result in degenerative alterations assuming the pH of the cytoplasm is low enough to allow the enzymes to exert lytic action. These findings support the "suicide-bag" (lysosomal death) concept of de Duve. Many authors doubt this mechanism of cell death and claim lysosomes rupture only following cell destruction.

The use of the photosensitizing weak base AO to induce photolytic damage to lysosomal membranes in living cells appears to be a valuable method to investigate the intactness of these membranes after various treatments that may affect the lysosomal vacuome.

VII. LYSOSOMAL IRON INFLUENCING THE EFFECT OF IONIZING RADIATION

Ionizing radiation interacting with normal or tumor tissues mainly results in radiolysis of water since water constitutes about 70% of soft tissues. In the presence of oxygen, this results in formation of hydroxyl radicals, superoxide anion radicals, and hydrogen peroxide, which are all reactive oxygen metabolites (Reactions 10, 3, and 4).

$$H_2O_2 + \text{ionizing radiation} \rightarrow OH^{\cdot} + H^+ + e^- \tag{10}$$

$$O_2 + e^- \rightarrow O_2^{\cdot -} \tag{3}$$

$$O_2^{\cdot -} + O_2^{\cdot -} + 2H^+ \rightarrow H_2O_2 + O_2 \tag{4}$$

The hydroxyl reaction is a highly aggressive oxygen-centered radical which reacts with virtually all organic compounds.

Formation of hydroxyl radicals within the nucleus of normal and malignant cells induces hydroxylation processes resulting in damage to the nucleic bases as well as to the DNA sugar and phosphate backbone. (See also Chapter 7.) This can cause mutations which, in turn, might destroy normal gene functions and induce cell death. Tumor cells are especially vulnerable because they usually have a higher mitotic rate than normal cells resulting in more destruction of the malignant cell population since DNA repair processes are less operative during DNA replication than during interface.

All cellular damage due to ionic radiation, however, is probably not due to DNA damage. Some cells are particularly vulnerable although they do not frequently divide. Such cells are mature lymphocytes, serous epithelial salivary gland cells, mast cells, and Kuppfer cells.[57,58] For these cells alternative mechanisms of cell damage must occur. Oral complications from salivary gland injury caused by ionizing radiation during treatment of head and neck tumors are well documented.[59] Many studies have shown unequivocally that the parotid gland (where saliva is produced by serous epithelial cells) is the most radiosensitive of the three major salivary glands.[58] Sublingual glands, which are almost purely mucous, are relatively radioresistant, while the radioresponse of the submandibular gland — a mixed gland containing both serous and mucous cells — is intermediate.[58] The apparent difference in radiosensitivity between serous and mucous epithelial cells has been convincingly demonstrated by the application of single doses of radiation to submandibular glands.

These experiments showed that pronounced degenerative alterations took place in the serous parenchyma while the mucous cells were affected only very slightly.[58] Our experiments[58] have shown that this radiosensitivity is related to the presence of secretory granules within the serous epithelial cells. It was possible to modulate the radiosensitivity of rat submandibulary salivary glands by treating the rats before radiation with atropine, which causes accumulation of secretory granules, or with secretagogues decreasing the number of granules. Increased amount of secretory granules within serous epithelial cells caused increased damage while cells depleted of secretory granules showed very little radiation damage. Using particle-induced X-ray emission (Pixe) spectroscopy it was possible to show that secretory granules are very rich not only in zinc, which is well known, but also in iron. A tempting hypothesis is that X-radiation gives rise to peroxidation of lipids within the membrane surrounding the secretory granule (see Reactions 5 to 7). Hydroperoxides formed may react with iron complexes containing both ferrous and ferric iron in such a way that alcoxyl and peroxyl radicals are produced which may further initiate peroxidation (see Reaction 8 and 9). Iron complexes are well known to catalyze fragmentation of peroxides (Figure 1), and the net results of such reactions may be destruction of the membranes around secretory granules with leakage to the cell sap of their content including amylase and other enzymes with the capacity to destroy the cell.

In additional studies on cultured mouse peritoneal macrophages (MPMs) it was possible to further substantiate this hypothesis.[59] Macrophages in culture were exposed to various concentrations of $FeCl_3$ in the medium (10 to 30 μM) for about 2 d, rinsed and exposed to X-radiation in doses between 10 and 40 Gy. Cell survival and production of malondialdehyde indicating lipid peroxidation and fragmentation of peroxides were then followed. Light and electron microscopic studies of macrophages exposed to different concentrations of Fe^{3+} in the medium revealed that the cytoplasm of the cells became filled with Perl's blue-stainable granules. It is likely that the iron present in the culture medium conjugates with serum proteins. Subsequently, the macromolecular iron-binding complexes are believed to become endocytosed by the cells and by fusing with lysosomes form the stainable granules. Since these granules have a size and distribution corresponding to that of acid phosphatase-containing granules (as revealed by cytochemical studies), the evidence suggests that at least the bulk of iron-positive granules represent lysosomes, and that the endocytotic vacuoles had fused with the lysosomes.[59]

The enhanced production of MDA following the combined exposure to 30 μM Fe^{3+} and 10 Gy — both of which individually failed to produce such

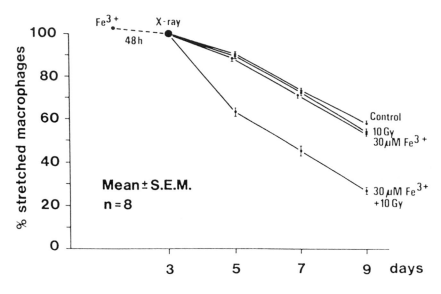

FIGURE 7. Survival rates of cultured macrophages after exposure to 30 μM Fe^{3+}, 10 Gy X-radiation, and 30 μM Fe^{3+} in combination with 10 Gy X-radiation, as compared to controls.

an effect — favors the assumption of iron-induced catalysis of lipid peroxidation. Moreover, while survival of the macrophages was largely unaffected by exposure of the cells to either 30 μM Fe^{3+} or the low dose of X-radiation (10 Gy), a remarkable decline in survival occurred following the combined treatment. These observations also suggest a potentiating action of small amounts of iron on the effects of radiation. Taken together, the findings of this study indicate a catalytic effect of the iron on induction of lipid peroxidation by free radicals produced during radiation of the cells and the surrounding medium (Figure 7).

Macrophages, both mobile and fixed ones like Kuppfer cells, are known to be radiosensitive; and since these cells phagocytose foreign material including red blood cells, their lysosomal vacuome becomes rich in iron. As shown in Reactions 9 and 10 iron may catalyze degradation of peroxidized lipids. This could place the lysosome membranes into a category of especially vulnerable structures after being exposed to $OH^{\cdot}$ produced during radiolysis of water and create the situation of leakage of lysosomal enzymes through damaged lysosomal membranes with resulting cell degeneration and cell death.

VIII. SUMMARY AND CONCLUSIONS

Iron, an essential metal with a multitude of important functions related to redox processes, is incorporated in very stable metalloorganic compounds during transportation and storage and in the functional state. Being a transition metal, iron is capable of catalyzing cleavage of peroxides causing formation of different lipid-oxygen radicals as well as the very aggressive hydroxyl radical. Interaction of Fe^{2+} and hydrogen peroxide results in Fenton chemistry and production of hydroxyl radicals which might initiate profound peroxidation and fragmentation reactions of a variety of macromolecular structures.

Lysosomes and acidified endosomes constitute cellular compartments where iron for short periods of time may exist in reactive form allowing for peroxidative processes. The importance was demonstrated in model systems of cultured cells subjected to oxidative stress and augmented amounts of $FeCl_3$ in the culture medium. This combination was considered to result in increased intracellular, mainly mitochondrial, production of hydrogen peroxide as well as increased intralysosomal concentration of iron. One of the results of this situation was dramatically increased lipofuscinogenesis. Additionally, increased oxidative stress accomplished by the addition of H_2O_2 in the μM ranges to the medium, resulted in upsetting of the proton gradient over the lysosomal membranes and ensuing leakage of lysosomal enzymes to the cytosol.

The pronounced radiosensitivity of some nondividing cells is thought to be due to the combined occurrence of iron and lytic enzymes within their lysosomes or secretory granules, subjecting the surrounding membranes of these organelles to iron-catalyzed fragmentation following peroxidative events. The latter are due to hydroxyl radicals formed as a consequence of radiolytic decomposition of water. Lysosomal membranes subjected to free-radical attack may thus be the weak link for cellular resistance to oxidative stress. Leakage of lysosomal contents to the cytosol may result in devastating irreversible intracellular alterations and death.

REFERENCES

1. **Sohal, R. S., Ed.,** *Age Pigments,* Elsevier, Amsterdam, 1981.
2. **Donato, H. J. and Sohal, R. S.,** Lipofuscin, in *Handbook of Biochemistry in Aging,* Florini, J., Ed., CRC Press, Boca Raton, FL, 1982, 221.
3. **Porta, E. and Hartroft, W. S.,** Lipid pigments in relation to aging and dietary factors (lipofuscin), in *Pigments in Pathology,* Wolman, M., Ed., Academic Press, New York, 1969, 191.
4. **Strehler, B. L.,** On the histochemistry and ultrastructure of age pigment, in *Advances in Gerontological Research,* Vol. 1, Strehler, B. L., Ed., Academic Press, New York, 1964, 343.
5. **Collins, V. P., Arborgh, B., Brunk, U. T., and Schellens, J. P. M.,** Phagocytosis and degradation of rat liver mitochondria by human glial cells, *Lab Invest.,* 42, 209, 1980.
6. **Sohal, R. S. and Wolfe, L. S.,** Lipofuscin: characteristics and significance, *Prog. Brain Res.,* 70, 171, 1986.
7. **Tappel, A. L.,** Lipid peroxidation and fluorescent molecular damage to membranes, in *Pathobiology of Cell Membrane,* Trump, B. and Arstila, A., Eds., Academic Press, New York, 1975, 145.

8. **Brunk, U. T. and Sohal, R. S.**, Mechanisms of lipofuscin formation, in *Membrane Lipid Oxidation,* Vol. 2, Vigo-Pelfrey, C., Ed., CRC Press, Boca Raton, FL, 1991, 191.
9. **Elleder, M.**, Chemical characterization of age pigments, in *Age Pigments,* Sohal, R. S., Ed., Elsevier, Amsterdam, 1981, 203.
10. **Wolfe, L. S., Gauthier, S., and Durham, H. D.**, Dolichols and phosphorylated dolichols in the neuronal ceroid lipofuscinosis, other lysosomal storage diseases and Alzheimer's disease. Induction of autolysosomes in fibroblasts, in *Lipofuscin-1987: State of the Art,* Nagy, I., Zs., Ed., Akademiai Kiado, Budapest and Elsevier, Amsterdam, 1988, 389.
11. **Ivy, G. O. and Gurd, J. W.**, A proteinase inhibitor model of lipofuscin formation, in *Lipofuscin-1987: State of the Art,* Nagy, I., Zs., Ed., Akademiai Kiado, Budapest and Elsevier, Amsterdam, 1988, 83.
12. **Marzabadi, M. R., Sohal, R. S., and Brunk, U. T.**, Mechanisms of lipofuscinogenesis: effect of the inhibition of lysosomal proteases and lipases under varying concentrations of ambient oxygen in cultured rat neonatal myocardial cells, *APMIS,* 99, 416, 1991.
13. **Brizzee, K. P., Cancilla, P. A., Sherwood, N., and Timiras, P. S.**, The amount and distribution of pigments in neurons and glia of the cerebral cortex, *J. Gerontol.,* 24, 127, 1969.
14. **Wolman, M.**, Lipid pigments (chromolipids): their origin, nature and significance, in *Pathobiology Annual,* Vol. 10, Joachim, H. M., Ed., Raven Press, New York, 1980, 253.
15. **Nandy, K.**, Properties of neuronal lipofuscin pigment in mice, *Acta Neuropathol.,* 19, 25, 1971.
16. **Pearse, A. G. E.**, *Histochemistry,* Vol. 2, 3rd ed., Williams & Wilkins, Baltimore, 1972.
17. **Björkerud, S.**, Isolated lipofuscin granules — a survey of a new field, *Adv. Gerontol. Res.,* 1, 257, 1964.
18. **Jolly, R. D., Barnes, A. B., and Palmer, D. N.**, Ovine ceroid-lipofuscinogenesis: chemical constituents of the lipopigment, their pathogenic significance and similarities to age pigment, *Adv. Biol. Sci.,* 64, 197, 1987.
19. **Hill, K. T. and Womersly, C.**, Critical aspects of fluorescent age-pigment methodologies: modification for accurate analysis and assessments in aquatic organisms, *Marine Biol.,* 109, 1, 1991.
20. **Ericsson, J. L. E.**, Mechanisms of cellular autophagy, in *Lysosomes in Biology and Pathology,* Vol. 2, Dingle, J. T. and Fell, H. B., Eds., North-Holland, Amsterdam, 1969, 345.
21. **Ohkuma, S., Moriyama, Y., and Takano, T.**, Identification and characterization of a proton pump on lysosomes by fluorescein isothiocyanate-dextran fluorescence, *Proc. Natl. Acad. Sci. U.S.A.,* 79, 2758, 1982.
22. **Brunk, U. T. and Collins, V. P.**, Lysosomes and age pigment in cultured cells, in *Age Pigments,* Sohal, R. S., Ed., Elsevier, Amsterdam, 1981, 243.
23. **Brunk, U.**, Distribution and shifts of ingested marker particles in residual bodies and other lysosomes, *Exp. Cell Res.,* 79, 1, 1973.
24. **de Duve, C.**, The lysosomes in retrospect, in *Lysosomes in Biology and Pathology,* Vol. 1, Dingle, J. T. and Fell, H. B., Eds., North-Holland, Amsterdam, 1969, 3.
25. **Goldfischer, S. and Bernstein, J.**, Lipofuscin (aging) pigment granules of the newborn human liver, *J. Cell Biol.,* 42, 253, 1969.
26. **Sohal, R. S., Marzabadi, M. R., Galaris, D., and Brunk, U. T.**, Effect of ambient oxygen concentration on lipofuscin accumulation in cultured rat heart myocytes — a novel *in vitro* model of lipofuscinogenesis, *Free-Radical Biol. Med.,* 6, 23, 1989.
27. **Brunk, U. and Ericsson, J. L. E.**, Electron microscopical studies on rat brain neurons. Localization of acid phosphatase and mode of formation of lipofuscin, *J. Ultrastruct. Res.,* 38, 1, 1972.

28. **Thaw, H. H., Brunk, U. T., and Collins, V. P.,** Influence of oxygen tension, pro-oxidants and antioxidants on the formation of lipid peroxidation products (lipofuscin) in individual cultivated human glial cells, *Mech. Ageing Dev.,* 24, 211, 1984.

29. **Marzabadi, M. R., Sohal, R. S., and Brunk, U. T.,** Effect of ferric iron and desferrioxamine on lipofuscin accumulation in cultured rat heart myocytes, *Mech. Ageing Dev.,* 46, 145, 1988.

30. **Halliwell, B. and Gutteridge, J. M. C.,** The importance of free radicals and catalytic metals in human diseases, *Mol. Aspects Med.,* 8, 89, 1985.

31. **Brunk, U. and Cadenas, E.,** The potential intermediate role of lysosomes in oxygen free-radical pathology, *APMIS,* 96, 3, 1988.

32. **Sohal, R. S.,** Quantification of lipofuscin: a critique of the current methodology, in *Advances in Age Pigment Research,* Totaro, E. J., Glees, P., and Pianti, F. A., Eds., Pergamon Press, Oxford, 1987, 85.

33. **Yin, D. and Brunk, U.,** Microfluorometric and fluorometric lipofuscin spectral discrepancies: a concentration-dependent metachromatic effect?, *Mech. Ageing Dev.,* 59, 95, 1991.

34. **Goldfischer, S.,** The localization of copper in the pericanalicular granules (lysosomes) of liver in Wilson's disease (hepatolenticular degeneration), *Am. J. Pathol.,* 46, 977, 1965.

35. **Lindquist, R. R.,** Studies on the pathogenesis of hepatolenticular degeneration. I. Acid phosphatase activity in copper-loaded rat livers, *Am. J. Pathol.,* 51, 471, 1967.

36. **Pihl, E.,** Ultrastructural localization of heavy metals by a modified sulfide-silver method, *Histochemie,* 10, 126, 1967.

37. **Brunk, U., Brun, A., and Sköld, G.,** Histochemical demonstration of heavy metals with the sulfide-silver method, *Acta Histochem.,* 31, 345, 1968.

38. **Haug, S. J. S.,** Electron microscopical localization of the zinc in hippocampal mossy fiber synapses by a modified sulfide-silver procedure, *Histochemie,* 8, 355, 1967.

39. **Brun, A. and Brunk, U.,** Histochemical indications for lysosomal localization of heavy metals in normal rat brain and liver, *J. Histochem. Cytochem.,* 18, 820, 1970.

40. **Ibata, Y. and Otsuka, N.,** Electron microscopic demonstration of zinc in the hippocampal formation using Timm's sulfide-silver technique, *J. Histochem. Cytochem.,* 17, 171, 1969.

41. **Miyawaki, H.,** Histochemistry and electron microscopy of iron containing granules, lysosomes and lipofuscin in mouse mammary glands, *J. Natl. Cancer Inst.,* 34, 601, 1965.

42. **Essner, E. and Novikoff, A. B.,** Human hepatocellular pigments and lysosomes, *J. Ultrastruct. Res.,* 3, 373, 1960.

43. **Timm, F.,** Zur Histochemie der schwermetalle. Das sulfid-silberverfahren, *Dtsch. Z. Ges. Gerichtl. Med.,* 46, 706, 1958.

44. **Timm, F., Naundorg, C., and Kraft, M.,** Zur histochemie und genese der chronischen quecksilbervergiftung, *Int. Arch. Gewerbepath. Gewerbehug.,* 22, 236, 1966.

45. **Malmström, B. and Neilands, J. B.,** Metalloproteins, *Annu. Rev. Biochem.,* 33, 331, 1964.

46. **de Duve, C. and Wattiaux, R.,** Functions of lysosomes, *Annu. Rev. Physiol.,* 28, 435, 1966.

47. **Bacon, R. B. and Britton, R. S.,** The pathology of hepatic iron overload: a free-radical-mediated process?, *Hepatology,* 2, 127, 1990.

48. **Chance, B., Sies, H., and Boveris, A.,** Hydroperoxide metabolism in mammalian organs, *Physiol Rev.,* 59, 527, 1979.

49. **Farber, J. L., Marlene, E. K., and Coleman, J. B.,** Biology of disease mechanisms of cell injury by activated oxygen species, *Lab. Invest.,* 62, 670, 1990.

50. **Halliwell, B. and Gutteridge, J. M. C.,** *Free Radicals in Biology and Medicine,* Clarendon Press, Oxford, 1989.

51. **de Duve, C., Barsy, T., Poole, B., Trouet, A., Tulkens, P., and van Hoof, F.,** Lysosomotropic agents, *Biochem. Pharmacol.,* 86, 180, 1974.
52. **Allison, A. C., Harington, J. S., and Birbeck, M.,** An examination of the cytotoxic effects of silica on macrophages, *J. Exp. Med.,* 209, 874, 1966.
53. **Ericsson, J. L. E. and Brunk, U. T.,** Alterations in lysosomal membrane as related to disease processes, in *Pathobiology of Cell Membrane,* Trump, B. F. and Arstila, A. U., Eds., Academic Press, New York, 1975, 217.
54. **Zdolsek, J., Zhang, H., Roberg, K., and Brunk, U.,** Oxidative stress, hydrogen peroxide and lysosomal integrity, manuscript.
55. **Zdolsek, L. M., Olsson, G. M., and Brunk, U. T.,** Photooxidative damage to lysosomes of cultured macrophages by acridine orange, *Photochem. Photobiol.,* 51, 67, 1990.
56. **Abok, K., Ericsson, J. L. E., and Brunk, U.,** Effects of iron on the stability of macrophage lysosomes, *Virchows Arch. B,* 43, 85, 1983.
57. **Abok, K., Rundquist, I., Forsberg, B., and Brunk, U. T.,** Dimethyl sulfoxide increases the survival and lysosomal stability of mouse peritoneal macrophages exposed to low-LET ionizing radiation and/or ionic iron in culture, *Virchows Arch. B,* 46, 307, 1984.
58. **Abok, K., Brunk, U. T., Jung, B., and Ericsson, J. L. E.,** Morphologic and histochemical studies on the differing radiosensitivity of ductular and acinar cells of the rat submandibular gland, *Virchows Arch. B,* 45, 433, 1984.
59. **Abok, K., Blomquist, E., Ericsson, J., and Brunk, U.,** Macrophage radiosensitivity in culture as a function of exposure to ionic iron, *Virchows Arch. B,* 42, 119, 1983.

Part IV
Roles for Iron in Cardiovascular Disease

9. Role of Iron in the Oxidative Modification of LDL

Sampath Parthasarathy

*Department of Medicine, University of California, San Diego,
La Jolla, California*

I. INTRODUCTION

The atherogenicity of low density lipoprotein (LDL)-associated choles-terol and the involvement of monocyte/macrophages in the development of early atherosclerotic foam cell lesions have been firmly established.[1] How-ever, the inability of LDL to generate foam cells *in vitro*[2] has led to the race in search of an LDL-derived progeny that would do so. A wide array of such modified low-density lipoproteins have since been identified. These include acetyl LDL, malondialdehyde LDL (MDA-LDL) and other aldehyde adducts of LDL, dextran sulfate complexed LDL, aggregated LDL, and oxidized LDL (ox-LDL).[1] Of these, there is considerable evidence to suggest that ox-LDL exists *in vivo* and prevention of oxidation of LDL may decrease the extent of atherosclerosis.[1] The atherogenicity of ox-LDL may be due to a multitude of potent biological effects (Table 1).[1,3-5] However, it remains to be established how oxidation of LDL influences the atherogenic process *in vivo*.

II. THE OXIDIZED LDL

Oxidation of LDL can be achieved by a variety of means. These include incubation with specific cell types and incubation with metal ions, notably copper and ferric iron, in the absence of any cells.[6-13] Although there appeared to be some confusion regarding the ability of iron to induce the oxidation of LDL in simple buffers,[11-13] an overwhelming majority of studies confirms that LDL can readily be oxidized by the inclusion of iron. However, the mechanism(s) by which either iron or copper induces lipid peroxidation in simple systems such as phosphate buffered saline remains to be elucidated. It is possible that during the isolation procedure LDL acquired low levels of peroxides that in the presence of metals caused rapid propagation of lipid peroxidation. Common to all these methods is the peroxidative decomposition of fatty acids associated with LDL lipids and covalent modification of the apoprotein B_{100} by the carbonyl products.[1,14,15] The apoprotein itself suffers a nonenzymatic, oxidative proteolysis during the oxidative process.[16] Oxi-dation of LDL by cells also may depend on the presence of trace metal ions because media that support oxidation often contain either ferric iron or copper. More importantly the oxidative modification of LDL is subject to inhibition by metal chelators.[6]

A. MECHANISM(S) OF OXIDATIVE MODIFICATION OF LDL

The cell-mediated modification of LDL has been extensively studied during the past few years, and as a result the following sequence of events has been suggested to be involved in the modification:[1]

1. Oxidation of phospholipids at the surface
2. Hydrolysis of the phospholipid peroxides by an intrinsic phospholipase A_2 activity

TABLE 1
Biological Effects of Oxidized LDL

Increased uptake by macrophages results.
Oxidized LDL is chemotactic for monocytes.
Oxidized LDL inhibits macrophage chemotaxis.
Oxidized LDL is cytotoxic to cultured cells.
Oxidized LDL inhibits endothelium-dependent relaxation.
Oxidized LDL induces differentiation of U937 cells and human monocytes.
Oxidized LDL increases TNF mRNA expression.
Minimally oxidized LDL enhances monocyte adhesion to endothelial cells.
Minimally oxidized LDL induces endothelial cell expression of granulocyte and macrophage
  colony-stimulating factors.
Minimally oxidized LDL stimulates macrophage chemotactic peptide-1 from both endothelial
  cells and smooth muscle cells.

3. Propagation of lipid peroxidation into the core
4. Oxidative nonenzymatic cleavage of apoprotein B_{100} and oxidative changes in amino acids
5. Breakdown of lipid peroxides into reactive aldehydes, e.g., malondialdehyde, 4-OH nonenal, hexanal, etc.
6. Derivatization of ϵ-amino groups of lysine residues with the aldehydes forming Schiff's bases

Charge or conformational changes resulting from these modifications alter the particle to such an extent that the receptor that recognizes native LDL does not recognize the ox-LDL.[1] ANother receptor, namely, acetyl LDL receptor that belongs to the scavenger receptor family that is in part involved in the recognition and internalization of ox-LDL has been purified and cloned.[17-19] However, additional receptors for ox-LDL have been suggested, at least on mouse peritoneal macrophages.[20]

B. OXIDATION OF LDL IN PLASMA

Oxidatively modified LDL, like acetyl LDL, when injected intravenously into animals disappears within minutes.[21] The sinusoidal endothelial cells of the liver very rapidly take up these lipoproteins from circulation.[22] This suggested that such LDL is likely to be present *in vivo* in the sequestered environment under the endothelial surface, and not in the plasma. However, oxidized LDL is not a single, homogeneous entity, and LDL oxidized to a lesser degree may be present in the plasma. In fact, the rate of clearance of oxidized LDL from the plasma appears to be related to the extent to which it is oxidized.[21] If LDL oxidized to a very low extent exists in the plasma, whether lipid peroxidation occured in the antioxidant-rich plasma or the peroxidized lipids made elsewhere in the body became associated with the lipoprotein, would be an important criteria in evaluating the mechanism(s) of oxidation of LDL. On the other hand, LDL subfractions that differ in their ability to be oxidized have been described.[23,24]

C. SUPEROXIDE ANION IN THE OXIDATION OF LDL

Many cell types that are associated with the atherosclerotic artery are capable of oxidatively modifying LDL. These include endothelial cells, smooth muscle cells, monocytes, and macrophages.[1] Studies on smooth muscle cell and monocyte-mediated modification of LDL have suggested that superoxide radicals may be involved in the modification of LDL.[8,25-27] Direct superoxide generation by specific enzymes as well as indirect extracellular generation of superoxide has been hinted.[28] The latter presumably results as a result of interaction of thiols with metal ions in the medium or via a lipoxygenase intermediate. The modification of LDL by smooth muscle cells and monocyte is readily inhibited by superoxide dismutase.

In contrast, the modification of LDL by endothelial cells or by resident peritoneal macrophages are poorly affected by superoxide dismutase.[29,30] Oxidation of LDL by these cells has been shown to be susceptible for inhibition by inhibitors of lipoxygenase reaction.

D. LIPOXYGENASE IN THE OXIDATION OF LDL

There is considerable evidence for the presence of oxidized LDL *in vivo.*[1] However, the cell types responsible for the oxidation of LDL in the body are open to speculation. Considering the finding that most of the oxidation specific immunostainable material centers around the macrophage-rich areas of the lesion, it is likely that these cells are intimately involved in the oxidative process. In addition to cell culture studies that suggested the involvement of lipoxygenases in the initiation of lipid peroxidation, earlier studies also showed that lipoxygenases can induce lipid peroxidation and oxidative modification of LDL.[31] Ylä-Herttuala et al.[32,33] probed human and Watanabe heritable hyperlipidemic (WHHL) rabbit arteries with specific antisense mRNA probes of various lipoxygenases and showed the presence of 15-lipoxygenase mRNA. Using antibodies to 15-lipoxygenase, they also demonstrated the enzyme protein. Increased levels of 15-lipoxygenase enzyme activity and products also have been reported in the atherosclerotic aorta.[34,35] Thus, there is suggestive evidence for the presence and involvement of an enzyme that can initiate the oxidation of LDL.

III. ROLE OF IRON IN THE OXIDATION OF LDL

The cell-induced oxidation of LDL is inhibited by antioxidants and metal chelators.[1] It is very likely that under the incubation conditions these agents act in the medium protecting the LDL from oxidation. This is also supported by the finding that LDL isolated from patients on antioxidant, treatment (probucol) is resistant to oxidation.[36] However, under *in vivo* conditions, the possibility that cell-associated antioxidants modulate lipid peroxidation intracellularly cannot be ignored. For example, all lipoxygenases contain an essential ferric iron atom that is very much involved in the catalytic mechanism.[37] It has been proposed that iron is involved in the generation of the fatty acid pentadienyl radical.[38] Antioxidants, such as vitamin E or hydroxamic acid derivatives, are suggested to reduce the ferric state of the iron to ferrous iron, thus inhibiting the enzyme activity.[39,40] This iron atom is presumably coordinated to histidine residues and is not readily removable by simple chelators such as ethylenediaminetetraacetic acid (EDTA). Currently most of the lipoxygenase inhibitors available fall in the major category of either an antioxidant or an *N*-hydroxy derivative.

Iron also may play an important role not only in the rapid propagation of lipid peroxidation but also in the decomposition of the peroxide to reactive aldehydes. It is frequently observed that oxidation of LDL in metal-containing media generated greater amounts of thiobarbituric acid products than oxidation in simple buffers, for example with AAPH, a free-radical generator.

In summary, the oxidation hypothesis that centers around the oxidative modification of LDL is an attractive candidate for defining the initiating mechanisms in atherogenesis. If this hypothesis is validated, redox metal ions (particularly iron) may play an important role. Involvement of specific iron-containing oxygenases in the development of the early atherosclerotic lesion may offer an important target for intervention.

REFERENCES

1. **Steinberg, D., Parthasarathy, S., Carew, T. E., Khoo, J. C., and Witzum, J. L.,** Beyond cholesterol: modifications of low density lipoprotein that increase its atherogenicity, *N. Engl. J. Med.,* 320, 915, 1989.
2. **Goldstein, J. L., Ho, Y. K., Basu, S. K., and Brown, M. S.,** Binding site on macrophages that mediates uptake and degradation of acetylated low density lipoprotein producing massive cholesterol deposition, *Proc. Natl. Acad. Sci. U.S.A.,* 76, 333, 1979.
3. **Berliner, J. A., Territo, M. C., Sevanian, A., Ramin, S., Kim, J. A., Bamshad, B., Esterson, M., and Fogelman, A. M.,** Minimally modified LDL stimulates monocyte endothelial cell interactions, *J. Clin. Invest.,* 85, 1260, 1990.
4. **Cushing, S. D., Berliner, J. A., Valente, A. J., Territo, M. C., Navab, M., Parhami, F., Gerrity, R., Schwartz, C. J., and Fogelman, A. M.,** Minimally modified low density lipoprotein induces monocyte chemotactic protein 1 in human endothelial cells and smooth muscle cells, *Proc. Natl. Acad. Sci. U.S.A.,* 87, 5134, 1990.
5. **Rajavashisht, T. B., Andalibi, A., Territo, M. C., Berliner, J. A., Navab, M., and Lusis, A. J.,** Induction of endothelial cell expression of granulocyte and macrophage colony-stimulating factors by modified low density lipoproteins, *Nature (London),* 344, 254, 1990.
6. **Steinbrecher, U. P., Parthasarathy, S., Leake, D. S., Witztum, J. L., and Steinberg, D.,** Modification of low density lipoproteins by endothelial cells involves lipid peroxidation and degradation of low density lipoprotein phospholipids, *Proc. Natl. Acad. Sci. U.S.A.,* 81, 3883, 1984.
7. **Morel, D. W., DiCarletto, P. E., and Chisolm, G. M.,** Endothelial and smooth muscle cells alter low density lipoprotein *in vitro* by free radical oxidation, *Arteriosclerosis,* 4, 357, 1984.

268

8. **Heinecke, J. W., Baker, L., Rosen, H., and Chait, A.,** Superoxide-mediated modification of low density lipoprotein by arterial smooth muscle cells, *J. Clin. Invest.,* 77, 757, 1986.

9. **Parthasarathy, S., Printz, D. J., Boyd, D., Joy, L., and Steinberg, D.,** Macrophage oxidation of low density lipoprotein generates a modified form recognized by the scavenger receptor, *Arteriosclerosis,* 6, 505, 1986.

10. **Hiramatsu, K., Rosen, H., Heinecke, J. W., Wolfbauer, G., and Chait, A.,** Superoxide initiates oxidation of low density lipoprotein by human monocytes, *Arteriosclerosis,* 7, 55, 1987.

11. **Kosugi, K., Morel, D. W., DiCarleto, P. E., and Chisolm, G. M.,** Toxicity of oxidized LDL to cultured fibroblast is selective for S phase of the cycle, *J. Cell. Physiol.,* 130, 311, 1987.

12. **Esterbauer, H., Rotheneder, M. D., Waeg, G., Striegl, G., and Jürgens, G.,** Biochemical, structural, and functional properties of oxidized low-density lipoprotein, *Chem. Res. Toxicol.,* 3, 77, 1990.

13. **Kuzuya, M., Yamada, K., Hayashi, T., Funaki, C., Naito, M., Asai, K., and Kuzuya, F.,** Oxidation of low density lipoprotein by copper and iron in phosphate buffer, *Biochim. Biophys. Acta,* 1084, 198, 1991.

14. **Esterbauer, H., Jürgens, G., Quehenberger, O., and Koller, E.,** Autoxidation of human low density lipoprotein: loss of polyunsaturated fatty acids and vitamin E and generation of aldehydes, *J. Lipid Res.,* 28, 495, 1987.

15. **Steinbrecher, U. P.,** Oxidation of human low density lipoproteins results in derivatization of lysine residues of apolipoprotein B by lipid peroxide decomposition products, *J. Biol. Chem.,* 262, 3603, 1987.

16. **Fong, L. G., Parthasarathy, S., Witztum, J. L., and Steinberg, D.,** Nonenzymatic degradation of apoprotein B-100 during the oxidative modification of low density lipoprotein, *J. Lipid Res.,* 28, 1466, 1987.

17. **Via, D. P., Dresel, H. A., Cheng, S. L., and Gotto, A. M., Jr.,** Murine macrophage tumors are a source of a 260,000-dalton acetyl-low density lipoprotein receptor, *J. Biol. Chem.,* 260, 7379, 1985.

18. **Kodama, T., Freeman, M., Rohrer, L., Zabrecky, A. J., Matsudaira, P., and Krieger, M.,** Type 1 macrophage scavenger receptor contains α-helical and collagen-like coils, *Nature (London),* 343, 532, 1990.

19. **Rohrer, L., Freeman, M., Kodama, T., Penman, M., and Krieger, M.,** Coiled-coil fibrous domains mediate binding by the macrophage scavenger receptor type II, *Nature (London),* 343, 570, 1990.

20. **Sparrow, C. P., Parthasarathy, S., and Steinberg, D. A.,** Macrophage receptor that recognizes oxidized low density lipoprotein but not acetylated low density lipoprotein, *J. Biol. Chem.,* 264, 2599, 1989.

21. **Steinbrecher, U. P., Witztum, J. L., Parthasarathy, S., and Steinberg, D.,** Decrease in reactive amino groups during oxidation of endothelial cell modification of LDL. Correlation with change in receptor-mediated catabolism, *Ateriosclerosis,* 7, 135, 1987.

22. **Nagelkerke, J. F., Havekes, L., van Hinsbergh, V. W., and van Berkel, T. J.,** *In vivo* catabolism of biologically modified LDL, *Arteriosclerosis,* 4, 256, 1984.

23. **Knipping, G., Rotheneder, M., Striegl, G., and Esterbauer, H.,** Antioxidants and resistance against oxidation of porcine LDL subfractions, *J. Lipid Res.,* 31, 1965, 1990.

24. **Shimano, H., Yamada, N., Ishibashi, S., Mokuno, H., Mori, N., Gotoda, T., Harada, K., Akanuma, Y., Murase, T., Yazaki, Y., and Takaku, F.,** Oxidation-labile subfractions of human plasma low density lipoprotein isolated by ion-exchange chromatography, *J. Lipid Res.,* 32, 763, 1991.

25. **Heinecke, J. W., Rosen, H., and Chait, A.,** Iron and copper promote modification of low density lipoprotein by human arterial smooth muscle cells in culture, *J. Clin. Invest.,* 74, 1890, 1984.

26. **Cathcart, M. K., McNally, A. K., Morel, D. W., and Chisolm, G. M., III,** Superoxide anion participation in human monocyte-mediated oxidation of low density lipoprotein and conversion of low density lipoprotein to a cytotoxin, *J. Immunol.,* 142, 1963, 1989.
27. **McNally, A. K., Chisolm, G. M., III, Morel, D. W., and Cathcart, M. K.,** Activated human monocytes oxidize low density lipoprotein by a lipoxygenase-dependent pathway, *J. Immunol.,* 145, 254, 1990.
28. **Heinecke, J. W., Rosen, H., and Chait, A.,** The role of sulfur-containing amino acids in superoxide production by arterial smooth muscle cells, *J. Biol. Chem.,* 262, 10098, 1987.
29. **Parthasarathy, S., Wieland, E., and Steinberg, D.,** A role for endothelial cell lipoxygenase in the oxidative modification of low density lipoprotein, *Proc. Natl. Acad. Sci. U.S.A.,* 86, 1046, 1989.
30. **Rankin, S. M., Parthasarathy, S., and Steinberg, D.,** Evidence for a dominant role of lipoxygenase(s) in the oxidation of LDL by mouse peritoneal macrophages, *J. Lipid Res.,* 32, 449, 1991.
31. **Sparrow, C. P., Parthasarathy, S., and Steinberg, D.,** Enzymatic modification of low density lipoprotein by purified lipoxygenase plus phospholipase A2 mimics cell-mediated oxidative modification, *J. Lipid Res.,* 29, 745, 1988.
32. **Ylä-Herttuala, S., Rosenfeld, M. E., Parthasarathy, S., Glass, C. K., Sigal, E., Witztum, J. L., and Steinberg, D.,** Colocalization of 15-lipoxygenase mRNA and protein with epitopes of oxidized low density lipoprotein in macrophage-rich areas of atherosclerotic lesions, *Proc. Natl. Acad. Sci. U.S.A.,* 87, 6959, 1990.
33. **Ylä-Herttuala, S., Rosenfeld, M. E., Parthasarathy, S., Sigal, E., Särkioja, T., Witztum, J. L., and Steinberg, D.,** Gene expression in macrophage-rich human atherosclerotic lesions. 15-Lipoxygenase and acetyl low density lipoprotein receptor messenger RNA colocalize with oxidation specific lipid-protein adducts, *J. Clin. Invest.,* 87, 1146, 1991.
34. **Henriksson, P., Hamberg, M., and Diczfalusy, U.,** Formation of 15-HETE as a major hydroxyeicosatetraenoic acid in the atherosclerotic vessel wall, *Biochim. Biophys. Acta,* 834, 272, 1985.
35. **Simon, T. C., Makheja, A. N., and Baily, J. M.,** Formation of 15-hydroxyeicosatetraenoic acid (15-HETE) as the predominant eicosanoid in aortas from Watanabe heritable hyperlipidemic rabbits, *Atherosclerosis,* 75, 31, 1989.
36. **Parthasarathy, S., Young, S. G., Witztum, J. L., Pittman, R. C., and Steinberg, D.,** Probucol inhibits the oxidative modification of low density lipoprotein, *J. Clin. Invest.,* 77, 641, 1986.
37. **Sigal, E.,** The molecular biology of mammalian arachidonic acid metabolism, *Am. J. Physiol.,* 260, L13, 1991.
38. **Nelson, M. J., Seitz, S. P., and Cowling, R. A.,** Enzyme bound pentadienyl and peroxy radicals in purple lipoxygenase, *Biochemistry,* 29, 6897, 1990.
39. **Nelson, M. J., Batt, D. G., Thompson, J. S., and Wright, S. W.,** Reduction of the active-site iron by potent inhibitors of lipoxygenases, *J. Biol. Chem.,* 266, 8225, 1991.
40. **Summers, J. B., Kim, K. H., Nazdiyasni, H., Holms, J. H., Ratajczyk, J. D., Stewart, A. D., Dyer, R. D., and Carter, G. W.,** Hydroxamic acid inhibitors of 5-lipoxygenase: quantitative structure-activity relationships, *J. Med. Chem.,* 33, 922, 1990.

10. The Role of Iron in Myocardial Reperfusion Injury

JAY L. ZWEIER

EPR Laboratories and Cardiology Division, The Johns Hopkins Medical Institutions, Francis Scott Key Medical Center, Baltimore, Maryland

I. INTRODUCTION

Ischemic heart disease remains the most important cause of morbidity and mortality in the U.S. Over the last decade acute revascularization with thrombolytic drugs has emerged as the standard treatment for patients with acute myocardial infarction.[1,2] While reperfusion of ischemic tissues limits ischemic damage, reperfusion itself initiates a chain of events which causes a new form of tissue damage. This damage has been termed "reflow" or "reperfusion" injury. Considerable evidence has emerged over the last decade which indicates that iron may play a key role in the pathogenesis of reperfusion injury in the heart.

This chapter will summarize the evidence for oxidative free-radical-mediated reperfusion injury in the postischemic heart and the evidence for iron-mediated Fenton chemistry in the pathogenesis of this injury.

II. REPERFUSION INJURY

Reperfusion injury in the heart is characterized by a unique histological picture with the formation of contraction bands in the contractile proteins, calcific granules within mitochondria as well as cell swelling and the disruption of sarcoplasmic and mitochondrial membranes.[1,2] A number of mechanisms have been proposed to mediate reperfusion injury. These include cellular calcium loading, the occurrence of a no reflow phenomenon due to cell swelling or formation of white cell plugs, and, perhaps most importantly, the formation of oxygen free radicals. The oxygen free-radical hypothesis is of particular importance because it can potentially explain each of the other three mechanisms of reperfusion injury. It has been demonstrated that exogenous free radicals cause cellular calcium loading with inhibition of the sarcoplasmic reticulum calcium ATPase and inhibition of the sodium-potassium ATPase leading to sodium-mediated calcium gain.[3] It is well known that oxygen radicals cause lipid peroxidation which can result in cell membrane breakdown causing cell swelling. It has been demonstrated that oxygen radicals result in the chemotaxis of neutrophils which, in turn, can lead to white cell plugging of capillaries. In addition, white cells which are chemotaxed and activated are potent sources of further oxygen radical generation.[4] A number of mechanisms have been proposed to cause oxygen free-radical generation in reperfused myocardium. These include the enzyme xanthine oxidase, mitochondrial oxidation, catecholamine oxidation, white cell activation, and iron or other transition metal redox cycling. A number of changes occur in ischemic tissues which predispose the tissue for subsequent oxidative reperfusion injury. It has been demonstrated that the enzyme xanthine dehydrogenase is converted to xanthine oxidase which is a potent generator of superoxide and hydrogen peroxide.[5] During ischemia the substrates for this reaction — hypoxanthine, xanthine, and inosine — accumulate. In addition, it has been shown that during ischemia cellular defenses against oxidative injury are impaired with lower activities of superoxide dismutase and glutathione peroxidase observed.[6] For each of these mechanisms iron also may be involved in modulating toxicity through the conversion of superoxide and hydrogen peroxide to the more reactive hydroxyl free radical.

III. FREE-RADICAL CHEMISTRY IN REPERFUSED TISSUE

Reduced forms of oxygen which can mediate cellular injury include the superoxide anion free radical, $O_2^{\cdot-}$, the one-electron reduced form of oxygen; hydrogen peroxide, H_2O_2, the two-electron reduced form of oxygen; and hydroxyl free radical, $OH^{\cdot}$, the three-electron reduced form of molecular oxygen. Both $O_2^{\cdot-}$ and $OH^{\cdot}$ are free radicals which are reactive in aqueous solution with the potential of reacting with biological macromolecules and inducing damage. H_2O_2 is also a potent but sluggish oxidizing agent and generates $O_2^{\cdot-}$ and $OH^{\cdot}$ in the presence of transition metal ions. $O_2^{\cdot-}$ spontaneously reacts with or dismutates in aqueous solution to yield H_2O_2 and O_2 by the reaction:

$$2O_2^{\cdot-} + 2H^+ \rightarrow H_2O_2 + O_2$$

In the presence of transition metals such as Fe^{3+} or Cu^{2+}, $O_2^{\cdot-}$ and H_2O_2 react to form the more reactive $OH^{\cdot}$ radical via the Fenton and Haber-Weiss reactions:

$$O_2^{\cdot-} + Fe^{3+} \rightarrow O_2 + Fe^{2+}$$
$$\underline{H_2O_2 + Fe^{2+} \rightarrow OH^{\cdot} + OH^- + Fe^{3+}}$$
$$\text{SUM:} \quad O_2^{\cdot-} + H_2O_2 \rightarrow OH^{\cdot} + OH^- + O_2$$

The superoxide-driven Fenton reaction can also be visualized as an iron redox cycle (Figure 1). Iron is ubiquitous in biological cells and tissues with low molecular weight chelates, hematin, or protein-bound iron (such as hemoglobin, myoglobin, or ferritin) present which can potentially catalyze the formation of $OH^{\cdot}$.[7-9]

The $OH^{\cdot}$ radical can react with fatty acids abstracting a hydrogen atom generating a carbon-centered alkyl radical, $R^{\cdot}$, on the fatty acid (Figure 2). In the polyunsaturated fatty acid shown, hydrogen abstraction would be followed by molecular rearrangement and oxygen uptake with the formation of the lipid or alkyl peroxy radical, $ROO^{\cdot}$.

IV. EVIDENCE FOR FREE-RADICAL-MEDIATED REPERFUSION INJURY

There are a large number of studies which have suggested that oxygen free radicals are important mediators of myocardial reperfusion injury. It has

Fe3+-chelate
·OH
·O2−
2H+ + 2·O2− → H2O2
Fe2+-chelate
O2

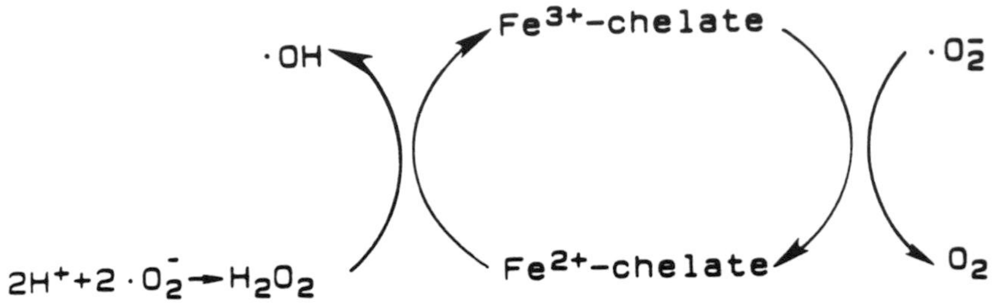

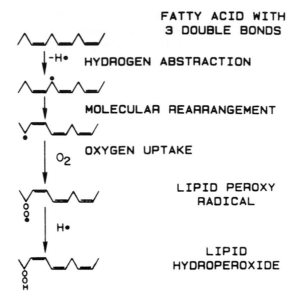

FIGURE 1. Iron redox cycling in the superoxide-driven Fenton reaction.

FATTY ACID WITH
3 DOUBLE BONDS
-H•
HYDROGEN ABSTRACTION
MOLECULAR REARRANGEMENT
OXYGEN UPTAKE
O2
LIPID PEROXY
RADICAL
H•
LIPID
HYDROPEROXIDE

FIGURE 2. Hydroxyl radical-mediated lipid peroxidation.

been demonstrated in a number of laboratories that superoxide dismutase can enhance the recovery of contractile function and decrease infarct size.[10-13] We have observed that superoxide dismutase administration on postischemic reperfusion enhances the recovery of contractile function in isolated perfused rabbit hearts.[14] Improved metabolic recovery is observed accompanying the improved functional recovery with higher concentrations of ATP and phosphocreatine PCr observed in the reperfused hearts as measured by phosphorus-31 NMR (Figure 3).

In the *in-vivo* canine model of regional ischemia, a number of laboratories have observed that administration of recombinant human superoxide dismutase decreases infarct size. With control reperfusion large contiguous hemorrhagic infarcts were observed while with SOD treatment smaller areas of patchy infarction were observed, (Figure 4).[15]

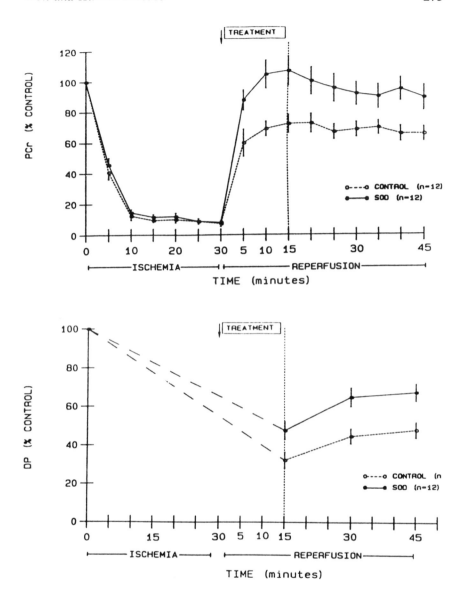

FIGURE 3. Graphs of the functional and metabolic recovery of isolated rabbit hearts reperfused in the presence or absence of SOD.

While many laboratories have observed protection with SOD, several others have not. A variety of reasons have been proposed to explain the varying protection observed with SOD. We have observed that the efficacy of SOD in preventing the generation of hydroxyl radicals derived from superoxide is modulated by the presence of iron.[16]

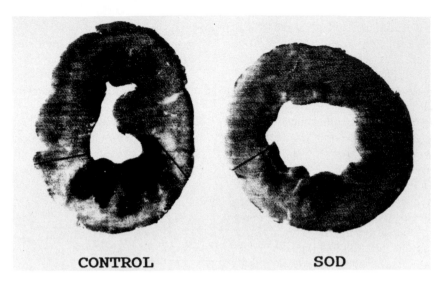

FIGURE 4. Histological sections through the left ventricles of canine hearts reperfused in the presence or absence of SOD.

V. EVIDENCE FOR IRON-MEDIATED REPERFUSION INJURY

A number of studies have been performed using the iron chelator deferoxamine. In isolated hearts it has been observed that deferoxamine treatment can markedly enhance the recovery of contractile function.[17] In these deferoxamine-treated hearts, higher coronary flows and an improved metabolic state were observed. Studies in the *in vivo* canine stunning model have also demonstrated that deferoxamine enhances the recovery of postischemic function.[18] To date the efficacy of deferoxamine in preventing postischemic injury has been observed in a number of laboratories. We will describe the results from several of these studies as follows.

In 1987 Ambrosio et al.[17] reported that deferoxamine administered at reflow could enhance the recovery of contractile function in the isolated postischemic rabbit heart. These experiments were performed in isolated perfused rabbit hearts subjected to 30 min of global 37°C ischemia with physiological measurements of hemodynamic parameters and phosphorous-31 NMR measurement of the bioenergetic state of the heart. These hearts were perfused retrograde at constant pressure, using a modified Langendorff technique. A balloon was placed within the left ventricle to measure left ventricular pressures. The hearts were perfused within 25 mm tubes placed within a ^{31}P probe of an NMR spectrometer. Simultaneous measurement of the contractile function and the bioenergetic state of the heart were thus obtained. Hearts were either reperfused in the presence or absence of deferoxamine. Hearts treated with deferoxamine showed significantly greater recovery of phosphocreatine concentrations and more rapid restoration of normal values of intracellular pH compared to untreated control hearts (Figure 5). This metabolic improvement was accompanied by preservation of myocardial function with higher left ventricular developed pressures and lower end diastolic pressures. The measured coronary flow also was observed to have enhanced recovery perhaps due to decreased vascular tone secondary to the prevention of cell swelling. Direct electron paramagnetic resonance (EPR) measurements of rapidly frozen tissue were performed and demonstrated that oxygen free-radical generation was quenched. It was hypothesized that the improved metabolic state observed in these hearts might reflect better preservation of mitochondria in deferoxamine-treated hearts with improved rates of aerobic metabolism in deferoxamine-treated myocardium. Subsequent studies demonstrated that intraischemic treatment with deferoxamine was as effective as treatment at reflow.[19]

Subsequently in 1990, van Jaarsveld et al.[20,21] reported that the impairment in mitochondrial function observed as a function of ischemia and reperfusion was decreased in deferoxamine-treated hearts. Isolated rat hearts were perfused and subjected to ischemia and reperfusion in the presence or absence of deferoxamine. Mitochondria were isolated from these hearts, and measurements of oxidative phosphorylation were performed. Significantly higher values of ADP/O ratio and rates of state three respiration were observed in hearts treated with deferoxamine.

Recently, Liu et al.[22] have utilized deferoxamine to study the role of iron on membrane phospholipid breakdown in the postischemic rat heart. Isolated Langendorff perfused rat hearts were subjected to 30 min of normothermic ischemia followed by reperfusion in the presence of deferoxamine. Deacylation and reacylation of membrane phospholipids was measured using [^{14}C]-arachidonic acid, and *de novo* phospholipid synthesis was evaluated using [^{3}H]glycerol, both labels perfused into the heart. In deferoxamine-treated hearts, the loss of [^{14}C]phosphatidylcholine and the accumulation of isotopically labeled lysophosphoglycerides and arachidonic acid was lower than in untreated hearts, while the incorporation of radioactive label into phospholipids was increased in the deferoxamine-treated hearts. They also observed that deferoxamine decreased the formation of malonaldehyde and the release of lactate dehydrogenase. In deferoxamine-treated hearts a higher recovery of high energy phosphate compounds was observed with decreased myocardial dysfunction. Together these results demonstrated that deferoxamine treatment prevents the degradation of membrane phospholipids during ischemia and reperfusion, as well as cellular, metabolic, and functional injury.

Several laboratories have studied the role of iron-mediated mechanisms of the cardiac injury in the setting of cardioplegia as is performed clinically in open heart surgery and heart transplantation. Bernard et al.[23] have performed studies evaluating the use of deferoxamine to enhance cardiac preservation during cardioplegic arrest. They subjected isolated working rat hearts to 30 min of low flow (75% reduction) ischemia followed by cardioplegic arrest at 15°C for 2 h followed by 30 min of normothermic reperfusion. Deferoxamine

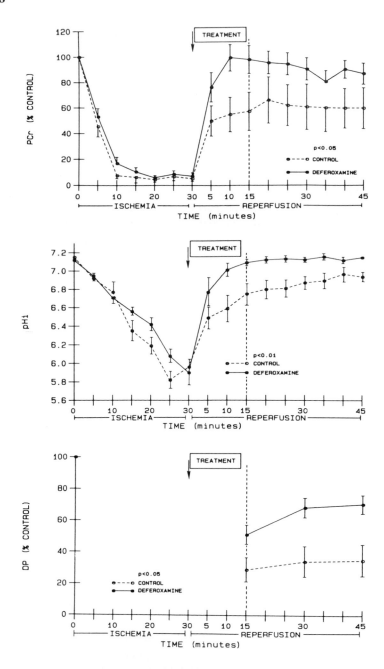

FIGURE 5. Graphs of the functional and metabolic recovery of isolated rabbit hearts reperfused in the presence or absence of deferoxamine.

was administered during the last 15 min of the low flow ischemia period. They observed that deferoxamine treatment resulted in higher recovery of coronary flow and ATP levels. More recently Menasch et al.[24] reported studies in which isovolumic buffer perfused rat hearts were subjected to longer periods of cardioplegic arrest of 5 h, followed by global ischemia at 15°C for 1 h, to simulate the surgical implantation procedure, followed by normothermic reperfusion for 1 h. They observed that improved functional recovery was observed with deferoxamine given as an additive to single dose cardioplegic solution at the end of the arrest period as well as within the perfusate during early reoxygenation. They observed that deferoxamine treatment enhanced the recovery of ventricular pressure development, left ventricular compliance, and coronary flow. Since they observed that deferoxamine had no inotropic effect, they hypothesized that its protective effect was most likely due to a decrease in catalytic iron required for free-radical production. Their results support the hypothesis that iron-mediated oxidative damage may contribute to the contractile failure which is sometimes observed in transplanted donor hearts.

Illes et al.[25] performed studies in an *in-vivo* canine cardioplegia model designed to simulate the cardioplegic cardiac arrest used in coronary bypass surgery. Hearts were subjected to 20 min of left anterior descending artery occlusion followed by 60 min of cardioplegic arrest in the presence of blood with or without deferoxamine and reperfusion with or without deferoxamine. Regional myocardial contractile function was measured by sonomicrometric measurements of regional stroke work. They observed that deferoxamine administered during cardioplegic arrest resulted in an improved recovery of contractile function and a prevention of postischemic myocardial stunning.

A number of studies have been published which report that deferoxamine can prevent myocardial stunning and decrease infarct size in *in-vivo* animal models. Bolli et al.[18] reported experiments in which open chest dogs were subjected to 15 min coronary occlusion and 4 h of reperfusion with defer-oxamine treatment beginning at either 2 min before reflow or 1 min after reflow. Additional animals were studied with iron-loaded deferoxamine administered 2 min before reflow, or vehicle control. To determine whether the protection afforded by deferoxamine was due to inhibition of free-radical generation, myocardial free-radical generation was assessed by intracoronary infusion of the spin trap α-phenyl-*N*-*tert*-butyl nitrone (PBN). They observed that deferoxamine treatment before reflow resulted in increased recovery of contractile function while treatment after reflow or treatment with iron-loaded deferoxamine afforded no protection. Deferoxamine pretreatment resulted in decreased production of PBN radical adducts measured upon reperfusion. It was suggested from these studies that a substantial portion of the damage responsible for myocardial stunning is caused by iron-catalyzed free-radical reactions that develop in the initial seconds of reperfusion. These results demonstrated that the attenuation of postischemic dysfunction by deferox-amine is associated with attenuation of free-radical reactions *in vivo*.

Recently, clinical evidence for the presence of oxidative reperfusion injury in the human heart has been reported. Ferreira et al.[26] report performing a study of 14 patients undergoing myocardial revascularization. Half of these patients received a cardioplegic solution containing deferoxamine, 1 g/l, and half received a control cardioplegic solution without deferoxamine. Myocardial biopsy samples were obtained before ischemia and during reperfusion. Chemiluminescence measurements were performed to indirectly access oxygen free-radical generation, and electron microscopic studies were performed to measure morphologically detectable injury. A twofold increase in tissue chemiluminescence was observed after reperfusion in the absence of deferoxamine while no increase occurred with deferoxamine treatment. The electron microscopic studies demonstrated a significant increase in severely damaged mitochondria in reperfusion biopsy samples. However, with deferoxamine treatment a better preservation of myocardial cells with less mitochondrial damage was seen. These results were interpreted to support the hypothesis that oxygen free radicals are responsible, in part, for the production of reperfusion injury in the human heart.

VI. MEASUREMENT OF FREE-RADICAL GENERATION IN THE POSTISCHEMIC HEART: EVIDENCE THAT IRON CAN MODULATE RADICAL GENERATION IN POSTISCHEMIC MYOCARDIUM

EPR spectroscopy can be applied to measure free-radical generation in the heart. In the EPR experiment the sample is placed in a magnetic field, H. It is irradiated with electromagnetic radiation usually in the microwave frequency range. The magnetic field, H, is varied, and the absorption of microwave energy, A, is measured as a function of H. Resonance is defined by the equation:

$$h\nu = g\beta H$$

where h is Plank's constant, ν is the microwave frequency, g is an empirical constant measured from the spectrum whose value serves to identify any given free radical, β is a constant called the Bohr magneton, and H is the applied magnetic field. For an isotropic electron or free radical the absorption function appears as a simple lorenzian or gaussian line as shown in Figure 6A(H). The usual convention is to display the first derivative absorption function as shown in Figure 6A'(H).

EPR spectroscopy can define the chemical structure of free radicals, the symmetry of the electron environment, and the presence of nuclei in the vicinity of the electron. For example, one can distinguish a simple isotropic free radical such as a delocalized carbon-centered semiquinone, from an oxygen-centered free radical such as ROO˙ from a nitrogen-centered free

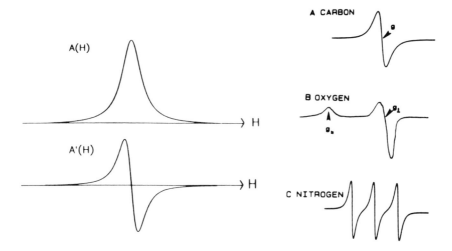

FIGURE 6. Left panel, absorption function and first derivative absorption function EPR line shapes; right panel, EPR spectra of different free radicals.

radical. The semiquinone radical gives rise to an isotropic signal as shown in Figure 6A while an oxygen-centered radical such as ROO˙ gives rise to an anisotropic spectrum with axial symmetry as shown in Figure 6B which is defined by two g values, $g_\parallel$ and $g_\perp$. A nitrogen-centered free radical such as a nitroxide shown in Figure 6C gives rise to a triplet signal due to hyperfine splitting from the nitrogen nucleus which has a spin of one. The magnitude of the hyperfine splitting is defined by the hyperfine coupling constant a_N.

Reactive oxygen free radicals can be measured by EPR spectroscopy in two different ways. Direct measurement of fast frozen samples can be performed at cryogenic temperatures, ≤ 77 K, or alternatively these radicals can be trapped using nitrone or other spin trap molecules and measured at room temperature or physiological temperatures. Each of these techniques has inherent advantages and disadvantages. Advantages of the direct rapid freeze measurement of free radicals include:

1. This is the most conclusive technique in that one directly measures radicals of interest.
2. At low temperatures, ≤ 77 K, the radicals measured are stable and can be studied for long periods of time.
3. One can study radical properties including power saturation and temperature stability which aid in identification.
4. There are no problems with artifact from added chemical-spin trap reagents.
5. Quantitative measurements can be performed on the actual primary radical.

Disadvantages of this technique include:

1. It is destructive. One sample yields information at only one time point. Therefore, one cannot simultaneously correlate radical concentrations and subsequent heart function.
2. There are technical difficulties in working at low temperature. The samples must be maintained at or below 77 K since warming will result in loss or alteration of radical signals.
3. This technique is often less sensitive than spin-trapping techniques.
4. Possible mechanical effects of tissue processing must be controlled.
5. Highly labile radicals such as OH˙ are not measureable.

Spin trapping techniques have a number of advantages including:

1. They have greater sensitivity with an integrative effect of the trap with respect to radical measurement.
2. Very labile radicals including OH˙ can be measured.
3. Assignment of radical signals is usually simple.
4. Measurements can be performed at physiological or room temperature.
5. The technique is nondestructive which allows for simultaneous measurements of radicals and correlation with organ function.

The spin-trapping technique also has disadvantages including:

1. Signals can be observed in the absence of radical generation due to impurities in the trap, light exposure, or nonspecific redox reactions of the trap.
2. Therefore, matched control measurements are always essential.
3. Trapping is not 100% efficient with the efficiency of radical trapping varying as a function of trap concentration.
4. The spin trap molecules in high concentrations can cause alterations in cells and tissues.

Thus, the direct low temperature and spin-trapping techniques for measuring free radicals have relative strengths and weaknesses. The combined use of both of these techniques can thus provide more information than the use of either technique alone.

A. DIRECT MEASUREMENTS

Langendorff-perfused rabbit hearts have been studied to determine whether there is measurable free-radical generation on postischemic reperfusion.[27] In this preparation the animals were anesthetized, the hearts removed, the aorta cannulated, the hearts perfused with a Krebs bicarbonate buffered perfusate at a constant pressure of 80 mmHg, and a left ventricular balloon inserted to measure contractile function. The balloon volume was adjusted to achieve a diastolic pressure in the range of 8 to 12 mmHg. The hearts were perfused for a period of at least 15 min prior to starting the experiments to allow for stabilization. Left ventricular developed pressures of approximately 110 mmHg were observed with intrinsic heart rate of 150 beats per minute (bpm). At the desired time the left ventricular balloon was removed and hearts were freeze-clamped using Wollenberger tongs cooled to 77 K. The freeze-clamped heart tissue was then ground to a granular powder under liquid nitrogen and the powder was transferred to precision EPR tubes. Mechanical processing of the tissue was minimized by limiting the duration of grinding to <1.5 min with a resulting frozen particle size of 1.5 to 2.5 mm diameter. In addition, care was taken to prevent exposure of the tissue to air. These steps minimized the generation of mechanically derived radicals which can be observed on excessive mechanical processing of tissues. In order to further verify that the observed radical signals were not due to processing artifact, samples were processed by the different technique of tissue extrusion using a stainless steel-funneled extrusion cylinder under liquid nitrogen. With this latter technique relatively large tissue fragments can be compacted into the shape of a cylindrical core ideal for EPR measurements.

Both of these tissue-processing techniques gave rise to identical EPR spectra, suggesting the absence of significant processing artifact. Great care was taken to maintain the tissue under liquid nitrogen at all times with both of these techniques. Quantitative EPR measurements were performed by comparison of the double integral of the observed signal with that of the commonly used free-radical standard potassium peroxylamine disulfonate in frozen aqueous solution in identical EPR tubes. In these measurements the EPR tubes were 3 mm on the inside diameter and were filled to a height more than sufficient to achieve the optimum critical filling of the TE102 resonator used. It is essential to achieve this identical filling of critical volume of the resonant cavity for accurate quantitative measurements. The measured tissue weights of these samples were all identical to within 10%. Care was taken to perform measurements with nonsaturating microwave power.

EPR spectra obtained from normally perfused control hearts exhibit a signal with a g value of 2.004 (Figure 7A). In ischemic hearts two additional components were observed and on postischemic reperfusion all three components markedly increased (Figure 7B and C). Temperature annealing studies were performed to separate out each of the component signals. If each component radical has different temperature stability, it should be possible to separate the observed signals by gradual warming of the sample. As shown in Figure 8 on warming of the reperfused heart tissue, sample for sample to $-80°C$ for 1 min, one of the components (shown in the subtraction spectrum A-B) disappears. On further warming to $-80°C$ for 1h, a second component (subtraction spectrum B—C) disappears leaving only one remaining component, the symmetric gaussian line shown in spectrum C.

Figure 9 shows the three component signals: A, a symmetric gaussian line at g = 2.004 indicative of an isotropic free radical; B, a signal with

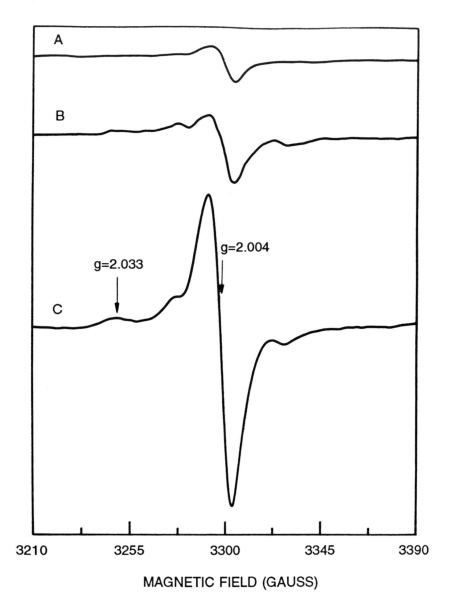

FIGURE 7. EPR spectra of control, ischemic, and reperfused heart tissue at 77 K. (A) From a normally perfused control heart; (B) from a heart subjected to 30 min ischemia; (C) from a heart subjected to 30 min ischemia followed by 15 s of reflow. Spectra were recorded with a microwave frequency of 9.246 GHz.

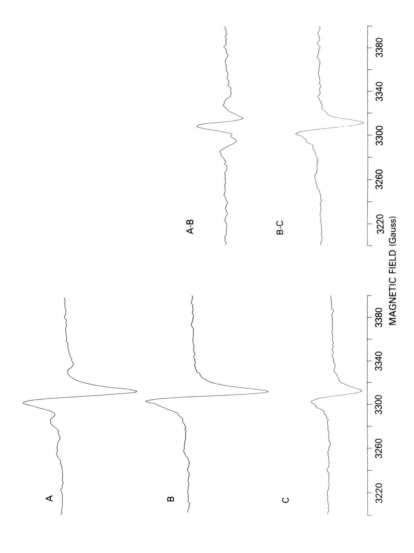

FIGURE 8. Temperature-annealing experiment performed to separate the overlapping EPR signals observed in a heart freeze clamped after 10 s of postischemic reflow.

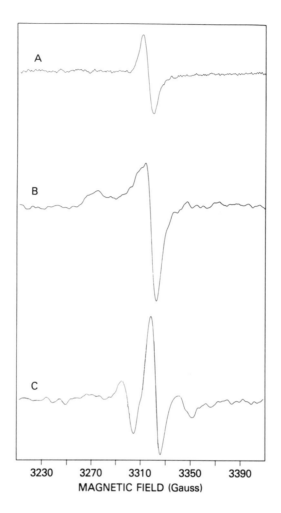

FIGURE 9. EPR spectra of the three component free-radical signals in heart tissue.

axial symmetry $g_\parallel$ = 2.003, $g_\perp$ = 2.005; and C, a triplet signal with g = 2.000 and hyperfine splitting a_N = 24 G. Signal A exhibits an identical g value, line width, power saturation, and temperature stability to that of a semiquinone free radical. This signal, which is observed in control hearts, may correspond to the signal arising from the one electron-reduced ubiquinone free radical that has been previously noted in cells and mitochondrial suspensions.[28] Signal B, which exhibits axial symmetry, is similar to signals previously reported for oxygen-centered free radicals. The observed g values are identical to those of the alkyl peroxy free radical, ROO˙. Signal C is a triplet suggestive of a nitrogen free radical such as a peroxyl amine, however, the identity of this radical is uncertain.

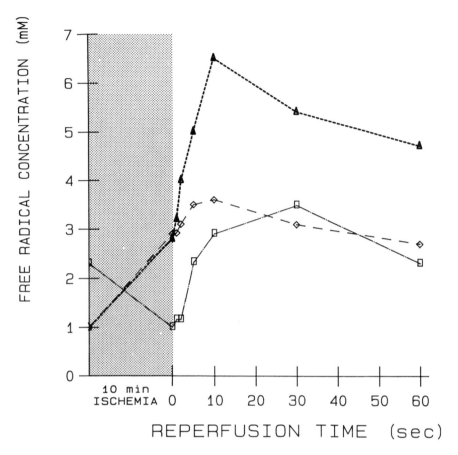

FIGURE 10. Time course of free-radical generation; each point corresponds to measurements performed on hearts freeze clamped at different points in time. □ , Signal A; △, Signal B; ◇, Signal C.

To determine the time course of free-radical generation during postischemic reperfusion, a series of hearts were freeze clamped after varying periods of reflow ranging from 1 to 60 s. The temperature annealing procedure described earlier was used to quantitate each of the three signals in each sample. Figure 10 shows the time course of each of three signals. In control hearts signal A was predominant with only small quantities of the other two signals. During ischemia signal B and signal C increased, while signal A decreased. After postischemic reperfusion with oxygenated perfusate, a dramatic increase in signal B, and to a lesser extent signal C, was observed with levels peaking at 10 s of reflow. Thus, on reperfusion with oxygenated perfusate, there is a burst of free-radical generation. On similar reperfusion with anoxic perfusate equilibrated with 95% N_2/5% CO_2, the levels of free radicals did not increase above the levels measured at the end of ischemia. In order to determine whether the oxygen radical ROO˙, signal B, is derived from the

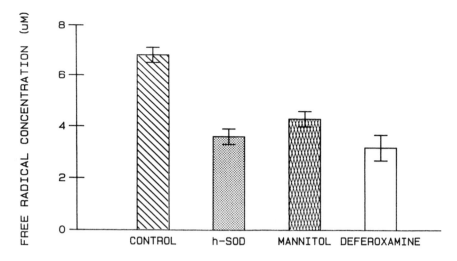

FIGURE 11. Effects of SOD, mannitol, and deferoxamine on the concentration of oxygen free radicals in the postischemic heart (N = 7).

superoxide free radical, experiments were performed reperfusing hearts with recombinant human superoxide dismutase, SOD.[29] With SOD administration on reperfusion the burst of oxygen free-radical generation was abolished. SOD denatured by the procedure of Hodgson and Fridovich[30] did not alter the observed radical concentrations.

Thus, direct low temperature EPR measurements demonstrate a burst of free-radical generation on reperfusion of ischemic myocardium. Peak radical concentrations are observed after only 10 to 15 s of reperfusion. Administration of SOD eliminates the reperfusion burst in oxygen radical generation, while the denatured enzyme has no effect. These observations confirm that O_2^- is actually generated in reperfused myocardium and suggest that the beneficial effect of SOD is actually due to the specific enzymatic scavenging of the superoxide free radical.

Additional experiments were performed in which hearts were reperfused in the presence of deferoxamine and hearts freeze clamped for direct EPR measurements. Deferoxamine treatment was found to be as effective as SOD at preventing oxygen free-radical generation (Figure 11).[31]

B. SPIN-TRAPPING MEASUREMENTS

Spin-trapping EPR studies were performed in isolated perfused rabbit hearts subjected to ischemia followed by reperfusion.[17] In these studies the nitrone spin trap molecule 5,5'-dimethyl-1-pyrroline-N-oxide (DMPO) was utilized to detect labile free radicals. DMPO reacts with primary radicals such as $OH^\cdot$, O_2^-, $R^\cdot$, and $RO^\cdot$ forming relatively stable EPR-detectable nitroxide radicals. Each of these radical adducts have different hyperfine coupling constants. Therefore, different trapped radicals give rise to different EPR

	a_N	a_H	a_H^{α}
DMPO–OOH	14.3	11.7	1.25
DMPO–OH	14.96	14.96	– – –
DMPO–R	15.86	22.86	– – –

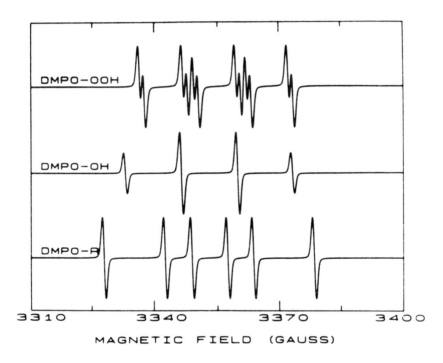

FIGURE 12. EPR spectra of different DMPO free-radical adducts and table showing the different hyperfine coupling constants of these adducts.

spectra. As shown below trapped O_2^-, OH·, and R· radicals give rise to distinctly different spectra (Figure 12).

After removal of the heart from the animal and cannulation, a 15 min period of control perfusion was allowed for the hearts to reach a stable left ventricular function with developed pressures of approximately 110 mmHg, as described earlier. Subsequently, perfusate containing 40 mM DMPO was administered for a period of 1 min and the effluent sampled in 10-s aliquots. No EPR signal was observable in either the DMPO containing perfusate

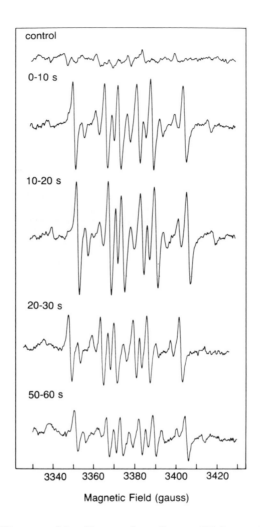

control

0-10 s

10-20 s

20-30 s

50-60 s

3340   3360   3380   3400   3420

Magnetic Field (gauss)

FIGURE 13. EPR spectra of the effluent perfusate from a rabbit heart perfused with 40 m*M* DMPO. Measurements were performed on effluent collected in 10-s samples prior to ischemia and upon reflow after 30 min ischemia.

solution or in any of the 10-s samples of effluent perfusate. After an additional 10 min, the hearts were subjected to 30 min of global ischemia followed by reperfusion in the presence of 40 m*M* DMPO. At the onset of reperfusion, perfusate was again sampled in 10-s aliquots and EPR measurements performed. After 10 to 20 s of reperfusion, a prominent EPR spectrum was observed (Figure 13). The observed spectrum was complex consisting of two major components, a 1:1:1:1:1:1 sextet and a smaller 1:2:2:1 quartet. Computer simulation of this spectrum demonstrated that the hyperfine couplings of the sextet signal were $a_N = 15.8$ G and $a_H = 22.8$ G most suggestive of DMPO-R, while the couplings of the quartet were $a_N = a_H = 14.9$ G indicative of DMPO-OH. On examination of the time course for the appearance of the spin trap signals, maximum intensity was observed at 10 to 20 s of reperfusion followed by a gradual decline over the next 1 to 2 min.

In order to determine whether the observed free-radical signals were derived from the superoxide free radical, additional experiments were performed reperfusing hearts after 30 min of ischemia with recombinant human superoxide dismutase in the presence of 25 mM DMPO. SOD was administered over the first 5 min of reperfusion. Perfusate was sampled in 10-s aliquots over the first minute of reperfusion, and a >80% decrease in both of the previously observed signals was noted in all aliquots. Administration of an identical concentration of inactivated SOD did not reduce the observed EPR signals. These results indicate that the DMPO-OH and DMPO-R signals are derived from the superoxide free radical.

In order to further determine whether superoxide derived free-radical generation on reperfusion actually leads to diminished contractile function, experiments were performed combining spin-trapping measurements of free-radical generation with subsequent assessment of recovered left ventricular function. It was again observed that treatment with active SOD resulted in a >80% decrease in the observed EPR signals, and this radical scavenging was accompanied by the recovery of considerably higher left ventricular-developed pressures with lower end diastolic pressures (Figure 14, Table 1). The denatured enzyme did not decrease the observed radical concentrations or result in improved functional recovery. While SOD markedly decreased concentrations of observed radicals, the scavenging was not complete. In order to determine whether this incomplete scavenging was due to competitive reactions with iron resulting in generation of OH˙, similar experiments were performed with perfusate pretreated to remove adventitial iron. On reperfusion after 30 min of ischemia with chelex treated perfusate, a fourfold decrease in the DMPO-R signal was observed with a twofold increase in the DMPO-OH signal suggesting that iron-mediated Fenton chemistry does occur (Figure 15A). When similar reperfusion was performed in the presence of SOD, complete scavenging was observed with no detectable EPR signal (Figure 15B). Simultaneous measurements of contractile function demonstrated once again that the decreases in total radical concentration were accompanied by improved contractile function (Table 1).

These experiments demonstrate that superoxide-derived OH˙ and R˙ free radicals are generated in the reperfused heart via Fenton chemistry. Simultaneous measurements of contractile function demonstrate that this radical generation is associated with the impairment in contractile function observed on postischemic reperfusion.

VII. CONCLUSION

In conclusion, there is much indirect evidence that oxygen free radicals are important mediators of reperfusion injury and that iron redox chemistry

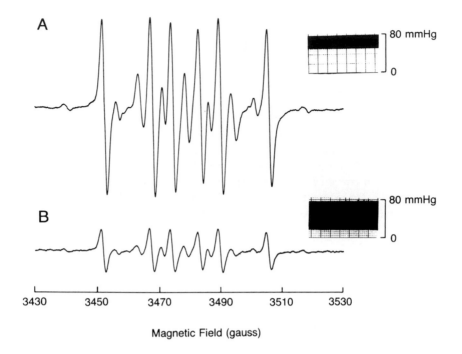

FIGURE 14. EPR spin-trapping experiment of hearts reperfused after 30 min of ischemia in the presence of enzymatically active recombinant human superoxide dismutase, (B), or identical concentrations of inactivated enzyme, (A). The spectra shown were recorded from measurements of perfusate sampled 10 to 20 s after the onset of reflow. The right insets show the recovered left ventricular function after 45 min of reperfusion.

TABLE 1

Reperfusion conditions	Free-radical concentration (μM)[a]		Contractile function	
	DMPO-OH	DMPO-R	LVDP[b]	EDP[c]
Denatured r-h-SOD	.12	.76	24	56
Active r-h-SOD	.02	.15	58	20
Chelexed perfusate	.24	.19	39	40
Chelexed perfusate + active r-h-SOD	0 (<.01)	0 (<.01)	68	16

[a] Measurements performed using 25 mM DMPO at 10 to 20 s of reperfusion.
[b] LVDP = maximum recovered left ventricular developed pressure (mmHg).
[c] EDP = end diastolic pressure (mmHg).

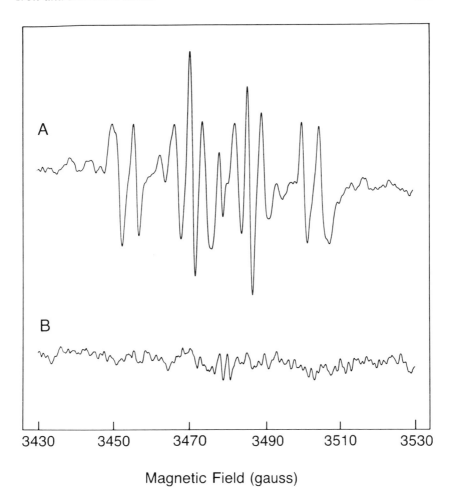

Magnetic Field (gauss)

FIGURE 15. EPR spin-trapping experiment of hearts reperfused with chelexed perfusate after 30 min of global ischemia. (A) Reperfused without SOD; (B) reperfused with active SOD.

is an important mechanism of this free-radical generation. Oxygen radical scavengers have been shown to decrease infarct size and enhance functional and metabolic recovery in reperfused myocardium. High affinity iron chelators such as deferoxamine have shown similar efficacy. EPR studies demonstrate that oxygen free radicals including $O_2^{\cdot-}$, $OH^{\cdot}$, and $ROO^{\cdot}$ as well as $R^{\cdot}$ are generated in reperfused myocardium. Simultaneous EPR measurements of free-radical generation along with measurements of contractile function demonstrate that oxygen radical scavenging decreases reperfusion injury. It has been demonstrated that high affinity iron chelators can quench free-radical generation and reperfusion injury in isolated hearts in *in vivo* animal models, and in the human heart. Therefore, there is much evidence that iron-mediated oxygen free-radical generation is an important mechanism of myocardial reperfusion injury.

REFERENCES

1. Whalen, D. A., Hamilton, D. G., Ganote, C. E., and Jennings, R. B., *Am. J. Pathol.*, 74, 381, 1974.
2. Kloner, R. A., Ganote, C. E., Whalen, D. A., and Jennings, R. B., *Am. J. Pathol.*, 74, 399, 1974.
3. Hess, M. S. and Manson, N. H., *J. Mol. Cell Cardiol.*, 16, 969, 1984.
4. Rosen, H. and Klebanoff, S. J., *J. Clin. Invest.*, 64, 1725, 1979.
5. McCord, J. M., *N. Engl. J. Med.*, 312, 159, 1985.
6. Guarnieri, C., Flamigni, F., and Caldarera, C. M., *J. Mol. Cell Cardiol.*, 12, 797, 1980.
7. Floyd, R. A., *Arch. Biochem. Biophys.*, 225, 263, 1983.
8. Floyd, R. A. and Lewis, C. A., *Biochemistry*, 22, 2645, 1983.
9. Gutteridge, J. M., *Biochem. J.*, 224, 761, 1984.
10. Shlafer, M., Kane, P. F., and Kirsh, M. M., *J. Thor. Cardiovasc. Surg.*, 83, 830, 1982.
11. Jolly, S. R., Kane, W. J., Bailie, M. B., Abrams, G. D., and Lucchesi, B. R., *Circ. Res.*, 54, 277, 1984.
12. Werns, S. W., Shea, M. J., Driscoll, E. M., Cohen, C., Abrams, G. D., Pitt, B., and Lucchesi, B. R., *Circ. Res.*, 56, 895, 1985.
13. Chambers, D. E., Parks, D. A., Patterson, G., Roy, R., McCord, J. M., Yashida, S., Parmley, L. F., and Downey, J. M., *J. Mol. Cell Cardiol.*, 17, 145, 1985.
14. Ambrosio, G. M., Weisfeldt, M. L., Jacobus, W. E., and Flaherty, J. T., *Circulation*, 75, 282, 1987.
15. Ambrosio, G., Becker, L. C., Hutchins, G. M., Weisman, H. F., and Weisfeldt, M. L., *Circulation*, 74, 1424, 1986.
16. Zweier, J. L., *J. Biol. Chem.*, 263, 1353, 1988.
17. Ambrosio, G., Zweier, J. L., Jacobus, W. E., Weisfeldt, M. L., and Flaherty, J. T., *Circulation*, 76, 906, 1987.
18. Bolli, R., Patel, B. S., Jeroudi, M. O., Li, X. Y., Triana, J. F., Lai, E. K., and McCay, P. B., *Am. J. Physiol.*, 259, H1901, 1990.
19. Williams, R. E., Zweier, J. L., and Flaherty, J. T., *Circulation*, 83, 1006, 1991.
20. van Jaarsveld, H., Potgieter, G. M., Kuyl, J. M., Barnard, H. C., and Barnard, S. P., *Clin. Biochem.*, 23, 509, 1990.
21. van Jaarsveld, H., Potgieter, G. M., Barnard, S. P., and Potgieter, S., *Adv. Exp. Med. Biol.*, 264, 361, 1990.
22. Liu, X. K., Prasad, M. R., Engelma, R. M., Jones, R. M., and Das, D. K., *Am. J. Physiol.*, 259, H1101, 1990.
23. Bernard, M., Menasche, P., Pietri, S., Grousset, C., Piwnica, A., and Cozzone, P. J., *Circulation*, 78, III164, 1988.
24. Menasche, P., Grousset, C., Mouas, C., and Piwnica, A., *J. Thor. Cardiovasc. Surg.*, 100, 13, 1990.
25. Illes, R. W., Silverman, N. A., Krukenkamp, I. B., del Nido, P. J., and Levitsky, S., *Circulation*, 80, III30, 1989.
26. Fereira, R., Burgos, M., Milei, J., Llesuy, S., Molteni, L., Hourquebie, H., and Boveris, A., *J. Thor. Cardiovasc. Surg.*, 100, 708, 1990.
27. Zweier, J. L., Flaherty, J. T., and Weisfeldt, M. L., *Proc. Natl. Acad. Sci. U.S.A.*, 84, 1404, 1987.
28. Onishi, T. and Trumpower, B., *J. Biol. Chem.*, 255, 3278, 1980.
29. Zweier, J. L., Rayburn, B. K., Flaherty, J. T., and Weisfeldt, M. L., *J. Clin. Invest.*, 80, 1728, 1987.
30. Hodgson, E. K. and Fridovich, L., *Biochemistry*, 14, 5294, 1975.
31. Zweier, J. L., Kuppusamy, P., Williams, R., Rayburn, B. K., Smith, D., Weisfeldt, M. L., and Flaherty, J. T., *J. Biol. Chem.*, 264, 18890, 1989.

11. Stored Iron as a Risk Factor for Ischemic Heart Disease

JEROME L. SULLIVAN

Veterans Affairs Medical Center, Charleston, South Carolina, and Department of Pathology and Laboratory Medicine, Medical University of South Carolina, Charleston, South Carolina

I. INTRODUCTION

The purpose of this chapter is to reexamine a theory on iron and heart disease that was first proposed a decade ago.[1] The core hypothesis of the theory is that iron depletion protects against ischemic heart disease (IHD). Since these ideas have been recently reviewed,[2-4] I will provide a brief account of the origin of the theory and then address some key points that have caused confusion. The theory was novel when it was proposed in 1981,[1] and its novelty evidently has not worn off, judging from the dismissive statements of some reviewers of recent manuscripts. One reviewer went so far as to proclaim the theory "dangerous". Preconceptions can cause a reviewer to be satisfied with superficial counterarguments that would otherwise not withstand critical scrutiny.

II. THEORY FORMATION

In considering a new theory, it is useful to know the path that was taken from the old to the new. This exercise will illuminate some of the conceptual underbrush that must be cleared. I first became interested in the question of sex difference in heart disease risk in the late 1970s. The remarkable degree of protection enjoyed by young women suggested that potent forces are at work. A preliminary look at the literature on the subject led to the surprising conclusion that very little is known for certain. The question was widely regarded as not an especially interesting one since the one sure fact was that sex is a "nonmodifiable" risk factor. Estrogens were thought to be the protective agent, though the mechanism of protection by estrogens was obscure and generally uninteresting. Increased cardiovascular mortality in men given pharmacological doses of estrogen[5] was disappointing but did not stimulate any significant inquiry into the possibility that women might be protected by some factor other than estrogen. My continued interest in the sex difference question was driven by the chance that sex might not be a nonmodifiable risk factor. Application of young women's protective mechanism to men and older women, if it were possible, might allow major improvement in our ability to prevent heart disease.

Early speculation was stimulated by anecdotal observations on anemia and coronary atherosclerosis. It has been noted that dilated, plaque-free coronary arteries are sometimes seen at autopsy in older patients who have been markedly anemic for a time before death. Entirely plaque-free coronaries in cases from older age groups are not typical. This suggested that marked anemia might be associated with reversal of coronary atherosclerosis. I am not aware of any experimental studies of this question at that time or since. This is still a potentially fruitful research area since a period of induced anemia under medical supervision is undoubtedly more benign than coronary bypass surgery. In any case, these observations pointed to a possible mechanism for the sex difference in heart disease risk. At the time I was unaware that the sex difference in hematocrit had been proposed in 1962[6] as the basis for low disease incidence in women. I subsequently became convinced that low hematocrit is not the explanation for reasons previously noted[1,2] and discussed as follows.

Initially I assumed, incorrectly, that the sex difference in hematocrit is caused by regular menstrual blood loss. The sex difference in hematocrit is actually much more dependent on the stimulation of erythropoiesis by androgens in men. This mechanism makes sense of the observation that hematocrit in women after menopause does not catch up to that in men.[7] Women become iron replete soon after cessation of menses[7] but their hematocrits do not appreciably increase. In my view, this simple bit of epidemiology excludes hematocrit as the basis for the sex difference in heart disease risk. Heart disease incidence increases soon after menopause despite a continuation of low hematocrits. Low hematocrit does not protect after menopause; thus, it is unlikely that it is the protective mechanism in menstruating women.

The other problem with low hematocrit as a possible protective mechanism is that the sex difference in hematocrit is small in comparison with the sex difference in heart disease risk. It seemed unreasonable to ascribe the basis for the 300 to 400% sex difference in disease risk to the 15 to 20% sex difference in hematocrit. However, given the marked dependence of blood viscosity on red cell concentration, this was not seen as impossible. After all, the small sex difference in monthly iron loss is associated with a 300 to 400% sex difference in iron stores and serum ferritin.

As an early alternative hypothesis I considered that the sex difference in iron stores might be the basis for the difference in heart disease risk independently of an effect on hematocrit. Awareness of the cardiomyopathy of massive iron overload kept this alternative alive, although a relationship between this lesion at the pathophysiology of IHD was, to say the least, unexplored ground. The heart lesion of hemochromatosis and thalassemia, nonetheless, was an important hint that iron might have cardioselective toxicity. The relationship between iron overload cardiomyopathy and IHD pathophysiology is a fundamental and as yet unresolved problem. New data accumulated since 1981 on protection against ischemic myocardial injury by the iron chelator deferoxamine[3,4] strongly support the possibility of a connection between iron cardiomyopathy and IHD (see the following discussion).

Another major stimulus to theorizing on the sex difference in IHD was publication of the Framingham Study data on menopause and heart disease.[8,9] The authors found that simple premenopausal hysterectomy with preservation of functioning ovaries was enough to eliminate protection against IHD. This is a profoundly significant finding and its importance was clearly recognized by the Framingham workers.[9] The Framingham investigators were not the first or last to publish data supporting this conclusion, but their study is the most rigorous to date (see detailed discussion in Reference 3). In my view this finding from a rigorous prospective study of heart disease still stands despite contrary explanations of a few less rigorous studies. There have been many flawed interpretations of data on menopause and heart disease over the years (see discussion in Reference 3). Presumably there would have been a more critical and searching review of the data if sex had not been seen as a "nonmodifiable" and therefore noninteresting risk factor.

The Framingham findings on menopause and heart disease have a dual significance. First, they argue against the estrogen hypothesis. Protection is lost after simple premenopausal hysterectomy despite continued ovarian function. Failure of the estrogen hypothesis leaves the effect of simple hysterectomy on heart disease in something of an explanatory void. Traditional risk factors do not account for the disease increase since they are not changed by simple premenopausal hysterectomy. The absence of a ready explanation may have helped to lead some thinkers to conclude incorrectly that menopause has no effect on heart disease. Second, loss of protection after surgical removal of only the uterus strongly suggests that a uterine, not an ovarian, function is responsible for protection against IHD. Perhaps the uterus has an unknown endocrine function that protects.[2,10] This is an entirely valid hypothesis, but why postulate an endocrine explanation? There is no reason for seeking a protective endocrine function of the uterus other than the habit of seeing all sex differences as endocrine differences.

At the time I became aware of the Framingham data on menopause and heart disease, I was preoccupied with the idea that monthly blood loss might protect young women by making them slightly anemic. The Framingham data were very exciting because they seemed to give strong support to the working hypothesis that monthly bleeding, an effect requiring an intact uterus, was protective. These data did nothing to discourage speculation on stored iron as a risk factor because it was clear that menstrual bleeding has a much stronger effect on iron stores than on hematocrit.

These data increased the level of speculative ferment, but did not decisively favor iron depletion over anemia as the protective factor. What finally crystallized the theory that iron depletion protects against IHD were the findings on acquisition of stored iron in men and women. Textbooks to this day give a static description of the level of iron stores in men and women. Typically the books say that the average adult man has about 1000 mg of stored iron and the average adult woman has about 300 mg. These numbers obscure the very different patterns of iron acquisition in men and women. In adolescence, there is essentially no sex difference in amount of stored iron. Very little iron is stored in either sex until after growth cessation. In men, beginning in late adolescence, storage iron is accumulated, assuming no cause of chronic blood loss is present. The textbook level of 1000 mg is not achieved for another decade or two. In women, menstrual iron losses generally prevent acquisition of stored iron. However, after age 45, on the average, women rapidly acquire iron stores at a rate similar to that seen much earlier in men. In the absence of illnesses causing chronic bleeding, men and older women continue to save excess iron into old age. Iron storage loads much in excess of 1000 mg are common in older men and women.

In over two years of thinking about gender and heart disease, these fundamental patterns of iron acquisition had escaped my full attention. The paper by Cook, Finch, and Smith[7] on the iron status of a population thus came as a revelation. They studied iron status in a large group of normal subjects and published a plot of serum ferritin as a function of age in men and women. The curves closely match plots of heart disease incidence as a function of age in men and women. They also conveniently showed a plot of hemoglobin level as a function of age in men and women demonstrating side by side with the ferritin graph that hemoglobin does not increase after menopause. The ferritin and hemoglobin data, the Framingham findings, and the cardiomyopathy of iron overload all came into focus in strong support of the hypothesis that iron depletion protects against IHD. The match between heart disease incidence and ferritin curves as a function of age in both men and women was seen as just too close to be a product of chance. The conspicuous similarity of these patterns can be seen in a plot of the sex ratios (M/F) of serum ferritin values and the incidence of IHD death as a function of age (Figure 1). The M/F ratios of some representative cholesterol values are shown for comparison.

Not only do the patterns match but, remarkably, the maximal male/female ratios for ferritin and heart disease are in essence numerically equal. The maximal sex differences occur at about age 45 for both iron stores and heart disease incidence. Before age 45 women have very little evidence of stored iron or IHD, while 45-year-old men have been acquiring both for more than two decades. At age 45, the male/female ratio for both serum ferritin and IHD death rate is approximately four. The similarity in the ratios may be a clue to the mechanism of protection by iron depletion.

In thinking through the implications of the hypothesis that iron depletion protects against IHD, it became apparent that it has considerable explanatory power. A theory should be evaluated for the range of phenomena it can explain. A contention that a theory "explains" a given phenomenon is not a claim that the postulated factor is the necessary, sufficient, and sole cause of the phenomenon. In crafting a new theory, it is desirable that the postulated factor behave in the predicted way in as broad a range of situations as possible. One seeks to explain as much as possible with the fewest possible hypotheses. In this sense the iron hypothesis has significant explanatory power.

The iron depletion hypothesis generalizes to a broad range of observations in addition to the sex difference in IHD risk.[1-3] One of the most important

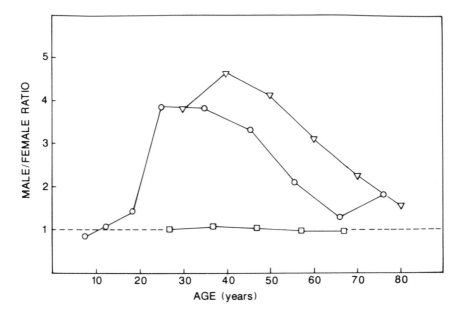

FIGURE 1. Effect of age on sex ratios of IHD death rates (∇),[11] median serum ferritin ($\circ$),[7] and total plasma cholesterol ($\square$)[12] in representative populations in the U.S. (From Sullivan, J. L., *Am. Heart J.*, 117, 1177, 1989. With permission.)

of these is the geographical distribution of IHD.[1-3,13] In general, iron deficiency is most severe and prevalent in regions of the world with lowest prevalence of IHD. A recent study by Lauffer[13] provides support for an international association between iron stores and mortality from coronary artery disease. In combined data from men and women the correlation between iron stores and cardiovascular mortality is positive and highly significant.

Other phenomena in which there appears to be decreased risk in association with lower levels of iron or increased risk with higher levels include the following: oral contraceptives decrease menstrual blood loss and increase heart disease risk. Oral contraceptive users are in essence perimenopausal with respect to their iron status and their risk of heart disease. Long-term regular use of some drugs or nutrients that can cause iron depletion may decrease heart disease risk. These include aspirin, cholestyramine, and fish oil. Vigorous exercise can cause occult iron losses sufficient to produce anemia.[14] Postmenopausal estrogen use in women with intact uteri is associated with periodic uterine bleeding and loss of iron that may explain some of the apparent protective effects against cardiovascular disease. There is a prominent circadian variation in the occurrence of myocardial infarctions that closely matches the well-known circadian rhythm of serum iron. Serum iron and incidence of myocardial infarction both peak around 9:30 a.m. These corollary hypotheses have been reviewed.[3,13,14]

III. OBJECTIONS TO THE THEORY: GENERAL COMMENTS

IHD research based on existing theories has not led to a successful, accepted preventive therapy despite massive and continuing expenditures of research funds. A cold-eyed look at the preventive interventions that have been tested to date[15] demonstrates that new theories are urgently needed and should not be lightly dismissed. Conventional theories on the causes of IHD impose habits of thought that may easily cause one to miss the point of a new theory. Criticisms couched in terms of other theories can be a source of much confusion in critical evaluations of a proposed theory.

One prevalent way of thinking about the pathophysiology of IHD, i.e., the cholesterol hypothesis, has dominated thinking for some time but has failed to yield a successful preventive therapy. The core hypothesis of the cholesterol paradigm is more than the statement that elevated plasma cholesterol causes IHD. It is important to avoid the error of thinking that IHD and atherosclerosis are interchangeable terms. A more accurate version is (1) that elevated plasma cholesterol causes atherosclerosis and (2) that atherosclerosis causes IHD. These hypotheses sharply restrict the scope of inquiry into two important questions: what causes IHD and what can be done to prevent IHD? Many of the objections to the present theory have been expressed in terms of these two component hypotheses of the cholesterol paradigm. Restricting the scope of inquiry is not in itself a deficiency of the cholesterol paradigm. It is clearly the proper function of a scientific paradigm to narrow the focus of investigation in order to make sense of an otherwise overwhelming array of phenomena. However, extensive studies[15] suggest that the cholesterol paradigm may not allow much additional progress in delaying and preventing IHD.

What is left out by the first hypothesis is the vast multiplicity of factors and processes besides cholesterol that contribute to atherosclerosis. For example, it recently has been shown that cholesterol-fed rabbits are almost free from atherosclerosis if the diet also contains butylated hydroxytoluene (BHT), an antioxidant.[16] BHT dramatically increases the plasma concentration of cholesterol in comparison with cholesterol-fed controls but, surprisingly, decreases aortic atherosclerosis. This experiment is a hint that the process of atherogenesis is far too complex and multifactorial to be comprehended by the simple hypothesis that elevated cholesterol causes atherosclerosis. (See Chapter 9.) It also suggests that the state of host antioxidant defenses is much more important than the cholesterol number in determining the rate of atherogenesis. (Iron depletion appears to enhance antioxidant defenses substantially.)

The second component of the cholesterol hypothesis (atherosclerosis causes IHD) obscures other processes that contribute to the clinical phenomena that we label "ischemic heart disease". Recent experimental work on the iron chelator deferoxamine and ischemia/reperfusion injury in the heart[3,4,17-27] shows that a period of total coronary occlusion can have very different consequences depending on the amount of deferoxamine present. Deferoxamine enhances postischemic ventricular function and suppresses otherwise fatal arrhythmias. This work suggests that a spontaneous coronary event may or may not result in a clinical presentation depending on the amount of iron available at the site of myocardial injury. (See also Chapter 10.) There are undoubtedly many other factors in addition to iron that can modify the effect of a given degree of coronary atherosclerosis.

The point of these comments is not to suggest that prevalent theories are completely devoid of merit. My purpose is to exhort the reader to consider the large gaps in our understanding of IHD and to maintain an open mind in evaluating the iron hypothesis. Using conventional theories as a guide for investigation has plainly failed to generate a successful preventive strategy.

IV. IRON OVERLOAD CARDIOMYOPATHY AND IHD

A criticism that has often been made against this theory is that there is no connection between the cardiomyopathy of iron overload and IHD. The serious cardiomyopathy seen frequently in patients with thalassemia or hemochromatosis appears distinct from the usual pathophysiology associated with IHD. However, a link between the two is suggested by the studies on deferoxamine and ischemic myocardial injury.[3,4,17-27] Deferoxamine can decrease myocardial injury, improve ventricular function, and suppress arrhythmias in hearts subjected to coronary artery ligation and reperfusion. Exogenous apotransferrin also improves cardiac contractile function after oxygen-radical mediated injury.[28] These studies[3,4,17-28] raise the possibility of a connection between the heart failure of massive iron overload and the pathological effects of myocardial ischemia. Deferoxamine appears at least equally effective in improving cardiac function in thalassemics with failing hearts as in reperfused hearts from animals with ''normal'' iron status. Perhaps, in subjects with massive iron overload, the myocardium is chronically in a postischemia-like state, in other words, at increased risk of fatal arrhythmias or pump failure. In those with massive iron overload the classical clinical picture of IHD may be obscured by the severe supervening cardiomyopathy. The deferoxamine experiments and the well-known beneficial effects of deferoxamine in patients with thalassemia suggest that similar iron-dependent mechanisms of myocardial injury may be acting in IHD and in the cardiomyopathy of iron overload.

V. MASSIVE IRON OVERLOAD VS. "NORMAL" IRON STORES

A related criticism is that massive iron overload damages the heart, but there is no evidence that the amounts of iron observed in normal iron replete subjects are harmful. The emphasis in this criticism is on the immense difference in amount of iron present in authentic hemochromatotics and subjects with "normal" iron stores. The textbook adult male has about 1 g stored whereas some homozygotes have 50 g. Part of the answer to this point is that nearly all of the storage iron in those with 1 or 50 g is very well stored indeed. The free, potentially destructive iron is in much smaller concentration even in massive overload. It is also clear that myocardial damage can occur in homozygotes at iron storage levels much more modest than 50 g. The minimum amount required for myocardial damage in hemochromatosis has not yet been defined.

There is now direct evidence that a normal load of storage iron may be harmful to the heart. The experiments on deferoxamine and myocardial injury in animals with normal iron status suggest that they have enough available iron to enhance myocardial injury. The experiments show that sequestration of this iron suppresses myocardial injury.

It has also been demonstrated recently that dietary iron depletion is equal to deferoxamine treatment in decreasing brain injury following ischemia/ reperfusion in an experimental model system.[29] These workers "were able to demonstrate a correlation between the level of iron and the degree of [brain] swelling following ischemia/reperfusion."[29] A dosage effect of iron level *in vivo* on brain injury is a very important finding of great relevance to this discussion (see also Chapter 12). A protective effect in myocardial injury has not yet been investigated to my knowledge. The findings in brain injury are a strong indication that iron depletion may also protect against myocardial injury.

VI. IRON AND ATHEROSCLEROSIS

The hypothesis that iron depletion protects against IHD does not specify that the mechanism of protection is a decrease in atherosclerosis. There is no *a priori* requirement that iron depletion must protect against IHD by a mechanism stipluated by the cholesterol hypothesis. However, it is equally clear that there are no studies to date that exclude an important role for iron in atherogenesis.

The following argument has been put forward: " . . . simple clinical observation suggests that these patients [with idiopathic hemochromatosis] do not suffer any increased incidence of atherosclerosis-related diseases such as strokes or myocardial infarction. This perhaps suggests that iron is not the metal that favours atherogenesis *in vivo*."[30] One of the chief weaknesses of this argument is that artherogenesis in hemochromatosis has simply not been critically investigated. A question of this importance must be addressed with much more rigor before the stated conclusion can be drawn. A more serious deficiency in the argument is that it dismisses a role for iron in atherogenesis without giving full consideration to possible mechanisms. If iron promotes atherogenesis, how much iron is needed for maximal stimulation? It may be that very little iron is required to maximally promote plaque formation. In that case, those with hemochromatosis might have no more coronary plaque than normal subjects who are merely iron replete.

Studies of atherogenesis in hemochromatosis cannot give a complete answer to the question of the role of iron. Adequate investigation of this problem must include studies of atherogenesis in iron-depleted subjects. It is becoming increasingly clear that iron depletion has a strong, stable antioxidant effect *in vivo*.[29,31-34] Antioxidant treatment with probucol or BHT can markedly decrease atherogenesis.[16,35,36] In addition, iron promotes low density lipoprotein modification *in vitro,* a process thought to promote plaque formation.[37] These findings, taken together indirectly but strongly, support the hypothesis that iron depletion inhibits atherogenesis *in vivo*. This hypothesis can be evaluated experimentally, e.g., in iron-depleted cholesterol-fed rabbits.

VII. ABSENCE OF FREE IRON IN NORMAL PLASMA

Iron-binding capacity in plasma greatly exceeds the plasma iron concentration in normal iron replete subjects. The absence of free iron in normal plasma has been cited as an argument against the theory presented here. This criticism holds that free iron must be present in plasma for myocardial injury to occur. Using very sensitive methods free plasma iron can be found in patients with homozygous hemochromatosis.

The absence of free iron in normal plasma does not tell us much about the availability of free iron in ischemic tissues. Clearly, there is much more stored iron in tissue in normal iron replete subjects than in those with iron depletion. The amount of free iron liberated from storage in ischemia/reperfusion situations is difficult to quantitate. Even if the total amount of free iron per unit weight of ischemic tissue is known, it is not usually possible to determine its concentration in every potential site of cellular injury. However, there is growing evidence that lowering the amount of storage iron *in vivo* decreases oxygen radical-mediated injury.[29,31-34] We cannot easily measure free iron in each cellular compartment, but we can experimentally decrease the amount of storage iron *in vivo* in all compartments and observe the resulting effects. These experiments suggest that there is excess, injury-promoting iron in normal iron replete subjects, even though no free iron can be detected in plasma.

VIII. IHD, IRON, AND THE BANTU

Iron deficiency is not universal among Third World peoples. In some cases, such as the Bantu (see Chapter 4), there are conditions that cause iron overload. Why do the iron-overloaded Bantu in Africa not have an increased incidence of IHD? The criticism that people in these situations do not have increased IHD is a variant on the question of relationship between the pathophysiology of IHD and that of iron overload cardiomyopathy. Other factors may further modify this relationship in the case of the Bantu. Bantu hearts could be protected from iron overload. One possibility is that widespread vitamin C deficiency protects their hearts from iron overload. Vitamin C supplements can provoke heart failure in iron-overloaded patients.[38] It is also possible that the Bantu have otherwise favorable risk factor profiles that compensate for their high iron levels, e.g., very low cholesterol levels.

IX. INTERNATIONAL DISTRIBUTIONS OF IHD AND IRON DEFICIENCY

The case of the Bantu is an example of the challenges of investigating the corollary hypothesis that some of the international differences in IHD incidence are explained by differences in iron level.[1-3,13] A preliminary retrospective study by Lauffer[13] suggests that there may be some significant international associations between coronary mortality and liver iron level. His study must be regarded as a preliminary and not the final analysis of this question. One of the major limitations of an analysis of existing data is the lack of an extensive data base on storage iron levels.

One of the reviewer's criticisms of Lauffer's preliminary study involves the possible confounding effects of dietary lipids:

> Given the real association between mean consumption of saturated fatty acids, mean level of serum LDL-cholesterol and coronary mortality rates, we generally find higher rates of coronary heart disease in populations that eat a substantial amount of meat than in those that get most of their protein from vegetable sources. Wouldn't we expect on that basis alone to find an ecological correlation between iron stores and coronary mortality?

Even "real" associations do not demonstrate cause and effect. Significant associations of both iron level and fat consumption with coronary mortality cannot by themselves prove a cause and effect relationship for either factor. Fat consumption could just as easily be the spurious association. Fat consumption changes do not explain the sex difference in IHD or the effect of menopause. Prospective studies involving hundreds of thousands of man-years of observation have also shown beyond reasonable doubt that improving the lipid risk profile has, at best, feeble effects on coronary mortality and may actually increase total mortality.[15] In considering whether iron or lipid associations are more important in determining the international distribution of IHD, due weight must be given to the evidence against lipids from prospective studies, real statistical associations notwithstanding. (See also the Introduction of this book and Chapter 19).

X. STORAGE IRON AND HEMATOCRIT

Some critics confuse hematocrit with iron level. In considering this hypothesis, it is important to distinguish the two clearly. There are much more epidemiological data available on hematocrit than on serum iron and ferritin. Low hematocrits have not been shown in epidemiological studies to be an especially strong protective factor in either sex. Those studies are not very relevant to the iron hypothesis since hematocrit is a very poor indicator of iron status in a population sample.

Normal hematocrits can be associated with stored iron loads ranging from zero to many hundreds of mg. On the other hand, abnormally low hematocrits are not specific for iron deficiency, i.e., only a fraction of anemias are caused by iron deficiency. Hematocrit therefore cannot be used as surrogate indicator of iron status in epidemiological studies. The proposed hypothesis is that iron depletion, not low hematocrit, protects against IHD.

XI. BEHAVIOR OF FERRITIN AS A RISK FACTOR

The epidemiological findings and the accumulating data on the protective effects of deferoxamine in myocardial injury are consistent with the iron depletion hypothesis. The hypothesis implies that ferritin is a risk factor for IHD but does not precisely define the epidemiological behavior of ferritin as a risk factor. The hypothesis focuses on protective effects of iron depletion, a state in which there is essentially no ferritin present. The hypothesis does not, and with available data, cannot adequately address the quantitative aspects of the relationship between ferritin and incidence IHD. The strength of serum ferritin as a risk factor for IHD may vary considerably over its clinically observed range.

The unresolved question involves the amount of iron required for promotion of IHD. Perhaps the key protective factor is the maintenance of iron depletion. Nearly maximal promotion of IHD may require relatively small amounts of storage iron. After iron sufficiency is achieved, further increments may be associated with progressively less added risk per additional milligram of storage iron. If this is the case, serum ferritin would behave as a strong risk factor, but only over the extreme low end of its observed range. (See also Section I.) This implies that iron repletion or iron sufficiency exerts a permissive effect in the development of IHD. As long as iron depletion or near iron depletion is maintained, the other risk factors may not promote IHD. It is clear from the BHT study[16] that even enormous concentrations of cholesterol may be rendered harmless if antioxidant defenses are strong enough.

Above the extreme low end of its observed range, serum ferritin may also be a significant, though weaker, risk factor. Clearly, there are many more iron-replete men and postmenopausal women without clinical evidence of IHD than those with it. If iron depletion is protective and if the other risk factors promote disease only in iron-replete subjects, serum ferritin may appear to be a risk factor only insofar as it is a marker for the number of years a given subject has been iron replete.

These considerations should be kept in mind in future epidemiological work on iron and heart disease. Care should be taken to design studies that do not overlook effects of iron depletion. A study of only iron-replete subjects would not be expected to reveal protective effects of iron depletion. A recent report by Riemersma and co-workers[39,40] is an example of such an oversight. They investigated the relationship between antioxidant vitamins and angina in a group of middle-aged Scottish men and included measurement of serum ferritin, iron, and iron-binding capacity (IBC). They concluded that iron, IBC, or ferritin did not contribute significantly to the explanation of angina risk[39,40] and noted the lack of significant differences in the means for these in the control and angina groups. The ferritin data confirm that very few, if any, of these men were iron depleted. These data thus do not invalidate the hypothesis that iron depletion protects against coronary heart disease.

An additional caveat for future epidemiological investigations concerns the study of spontaneously iron-depleted subjects. Any iron-depleted men in the Riemersma study[39,40] were most likely in this category. In affluent societies there are few causes of iron depletion in completely healthy adult subjects. Menstrual blood loss and regular frequent blood donation are by far the most common causes in Western countries. Middle-aged men with low ferritin are unusual. In this group low ferritin is often an important sign of poor health. Low ferritins can be associated with chronic occult blood loss, chronic malabsorption, or chronic use of certain drugs. A study of IHD incidence in spontaneously iron-depleted subjects might be invalid because of high prevalences of these disorders, especially if all cause mortality is one of the end points of interest.

XII. SPURIOUS ASSOCIATIONS

The following criticism has been made: "One cannot prove guilt by association. Mortality from coronary disease mirrors the prevalence of TV antennas yet no one would invoke a causal relationship on this evidence." This reviewer's TV antenna hypothesis is deeply flawed. Among its numerous other problems is the following: the TV antenna hypothesis fails to explain the sex difference in IHD. Men and women are equally exposed to TV antennas yet men have more disease. It also does not explain the effect of menopause. Postmenopausal women generally continue to have their customary exposure to TV antennas, but suffer a marked escalation in their incidence of IHD.

The sex difference is a particularly important experiment of nature in sorting through associations between IHD and various risk factors. In contrast to TV antennas, iron levels show both an international distribution and age- and sex-dependent fluctuations expected of a strong risk factor.

XIII. THE ONLY CAUSE?

The following question has been posed: does the author really believe that iron is both the necessary and sufficient and only cause? This critic seriously overstates my case. I am not suggesting that iron is the only cause of IHD. The hypothesis states that "iron depletion protects against IHD". Framed in this way, the hypothesis is testable. Suppose for the sake of argument that the hypothesis were unambiguously confirmed. Would the pathophysiology of IHD then be completely defined? Obviously it would not be. Confirmation of the hypothesis would clearly not exclude other contributing causes. The hypothesis does not specify a particular pathophysiological mechanism.

XIV. EXPERIMENTAL VERIFICATION

The hypothesis that iron depletion protects against IHD can be tested experimentally.[1-3] Testability is an important feature of the hypothesis and distinguishes it from mere speculation. If the hypothesis is correct, blood donors who give blood often enough to make themselves chronically iron depleted should have a significantly lower incidence of IHD. Experimental designs have been proposed.[41] It is not appropriate to discard the hypothesis prematurely because these lengthy, expensive studies have not yet been done.

XV. ESTABLISHED MECHANISMS

The epidemiological phenomena that the hypothesis seeks to explain do not reveal the mechanism(s) of protection. The hypothesis that iron depletion protects against IHD is often criticized because of a perceived lack of plausible mechanisms. This is a weak criticism since the criteria of plausibility depend on the assumptions of conventional theories of IHD. It is also becoming less relevant as data accumulate on the protective effects of deferoxamine in myocardial injury[3,4,17-27] (see Chapter 10).

The effects of iron depletion *in vivo* are pervasive and complex. There have been no organized studies of the impact of these phenomena on myocardial injury or atherogenesis. Reexamination of what is known about the effects of iron depletion suggests many possible mechanisms of protection.[1-3] Protection against IHD by iron depletion may be a multifactorial effect. On the other hand, there may be one particular effect that dominates. The epidemiology does not help in sorting through possible mechanisms.

The growing body of work on deferoxamine and heart injury suggests that the antioxidant effects of iron depletion *in vivo* may be especially important. It is, however, too early to rule out unexpected mechanisms not based on antioxidant effects. Iron not only affects antioxidant defenses but also is an important nutrient. Perhaps some of the cellular elements of atheromata are stimulated to proliferate above some threshold level of iron. The monocyte/macrophage is an important cell both in iron metabolism and in atherogenesis.[42] Does iron depletion suppress monocyte/macrophage growth within atherosclerotic plaque? Regulation of monocyte/macrophage proliferation by iron would not be a surprising finding. (See also Chapter 5.) Stimulation of monocyte/macrophage proliferation by excess iron would serve to boost the number of iron storage sites to accommodate the increase.

It should also be recalled that established mechanisms are not a requirement for true progress in preventive medicine. Effective methods for prevention of scurvy and puerperal sepsis were available long before the pathophysiology was understood. In both cases criticisms based on entrenched theories delayed full acceptance of these methods, causing much needless suffering and premature death.

XVI. CONCLUDING REMARKS

A very low incidence of IHD in menstruating women is not seen only in normal women. Even young women with heterozygous familial hypercholesterolemia are almost entirely free from clinically evident IHD.[2,3,43,44] Menstruating heterozygotes are protected despite higher levels of plasma cholesterol and more tendon xanthomas than affected young men. Female heterozygotes are clearly susceptible to heart disease since they have a marked excess of disease after menopause. The young male heterozygotes develop heart disease, the young heterozygous women do not.

This is a profoundly hopeful finding. It suggests that there is some physiological mechanism for avoiding the consequences of extraordinary levels of cholesterol. It is becoming increasingly clear that this phenomenon cannot be explained by conventional theories. Discovery of the mechanism should be given the highest priority. The absence of an explanation for such a striking anomaly should compel a more thorough examination of the underlying assumptions of existing theories. The hypothesis that iron depletion protects against IHD offers both an explanation of the low incidence of IHD in menstruating heterozygotes and a potential preventive therapy (see Chapter 19).

NOTE ADDED IN PROOF

A recent study provides the first empirical evidence from a prospective human study that serum ferritin is a strong risk factor for acute myocardial infarction and hypertension.[45] Baseline examinations were done on 1931 Finnish men between March 1984 and December 1989 as part of the Kuopio Ischaemic Heart Disease Risk Factor Study. In a Cox model adjusting for multiple risk factors, an increment of 10% in serum ferritin concentration was associated with a 10% elevation in acute myocardial infarction risk ($z = 2.73$, $p < 0.01$).

REFERENCES

1. **Sullivan, J. L.,** Iron and the sex difference in heart disease risk, *Lancet,* 1, 1293, 1981.
2. **Sullivan, J. L.,** The sex difference in ischemic heart disease, *Persp. Biol. Med.,* 26, 657, 1983.
3. **Sullivan, J. L.,** The iron paradigm of ischemic heart disease, *Am. Heart J.,* 117, 1177, 1989.
4. **McCord, J. M.,** Is iron sufficiency a risk factor in ischemic heart disease?, *Circulation,* 83, 1112, 1991.
5. Coronary Drug Project Research Group, Findings leading to the discontinuation of 2.5 mg/day estrogen group, *JAMA,* 226, 652, 1973.
6. **Stokes, J.,** Haematological factors as related to the sex difference in coronary-artery disease, *Lancet,* 2, 25, 1962.
7. **Cook, J. D., Finch, C. A., and Smith, N. J.,** Evaluation of the iron status of a population, *Blood,* 48, 449, 1976.
8. **Kannel, W. B., Hjortland, M. C., McNamara, P. M., and Gordon, T.,** Menopause and the risk of cardiovascular disease: the Framingham Study, *Ann. Intern. Med.,* 85, 447, 1976.
9. **Gordon, T., Kannel, W. B., Hjortland, M. C., and McNamara, P. M.,** Menopause and coronary disease: the Framingham Study, *Ann. Intern. Med.,* 89, 157, 1978.
10. **Seely, S.,** Possible reasons for the comparatively high resistance of women to heart disease, *Am. Heart J.,* 91, 275, 80, 1976.
11. Division of Vital Statistics, National Center for Health Statistics, Chartbook for the conference on the decline in coronary heart disease mortality, Government Printing Office, Washington, D.C., 1978, 13.
12. **Braunwald, E.,** *Heart Disease. A Textbook of Cardiovascular Medicine,* W. B. Saunders, Philadelphia, 1254, 1980.
13. **Lauffer, R. B.,** Iron stores and the international variation in mortality from coronary artery disease, *Med. Hypotheses,* 35, 96, 1991.
14. **Lauffer, R. B.,** Exercise as prevention: do the health benefits derive in part from lower iron levels?, *Med. Hypotheses,* 35, 103, 1991.
15. **McCormick, J. and Skrabanek, P.,** Coronary heart disease is not preventable by population interventions, *Lancet,* 2, 839, 1988.
16. **Bjorkhem, I., Henriksson-Freyschuss, A., Breuer, O., Diczfalusy, U., Berglund, L., and Henriksson, P.,** The antioxidant butylated hydroxytoluene protects against atherosclerosis, *Arteriosclerosis Thromb.,* 11, 15, 1991.
17. **Babbs, C. F.,** Role of iron ions in the genesis of reperfusion injury following successful cardiopulmonary resuscitation: preliminary data and a biochemical hypothesis, *Ann. Emerg. Med.,* 14, 777, 1985.
18. **Myers, C. L., Weiss, S. J., Kirsh, M. M., and Shlafer, M.,** Involvement of hydrogen peroxide and hydroxyl radical in the "oxygen paradox". Reduction of enzyme leakage by catalase, allopurinol or deferoxamine, but not by superoxide dismutase, *J. Mol. Cell Cardiol.,* 17, 675, 1985.
19. **Myers, C. L., Weiss, S. J., Kirsh, M. M., Shepard, B. M., and Shlafer, M.,** Effects of supplementing hypothermic crystalloid cardioplegic solution with catalase, superoxide dismutase, allopurinol, or deferoxamine on functional recovery of globally ischemic and reperfused isolated hearts, *J. Thorac. Cardiovasc. Surg.,* 91, 281, 1986.
20. **Bernier, M., Hearse, D. J., and Manning, A. S.,** Reperfusion-induced arrhythmias and oxygen-derived free radicals. Studies with antifree radical interventions and a free-radical generating system in the isolated perfused rat heart, *Circ. Res.,* 58, 331, 1986.
21. **Bolli, R., Patel, B. S., Zhu, W-X., O'Neill, P. G., Hartley, C. J., Charlat, M. L., and Roberts, R.,** The iron chelator desferrioxamine attenuates postischemic ventricular dysfunction, *Am. J. Physiol.,* 253, H1372, 1987.

22. **Ambrosio, G., Zweier, J. L., Jacobus, W. F., Weisfeldt, M. L., and Flaherty, J. T.,** Improvement of postischemic myocardial dysfunction and metabolism induced by administration of deferoxamine at the time of reflow: the role of iron in the pathogenesis of reperfusion injury, *Circulation,* 76, 906, 1987.

23. **Menasche, P., Pasquier, C., Bellucci, S., Lorente, P., Jaillon, P., and Piwnica, A.,** Deferoxamine reduces neutrophil-mediated free-radical production during cardiopulmonary bypass in man, *J. Thorac. Cardiovasc. Surg.,* 96, 582, 1988.

24. **Farber, N. E., Vercellotti, G. M., Jacob, H. S., Pieper, G. M., and Gross, G. J.,** Evidence for a role of iron-catalyzed oxidants in functional and metabolic stunning in the canine heart, *Circ. Res.,* 63, 351, 1988.

25. **Reddy, B. R., Kloner, R. A., and Pryzklenk, K.,** Early treatment with deferoxamine limits myocardial ischemic/reperfusion injury, *Free Radical Biol. Med.,* 7, 45, 1989.

26. **Lesnefsky, E. J., Repine, J. E., and Horwitz, L. D.,** Deferoxamine pretreatment reduces canine infarct size and oxidative injury, *J. Pharmacol. Exp. Ther.,* 253, 1103, 1990.

27. **Maruyama, M., Pieper, G. M., Kalyanaraman, B., Hallaway, P. E., Hedlund, B. E., and Gross, G. J.,** Effects of hydroxyethyl starch conjugated deferoxamine on myocardial functional recovery following coronary occlusion and reperfusion in dogs, *J. Cardiovasc. Pharmacol.,* 17, 166, 1991.

28. **Tiede, R., Sareen, S., and Singal, P. K.,** Transferrin delays oxygen radical induced cardiac-contractile failure, *Can. J. Physiol. Pharmacol.,* 68, 480, 1990.

29. **Patt, A., Horesh, I. R., Berger, E. M., Harken, A. H., and Repine, J. E.,** Iron depletion or chelation reduces ischemia/reperfusion-induced edema in gerbil brains, *J. Pediatr. Surg.,* 25, 224, 1990.

30. **Halliwell, B.,** Current status review: free radicals, reactive oxygen species and human disease: a critical evaluation with special reference to atherosclerosis, *Br. J. Exp. Pathol.,* 70, 737, 1989.

31. **Sullivan, J. L., Till, G. O., and Ward, P. A.,** Iron depletion decreases lung injury after systemic complement activation, *Fed. Proc.,* 45, 452, 1986.

32. **Sullivan, J. L., Till, G. O., Ward, P. A., and Newton, R. B.,** Nutritional iron restriction diminishes acute complement-dependent lung injury, *Nutr. Res.,* 9, 625, 1989.

33. **Andrews, F. J., Morris, C. J., Lewis, E. J., and Blake, D. R.,** Effect of nutritional iron deficiency on acute and chronic inflammation, *Ann. Rheum. Dis.,* 46, 859, 1987.

34. **Chandler, D. B., Barton, J. C., Briggs, D. D., Butler, T. W., Kennedy, J. I., Grizzle, W. E., and Fulmer, J. D.,** Effect of iron deficiency on bleomycin-induced lung fibrosis in the hamster, *Am. Rev. Respir. Dis.,* 137, 85, 1988.

35. **Kita, T., Nagano, Y., Yokode, M., Ishii, K., Kume, N., Ooshima, A., Yoshida, H., and Kawai, C.,** Probucol prevents the progression of atherosclerosis in Watanabe heritable hyperlipidemic rabbit, an animal model for familial hypercholesterolemia, *Proc. Natl. Acad. Sci. U.S.A.,* 84, 5928, 1987.

36. **Carew, T. E., Schwenke, D. C., and Steinberg, D.,** Antiatherogenic effect of probucol unrelated to its hypocholesterolemic effect: evidence that antioxidants *in vivo* can selectively inhibit low density lipoprotein degradation in macrophage-rich fatty streaks and slow the progression of atherosclerosis in the Watanabe heritable hyperlipidemic rabbit, *Proc. Natl. Acad. Sci. U.S.A.,* 84, 7725, 1987.

37. **Steinberg, D., Parthasarathy, S., Carew, T. E., Khoo, J. C., and Witztum, J. L.,** Beyond cholesterol. Modifications of low-density lipoprotein that increase its atherogenicity, *N. Engl. J. Med.,* 320, 915, 1989.

38. **Nienhuis, A. W.,** Vitamin C and iron, *J. Engl. J. Med.,* 304, 170, 1981.

39. **Riemersma, R. A., Wood, D. A., MacIntyre, C. C. A., Elton, R. A., Gey, K. F., and Oliver, M. F.,** Risk of angina pectoris and plasma concentrations of vitamins A, C, and E and carotene, *Lancet,* 337, 1, 1991.

40. **Riemersma, R. A., Wood, D. A., MacIntyre, C. C. A., Elton, R. A., Gey, K. F., and Oliver, M. F.,** Anti-oxidants and pro-oxidants in coronary heart disease, *Lancet,* 337, 677, 1991.

41. **Sullivan, J. L.,** Blood donation may be good for the donor. Iron, heart disease, and donor recruitment, *Vox Sang,* 61, 161, 1991.

42. **Weinberg, E. D.,** Roles of iron in functions of activated macrophages, *J. Nutr. Immunol.,* 1, 41, 1992.

43. **Stone, N. J., Levy, R. I., Fredrickson, D. S., and Verter, J.,** Coronary artery disease in 116 kindred with familial type II hyperlipoproteinemia, *Circulation,* 49, 476, 1974.

44. **Hill, J. S., Hayden, M. R., Frohlich, J., and Pritchard, P. H.,** Genetic and environmental factors affecting the incidence of coronary artery disease in heterozygous familial hypercholesterolemia, *Arteriosclerosis Thromb.,* 11, 290, 1991.

45. **Salonen, J. T., Salonen, R., Nyyssonen, K., and Korpela, H.,** Iron sufficiency is associated with hypertension and excess risk of myocardial infarction: The Kuopio Ischaemic Heart Disease Risk Factor Study (KIHD), *Circulation,* 85, 864, 1992.

12. Iron and Stroke

Lance S. Terada, Irene R. Willingham, and John E. Repine

Webb-Waring Lung Institute and the Departments of Medicine and Neurosurgery, University of Colorado Health Sciences Center, Denver, Colorado

I. INTRODUCTION

Stroke or cerebrovascular insufficiency is a major cause of morbidity and mortality in our society today. Each year more than 1 million people in the U.S. alone are subjected to stroke or central nervous system (CNS) trauma. Besides supportive treatment, no specific therapies currently exist, largely because of a lack of understanding of the fundamental mechanisms responsible for neuronal cell death.

Great interest has emerged recently in the potential role of iron in the genesis of cerebrovascular diseases. In stroke syndromes, the brain appears to be particularly sensitive to iron-mediated oxidative damage because of its high levels of polyunsaturated lipids which are vital for neural transmission, its acidic environment during ischemia, and its high metabolic rate. The ability of excess iron to facilitate peroxidation of brain lipids has been amply demonstrated. Addition of exogenous Fe(II) to oxygen-exposed brain homogenates, for instance, increases lipid peroxidation 10- to 20-fold.[1] Similarly, subpial injection of $FeCl_2$ into rat brains causes lipid peroxidation.[2] In addition, exogenous hemoglobin increases lipid peroxidation *in vitro* and *in vivo*[3] and causes seizures *in vivo*.[4] Deferoxamine abrogates hemoglobin-induced formation of peroxides, suggesting a role for free iron in this process.[3]

It is likely that organic and oxygen free radicals generated during or following brain ischemia in large part mediate or promote the adverse oxidative effects of iron in the CNS. Iron and free radicals potentially interact to promote lipid peroxidation by several means. (See also Chapter 7.) Iron can serve to catalyze the Haber-Weiss reaction, which results in the formation of the extremely potent oxidant hydroxyl radical (OH·), an efficient initiator of lipid peroxidation. This reaction requires H_2O_2 and O_2^- (Reactions 1 and 2):

$$Fe^{III} + O_2^- \rightarrow Fe^{II} + O_2 \tag{1}$$

$$Fe^{II} + H_2O_2 \rightarrow Fe^{III} + OH^- + \cdot OH \tag{2}$$

Alternatively, ferryl iron, another strong oxidant, may also result from the oxidation of Fe(II) by H_2O_2 (Reaction 3):

$$Fe^{II} + H_2O_2 \rightarrow Fe^{III} OH + OH^-$$

$$or \rightarrow Fe^{IV} (OH^-)_2 \tag{3}$$

O_2^- itself may be generated by the autooxidation of either free iron[5] or hemoglobin-complexed iron.[6] Further, reduction of Fe(III) may also be driven by organic radicals such as semiquinones, as well as ascorbate or thiols. Hence, these compounds may also participate in iron-mediated oxidative brain injury.[7] Interestingly, hemoglobin-bound iron may itself act as a biological

Fenton reagent in the formation of $OH^{\cdot}$.[8] The importance of hemoglobin-derived iron in CNS disease is further highlighted by the association of familial idiopathic epilepsy with low levels of the hemoglobin-clearing protein haptoglobin.[9]

Once formed, $OH^{\cdot}$ can easily abstract hydrogen from unsaturated fatty acids (Equation 4) and initiate a chain reaction resulting in peroxidated lipids (Equations 5 and 6):

$$RH + OH^{\cdot} \rightarrow R^{\cdot} + H_2O \tag{4}$$

$$R^{\cdot} + O_2 \rightarrow ROO^{\cdot} \tag{5}$$

$$ROO^{\cdot} + RH \rightarrow ROOH + R^{\cdot} \tag{6}$$

In addition, ferrous or ferric iron can initiate peroxidation chain reactions from existing lipid peroxides by the formation of alkoxyl or peroxyl radicals[5] (Equations 7 and 8):

$$ROOH + Fe^{II} \rightarrow RO^{\cdot} + OH^- + Fe^{III} \tag{7}$$

$$ROOH + Fe^{III} \rightarrow ROO^{\cdot} + Fe^{II} + H^+ \tag{8}$$

Hence, CNS iron may promote both initiation and dissemination of lipid peroxidation in the presence of even relatively small quantities of oxygen free radicals. The acidic environment of the ischemic brain also increases the accessibility of reactive iron by promoting the release of iron from ferritin and transferrin. In addition, O_2^- allows the reductive mobilization of Fe(III) from intracellular ferritin,[10] and H_2O_2 increases the release of free iron from hemoglobin.[11] Therefore, the simultaneous presence of reduced oxygen metabolites and iron may conceptually synergize to greatly enhance oxidative damage to the ischemic brain. One must, therefore, consider oxygen metabolites and iron as coconspirators in the pathogenesis of stroke, and their relative roles should be studied in tandem.

II. SOURCE OF O_2 METABOLITES IN STROKE

Increasing evidence that reduced O_2 metabolites participate in ischemic cerebrovascular disease is available in a number of experimental models. The precise molecular source of oxygen radicals is unknown but of primary importance for several reasons. First, specific inhibitors of radical generation may be designed to obviate the potential therapeutic limitations of iron chelators or nonspecific scavengers. Second, appropriate delivery of radical scavengers may be better targeted to act at critical sites. This is currently a therapeutic stumbling block. For instance, liposome-encapsulated superoxide dismutase (SOD)[12] or polyethylene glycol-conjugated SOD[13] but not native SOD[14,15] decrease brain edema and infarct volume following cerebrovascular occlusion. Third, identification of distinct radical-generating enzymes will allow assessment of genetic predisposition for cerebrovascular disease and open the door for specific gene therapy.

Accordingly, we investigated the specific contribution of xanthine oxidase (XO) in ischemic brain injury. XO is a purine catabolic enzyme which under normal conditions appears to exist largely as an NAD^+-consuming dehydrogenase (XD). Ischemia causes the breakdown of high energy phosphates to hypoxanthine, the substrate for XO, and may also promote the proteolytic conversion of XD to XO.[16] Upon reperfusion, molecular oxygen serves as an efficient electron acceptor for XO, with the subsequent formation of O_2^- and H_2O_2.

In most organs, XO appears to be highly concentrated within the microvascular endothelium.[17] Conceptually, this places XO at a location critical to the maintenance of the blood-brain barrier, and uncontrolled production of reactive O_2 metabolites by XO might easily facilitate accumulation of brain edema during or following ischemia. However, very low or undetectable levels of XO activity in brain have been reported.[18] Indeed, histological studies have suggested the absence of immunoreactive XO in brain capillary endothelium despite its abundance in the microvascular endothelium of most other organs.[19] Physiological studies have been similarly difficult to interpret. Although some investigators have found that treatment with an XO inhibitor, allopurinol, decreases infarct volume and edema following stroke,[20] others have not found protection from brain edema except at high doses of allopurinol.[21] In these studies, the presence of XO activity in brain and the effect of allopurinol on XO activity was not investigated.

We, therefore, isolated brain microvascular endothelial cells (EC) from cows and grew them in pure culture.[22] We found that brain EC in culture had high basal levels of XO and XD activities (Table 1). Surprisingly, although brain tissue has considerably lower XO and XD activities than lung tissue,[23] cultured brain EC had relatively high specific activities comparable to cultured lung EC. By comparison, whole brain homogenate and cultured glial cells had very low XO and XD activities, consistent with the explanation that XO activity is focally concentrated within brain capillary EC. Furthermore, cultured brain EC spontaneously released O_2^-, and tungsten treatment decreased both XO activity and O_2^- release (Figure 1). Thus, in brain, XO appears to be able to generate focally high quantities of O_2 metabolites capable of reacting with iron, and in addition is precariously positioned at the blood-brain barrier, which excludes the massive amounts of iron associated with hemoglobin.

We next tested the role of XO-derived oxidants in facilitating iron-mediated reperfusion induced cerebral edema by studying unilateral hemispheric ischemia reperfusion in gerbils.[24] Gerbils were subjected to unilateral carotid artery occlusion for 3 h followed by 3 h of cerebral reperfusion. Because

TABLE 1
Xanthine Oxidase and Xanthine Dehydrogenase Activities of Brain and Lung Cells

Source	XO activity (mU/g protein)	XD activity (mU/g protein)
Brain cortex	2 ± 1[a]	20 ± 1
Brain EC	52 ± 5	382 ± 46
Glia	17 ± 1	64 ± 4
Lung EC	43 ± 4	320 ± 27

[a] Each value is the mean ± SEM of 3 to 5 individual determinations.

Taken from Terada et al., *J. Cell. Physiol.*, 148, 191, 1991. With permission.

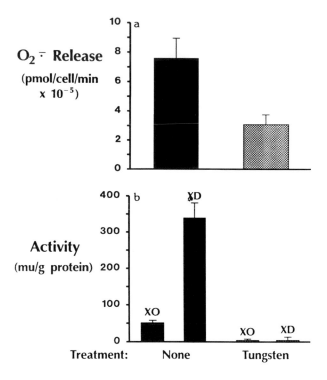

FIGURE 1. (a) Brain endothelial cells grown on control media released more ($p < 0.05$) O_2^- than EC grown in tungsten-enriched media. (b) Tungsten treatment decreased ($p < 0.05$) both XO and XD activity in brain EC compared to control EC. (From Terada et al., *J. Cell. Physiol.*, 148, 191, 1991. With permission.)

TABLE 2

Effect of Tungsten or Allopurinol Treatment on Gerbil Brain and Liver XO or Total Enzyme (XO + XD) Activities

Treatment	Brain XO activity	Brain XO + XD activity	Liver XO activity	Liver XO + XD activity
Saline	9 ± 1[a]	48 ± 3	35 ± 3	552 ± 10
Tungsten (4 week)	5 ± 5	17 ± 2	5 ± 2	153 ± 20
Tungsten (5 week)	0	8 ± 2	0	2 ± 1
Tungsten (6 week)	0	0	0	0
Allopurinol	7 ± 5	37 ± 4	18 ± 1	216 ± 26

[a]   Each value is the mean ± SEM of 2 to 10 individual determinations.

Taken and modified from Patt et al., *J. Clin. Invest.*, 81 1556, 1988. With permission.

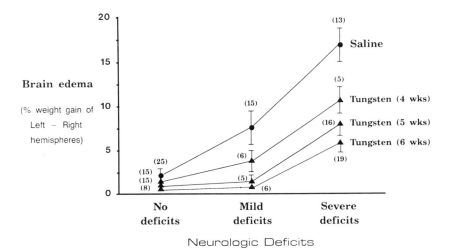

FIGURE 2.   Brain edema in symptomatic gerbils subjected to temporary unilateral carotid artery occlusion progressively decreased ($p < 0.05$) in gerbils fed a tungsten-enriched diet, compared with saline-treated controls. (From Patt et al., *J. Clin. Invest.*, 81, 1556, 1988. With permission.)

gerbils possess a variably collateralized cerebral circulation, variable degrees of neurological deficits resulted.

We found that gerbils fed a tungsten-enriched diet had progressively less brain XO and XD activities over a 4 to 6 week period (Table 2). In contrast, gerbils fed an allopurinol-supplemented diet did not have decreased brain XO and XD activities, despite having decreased liver XO and XD activities. In parallel, brain edema following carotid occlusion-release progressively decreased in symptomatic gerbils fed tungsten for 4 to 6 weeks (Figure 2).

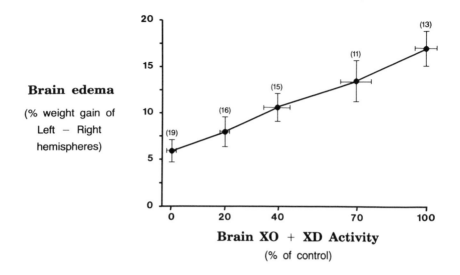

FIGURE 3. Brain edema increased as a function of brain XO + XD activity in gerbils subjected to temporary unilateral carotid artery occlusion. (From Patt et al., *J. Clin. Invest.*, 81, 1556, 1988. With permission.)

Therefore, the severity of brain edema correlated well with levels of XO + XD activity (Figure 3). Moreover, brain edema in allopurinol-fed gerbils was the same as control values, underscoring the association between brain edema and XO levels.

Subsequently, we tested the hypothesis that XO contributes to brain edema by generation of oxidants. H_2O_2 generation was assessed by quantifying the H_2O_2-dependent inactivation of catalase by aminotriazole. Brain H_2O_2 levels following carotid occlusion-release progressively decreased in symptomatic gerbils fed tungsten for 4 to 6 weeks (Figure 4). Again, brain XO + XD activities predicted brain H_2O_2 levels (Figure 5), further implicating XO as a principal source of O_2 metabolites in cerebral ischemia reperfusion. Brain edema and H_2O_2 levels were also measured in the presence of the small, diffusable molecule dimethylthiourea (DMTU), which scavenges H_2O_2 and is consumed in the process.[25] Treatment with DMTU decreased both brain edema and H_2O_2 levels (Figures 6 and 7), whereas treatment with urea — a nonscavenging analogue of DMTU — had no effect. Consistent with the overall hypothesis that iron promotes brain edema through oxidative processes, brain edema correlated well with brain H_2O_2 generation (Figure 8). Most significantly, survival of gerbils subjected to carotid occlusion-release was 100% following treatment with DMTU or tungsten, a striking improvement compared with untreated controls or gerbils treated with urea or allopurinol (Figure 9). To summarize, XO is present and focally concentrated in the brain microvascular endothelium, and XO-derived H_2O_2 appears to participate in the development of brain edema and mortality following temporary unilateral carotid artery occlusion.

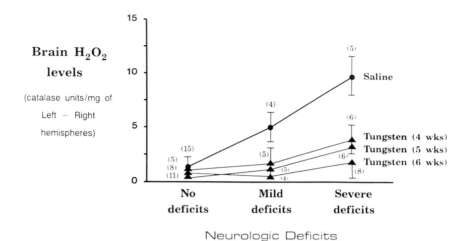

FIGURE 4. Brain H_2O_2 levels in symptomatic gerbils undergoing temporary unilateral carotid artery occlusion decreased ($p < 0.05$) in gerbils fed a tungsten-enriched diet, compared with saline-treated controls. (From Patt et al., *J. Clin. Invest.*, 81, 1556, 1988. With permission.)

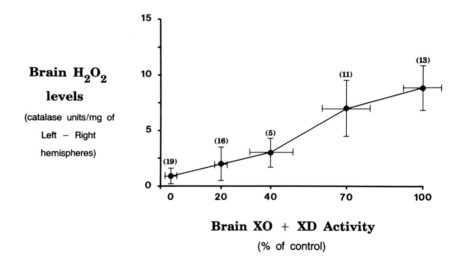

FIGURE 5. Brain H_2O_2 levels increased as function if brain XO + XD activity in gerbils were subjected to temporary unilateral carotid artery occlusion. (From Patt et al., *J. Clin. Invest.*, 81, 1556, 1988. With permission.)

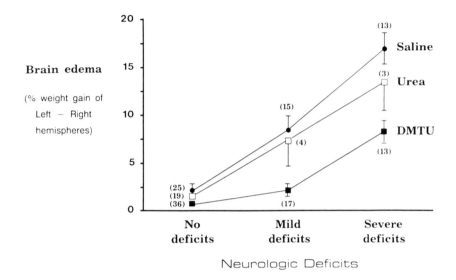

FIGURE 6. Brain edema in symptomatic gerbils undergoing temporary unilateral carotid artery occlusion was decreased ($p < 0.05$) following treatment with the H_2O_2 scavenger DMTU compared with saline or urea treatment. (From Patt et al., *J. Clin. Invest.*, 81, 1556, 1988. With permission.)

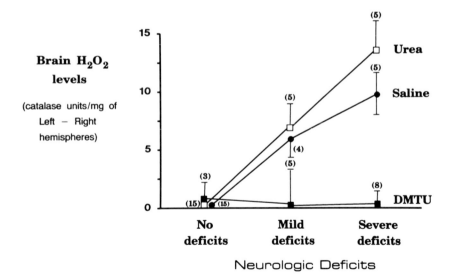

FIGURE 7. Brain H_2O_2 levels in symptomatic gerbils subjected to unilateral temporary carotid artery occlusion were decreased following treatment with DMTU compared with saline or urea treatment. (From Patt et al., *J. Clin. Invest.*, 81, 1556, 1988. With permission.)

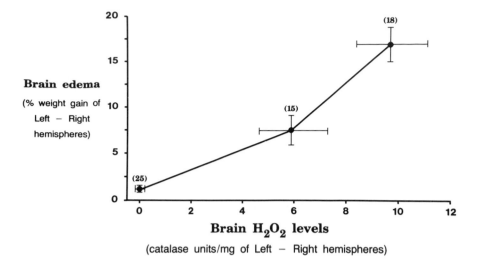

FIGURE 8. Brain edema increased as a function of brain H_2O_2 levels in gerbils subjected to unilateral temporary carotid artery occlusion. (From Patt et al., *J. Clin. Invest.*, 81, 1556, 1988. With permission.)

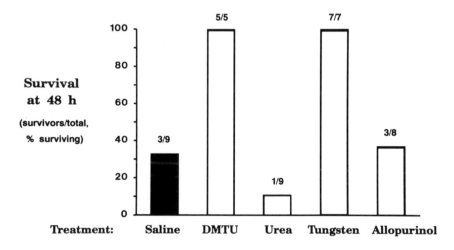

FIGURE 9. Survival of gerbils undergoing temporary unilateral carotid artery occlusion was greater in gerbils fed a tungsten diet or treated with DMTU than gerbils treated with saline, urea, or allopurinol. Tungsten but not allopurinol decreased brain XO levels (see Table 2). (From Patt et al., *J. Clin. Invest.*, 81, 1556, 1988. With permission.)

III. EVIDENCE FOR PARTICIPATION OF IRON IN STROKE

Despite the theoretical importance of iron in oxidative brain injury, very little direct evidence exists to implicate iron in stroke. We addressed this concern by testing the hypothesis that endogenous iron contributes to cerebral ischemia-reperfusion injury. The contribution of iron was assessed by decreasing redox active brain iron using two independent methods.[26] First, gerbils were subjected to a low-iron diet to deplete endogenous brain iron, and, second, iron-replete gerbils were treated with the iron chelator deferoxamine. Gerbils were again subjected to temporary unilateral carotid artery occlusion, and the severity of neurological deficits was correlated with brain edema.

Gerbil brains had reduced serum iron levels after 6 weeks of treatment with a low-iron diet when compared with gerbils fed a standard diet (Figure 10). In addition, gerbils had markedly reduced brain iron levels after 8 weeks of low-iron diet compared with gerbils fed a control diet. Conversely, gerbils with low brain iron levels were not anemic and did not have lowered activity of the O_2 metabolite-producing ferro-enzyme xanthine oxidase (XO).

Gerbils without neurological deficits did not develop brain edema. However, gerbils with mild or severe neurological deficits had graded increases in brain edema (Figure 11). Depletion of brain iron by feeding gerbils a low-iron diet for 8 weeks attenuated brain edema following cerebral ischemia reperfusion. Furthermore, feeding gerbils an iron-deficient diet for only 6 weeks did not decrease brain edema despite lowering serum iron levels. Thus, it appears that tissue iron levels may be more important than serum levels in determining cerebral ischemia-reperfusion injury.

In parallel, gerbils fed a control diet but given a single dose of deferoxamine just prior to cerebral reperfusion also had less brain edema when neurological deficits were present (Figure 12). Preloading of deferoxamine with iron, eliminating the chelating capacity of the compound, also abrogated the protective effect of deferoxamine. Hence, the salutory effects of deferoxamine appear to be directly related to the ability of deferoxamine to sequester reactive iron, and not to spurious effects on, for instance, scavenging of radicals.

In unilateral hemispheric ischemia-reperfusion, therefore, brain iron and XO-derived oxidants appear to have a mechanistic link with development of cerebral edema. It is highly probable that iron and O_2 metabolites interact as previously discussed to oxidatively modify lipids, proteins, and nucleic acids, with resultant loss of blood-brain barrier function, formation of cerebral edema, and ultimately neuronal cell death (Figure 13). It is particularly noteworthy in the preceding experiments that depletion of brain iron or suppression of XO-derived H_2O_2 in the ischemic-reperfused brain affords significant protection from brain edema and mortality even in gerbils with severe temporary symptoms during carotid occlusion. That is, specific treatment strategies were

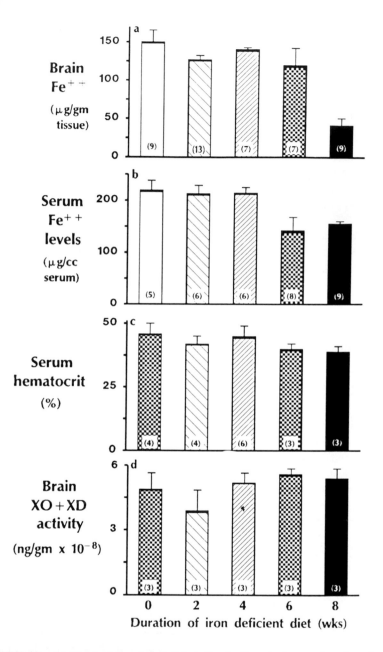

FIGURE 10. (a) Gerbils fed an iron-deficient diet for 8 weeks but not 0 to 6 weeks had decreased ($p < 0.05$) brain iron levels. (b) Serum iron levels were decreased ($p < 0.05$) after 6 to 8 weeks of a low-iron diet. (c) and (d) Blood hematocrit and brain XO + XD activity were unchanged after up to 8 weeks of an iron-deficient diet. (From Patt et al., *J. Pediatr. Surg.*, 25, 224, 1990. With permission.)

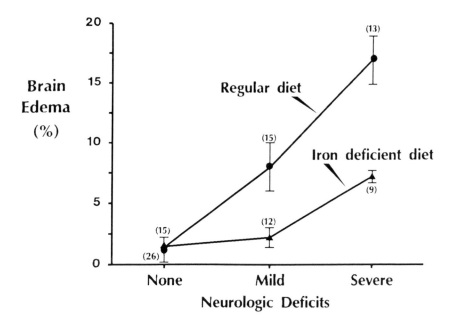

FIGURE 11. Brain edema (percent weight gain of left-right hemispheres) was decreased ($p < 0.05$) in symptomatic gerbils fed an iron-deficient diet compared with gerbils fed a control diet, following unilateral carotid artery occlusion-release. (From Patt et al., *J. Pediatr. Surg.*, 25, 224, 1990. With permission.)

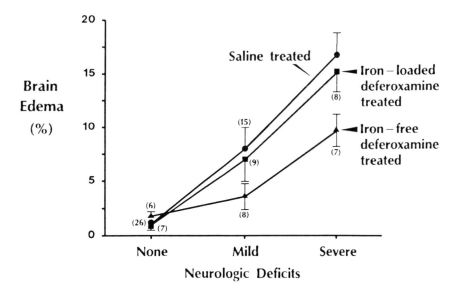

FIGURE 12. Brain edema was decreased ($p < 0.05$) in symptomatic gerbils treated with the iron chelator deferoxamine compared with saline-treated controls, following unilateral carotid artery occlusion-release. Treatment with iron-loaded deferoxamine had no effect ($p > 0.05$). (From Patt et al., *J. Pediatr. Surg.*, 25, 224, 1990. With permission.)

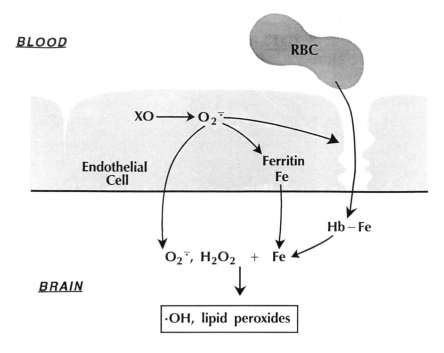

FIGURE 13. Schematic of brain endothelium during stroke. Endothelial cell XO generates oxygen metabolites which mobilize ferritin iron and disrupt the blood-brain barrier. Hemoglobin iron enters brain parenchyma and reacts with XO-derived oxygen metabolites with consequent brain injury.

successful in minimizing long-term sequellae even in severely ischemic brains. The clinical implications for salvage of neuronal tissue that has already been rendered ischemic are considerable.

IV. CONCLUSIONS

The importance of iron in stroke syndromes and the cooperative effects of iron and oxygen metabolites in precipitating oxidative injury to the ischemic brain have only recently been appreciated. Particularly when the cerebral endothelium has been disrupted by ischemia or other insults, red cell or serum iron will have access to the lipid-rich neuronal environment with potentially disastrous consequences. Preventative or therapeutic strategies need to be developed with these considerations in mind.

The basic mechanism of oxidative damage to the brain appears to be responsible for other forms of cerebrovascular injury besides primary ischemia. For instance, irradiation-induced alterations in cerebral blood flow are improved by inhibition of XO activity,[27] and the vasculopathy associated with viral cerebritis may also be linked to XO-derived oxygen metabolites.[28] XO activity is increased in human brain tumors,[29] and $O_2^{\cdot-}$ has been postulated to be responsible for peritumoral brain edema.[30] O_2^- production is also increased in experimental models of cranial trauma.[31] Furthermore, cold-induced brain edema and infarction are decreased in transgenic mice which express threefold higher levels of Cu/Zn SOD than control mice.[32] Free-radical products of monoamine oxidase B have recently been implicated in the development of Parkinson's disease[33] (see Chapter 14) and excessive oxidant production in the brain has been well documented in hyperoxic brain injury.[34,35] Finally, the oxidative effects of hemoglobin-associated iron appear to have a powerful effect on cerebral vasoreactivity and vascular remodeling. O_2^- may be more important than prostanoids in modulating arachidonic acid-induced vasoreactivity.[36] Hemoglobin also appears to inhibit both endothelium-dependent and endothelium-independent relaxation of cerebral vasculature.[37-39] The mechanism of this vasoconstrictive effect probably involves the generation of free radicals,[40] and cerebral vessels appear to be much more sensitive to hemoglobin-induced constriction than arteries of other vascular beds.[41] In addition to vasoconstriction, hemoglobin may also have local effects which promote excessive vessel wall remodeling, further increasing the risk of cerebral infarction.[42]

Clearly, many facets of the role of iron in initiating and amplifying oxidative injury to the brain are not yet understood. However, it is clear that iron must be tightly regulated within the brain parenchyma, and that the interaction between iron and free radicals has a broad ranging impact on a variety of central nervous system diseases. Specific therapies targeted at reducing the oxidative influence of reactive iron will bear significantly on a great number of diseases.

ACKNOWLEDGMENTS

This work was supported in part by grants from the National Institutes of Health (K08 HL02375, P50 HL40784); American Lung Association; Swan, Hill, Kleberg, Donner; and American Express Foundations.

REFERENCES

1. **Zaleska, M. M. and Floyd, R. A.,** Regional lipid peroxidation in rat brain *in vitro:* possible role of endogenous iron, *Neurochem. Res.,* 10, 397, 1985.
2. **Willmore, L. J. and Rubin, J. J.,** Formation of malonaldehyde and focal brain edema induced by subpial injection of $FeCl_2$ into rat isocortex, *Brain Res.,* 246, 113, 1982.
3. **Sadrzadeh, S. M., Anderson, D. K., Panter, S. S., Hallaway, P. E., and Eaton, J. W.,** Hemoglobin potentiates central nervous system damage, *J. Clin. Invest.,* 79, 662, 1987.
4. **Rosen, A. D. and Frumin, N. V.,** Focal epileptogenesis after intracortical hemoglobin injection, *Exp. Neurol.,* 66, 277, 1979.

5. **Braughler, J. M. and Hall, E. D.**, Central nervous system trauma and stroke. I. Biochemical considerations for oxygen radical formation and lipid peroxidation, *Free Radical Biol. Med.*, 6, 289, 1989.

6. **Misra, H. P. and Fridovich, I.**, The generation of superoxide radical during the autoxidation of hemoglobin, *J. Biol. Chem.*, 247, 6960, 1972.

7. **Sadrzadeh, S. M. H. and Eaton, J. W.**, Hemoglobin-mediated oxidant damage to the central nervous system requires endogenous ascorbate, *J. Clin. Invest.*, 82, 1510, 1988.

8. **Sadrzadeh, S. M. H., Graf, E., Panter, S. S., Hallaway, P. E., and Eaton, J. W.**, Hemoglobin: a biologic Fenton reagent, *J. Biol. Chem.*, 259, 14354, 1984.

9. **Panter, S. S., Sadrzadeh, S. M. H., Hallaway, P. E., Haines, J. I., Anderson, V. E., and Eaton, J. W.**, Hypohaptoglobinemia associated with familial epilepsy, *J. Exp. Med.*, 161, 748, 1985.

10. **Biemond, P., Swaak, A. J., Beindorff, C. M., and Koster, J. F.**, Superoxide-dependent and -independent mechanisms of iron mobilization from ferritin by xanthine oxidase. Implications for oxygen-free-radical-induced tissue destruction during ischaemia and inflammation, *Biochem. J.*, 239, 169, 1986.

11. **Gutteridge, J. M. C.**, Iron promoters of the Fenton reaction and lipid peroxidation can be released from haemoglobin by peroxides, *FEBS Lett.*, 201, 291, 1986.

12. **Chan, P. H., Fishman, R. A., Wesley, M. A., and Longar, S.**, Pathogenesis of vasogenic edema in focal cerebral ischemia. Role of superoxide radicals, *Adv. Neurol.*, 52, 177, 1990.

13. **Liu, T. H., Beckman, J. S., Freeman, B. A., Hogan, E. L., and Hsu, C. Y.**, Polyethylene glycol-conjugated superoxide dismutase and catalase reduce ischemic brain injury, *Am. J. Physiol.*, 256, H589, 1989.

14. **Schurer, L., Grogaard, B., Gerdin, B., and Arfors, K. E.**, Effects of neutrophil depletion and superoxide dismutase on postischemic hypoperfusion or rat brain, *Adv. Neurol.*, 52, 57, 1990.

15. **Agee, J. M., Flanagan, T., Blackbourne, L. H., Kron, I. L., and Tribble, C. G.**, Reducing postischemic paraplegia using conjugated superoxide dismutase, *Ann. Thorac. Surg.*, 51, 911, 1991.

16. **McCord, J. M.**, Oxygen-derived free radicals in post-ischemic tissue injury, *N. Engl. J. Med.*, 312, 159, 1985.

17. **Jarasch, E.-D., Grund, C., Bruder, G., Heid, H. W., Keenan, T. W., and Franke, W. W.**, Localization of xanthine oxidase in mammary-gland epithelium and capillary endothelium, *Cell*, 28, 67, 1981.

18. **Stirpe, F. and Della Corte, E.**, The regulation of rat liver xanthine oxidase: conversion *in vitro* of the enzymatic activity from dehydrogenase (Type D) to oxidase (Type O), *J. Biol. Chem.*, 244, 3855, 1969.

19. **Jarasch, E.-D., Bruder, G., and Heid, H. W.**, Significance of xanthine oxidase in capillary endothelial cells, *Acta Physiol. Scand.*, 126 (Suppl. 548), 39, 1986.

20. **Martz, D., Rayos, G., Schielke, G. P., and Betz, A. L.**, Allopurinol and dimethylthiourea reduce brain infarction following middle cerebral artery occlusion in rats, *Stroke*, 20, 488, 1989.

21. **Betz, A. L., Randall, J., and Martz, D.**, Xanthine oxidase is not a major source of free radicals in focal cerebral ischemia, *Am. J. Physiol.*, 260, H563, 1991.

22. **Terada, L. S., Willingham, I. R., Rosandich, M. E., Leff, J. A., Kindt, G. W., and Repine, J. E.**, Generation of superoxide anion by brain endothelial cell xanthine oxidase, *J. Cell Physiol.*, 148, 191, 1991.

23. **Parks, D. A. and Granger, D. N.**, Xanthine oxidase: biochemistry, distribution and physiology, *Acta Physiol. Scand.*, 126 (Suppl. 548), 87, 1986.

24. **Patt, A., Harken, A. H., Burton, L. K., Rodell, T. C., Piermattei, D., Schorr, W. J., Parker, N. B., Berger, E. M., Horesh, I. R., Terada, L. S., Linas, S. L., Cheronis, J. C., and Repine, J. E.**, Xanthine oxidase-derived hydrogen peroxide contributes to ischemia reperfusion-induced edema in gerbil brains, *J. Clin. Invest.*, 81, 1556, 1988.

25. **Toth, K. M., Harlan, J. M., Beehler, C. J., Berger, E. M., Parker, N. B., Linas, S. L., and Repine, J. E.,** Dimethylthiourea prevents hydrogen peroxide and neutrophil mediated damage to lung endothelial cells *in vitro* and disappears in the process, *Free Radical Biol. Med.,* 6, 457, 1989.

26. **Patt, A., Horesh, I. R., Berger, E. M., Harken, A. H., and Repine, J. E.,** Iron depletion or chelation reduces ischemia/reperfusion-induced edema in gerbil brains, *J. Pediatr. Surg.,* 25, 224, 1990.

27. **Cockerham, L. G., Arroyo, C. M., and Hampton, J. D.,** Effect of 4-hydroxypyrazolo (3,4-d) pyrimidine (allopurinol) on post-irradiation cerebral blood flow: implications of free radical involvement, *Free Radical Biol. Med.,* 4, 279, 1988.

28. **Boyes, B. E., Walker, D. G., McGeer, E. G., and O'Kusky, J. R.,** Increased uric acid in the developing brain and spinal cord following cytomegalovirus infection, *J. Neurochem.,* 53, 1719, 1989.

29. **Kokoglu, E., Belce, A., Ozyurt, E., and Tepeler, Z.,** Xanthine oxidase levels in human brain tumors, *Cancer Lett.,* 50, 179, 1990.

30. **Ikeda, Y., Anderson, J. H., Wunderlich, C. C., Hilton, J., and Long, D. M.,** Effect of superoxide dismutase in rabbits with peritumoral edema, *Adv. Neurol.,* 52, 441, 1990.

31. **Kontos, H. A. and Wei, E. P.,** Superoxide production in experimental brain injury, *J. Neurosurg.,* 64, 803, 1986.

32. **Chan, P. H., Yang, G. Y., Chen, S. F., Carlson, E., and Epstein, C. J.,** Cold-induced brain edema and infarction are reduced in transgenic mice overexpressing CuZn-superoxide dismutase, *Ann. Neurol.,* 29, 482, 1991.

33. **Tetrud, J. W. and Langston, J. W.,** The effect of deprenyl (selegiline) on the natural history of Parkinson's disease, *Science,* 245, 519, 1989.

34. **Yusa, T., Beckman, J. S., Crapo, J. D., and Freeman, B. A.,** Hyperoxia increases H_2O_2 production by brain *in vivo, J. Appl. Physiol.,* 63, 353, 1987.

35. **Jamieson, D.,** Oxygen toxicity and reactive oxygen metabolites in mammals, *Free Radical Biol. Med.,* 7, 87, 1989.

36. **Kontos, H. A., Wei, E. P., Povlishock, J. T., and Christman, C. W.,** Oxygen radicals mediated the cerebral arteriolar dilation from arachidonate and bradykinin in cats, *Circ. Res.,* 55, 295, 1984.

37. **Kanamaru, K., Waga, S., Kojima, T., Fujimoto, K., and Niwa, S.,** Endothelium-dependent relaxation of canine basilar arteries, *Stroke,* 18, 938, 1987.

38. **Toda, N.,** Hemolysate inhibits cerebral artery relaxation, *J. Cereb. Blood Flow Metab.,* 8, 46, 1988.

39. **Fujiwara, S., Kassell, N. F., Sasaki, T., Nakagomi, T., and Lehman, R. M.,** Selective hemoglobin inhibition of endothelium-dependent vasodilation of rabbit basilar artery, *J. Neurosurg.,* 64, 445, 1986.

40. **Steele, J. A., Stockbridge, N., Maljkovic, G., and Weir, B.,** Free radicals mediate actions of oxyhemoglobin on cerebrovascular smooth muscle cells, *Circ. Res.,* 68, 416, 1991.

41. **Tanishima, T.,** Cerebral vasospasm: contractile activity of hemoglobin in isolated canine basilar arteries, *J. Neurosurg.,* 53, 787, 1980.

42. **Mayberg, M. R., Okada, T., and Bark, D. H.,** The role of hemoglobin in arterial narrowing after subarachnoid hemorrhage, *J. Neurosurg.,* 72, 634, 1990.

Part V
Roles for Iron in Other Common Diseases

13. Iron and Cancer

RICHARD G. STEVENS

*Pacific Northwest Laboratory, Richland, Washington**

* Supported by the United States Department of Energy under contract DE-AC06-76RLO 1830.

I. INTRODUCTION

Body iron level is an important characteristic of health status. The impairment of health due to severe iron deficiency has been examined extensively. However, potential dangers of iron excess have not received much attention except in conditions of severe iron overload such as hemochromatosis. Moderate elevations in body iron stores may increase the risk of cancer by at least two possible mechanisms (reviewed in Reference 1). First, iron can catalyze the production of oxygen radicals[2] which may deplete available reducing equivalents rendering the cell more susceptible to the radicals produced by other agents such as toxic chemicals or radiation. Iron bound to DNA may be particularly effective in increasing the ability of radiation or chemicals to damage DNA. Second, iron may be a limiting nutrient to the growth and replication of a transformed cell in the human body,[3] thus, high iron stores may increase the chances that a transformed cell will survive to become a clinically detectable neoplasm. Because Western diet includes high amounts of available iron and because dietary increases in animal protein have been occurring throughout the world, the biological consequences of moderately elevated iron stores deserve attention.

The issue is whether moderate elevations in iron stores increase cancer risk. However, the definition of ''moderate'' is not clear. Severe iron deficiency is bad for health. It is also clear that severe iron overload increases risk of cancer and heart disease, and leads to early death (see Section V). At what point then, starting from severe iron deficiency, does increasing body iron stores cease to be a benefit and begin to become a detriment?

II. IRON AND OXYGEN RADICALS

Halliwell and Gutteridge[4] discuss the putative effects of oxygen radicals in a variety of disease processes and stress the role of iron. Oxygen radicals include the hydroxyl radical and superoxide anion.[2] These are highly toxic species produced intracellularly by reactions that can be catalyzed by iron. Oxygen radicals are believed to be some of the primary intermediates in the development of radiobiological damage. They have also been implicated in the cellular activation of carcinogens, the toxicity of several xenobiotics, and the deleterious effects of aging. Oxygen radicals can damage DNA extensively by inducing strand breakage and degradation of deoxyribose; they can induce lipid peroxidation, and they may play an important role in carcinogenesis and other disease processes.

Although neither free ferrous (Fe^{2+}) nor ferric (Fe^{3+}) ions are thought to exist in tissue in significant concentrations, iron can exist in a variety of iron complexes, e.g., Fe^{3+}-ADP.[5,6] Graf et al.[6] analyzed the ability of 12 different iron complexes to catalyze the Fenton reaction. They found that there is a requirement for at least one free iron coordination site for the iron complex to successfully produce hydroxyl radicals from hydrogen peroxide. For example, while iron complexes of adenosine di- and tri-phosphate were efficient, iron bound to phytate (naturally occurring in plant fiber) or Desferal® (desferrioxamine B methanesulfonate) was ineffective. Whether the Fenton reaction per se accounts for iron-mediated damage *in vivo* is not unequivocally clear,[2,7] although oxygen radicals are believed to be important.

Balla et al.[8] loaded cultured endothelial cells with chelated iron using 8-hydroxyquinoline. These iron-loaded cells were very sensitive to killing by (1) stimulated granulocytes, (2) menadione, and (3) H_2O_2. As little as 7 μmol/l H_2O_2 resulted in 50% reduction of survival of the iron-loaded cells, whereas untreated cells readily survived H_2O_2 concentrations of 2 mM, more than 100-fold greater. The authors concluded that iron sensitized the cells to killing by H_2O_2. Teicher et al.[9] showed that some complexes of Fe^{3+} increase killing of hypoxic EMT6 cells (a mammary tumor line) by γ-irradiation. Their purpose was to study whether these compounds might be clinically useful as radiosensitizers.

III. IRON AND DNA DAMAGE

Iron bound to DNA may be an important determinant for survival and mutation. Using isolated calf thymus DNA, Blakely et al.[10] showed that trace amounts of transition metals, namely, iron and copper, bound to DNA are necessary for H_2O_2-induced damage to occur; DNA pretreated with metal-ion chelators and extensively dialyzed was not susceptible to H_2O_2-induced damage. Imlay and Linn[11] found that a major source of the toxicity of hydrogen peroxide to *Escherichia coli* is mediated by DNA damage from Fenton reactions catalyzed by iron. These reactions are efficient enough to suggest a new technology for DNA cleavage. Oligodeoxynucleotide-EDTA-Fe^{2+} has been used to complex with DNA and cleave nonenzymatically at sequence-specific sites by exploiting Fenton chemistry.[12] Loeb et al.[13] incubated phage with iron, transfected it to *E. coli,* and observed mutation and inactivation of the phage. They speculated that free iron localized in cellular DNA may be an important cause of somatic mutation in humans. Following this work, McBride et al.[14] showed that the mutation of phage DNA by iron is not randomly distributed. The vast majority of mutations were single-base substitutions, primarily guanine to cytosine transversions. In addition, iron released from ferritin may play a role in lipid peroxidation,[15] and radiolytic products of water may accelerate the release of iron from ferritin.[16]

Transition metal ions may greatly influence the yields and types of DNA damage due to the production of hydroxyl radicals in close proximity to the DNA.[10] In fact, the proximity of these site-specific reactions to DNA targets makes scavenging extremely unfavorable even when the scavenger is present in high concentrations.

Ward et al.[17] has provided evidence that double-strand breaks in DNA are required to cause cell death. They used H_2O_2 at 0°C to produce single-strand breaks and asserted that these breaks resulted from metal-catalyzed oxidation of the H_2O_2 to the hydroxyl radical. At 0°C, they speculated, the reduction of the ferric back to the ferrous form was slow, and thus only one molecule at a time could cause damage. At 37°C, H_2O_2 was much more lethal. The authors suggested a mechanism whereby H_2O_2 diffuses to DNA where it can be oxidized by a DNA-ferrous iron adduct to a hydroxyl radical;[18-20] the ferric iron can be reduced once again to ferrous by another H_2O_2 molecule, and then react with a third to produce the double-strand break and cell death. Further work[21] suggested the importance of repair processes in H_2O_2 toxicity at 37°C. Repair plays a particularly vital role in survival after irradiation, and the repair capability of cells in response to radiation is now known to be considerably more complex (e.g., multiple repair processes, including additional fast and slow ones, operate simultaneously) than previously assumed or understood.[22]

IV. ANIMAL STUDIES

Weinberg[3] evaluated the possibility that an important defense against infection was the withholding of iron, an essential nutrient for invading pathogens (see Chapter 6). When challenged by a pathogen, the response of the host often includes a reduction of serum iron, a block in iron uptake by the gut, and a fever; each of these, Weinberg argues, is designed to limit the ability of the pathogen to acquire the iron necessary for its growth and spread. By slowing the pathogen, the body's immune defense mechanisms have a better chance of defeating the invader. By analogy, Weinberg also argues that a transformed cell may also be restricted by a lack of available iron, and encouraged by an iron excess. In order to test the hypothesis that excess iron would increase cancer cell growth, Bergeron et al.[23] inoculated a leukemia cell line (L1210) intraperitoneally into two groups of DBA-2 mice: one group received supplemental iron injections and the other did not. The group receiving iron died sooner and yielded larger tumor load from the peritoneum than the group not receiving iron. These results were consistent with the idea that increased iron increased the ability of cancer cells to survive and flourish.

Hann et al.[24] also examined the effects of iron on growth of transplanted cancer cells; only their experiments focused on iron deficiency as protective. Three different strains of mice (BALB/c, C3H/He, and DBA/2) were divided into groups of 15 either on a low-iron diet (5 mg/kg diet) or normal iron diet (312 mg/kg diet). Each group was then inoculated with tumor cells (CA07-A [colon cancer] into BALB/c, HE129 [hepatoma] into C3H/He, and M119 [breast cancer] into DBA/2). Although all mice developed tumors, the tumors grew more slowly (smaller in size at each weekly interval) in the mice on an iron-restricted diet. The authors stated that there were no obvious behavioral activity or appearance differences between the low- and normal iron groups.

The low-iron BALB/c mice were smaller than their normal iron counterparts; the reverse was true for the C3H/He and DBA/2 mice. The authors concluded that iron restriction reduced the ability of tumor cells to flourish.

In order to determine whether iron might increase the induction of cancer *de novo,* Thompson et al.[25] administered 1-methyl-1-nitrosourea (MNU) to a group of rats receiving normal rat chow, to a group of rats receiving a low-iron diet, and to a group of rats receiving an iron-supplemented diet. The group of rats receiving dietary iron supplementation suffered the greatest mammary-tumor burden, whereas the group of rats receiving an iron-restricted diet had fewer tumors than the group of rats on the normal diet (although this latter effect may have resulted simply from reduced body weight in the rats on an iron-restricted diet). These results were consistent with either an effect of iron on the survival of a cancer cell induced by MNU or an effect of iron in sensitizing a normal mammary epithelial cell to the effects of MNU by, for example, increasing oxidative stress in the cells.

Siegers et al.[26] examined dimethylhydrazine-induced (DMH) colon tumorigenesis in NMRI mice. Four groups of mice were treated as follows: (1) 20 mg/kg DMH subcutaneously and normal diet, (2) 20 mg/kg DMH subcutaneously and iron-enriched diet (3.5% Fe-fumarate), (3) 40 mg/kg DMH subcutaneously and normal diet, and (4) 40 mg/kg DMH subcutaneously and normal diet plus desferrioxamine (a potent iron chelator). Group two had significantly more animals with colonic tumors and more tumors per animal than group one; excess iron increased colon tumorigenesis by DMH. Groups three and four had too many tumors to count, and desferrioxamine did not have an obvious protective effect. In all groups the vast majority of tumors were adenomas with only a handful of carcinomas. The authors speculated that iron led to an increase in the proliferation of the colonic stem cells at risk and thereby to an increase in the effectiveness of DMH in tumor induction.

Smith et al.[27] used C57BL/10ScSn mice to show that iron-dextran injection increased sensitivity to liver carcinogenesis by the chemical hexachlorobenzene (HCB). A different strain of mice (DBA/2) was much less susceptible to potentiation of HCB carcinogenesis by iron. The authors speculated that increases in oxidative stress by iron accounted for the results.

V. GENETIC SUSCEPTIBILITY

Genetic susceptibility to oxidative damage may, in part, result from genetic variations in the absorption (e.g., hemochromatosis gene product); transport (e.g., transferrin variants); or intracellular processing (e.g., ferritin variants) of iron.

Hemochromatosis is a clinically defined condition in which there is a morbid increase in body iron stores. (See Chapter 4.) Those with hemochromatosis suffer severe health consequences and early death. The predisposition to hemochromatosis is genetically determined and the gene is located on chromosome 6 between the HLA-A and -B loci.[28] The hemochromatosis gene product is unknown but it apparently affects uptake of iron from the gut, perhaps coding for an iron transport protein in the intestinal wall. Kravitz et al.[29] reported a transferrin saturation of 93 and 83.7% in male and female hemochromatosis homozygotes, respectively, compared to only 32.8 and 30.2% in normal males and females, respectively. Obligate heterozygotes had intermediate transferrin saturations of 42.6 and 40.1%, respectively. Since the gene frequency of the abnormal hemochromatosis allele has been estimated to be 0.067 from a study of blood donors in Utah,[30] it is estimated that approximately 12 to 14% of the population may be heterozygotes. This raises the possibility that a large segment of the normal population may be at genetically determined increased risk of oxidative stress due to chronically higher body iron stores (as reflected in higher transferrin saturation) resulting from the hemochromatosis gene (in either the homozygous or heterozygous state).

Hemochromatosis victims suffer high risks of liver cancer, cardiomyopathy, and cirrhosis.[31] Iron stores also increase in patients given multiple transfusions to treat severe anemias. For example, patients with thalassemia die at an early age of heart disease, infection, liver disease, or cancer.[32] Treatment with the iron chelator desferrioxamine was initiated in 1975 in Italy; and since that time, survival of thalassemic children has improved significantly. Thus in both hemochromatosis and thalassemia, iron overload can induce severe physical harm.

VI. EPIDEMIOLOGICAL STUDIES

There have been only a handful of epidemiological studies that have investigated the association of body iron stores and risk of cancer. In each of these a surrogate for iron stores has been used because the actual measurement of liver or marrow stainable iron cannot be done in the large study size necessary to have any epidemiological validity. In fact, it is not clear what "high body iron stores" means, and some of the stainable iron may not have etiologic significance for cancer. Given the two mechanisms by which "high" iron might increase cancer risk as stated in the introduction, the definitions of high iron that can be stated are (1) relatively high intracellular iron content, particularly that iron associated with DNA, with ferritin, and with nonspecific iron complexes (e.g., Fe^{3+}-ADP); and (2) high iron content of blood and interstitial fluid in a form that can be utilized by cancer cells (e.g., high transferrin saturation).

It is very expensive and rarely feasible to perform a prospective study in which a large group of healthy people are given a series of tests then followed for years to determine whether the test outcomes are related to disease. Therefore, existing data bases are often used. In these, however, the measure of body iron stores is usually not optimum. Ideally, a serum ferritin measurement would be used.[33] If only medical records are available total iron-binding capacity (TIBC) is often recorded and sometimes serum iron. From these, a crude estimate of transferrin saturation can be calculated. If stored serum is also available, then it may be possible to test for the concentrations of the ferritin and transferrin proteins (not to be confused with transferrin saturation).

Serum ferritin and transferrin, TIBC, and transferrin saturation have each been used in studies of iron and cancer. In general, among healthy individuals, when body iron stores are high, transferrin saturation and serum ferritin are high, and TIBC and serum transferrin are low. These assumed relationships form the basis for the studies done to date.[34]

Four studies have been consistent with the hypothesis that high body iron stores increase the risk of cancer, or general mortality, in men[35-37] or in women.[38] One study from Finland that has only been presented in abbreviated form found no relationship between transferrin saturation and cancer risk.[39] However, a more detailed analysis of this study does show an increased risk of certain types of cancer in men with high transferrin saturation (D. Stipp, "Is Popeye doomed?" *The Wall Street Journal*, Jan. 17, 1992, p. B3).

A study was undertaken of the relationship of serum ferritin and transferrin and later risk of primary liver cancer or of death from cancer in general.[36] The study of liver cancer was motivated by the hypothesis stated by Blumberg et al.[40] that those carriers of hepatitis B virus who develop primary hepato-cellular carcinoma (PHC) have higher iron stores than those carriers who do not because iron is a necessary nutrient to cancer cells. The study of cancer, in general, was motivated both by the notion that iron is a nutrient and by the fact that iron can catalyze the production of oxygen radicals. Beasley and colleagues[41] enrolled 21,513 male Chinese government workers in Taiwan in a prospective study of the health effects of hepatitis B virus. A blood sample was taken and stored on each worker, and the cohort was followed prospectively for incidence of PHC and for death from any cause. Among these men, 239 had died of cancer or were alive with a diagnosis of PHC as of July, 1983. For the study of iron-binding proteins and cancer risk, two controls for each case were chosen from the cohort who were alive and free of PHC at the date of death from cancer, or at diagnosis of PHC. The controls were matched on age and serum hepatitis B surface antigen status. For cancer death excluding PHC, serum transferrrin was significantly lower among cases than controls, and serum ferritin was higher though not significantly so. These results were consistent with the hypothesis that high body iron stores increase cancer risk. For PHC, the serum ferritin was significantly higher among cases; serum transferrin was also higher although not significantly so. In addition, serum albumin was significantly lower among cases. This intriguing finding has been made in a number of studies,[42,43] and holds even after adjustment for smoking which could act as a confounder.[44]

In 1988, Stevens et al.[37] published the results of an analysis of cancer incidence in the first National Health and Nutrition Examination Survey

(NHANES) population. During the period from 1971 to 1975 a probability sample of the U.S. population was identified. On each of 14,407 identified subjects an extensive dietary questionnaire was administered, a medical examination was performed, anthropometric measurements were made, and a number of biochemical tests were done on serum and urine. Among the serum tests were serum iron and TIBC. From these transferrin saturation was calculated. Neither serum ferritin nor transferrin was determined. Among 3355 men for whom complete information was available and who remained alive and not diagnosed with cancer within 4 years of the biochemical tests, there were a significant association of serum iron and transferrin saturation, and an inverse association of TIBC with risk of cancer over an approximately 10-year follow-up period. In particular, cancers of the lung, colon, bladder, and esophagus appeared most strongly related to transferrin saturation. For cancer of the colon, risk in each quartile of transferrin saturation relative to a baseline of 1.0 for those under 22.8% increased to 1.76 in those 22.9 to 29.1%, to 3.11 in those 29.2 to 36.7%, and to 4.69 in those greater than 36.7%. This striking result was consistent with the prediction of Graf and Eaton[44a,45] who speculated that dietary phytate consumption would reduce risk of colon cancer by virtue of binding iron. The result was based on only 12 cases, however, and only provides the basis for investigating this relationship further in other population samples. Another finding of the NHANES study was significantly lower serum albumin in cancer cases than in controls.

The NHANES study has contributed to a heated controversy on the effects of moderate elevations in body iron stores. Those who have fought for iron fortification of food in order to avoid anemia dislike the results and fear the study will undermine their work. Their criticisms have been articulated by Yip and Williamson[46] in a letter responding to the study in the *New England Journal of Medicine*.

Yip and Williamson[46] criticized the NHANES study on three grounds. They claim that "inflammatory processes" could have invalidated the conclusions, and they cite a paper by Yip and Dallman[47] as evidence. Yet in that paper, Table 2 shows an inverse relationship between erythrocyte sedimentation rate (their measure of "inflammation") and transferrin saturation in the NHANES I men aged 60 to 74. Therefore, "inflammatory processes" should have reduced the ability of the NHANES study to detect a true effect of transferrin saturation on cancer risk if one, in fact, existed. In addition, serum iron in NHANES was higher in cancer cases than in controls, arguing against inflammation as accounting for the results.

Not mentioned by Yip and Williamson is the possibility that the observed low albumin in NHANES might also mean low serum transferrin which could lead to higher transferrin saturation as an artifact not necessarily reflecting higher iron stores. Since serum transferrin was not measured in NHANES, it is not possible to evaluate this possibility in the NHANES study.

Yip and Williamson then questioned the definition of high body iron stores in the NHANES study, claiming that "high" should be at least 50%

transferrin saturation, not the 36.8% used. Nevertheless, in the NHANES study, high iron stores were not used in an effort to define a clinical condition that required further tests and possible treatment based on transferrin saturation. The 36.8% was simply the cutoff for the top quartile of transferrin saturation among men in the NHANES I data base. The purpose was to determine whether quantitative increases in transferrin saturation were associated with corresponding increases in cancer risk among otherwise healthy people (i.e., not obviously sick). Clearly, there is variability in transferrin saturation measurements from day to day and test to test. The greater the variability, the less the reported transferrin saturation reflects body iron stores and the less the study is able to detect a true effect of body iron stores should it exist. Therefore, the significant association reported in the NHANES study may, in fact, reflect a stronger true association of body iron stores and risk of cancer.

Yip and Williamson apparently see body iron stores as either high or not high and that there is a specific level of transferrin saturation that distinguishes the two. From the point of view of a physician who must decide whether to treat iron overload, this may be a necessary view. However, body iron level is a continuous variable, and the intent of the NHANES study was to examine whether moderate elevations in iron stores might increase cancer risk, not simply whether those people clinically defined as iron overloaded are at increased risk.

Finally, Yip and Williamson[46] questioned the NHANES statistical analysis. This is a technical point which is dealt with by Korn and Graubard.[48] Their conclusion is that the NHANES analyses as presented are not invalidated by different analytic methods.

However, it is important to state that the NHANES study is by no means definitive. No one epidemiological study can be. A number of studies will be required before it becomes clear whether, and to what extent, moderate elevations in body iron stores increase cancer risk.

VII. IRON AND RADIATION SENSITIVITY

Exposure of human populations to radiation, whether from occupational, medical, or environmental sources, underscores the need to identify characteristics of the individual that influence risk of radiation injury. Tissue iron level may be one such characteristic. Epidemiological studies support the hypothesis that increased body iron stores increase the risk of cancer,[34,37] although studies to identify a possible interaction of iron and radiation exposure in human cancer etiology have not yet been done.

An effect of body iron stores on sensitivity to radiation injury would have important implications for: (1) second malignant neoplasms arising from radiation therapy, (2) diagnostic radiation exposure, (3) occupational radiation and residential radon exposures, and (4) exposure of astronauts and airline crews to cosmic radiation. In all these instances, the relative capacity of the individual to scavenge oxygen radicals may influence cancer risk associated with radiation exposure, and this capacity may be closely related to iron metabolism. While nutritional antioxidants have been receiving a great deal of attention in this regard, the "oxidant" iron has received very little.

Repine et al.[49] showed that dimethyl sulfoxide (DMSO) prevented 80% of single-strand breaks by γ-rays in isolated DNA, and 100% of single-strand breaks induced by an iron/H_2O_2 system. They concluded that since DMSO can scavenge OH·, 80% of the damage done to DNA by γ-rays is mediated by production of OH· whereas 100% of DNA damage from iron/H_2O_2 results from production of OH·. However, Blakely et al.[10] showed that DMSO reduced the yield of base damage products from hydrogen peroxide added to isolated DNA without added iron by only 40 to 60%.

Whiting et al.[51] showed that ferritin ($\sim$19% iron by weight) in the growth medium of CHO cells was clastogenic at added concentrations of 15 to 170 μg/ml, and cytotoxic at higher concentrations. Apoferritin (the iron-free protein) had no effect at comparable concentrations. At similar iron concentrations, other iron complexes (e.g., cysteine, glycine, histidine, EDTA) in the growth medium were much less clastogenic and cytotoxic than ferritin.

We recently completed an experiment to determine whether ferritin could increase sensitivity of mammalian cells to X-ray exposure.[50] Stationary-phase Chinese hamster ovary (CHO) cells were cultured in medium containing ferritin ($\sim$19% iron by weight) added at concentrations ranging from 0 to 128 μg/ml. One set of cultures was unirradiated, and another set was exposed to 4.0 Gy of X-rays. Clonogenic cell survival was assessed in each set of cultures. In the absence of added ferritin, 4.0 Gy killed approximately 50% of the cells. In the absence of radiation, ferritin was not toxic at less than 48 μg/ml; above 48 μg/ml, toxicity increases with concentration. Apoferritin was not toxic at any concentration tested (up to 1000 μg/ml). Although 32 μg/ml ferritin was not toxic, it reduced the survival after X-irradiation by an additional 75%; only $\sim$12% survived after 4 Gy compared to the 50% that survived after 4 Gy in the absence of added ferritin. These results indicate that a sublethal concentration of ferritin can be a potent radiosensitizer.

The results of our initial experiments can be compared with the results of Whiting et al.[51] In their system, 30 to 33 μg/ml ferritin was also not toxic, yet did yield observable chromosomal aberrations in $\sim$16% of cells. Ferritin added at 30 to 33 μg/ml yields an iron concentration in the growth medium of approximately 1×10^{-4} M; iron complexes of glycine, histidine, and EDTA added to give the same final iron concentration yielded no additional aberrations over the background (i.e., in <1% of cells). In addition, 1×10^{-4} M ferrous sulfate had no effect; aberrations began to appear at iron concentrations of 3×10^{-3} M. If our research demonstrates that ferritin and transferrin are more effective radiosensitizers than ferrous sulfate, then a possible implication for humans is that heme iron, that form of iron most easily absorbed from the diet,[52] is also most effective at increasing sensitivity to radiation injury.

Ferritin is the iron storage protein in tissue, although it is also found in serum at low concentration (~15 to 300 ng/ml[53]); normal serum contains ~1 to 2 μg/ml iron, but it is primarily bound to transferrin.[54] Our growth medium contains 10% fetal calf serum, or ~0.1 to 0.2 μg/ml iron. Since the ferritin used by us was ~19% iron by weight, 32 μg/ml ferritin represents ~6 μg/ml iron. Thus, even though ferritin added at 32 μg/ml increases the iron content of the medium 30- to 60-fold, this represents only a 3- to 6-fold increase in the iron concentration of the milieu surrounding cells in serum and tissue. Yet as we have shown, this moderate elevation in iron added as ferritin is a potent radiosensitizer to CHO cells.

This is the first report to our knowledge that ferritin can alter susceptibility of mammalian cells to ionizing radiation killing. Iron added as ferritin represents a physiological manipulation of iron level, and not an exotic or heroic experimental paradigm. The results, therefore, are not as far removed from possible implications for human radiation sensitivity as results from experiments utilizing xenobiotics to sensitize cells.

VIII. PROGNOSIS AFTER CANCER DIAGNOSIS

Manipulation of iron may play an important role in cancer therapy.[55,56] DeSousa et al.[57] examined survival in children with acute lymphocytic leukemia and found that those with transferrin saturation of less than 36% at entry into their study had significantly better survival than those with transferrin saturation greater than 36%. This was true after controlling for risk group, FAB classification, or presence of organomegaly. It was also observed in all subgroups.

As mentioned earlier in Section I, there is some evidence that iron-loaded cancer cells may be more susceptible to radiation therapy.[9] Based on oxidative mechanisms, it makes sense to build a compound that will seek out cancer cells and deliver a redox active substance to them before radiotherapy. Iron is effective as such, but may be a poor choice because it is also a necessary nutrient for the very cells one is attempting to kill.

IX. OTHER STUDIES

Lee et al.[58] found a significant effect of dietary red meat intake, no effect of fat, and a protective effect of soya protein on risk of breast cancer in young women in Singapore. Iron availability may account for these results.[59] Red meat contains the most readily absorbed form of dietary iron.[52] In addition, there is some animal evidence in support of a role for iron in mammary-tumor induction as cited in Section IV.[25] The protective effect of soya protein seen in the Lee et al.[58] study may also be related to iron metabolism. Soybeans are a source of phytate, a constituent of most cereals, nuts, and legumes that avidly binds iron in such a way that it is incapable of catalyzing the production of oxygen radicals.[45] The protective effect of soya protein may be shared by increased intakes of other plant products that are high in phytate but either not consumed in quantity in Singapore or not assessed in the questionnaire administered by Lee et al.[58]

Willett et al.[60] reported that red meat intake was significantly related to risk of colon cancer in a prospective study of 88,751 women followed from 1980 to 1986. The risk of colon cancer in women who reported consuming red meat every day relative to those who reported consuming it less than once a month was 2.5. Willett et al.[61] later suggested iron as a possible reason for their reported association of red meat with colon cancer risk. Dietary fat was not related to risk after taking account of red meat intake. As noted previously, red meat is a particularly good source of iron. In addition, there has been a report that high dietary iron increases colon tumorigenesis in mice by dimethylhydrazine[26] (see Section IV).

The effect of phytate on risk of breast cancer, if there is an effect, would be indirect; it might remove dietary iron from the potential for absorption. However, the effect of phytate on risk of colon cancer as hypothesized by Graf and Eaton[44a] would be directly mediated at the colonic epithelium; unbound iron may produce oxidative damage to the tissue, whereas iron bound by phytate would be unavailable for oxidative reactions.

X. CONCLUSION

The very quality that makes iron so useful to organisms, its redox cycling capacity, also makes it very dangerous to biological molecules, organelles, and membranes. Playing with iron is almost literally playing with fire. As with fire, however, iron can be a great benefit to life. Aerobes have developed complex mechanisms for using iron while avoiding self-destruction; these include iron-binding proteins and antioxidant defense systems. In humans, iron regulation is again very complex. Iron is well conserved in the body; presumably this has resulted from evolution through times of limited dietary iron availability and scarcity of meat. An important question in this age of abundant iron-rich foods is whether moderate elevations in body iron stores lead to long-term consequences such as cancer.

REFERENCES

1. **Stevens, R. G. and Kalkwarf, D. R.,** Iron, radiation, and cancer, *Environ. Health Perspec.,* 87, 291, 1990.
2. **Halliwell, B. and Gutteridge, J. M. C.,** Role of free radicals and catalytic metal ions in human disease: an overview, *Methods Enzymol.,* 186, 1, 1990.
3. **Weinberg, E. D.,** Iron withholding: a defense against infection and neoplasia, *Physiol. Rev.,* 64, 65, 1984.
4. **Halliwell, B. and Gutteridge, J. M. C.,** Oxygen free radicals and iron in relation to biology and medicine: some problems and concepts, *Arch. Biochem. Biophys.,* 246, 501, 1986.
5. **Floyd, R. A.,** Direct demonstration that ferrous ion complexes of di- and tri-phosphate nucleotides catalyze hydroxyl free radical formation from hydrogen peroxide, *Arch. Biochem. Biophys.,* 225, 263, 1983.
6. **Graf, E., Mahoney, J. R., Bryand, R. G., and Eaton, J. W.,** Iron-catalyzed hydroxyl radical formation, *J. Biol. Chem.,* 259, 3620, 1984.
7. **Winterbourn, C. C.,** The ability of scavengers to distinguish ˙OH production in the iron-catalyzed Haber-Weiss reaction: comparison of four assays for ˙OH, *Free Radical Biol. Med.,* 3, 33, 1987.
8. **Balla, G., Vercellotti, G. M., Eaton, J. W., and Jacob, H. S.,** Iron loading of endothelial cells augments oxidant damage, *J. Lab. Clin. Med.,* 116, 546, 1990.
9. **Teicher, B. A., Jacobs, J. L., Cathcart, K. N. S., Abrams, M. J., Vollano, J. F., and Picker, D. H.,** Some complexes of cobalt(III) and iron(III) are radiosensitizers of hypoxic EMT6 cells, *Radiat. Res.,* 109, 36, 1987.
10. **Blakely, W. F., Fuciarelli, A. F., Wegher, B. J., and Dizdaroglu, M.,** Hydrogen peroxide-induced base damage in deoxyribonucleic acid, *Radiat. Res.,* 121, 338, 1990.
11. **Imlay, J. A. and Linn, S.,** DNA damage and oxygen radical toxicity, *Science,* 240, 1302, 1988.
12. **Dreyer, G. B. and Dervan, P. B.,** Sequence-specific cleavage of single-stranded DNA: oligodeoxynucleotide-EDTA·FE(II), *PNAS,* 82, 968, 1985.
13. **Loeb, L. A., James, E. A., Waltersdorph, A. M., and Klebanoff, S. J.,** Mutagenesis by autoxidation of iron with isolated DNA, *Proc. Natl. Acad. Sci.,* 85, 3918, 1988.
14. **McBride, T. J., Preston, B. D., and Loeb, L. A.,** Mutagenic spectrum resulting from DNA damage by oxygen radicals, *Biochemistry,* 30, 207, 1991.
15. **Minotti, G. and Aust, S. D.,** The role of iron in oxygen radical mediated lipid peroxidation, *Chem.-Biol. Interact.,* 71, 1, 1989.
16. **Reif, D. W., Schubert, J., and Aust, S. D.,** Iron release from ferritin and lipid peroxidation by radiolytically generated reducing radicals, *Arch. Biochem. Biophys.,* 264, 238, 1988.
17. **Ward, J. F., Blakely, W. F., and Joner, E. I.,** Mammalian cells are not killed by DNA single-strand breaks caused by hydroxyl radicals from hydrogen peroxide, *Radiat. Res.,* 103, 383, 1985.
18. **Floyd, R. A.,** DNA-ferrous iron catalyzed hydroxyl free radical formation from hydrogen peroxide, *Biochem. Biophys. Res. Commun.,* 99, 1209, 1981.
19. **Lesko, S. A., Drocourt, J.-L., and Yang, S.-U.,** Deoxyribonucleic acid-protein and deoxyribonucleic acid interstrand cross-links induced in isolated chromatin by hydrogen peroxide and ferrous ethylenediaminetetraacetate chelates, *Biochemistry,* 21, 5010, 1982.
20. **Larramendy, M., Mello-Filho, A. C., Martins, E. A., et al.,** Iron-mediated induction of sister-chromatid exchanges by hydrogen peroxide and superoxide anion, *Mutation Res.,* 178, 57, 1987.
21. **Ward, J. F., Evans, J. W., Limoli, C. L., and Calabro-Jones, P. M.,** Radiation and hydrogen peroxide induced free radical damage to DNA, *Br. J. Cancer,* 55 (Suppl. 8), 105, 1987.

346

22. **Nelson, J. M., Brady, L. A., Metting, N. F., and Roesch, W. C.**, Multiple components of split-dose repair in plateau-phase mammalian cells: a new challenge for phenomenological modelers, *Radiat. Res.*, 121, 154, 1990.

23. **Bergeron, R. J., Streiff, R. R., and Elliott, G. T.**, Influence of iron on *in vivo* proliferation and lethality of L1210 cells, *J. Nutr.*, 115, 369, 1985.

24. **Hann, H. L., Stahlhut, M. W., and Blumberg, B. S.**, Iron nutrition and tumor growth: decreased tumor growth in iron-deficient mice, *Cancer Res.*, 48, 4168, 1988.

25. **Thompson, H. J., Kennedy, K., Witt, M., and Juzefyk, J.**, Effect of dietary iron deficiency or excess on the induction of mammary carcinogenesis by 1-methyl-1-nitrosourea, *Carcinogenesis*, 12, 111, 1991.

26. **Siegers, C. P., Bumann, D., Baretton, G., and Younes, M.**, Dietary iron enhances the tumor rate in dimethylhydrazine-induced colon carcinogenesis in mice, *Cancer Lett.*, 41, 251, 1988.

27. **Smith, A. G., Cabral, J. R. P., Carthew, P., Francis, J. E., and Manson, M. M.**, Carcinogenicity of iron in conjunction with a chlorinated environmental chemical, hexachlorobenzene, in C57BL/10ScSn mice, *Int. J. Cancer*, 43, 492, 1989.

28. **Edwards, C. O., Griffen, L. M., Dadone, M. M., et al.**, Mapping the locus for hereditary hemochromatosis: localization between HLA-B and HLA-A, *Am. J. Hum. Genet.*, 38, 805, 1986.

29. **Kravitz, K., Skolnick, M., Cannings, C., et al.**, Genetic linkage between hereditary hemochromatosis and HLA, *Am. J. Hum. Genet.*, 31, 601, 1979.

30. **Edwards, C. O., Griffen, L. M., Goldgar, D., et al.**, Prevalence of hemochromatosis among 11,065 presumably healthy blood donors, *N. Engl. J. Med.*, 318, 1355, 1988.

31. **Niederau, C., Fischer, R., Sonnenberg, A., et al.**, Survival and causes of death in cirrhotic and noncirrhotic patients with primary hemochromatosis, *N. Engl. J. Med.*, 313, 1256, 1985.

32. **Zurlo, M. G., DeStefano, P., Borgna-Pignatti, C., et al.**, Survival and causes of death in thalassemia major, *Lancet*, 2, 27, 1989.

33. **Lipschitz, D. A., Cook, J. D., and Finch, C. A.**, A clinical evaluation of serum ferritin as an index of iron stores, *N. Engl. J. Med.*, 290, 1213, 1974.

34. **Stevens, R. G.**, Iron and the risk of cancer, *Med. Oncol. Tumor Pharmacother.*, 7, 177, 1990.

35. **Stevens, R. G., Kuvibidila, S., Kapps, M., Friedlaender, J. S., and Blumberg, B. S.**, Iron-binding proteins, hepatitis B virus, and mortality in the Solomon Islands, *Am. J. Epidemol.*, 118, 550, 1983.

36. **Stevens, R. G., Beasley, R. P., and Blumberg, B. S.**, Iron-binding proteins and risk of cancer in Taiwan, *J. Natl. Cancer Inst.*, 76, 605, 1986.

37. **Stevens, R. G., Jones, D. Y., Micozzi, M. S., and Taylor, P. R.**, Body iron stores and the risk of cancer, *N. Engl. J. Med.*, 319, 1047, 1988.

38. **Selby, J. V. and Friedman, G. D.**, Epidemiological evidence of an association of body iron stores and risk of cancer, *Int. J. Cancer.*, 41, 677, 1988.

39. **Takkunen, H., Reunanen, A., Knekt, P., and Aromaa, A.**, Body iron stores and the risk of cancer, *N. Engl. J. Med.*, (letter), 320, 1013, 1989.

40. **Blumberg, B. S., Lustbader, E. D., and Whitford, P. L.**, Changes in serum levels due to infection with hepatitis B virus, *Proc. Natl. Acad. Sci.*, 78, 3222, 1981.

41. **Beasley, R. P., Lin, C. C., Hwang, L. Y., et al.**, Hepatocellular carcinoma and hepatitis B virus, *Lancet*, 2, 1129, 1981.

42. **Stevens, R. G. and Blumberg, B. S.**, Serum albumin and mortality, *Lancet*, 335, 351, 1990.

43. **Stevens, R. G. and Blumberg, B. S.**, Serum albumin and cancer risk, in *Nutrition and Cancer Prevention: Investigating the Role of Macronutrients*, Micozzi, M. S. and Moon, T. E., Eds., Marcel Dekker, 1992, 283.

44. **Stram, D. O., Akiba, S., Neriishi, K., Stevens, R. G., and Hosoda, Y.,** Smoking and serum proteins in atomic-bomb survivors in Japan, *Am. J. Epidemiol.,* 131, 1038, 1990.

44a. **Graf, E. and Eaton, J. W.,** Dietary suppression of colonic cancer: fiber or phytate?, *Cancer,* 56, 717, 1985.

45. **Graf, E. and Eaton, J. W.,** Antioxidant functions of phytic acid, *Free Radical Biol. Med.,* 8, 61, 1990.

46. **Yip, R. and Williamson, D. F.,** Correspondance, *N. Engl. J. Med.,* 320, 1012, 1989.

47. **Yip, R. and Dallman, P. R.,** The roles of inflammation and iron deficiency as causes of anemia, *Am. J. Clin. Nutri.,* 48, 1295, 1988.

48. **Korn, E. L. and Graubard, B. I.,** Epidemiological studies utilizing surveys: accounting for the sampling design, *Am. J. Public Health,* 81, 1166, 1991.

49. **Repine, J. E., Pfenninger, O. W., Talmage, D. W., Berger, E. M., and Pettijohn, D. E.,** Dimethylsulfoxide prevents DNA nicking mediated by ionizing radiation or iron/hydrogen peroxide generated hydroxyl radical, *Proc. Natl. Acad. Sci.,* 78, 1001, 1981.

50. **Nelson, J. M. and Stevens, R. G.,** Ferritin-iron increases killing of chinese hamster ovary cells by x irradiation, *Cell Prolif.,* 24, 411, 1991.

51. **Whiting, R. F., Wei, L., and Stich, H. F.,** Chromosome-damaging activity of ferritin and its relation to chelation and reduction of iron, *Cancer Res.,* 41, 1628, 1981.

52. **Cook, J. D.,** Adaptation in iron metabolism, *Am. J. Clin. Nutr.,* 51, 301, 1990.

53. **Jacobs, A.,** Ferritin: an interim reviews, *Curr. Top. Hematol.,* 5, 25, 1985.

54. **Huebers, H. A. and Finch, C. A.,** The physiology of transferrin and transferrin receptors, *Physiol. Rev.,* 67, 520, 1987.

55. **Cazzola, M., Bergamaschi, G., Dezza, L., and Arosio, P.,** Manipulations of cellular iron metabolism for modulating normal and malignant cell proliferation: achievements and prospects, *Blood,* 75, 1093, 1990.

56. **DeSousa, M. and Brock, J. H., Eds.,** *Iron in Immunity, Cancer and Inflammation,* John Wiley & Sons, Chichester, England, 1989.

57. **DeSousa, M., Potaznik, D., and Groshen, S. C. B.,** Body iron stores and risk of cancer (letter), *N. Engl. J. Med.,* 320, 1014, 1989.

58. **Lee, H. P., Gourley, L., Duffy, S. W., Estève, J., Lee, J., and Day, N. E.,** Dietary effects on breast-cancer risk in Singapore, *Lancet,* 337, 1197, 1991.

59. **Stevens, R. G.,** Dietary effects on breast cancer, *Lancet,* 338, 186, 1991.

60. **Willett, W. C., Stampfer, M. J., Colditz, G. A., Rosner, B. A., and Speizer, F. E.,** Relation of meat, fat, and fiber intake to the risk of colon cancer in a prospective study among women, *N. Engl. J. Med.,* 323, 1664, 1990.

61. **Willett, W. C., Stampfer, M. J., Colditz, G. A., Rosner, B. A., Speizer, F. E.,** Correspondence, *N. Engl. J. Med.,* 326, 201, 1992.

14. Brain Iron and Nigrostriatal Dopamine Neurons in Parkinson's Disease*

D. BEN-SHACHAR and M. B. H. YOUDIM

Rappaport Family Research Institute, Department of Pharmacology, Faculty of Medicine, Technion, Haifa, Israel

* Adapted from Ben-Shachar, D. and Youdim, M. B. H., Selectivity of melanized nigrostriatal dopamine neurons to degeneration in Parkinson's disease may depend on iron-melanin interaction, *J. Neural Transm.*, Suppl. 29, 251, 1990. With permission.

I. INTRODUCTION

Despite the many attempts to explain the neurodegenerative aspects of Parkinson's disease (PD) the etiology of this disorder remains obscure. On occasion the presence of endogenous (6-hydroxydopamine-like) or exogenous N-methyl-4-phenyl-1,2,3,6-tetrahydropyridine (MPTP) neurotoxins have been implicated. However, attempts to verify the presence of such compounds in the environment or the substantia nigra (SN) so far have met with little success. This does not mean that such a line of research should be abandoned. However, recent advances in the chemical pathology of PD indicate that other factors including metal-induced oxidative stress, may be involved.[1,2]

The nigrostriatal dopamine neurons of basal ganglia are very sensitive to chemical insult, some of which are endogenous in origin. Among these are the generation of oxygen free radicals and H_2O_2, resulting from autooxidation of dopamine to melanin and oxidative deaminated products of dopamine.[3] The ability to dispose adequately of the cytotoxic oxygen radicals and H_2O_2 is dependent on normal functioning of oxygen radical scavenger systems, such as reduced glutathione, glutathione peroxidase, superoxide dismutase, and ascorbate, known to be present in relatively high concentrations in the basal ganglia. The reduction in any of these could be highly damaging to the dopamine neurons as has been reported on several occasions.[4] This led Perry et al.[5] to suggest that PD is an abnormality or deficiency of oxygen free-radical scavenging processes in the basal ganglia. On the other hand, the excessive formation of cytotoxic oxygen free radicals, which in turn can be deleterious to the cell membrane, must also be considered. Thus, ultimately, the balance between production and disposition of free radicals formed from H_2O_2 may be the important factor in the pathogenesis of PD.[6]

Metals have been implicated in the pathogenesis of neurological disorders, and their role in oxygen free-radical formations has been well documented.[7-10] Iron, more than any other metal, is cited as being involved in oxygen free-radical formation and induction of lipid peroxidation via its interaction with H_2O_2 (Fenton reaction). The unique distribution of iron and its high concentration in the extrapyramidal regions warrants closer attention.[11,12] Thus, the high concentration of iron found in melanin-rich substantia nigra would suggest compartmentation of the metal. Recent biochemical[4,13-17] and MRI[18] analysis of iron in Parkinsonian brains has clearly shown a selective and highly significant increase of iron in the SN. The selective increase of iron in SN is thought to be responsible for the selective elevation of basal lipid peroxidation in this region of Parkinsonian brain[19,20] and the neurodegeneration of melaninized dopamine neurons.[2] The observations that other brain regions high in iron content (e.g., globus pallidus), but low in neuromelanin, do not show altered chemical pathology with regard to iron or lipid peroxidation is supportive of the hypothesis.

Iron is normally stored in its inactive form, either bound to ferritin or hemosiderin, such as that found in the liver. Although histochemically the presence of ferritin in the rat brain can be demonstrated,[12] we have not been able to observe appreciable concentrations of ferritin- or hemosiderin-bound iron in iron-rich brain areas of SN, globus pallidus, ventral pallidum, and caudate nucleus by a more direct method.[21] Indications are that the high amounts of iron present in these regions are either chelated by, or bound to, other proteins or small soluble molecules. The most telling and obvious candidate for such a molecule in the SN could be neuromelanin, which is present in relatively high amounts.

II. IRON-MELANIN INTERACTION

In normal circumstances melanin is considered a radical scavenger and protective of SN. However, melanin has a number of very important properties that could directly involve it in altering the amount, rate of formation, and distribution of reactive cytotoxic hydroxyl ($OH^.$) radicals as a result of its interaction with free iron in the SN. The substantial amount of free catechols, quinoline, and hydroxyl groups present in the polymer nature of melanin makes it an avid ion-exchange resin for highly efficient chelation of transition metals, especially iron, and the promotion of lipid peroxidation.[22-24] If melanin potentially acts as a modulator of nigrostriatal dopamine neuron neurodegeneration, resulting from its ability to induce membrane lipid peroxidation in the SN, then, under favorable conditions, all the components necessary to accumulate iron and alter its redox state need to be available for the generation of $OH^.$. Indeed the presence of melanin and the formation of H_2O_2 from dopamine deamination and autooxidation are highest in SN.

We have recently shown that dopamine melanin has two high affinity binding sites with K_D values of 13 and 200 nM for $^{59}Fe^{3+}$ and B_{max} values of 1.13 and 27.4 nmol/mg melanin[25] (Figure 1). These binding sites are specific since other drugs (e.g., flunitrazepam, spiperone, dopamine, and haloperidol) do not bind as effectively to dopamine melanin. Examination of a large number of psychotropic and nonpsychotropic agents, including MPTP and 1-methyl-4-phenylpyridine MPP^+ for their ability to inhibit the binding of $^{59}Fe^{3+}$ to dopamine melanin, shows that only the drugs with iron-chelating properties (e.g., desferrioxamine, *o*-phenanthroline) are effective inhibitors. By contrast, dopamine increased the binding of $^{59}Fe^{3+}$ to dopamine melanin. This action could be of great significance because dopamine could mobilize iron to bind to melanin in the SN since it is involved in the formation of melanin.[25] The binding of $^{59}Fe^{3+}$ is dependent on the pH and concentration of melanin. Although neuromelanin from substantia nigra was not examined for its capacity to bind $^{59}Fe^{3+}$, the role of protein in $^{59}Fe^{3+}$ binding can be excluded. Other studies have clearly shown a negligible role for protein in metal- and drug-binding capacity of melanin.[22] It is generally accepted that melanin is an effective radical scavenger and protects the nigrostriatal do-

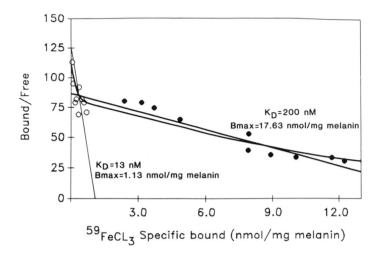

FIGURE 1. Scatchard plot of specific $^{59}FeCl_3$ binding to dopamine melanin. The computer-fitted curve demonstrates at least two binding sites.

pamine neurons from biochemical insult. However, this notion may now have to be altered because of our recent observations which indicate the participation of melanin in membrane lipid peroxidation and possible neurodegeneration. Fe^{3+}, but not dopamine melanin, promotes the lipid peroxidation of rat brain cortical membrane preparation. High melanin concentration can be inhibitory (Figure 2). In contrast, melanin has a synergistic action on this lipid peroxidation property of Fe^{3+}. This process can effectively be inhibited by iron chelators such as deferrioxamine, *o*-phenanthroline, and chlorpromazine (Figure 2).[25] The recent elegant studies of Pilas et al.[24] show that, with Fe^{2+}, melanin decreases the yield of OH˙ due to the binding of Fe^{2+} by melanin. Furthermore, they show that Fe^{2+} bound to melanin does not decompose H_2O_2 efficiently to OH˙. By contrast, melanin substantially increases the rate of OH˙ production if the predominant form of iron is Fe^{3+}. This was attributed to the ability of melanin to reduce Fe^{3+} to Fe^{2+}, thus driving the Fenton reaction. Hydroxyl radical production in the presence of melanin was significantly greater if the Fe^{3+} was chelated with endogenous chelators, e.g., ADP.[24,26,27]

The predominant increase of Fe^{3+} [4] and the elevation of basal lipid peroxidation in SN of Parkinsonian brains[20] have led Youdim et al.[1] to suggest that PD could be a progressive siderosis of SN. Furthermore, they suggest that iron chelators with the ability to cross the blood-brain barrier may be an alternative approach for the prevention or retardation of neurodegeneration. In this connection drugs (including iron chelators) that were able to inhibit the binding of Fe^{3+} to dopamine melanin are effective inhibitors of Fe^{3+} and

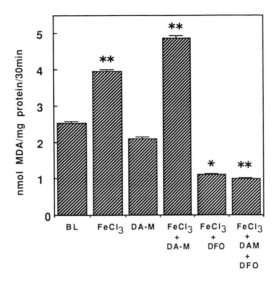

FIGURE 2. The effect of iron and dopamine melanin on rat cerebral cortex lipid peroxidation as measured by the formation of malondialdehyde (MDA) and its inhibition by iron chelator desferrioxamine (DFO). $FeCl_3$, 100 μM; dopamine melanin (DA-M), 3 $\mu g/0.25$ ml; desferrioxamine (DFO), 10 μM. The results are mean $\pm$ SEM; n = 4; *$p < 0.01$; **$p < 0.001$.

Fe^{3+} melanin-induced lipid peroxidation (Figure 2). These results are compatible with what has already been discussed regarding the optimal ratio of $Fe^{2+}:Fe^{3+}$ required for lipid peroxidation initiation and the relative ratio of $Fe^{2+}:Fe^{3+}$ present in Parkinsonian SN.[4,28,29] Therefore, depending on the state of iron in SN, melanin can either decrease or increase the production of $OH^{\cdot}$, thus being protective or destructive of the SN. Thus, the conditions necessary for participation of H_2O_2 and neuromelanin in lipid peroxidation and neuro-degeneration exist in the SN of Parkinsonian brains where Fe^{3+} is elevated (Figure 3). In the presence of diminished glutathione peroxidase activity and reduced glutathione (GSH)[4] the excess available H_2O_2 would be available to interact with iron and melanin to drive the Fenton reaction and alter the redox state of iron between its two forms. The net effect would be liberation of cytotoxic hydroxyl radical and lipid peroxidation (Figure 3). The report of increased basal lipid peroxidation in SN of Parkinsonian subjects is supportive of this hypothesis.[20]

III. 6-HYDROXYDOPAMINE MODEL OF PARKINSON'S DISEASE AND NIGROSTRIATAL IRON

The present hypotheses concerning the etiology of Parkinson's disease suggest that the metabolically active basal ganglia can generate a substantial amount of H_2O_2 from oxidation of dopamine (see Figure 3). In the condition of reduced glutathione peroxidase activity in SN, as is the case in PD, the

354

Selectivity of melaninized nigra-striatal dopamine neurons

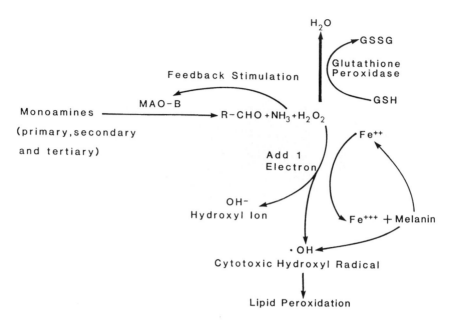

FIGURE 3. The reaction pathway illustrating the ability of hydrogen peroxide and melanin to alter the redox state of iron between its two valencies with resultant formation of cytotoxic hydroxyl radical and induction of lipid peroxidation.

H_2O_2 could interact with decompartmentalized iron (Fenton reaction), selectively increased in the SN zona compacta,[16,25,30] to generate cytotoxic oxygen free radicals of the hydroxyl type, leading to oxidative stress. Such radicals could theoretically induce the degeneration of nigrostriatal dopamine neurons. If this hypothesis is correct then chelation of iron may be one procedure by which the formation of cytotoxic oxygen radical can be prevented and the dopamine neurons protected against degeneration.[1] Iron chelation by iron chelators has been shown to reduce iron overload-induced tissue damage in the cardiovascular system and to protect against ischemia-induced brain injury.[31,32] These findings have led Youdim et al.[1] to propose that the SN zona compacta of Parkinsonian brains in a state of siderosis, where the iron and ferritin accumulate in the microglia and astrocytes,[17] could be damaged in a similar fashion.

At present it is difficult to validate that the accumulated iron in zona compacta of Parkinsonian brains is responsible for the state of oxidative stress in SN[33,34] and the initiation of dopaminergic neurodegeneration.[33] However, recent studies on animal models of PD clearly indicate that *in vivo* iron can participate in the neurodegeneration. The dopaminergic neurotoxin 6-hydroxydopamine (6-OHDA) is thought to owe its neurotoxicity to generation of

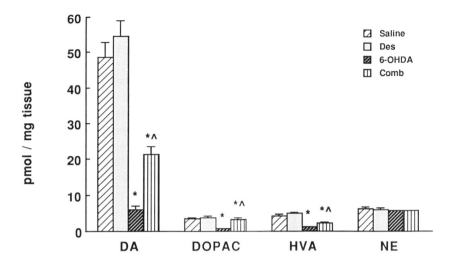

FIGURE 4. The effects of intraventricular injection of 6-hydroxydopamine (6-OHDA) on striatal dopamine metabolism and its protection by desferrioxamine (Des). DA, dopamine; DO-PAC, dihydroxyphenylacetic acid; HVA, homovanillic acid; NE, norepinephrine; Comb, 6-OHDA + Des; $*p < 0.001$; $\wedge p < 0.005$. (From Ben-Shachar, D., Eshel, G., Finberg, J. P. M., and Youdim, M. B. H., *J. Neurochem.*, 56, 1441, 1991. With permission.)

oxygen free radicals and lipid peroxidation[35-39] before or after uptake by the nigrostriatal dopamine neuron cell bodies. This was presumed to occur as a consequence of the involvement of a metal, since catecholamine can interact with transition metals (e.g., iron or copper) to form semiquinones and H_2O_2. Indeed it has been shown that 6-OHDA releases iron from its binding site in ferritin,[40] and its neurotoxicity has been attributed partly to this. Such a finding is also compatible with lung cytotoxicity of paraquat and diquat, where the latter compounds can also decompartmentalize iron from its binding sites in ferritin without altering the structure of ferritin and induce lung toxicity.[41] Animal studies using the iron chelator desferrioxamine (desferal) have shown that while the pretreatment of rats and mice with this chelator can block the cytotoxicity of paraquat,[6,42] iron potentiates its cytotoxicity. The effect of desferrioxamine on 6-OHDA-induced lesions of nigrostriatal dopamine neurons in rats examined so far has demonstrated for the first time that this iron chelator prevents (inhibits) the 6-OHDA-induced degeneration of nigrostriatal dopamine neurons.[25,43] This has been examined behaviorally, histologically, and biochemically. Thus, desferrioxamine pretreatment prevents the loss of dopamine (DA) from the neurons (Figure 4) and the behavioral changes (Figure 5) resulting from intraventricular 6-OHDA treatment, via protection of these neurons. The metabolites of DA, namely, dihydroxyphenylacetic acid (DOPAC) and homovanillic acid (HVA), are similarly affected. Desferrioxamine treatment alone does not produce significant changes in any of the parameters examined, including the behavior of these animals[43] (Figures 4

356

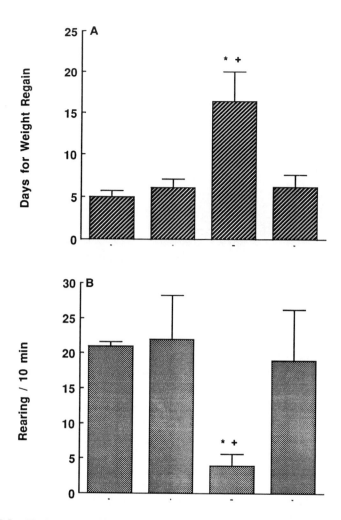

FIGURE 5. The behavioral responses of rats 4 weeks after a single intraventricularly administered injection with 6-OHDA or desferrioxamine and their combination. See Figure 4 for details. (From Ben-Shachar, D., Eshel, G., Finberg, J. P. M., and Youdim, M. B. H., *J. Neurochem.*, 56, 1441, 1991. With permission.)

and 5). The results indicate that, even though desferrioxamine does not completely protect the dopamine neurons, animal behavior and function of dopamine are normalized.

Further evidence supporting the neurotoxic action of ionic iron has come from *in vivo* experiments in rats where different doses (1 to 50 μg/5 μl) of Fe^{3+} have been injected alone or in combination with desferrioxamine into the right substantia nigra. Three weeks after such an operation the animal behavioral parameters examined showed that at higher iron (20 to 50 μg) doses there were significant ($p < 0.001$) reductions in spontaneous locomotor

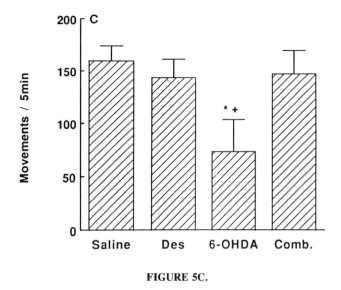

FIGURE 5C.

activity and sniffing, with increased episodes of freezing (Figure 6). Examination of right and left striatal dopamine, noradrenaline, serotonin, and their metabolites indicated a reduction of more than 90% in dopamine content of the right striatum without an alteration in the neurotransmitters, noradrenaline or serotinin, metabolisms (Figure 7).[44] The results indicate the selective vulnerability of the dopamine neurons and not the others. In desferrioxamine-pretreated rats, Fe^{3+} was not as effective in producing lesions of dopamine neurons.[44a]

The ability of intranigral iron injection to initiate degeneration of dopamine neurons, the reduction of striatal dopamine content, and the altered behavioral responses evident at higher iron dosage suggest that iron could be the cytotoxin responsible for the degeneration of nigrostriatal dopamine neurons. These parameters are persistent for at least 3 weeks after a single injection. The turnover of iron in the rat brain[45,46] is extremely slow, and this tissue has a capacity to sequester iron to a very high degree. Thus, more than 90% of iron which is deposited in the brain of a newborn rat (10-d-old) is still present in the brain of an adult (80-d-old).[46] The histochemical studies of Olanow,[47] in which they infused iron into the SN, have shown that 4 months after its injection iron is still present in the substantia nigra. Indeed the iron is accumulated in the pars compacta,[47] the nigral region in which we have identified a selective increase of iron in Parkinsonian brains.[16,17] Thus, iron can be heavily retained in the brain and may be damaging to the dopamine neuron selectively. These animal studies further contribute to and support the notion that ionic iron can be highly cytotoxic and cause cellular death via oxidative stress.

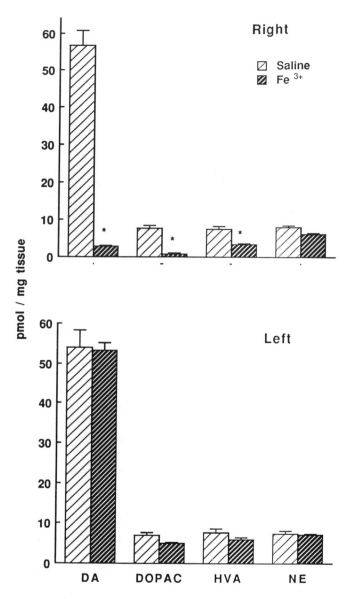

FIGURE 6. The effects of a single Fe^{3+} (50 μg/5 μl) injection into the right substantia nigra on dopamine metabolism in the right and left striatum 4 weeks later. See Figure 4 for details. *$p < 0.001$. (From Ben-Shachar, D. and Youdim, M. B. H., *J. Neurochem.*, 57, 2133, 1991. With permission.)

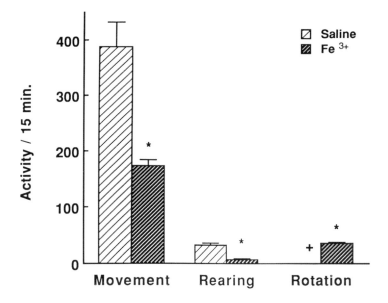

FIGURE 7. The behavior of rats in response to a single dose (50 μg/5 μl) of Fe^{3+} injection into the right substantia nigra 4 weeks later. +, No rotation; *$p < 0.001$. (From Ben-Shachar, D. and Youdim, M. B. H., *J. Neurochem.*, 57, 2133, 1991. With permission.)

In the final analysis the validity of these experiments is measured by the notion whether similar processes are operative in Parkinson's disease as a consequence of iron accumulation in the zona compacta.[16] This is an open question and needs further experimental evidence.

IV. IRON MELANIN AND PARKINSON'S DISEASE

Mann and Yates[48] showed that the more heavily pigmented neurons of the SN appear to be preferentially lost in PD and during the course of aging, when both iron and melanin are known to increase. In comparing the SN of control and Parkinsonian brains, Hirsch et al.[49] demonstrated the greater vulnerability of the population of dopamine neurons containing neuromelanin to the neurodegenerative process of PD. Their studies also showed a direct relationship between the distribution of pigmented neurons normally present and the distribution of cell loss in the SN of individuals dying with the disease. The interaction of iron with melanin, the excessive accumulation of this metal in the SN, and the increase of lipid peroxidation go some way to explain the selectivity and vulnerability of melaninized dopamine neurons to neurodegeneration.

The questions uppermost in our mind are how and why the SN should accumulate high-iron content and whether the iron is deposited within the neuromelanin-containing dopamine neurons in association with melanin, (see Note Added in Proof) thus making the neurons more vulnerable to neurodegeneration.[2] It remains to be established whether the ratio of iron to melanin during the course of aging has a direct bearing on the neurodegenerative process.

The present findings regarding the interaction of iron with melanin may also explain manganese-induced Parkinsonism in manganese miners, since melanin can also bind manganese. The alteration in redox states of manganese is also thought to generate free radicals and contribute to its dopaminergic neurotoxicity.[50] The ability of iron chelators to displace iron from melanin predicts that future therapeutic approaches for Parkinson's disease may include the use of metal chelators in a fashion similar to that used for the treatment of Wilson's disease.

V. CONCLUSIONS

The recent studies on the chemical pathology of Parkinson's disease show selective increases of iron and lipid peroxidation and decreased glutathione (GSH)-oxidizing capacity in the substantia nigra (SN). These changes are indicative of oxidative stress, possibly due to the accumulation of iron in the SN. The melaninized dopamine neurons are vulnerable to degeneration. The investigation of the interaction of iron with dopamine melanin demonstrates the presence of two relatively high affinity binding sites for $^{59}Fe^{3+}$ on dopamine melanin. Interaction of Fe^{3+} with dopamine melanin results in potentiation of lipid peroxidation of rat cerebral cortex as compared to that induced by Fe^{3+}. Only compounds with the ability to chelate iron are able to inhibit the binding of Fe^{3+} to melanin and the resultant lipid peroxidation. Therapeutic use of iron chelators, with the ability of crossing the blood-brain barrier, as agents for retarding the oxidative stress and Parkinson's disease is envisaged. This is valid since in animal models of Parkinson's disease using 6-hydroxydopamine, the iron chelator desferrioxamine is protective.

NOTE ADDED IN PROOF

Our most recent studies have shown the presence of iron in association with neuromelanin in remaining dopamine neurons of substantia nigra pars compacta of Parkinsonian brains and not in control brains.[51] The binding of iron to human neuromelanin is identical to that observed with synthetic dopamine melanin.

ACKNOWLEDGMENTS

This work was supported by grants from Technion Research and Development Fund in Haifa and Israel Center for Psychobiology in Jerusalem.

REFERENCES

1. **Youdim, M. B. H., Ben-Shachar, D., and Riederer, P.**, Is Parkinson's disease a progressive siderosis of substantia nigra resulting in iron and melanin induced neurodegeneration?, *Acta Neurol. Scand.*, 126, 47, 1989.

2. **Youdin, M. B. H., Ben-Shachar, D., and Riederer, R.**, Iron in brain function and dysfunction with emphasis on Parkinson's disease, *Eur. Neurol.*, 31 (Suppl. 1), 34, 1991.

3. **Cohen, G.**, in *Handbook of Neurochemistry*, Vol. 4, Lajtha, A., Ed., Plenum Press, New York, 1985, 315.

4. **Riederer, P., Sofic, E., Rausch, W. D., Schmidt, B., Reynolds, G. P., Kellinger, K., and Youdim, M. B. H.**, Transition metals, ferritin, glutathione and ascorbic acid in Parkinsonian brain, *J. Neurochem.*, 52, 515, 1989.

5. **Perry, T. L. and Young, V. N.**, Idiopathic Parkinson's disease, progressive supranuclear palsy and abnormal glutathione metabolism in the substantia nigra of patients, *Neurosci. Lett.*, 67, 269, 1986.

6. **Youdim, M. B. H.**, Iron in the brain: implications for Parkinson's and Alzheimer's diseases, *Mount Sinai J. Med.*, 55, 97, 1988.

7. **Slater, T. F.**, Free-radical mechanisms in tissue injury, *Biochem. J.*, 222, 1, 1984.

8. **Halliwell, B. and Gutteridge, J. M.**, Oxygen toxicity, oxygen radicals, transition metals and disease, *Biochem. J.*, 219, 1, 1984.

9. **Halliwell, B. and Gutteridge, J. M. C.**, Oxygen radicals and the nervous system, *TINS*, 8, 22, 1985.

10. **Halliwell, B. and Gutteridge, J. M.**, Oxygen free radicals and iron in relation to biology and medicine: some problems and concepts, *Arch. Biochem. Biophys.*, 246, 501, 1986.

11. **Youdim, M. B. H.**, Brain iron metabolism in relation to dopaminergic neurotransmission, in *Handbook of Neurochemistry*, Vol. 10, Lajtha, A., Ed., Plenum Press, New York, 1985, 731.

12. **Hill, J. M.**, in *Brain Iron: Neurochemical and Behavioural Aspects*, Youdim, M. B. H., Ed., Taylor & Francis, London, 1988, 1.

13. **Earle, K. M.**, Trace metals in Parkinsonian brains, *J. Neuropathol. Exp. Neurol.*, 27, 1, 1968.

14. **Dexter, D. T., Wells, F. R., Agid, F., Agid, Y., Lees, A. J., Jenner, P., and Marsden, C. D.**, Increased nigral iron content in postmortem Parkinsonian brain, *Lancet*, 2, 121, 1987.

15. **Sofic, E., Riederer, P., Heinsen, H., Beckmann, H., Reynolds, G. P., Hebenstreit, G., and Youdim, M. B. H.**, Increased iron(III) and total iron content in post motem substantia nigra of Parkinsonian brain, *J. Neural. Transm.*, 74, 199, 1988.

16. **Sofic, E., Paulus, W., Jenninger, K., Riederer, P., and Youdim, M. B. H.**, Selective increase of iron in substantia nigra zona compacta of Parkinsonian brains, *J. Neurochem.*, 56, 978, 1991.

17. **Jellinger, K., Paulus, W., Grundke-Iqbal, I., Riederer, P., and Youdim, M. B. H.**, Brain iron and ferritin in Parkinson's and Alzheimer's diseases, *J. Neural. Transm.*, 2, 327, 1990.

18. **Drayer, B. P., Olanow, W., Burger, P., Johnson, G. A., Herfkens, R., and Riederer, P.**, Parkinson plus syndrome: diagnosis using high field MR imaging of brain iron, *Radiology*, 159, 493, 1986.

19. **Dexter, D. T., Carter, C., Agid, F., Agid, Y., Lees, A. J., Jenner, P., and Marsden, C. D.**, Lipid peroxidation as cause of nigral cell death in Parkinson's disease, *Lancet*, 1, 639, 1986.

20. **Dexter, D. T., Carter, C. J., Wells, F. R., Javoy-Agid, F., Agid, Y., Lees, A., and Marsden, C. D.**, Basal lipid peroxidation in substantia nigra is increased in Parkinson's disease, *J. Neurochem.*, 52, 381, 1989.

21. **Iancu, T., Ben-Shachar, D., Hill, J. M., and Youdim, M. B. H.**, unpublished data, 1988.

362

22. **Bruenger, F. W., Stover, B. J., and Atherton, D. R.,** The incorporation of various metal ions *in vivo* and *in vitro* produced melanin, *Radiat. Res.,* 32, 1, 1967.

23. **Larsson, B. and Tjalve, H.,** Studies on the mechanism of drug binding to melanin, *Biochem. Pharmacol.,* 28, 1181, 1979.

24. **Pilas, B., Sana, T., Kalyanaraman, B., and Swartz, H. M.,** The effect of melanin on iron associated decomposition of hydrogen peroxide, *Free Radical Biol. Med.,* 4, 285, 1988.

25. **Ben-Shachar, D., Riederer, P., and Youdim, M. B. H.,** Iron-melanin interaction and lipid peroxidation: implication for Parkinson's disease, *J. Neurochem.,* in press, 1991.

26. **Potts, A. M. and Au, P. C.,** The affinity of melanin for inorganic ions, *Exp. Eye Res.,* 22, 487, 1976.

27. **Masson, H. S., Ingram, D. J., and Allen, B.,** The free radical property of melanins, *Arch. Biochem. Biophys.,* 86, 225, 1960.

28. **Braughler, J. M., Duncan, L. A., and Chase, R. L.,** The involvement of iron in lipid peroxidation. Importance of ferric to ferrous ratio in initiation, *J. Biol. Chem.,* 261, 10282, 1986.

29. **Minotti, G. and Aust, G. D.,** The requirement for iron(III) in the initiation of lipid peroxidation by iron(II) and hydrogen peroxide, *J. Biol. Chem.,* 262, 1098, 1987.

30. **Scalia, M., Geremia, E., Corsaro, C., Santoro, C., Baratha, D., and Sichel, G.,** Lipid peroxidation in pigmented and unpigmented liver tissues: protection role of melanin, *Pigment Cell Res.,* 3, 115, 1990.

31. **Wolfe, L., Olivier, N., and Sallan, D.,** Prevention of cardiac disease by subcutaneous desferrioxamine in patients with thalassemia major, *N. Engl. J. Med.,* 312, 1600, 1985.

32. **Krause, G. S., Kumar, K., White, B. C., Aust, S. D., and Weigenstein, J. G.,** Ischemia, resuscitation and reperfusion: mechanism of tissue injury and prospects for protection, *Am. Heart J.,* 3, 768, 1986.

33. **Youdim, M. B. H. and Ben-Shachar, D.,** The neurotoxic component of Parkinson's diseases may involve iron-melanin interaction and lipid peroxidation in the substantia nigra, in *Early Markers in Parkinson's and Alzheimer's Diseases,* Dostert, P., Riederer, R., Strolin Benedetti, M., and Roncucci, R., Eds., Springer-Verlag, Berlin, 1990, 111.

34. **Youdim, M. B. H., Ben-Shachar, D., and Riederer, P.,** The role of monoamine oxidase iron-melanin interaction and intracellular calcium in Parkinson's disease, *J. Neural. Transm.,* Suppl. 32, 239, 1990.

35. **Cohen, G., Heikkila, R. E., Allis, B., Cabbit, F., Dembiec, D., MacNamee, D., Mytilineou, C., and Winston, B.,** Destruction of sympathetic nerve terminals by 6-hydroxydopamine: protection by 1-phenyl-3-(2-thiazolyl)-2-thiourea, diethyldithiocar-bamate, methimazone, cysteamine, ethanol and *n*-butanol, *J. Pharmacol. Exp. Ther.,* 199, 336, 1976.

36. **Heikkila, R. E. and Cohen, G.,** Further studies on generation of hydrogen peroxide by 6-hydroxydopamine: potentiation by ascorbic acid, *Mol. Pharmacol.,* 8, 241, 1972.

37. **Sachs, C. H. and Jonsson, G.,** Mechanism of action of 6-hydroxydopamine, *Pharmacology,* 24, 1, 1975.

38. **Graham, D. G.,** Oxidative pathways for catecholamines in the genesis of neuromelanin and cytotoxic quinones, *Mol. Pharmacol.,* 14, 633, 1978.

39. **Graham, D. G., Tiffany, S. M., Bell, W. R., and Gutknecht, W. F.,** Autooxidation versus covalent binding quinones as mechanism of toxicity of dopamine, 6-hydroxydo-pamine and related compounds towards C1300 neuroblastoma cells *in vitro, Mol. Pharmacol.,* 14, 644, 1978.

40. **Monteiro, H. P. and Winterbourn, C. C.,** 6-Hydroxydopamine releases iron from ferritin and promotes ferritin-dependent lipid peroxidation, *Biochem. Pharmacol.,* 38, 4177, 1989.

41. **Thomas, C. C. and Aust, S. D.,** Reductive release of iron from ferritin by cation free radicals or paraquat and other bipyridils, *J. Biol. Chem.,* 261, 13064, 1986.

42. **Kohen, R. and Chevion, M.,** Paraquat toxicity is enhanced by iron and reduced by desferrioxamine in laboratory mice, *Biochem. Pharmacol.,* 34, 1841, 1985.

43. **Ben-Shachar, D., Eshel, G., Finberg, J. P. M., and Youdim, M. B. H.,** The iron chelator desferrioxamine (desferal) retards 6-hydroxydopamine-induced degeneration of nigrostriatal dopamine neurons, *J. Neurochem.,* 56, 1441, 1991.

44. **Ben-Shachar, D. and Youdim, M. B. H.,** Intranigral iron injection induces behavioural and biochemical Parkinsonism in rats, *J. Neurochem.,* 57, 2133, 1991.

44a. **Ben-Shachar, D.,** unpublished data.

45. **Ben-Shachar, D., Ashkenazi, R., and Youdim, M. B. H.,** Long term consequences of early iron-deficiency on dopaminergic neurotransmission in rats, *Int. J. Dev. Neurosci.,* 4, 81, 1986.

46. **Dwork, A. J., Lawler, G., Zybert, P. A., Durkin, M., Osman, M., Willson, N., and Barkai, A. I.,** An autoradiographic study of uptake and distribution of iron by the brain of young rat, *Brain Res.,* 518, 31, 1990.

47. **Olanow, W.,** personal communication, 1991.

48. **Mann, D. M. and Yates, P. O.,** Possible role of neuromelanin in the pathogenesis of Parkinson's disease, *Mech. Aging Dev.,* 21, 193, 1983.

49. **Hirsch, E., Graybiel, A. M., and Agid, Y. A.,** Melanized dopaminergic neurons are differentially susceptible to degeneration in Parkinson's disease, *Nature (London),* 334, 345, 1988.

50. **Liccione, J. J. and Maines, M. D.,** Selective vulnerability of glutathione metabolism and cellular defense mechanism in rat striatum to manganese, *J. Pharm. Exp. Ther.,* 247, 156, 1988.

51. **Jellinger, K., Kingel, E., Riedener, P., Youdin, M. B. H., and Ben-Shachar, D.,** Iron ferritin and neuromelanin in Parkinson's disease, *Adv. Neurol.,* in press.

15. Proteins of Iron Regulation in the Brain in Alzheimer's Disease

JAMES R. CONNOR

Department of Neuroscience and Anatomy, Pennsylvania State University, M.S. Hershey Medical Center, Hershey, Pennsylvania

I. INTRODUCTION

Alzheimer's disease (AD) is a neurodegenerative disease of unknown etiology associated with memory loss and dementia. Currently, Alzheimer's disease is a major health problem in the world, and the significance of this disease increases annually as the geriatic community becomes a higher percentage of the world population. Many possible causes of Alzheimer's disease have been put forth which include genetic, viral, and environmental (toxicological). Much has been written on the subject of AD, and the reader may find many excellent reviews on the general features of the disease.[1-3] This chapter will discuss one of the hypotheses regarding the pathogenesis of AD which is the role of toxic metals. Specifically, the focus of this chapter will be on iron imbalance in the brain in AD.

The importance of iron for normal neurological function is well established.[4] Iron is essential for oxidative reactions, and the brain has the highest rate of oxidative metabolism of any organ with little tolerance for hypoxia.[5] Abnormalities in oxidative metabolism have been suggested to play a role in AD.[6]

A wide range of neurological deficits have been reported in AD and the attraction of studying iron homeostasis in AD is that many of the known abnormalities that occur in the AD brain could result from either a local inadequate iron supply, perhaps not so much the result of low-iron levels as a result of untimely iron delivery. Prominent examples of how iron imbalance (not just iron deficiency, but also excess iron) could influence changes seen in AD include decreases in some mitochondrial enzymes,[6] which would lead to decreased cell activity, and the susceptibility of cholinergic neurotransmission, a well-known defect in AD, to impairment of oxidative metabolism.[4]

The specific functions for which iron is required in the brain are not well delineated. Neurons and glia, as do all cells, require iron for many aspects of their cell physiology including the cytochrome oxidase system, NADPH reductase activity, and as a co-factor for a number of enzymes including ribonucleotide reductase, the rate-limiting step in DNA synthesis.[7] More specific to neurological activity, iron is involved in the function and synthesis of the neurotransmitters dopamine, serotonin,[8] and possibly γ-aminobutyric acid (GABA).[9] Iron is also involved in the synthesis and degradation of fatty acids[10] and cholesterol.[11] These latter substances are important components of cell membranes and are especially high in myelin, the lipid-rich substance which insulates axons and forms the white matter of the brain.[12] Recent reports that cholesterol is decreased in the brain in AD[13] coupled with the knowledge that the brain is responsible for synthesizing its own cholesterol[12] are potentially significant to the story on iron imbalance in AD.

Perhaps equally as important as its role in normal activity is the role of iron as a significant component of oxidative injury. (See Chapter 7.) By virtue of its reactive ability with hydrogen peroxide and oxygen, free iron is known to initiate lipid peroxidation[14,15] leading to membrane damage and ultimately cell death. Because of its high lipid content, the brain is especially susceptible to oxidative injury.[16] Iron is a critical factor in the induction of events leading to lipid peroxidative damage in the brain.[17] Consequently, iron must both be available to cells and stringently regulated. An imbalance of iron and/or the iron regulatory proteins in the brain could result in substantial damage to neurons and glia leading to neurodegeneration and neurological dysfunction.

The potential for an imbalance of iron homeostasis in the brain will be examined in this chapter from the relatively novel view of proteins which regulate iron in the brain rather than only from the viewpoint of the metal itself. In addition to regulating iron, the proteins to be discussed in this chapter also contribute to transport and homeostasis of other metals in the brain such as manganese.[18] Some discussion will be allotted to the relationship of iron-binding proteins and aluminum which has been suggested to play a role in AD.

II. IRON HISTOCHEMISTRY

A. NORMAL

Studies on iron in the brain date back to at least 1886[19] but the first systematic study of brain iron is generally attributed to Spatz in 1922.[21] The first studies on iron in the brain determined its gross distribution and found that iron is particularly high in the extrapyramidal system[20-23] which is involved in motor function.

The predominant cell type in the brain which contains iron are the oligodendrocytes.[23-26] These cells are small and round and rarely exhibit iron-containing processes (Figure 1). Iron-positive oligodendrocytes are found in both gray and white matter in cortical as well as in subcortical regions. To date, the only known function of oligodendrocytes is to produce myelin, the lipid-rich substance which insulates axons. Because oligodendrocytes have relatively high lipid levels and concomitant relatively higher requirements for iron in conjunction with fatty acid synthesis and degradation, the working hypothesis is that high intracellular iron levels are required to initiate and support myelination. However, the possibility that oligodendrocytes may have a larger role in iron regulation in the nervous system cannot be discounted.[27] For example, iron-containing oligodendrocytes, in addition to being found in myelinated tracts, are found in perineuronal "satellite" positions and also in close association with blood vessels. It is tempting to speculate that a function of the perineuronal oligodendrocytes is to provide essential nutrients such as iron to adjacent neurons.

In subcortical gray matter, the predominant cell type to stain for iron is similar in morphological appearance to oligodendrocytes in the cerebral cortex. Iron-containing cells are particularly abundant in the basal ganglia and amygdala. A few of the iron-positive cells in the basal ganglia in human tissue are astrocytes.

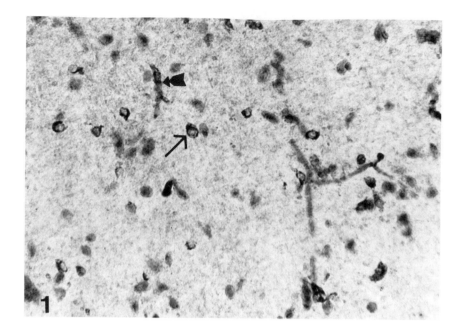

FIGURE 1. Iron-positive cells in the normal human cerebral cortical gray matter are small and round (e.g., at thin arrow). The reaction product is generally confined to one pole of the perikaryal cytoplasm. The walls of blood vessels are also positive for iron (thick arrow). (Magnification × 300.)

In human white matter, the iron reaction is intense and the iron-containing cells are grouped into patches (Figure 2). The iron-positive cells are typical of interfascicular oligodendrotcytes (Figure 3). The significance of the patches of iron-containing cells in the white matter is not known. Counterstained sections demonstrate that the patches are not a simple reflection of the normal cell pattern in the white matter, nor do cells in white matter containing transferrin (the iron mobilization protein) have the same distribution.[25,26] The patches of iron-containing cells in the white matter are also worthy of continued study and are particularly exciting in view of the patchy occurrence of plaques in the white matter in multiple sclerosis. Iron is reportedly a component of the plaques seen in multiple sclerosis.[28]

Also within the subcortical white matter in both rat and human brains, many iron-containing cells are clearly associated with blood vessels[24] (Figure 4). The pattern of perivascular containing iron cells in white matter is likely to be related to the uptake of iron into this part of the brain. In addition to the perivascular iron-containing cells, the walls of many blood vessels are lined with iron (Figure 1). The blood vessel staining most likely reflects the continuous uptake of iron from the plasma into the brain even in adulthood.[29,30]

The intracellular localization of iron cannot be determined ultrastructurally because the harsh treatment of the Perls' reaction destroys intracellular or-

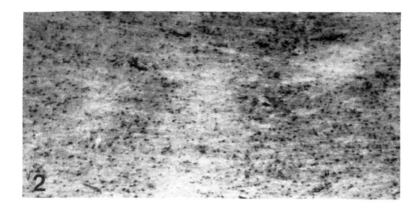

FIGURE 2. A low power micrograph demonstrating both the intensity of the iron stain and the patchy appearance of the white matter which occurs normally in the human. (Magnification × 75.)

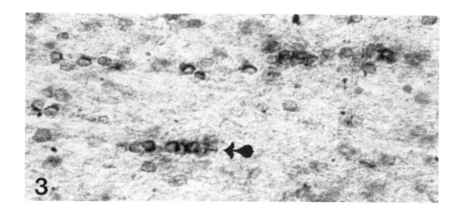

FIGURE 3. A higher magnification of the white matter than in Figure 2 reveals the presence of iron-containing cells aligned in rows (arrow) and other scattered iron-positive cells occurring singly. As in the gray matter, the reaction product is confined to the soma and few iron-positive processes are seen. (Magnification × 300.)

ganelles.[24] The reaction product for iron within cells is homogeneously distributed and does not appear as granules which suggests the iron is not concentrated in any particular organelle. However, caution must be used with this interpretation because the intracellular organelles may have been lysed during the treatment.

The amount of histochemically detectable iron in the white matter in reports from our laboratory is not consistent with many of the early histochemical studies of iron and the established view of iron distribution in the

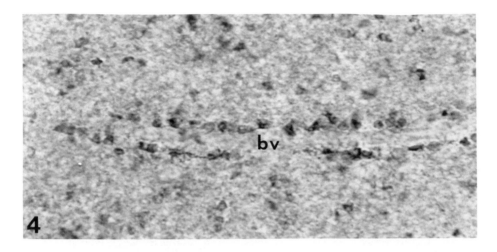

FIGURE 4.   Iron-positive cells aligning either side of a blood vessel (bv) in a normal human brain which is coursing through the center of this micrograph. (Magnification × 250.)

brain. Thus, some explanation is warranted. Quantitative studies have indicated that higher levels of iron are present in white matter than the histochemical studies would suggest. Bulk brain analysis revealed 42.4 μg/g wet weight of iron in the white matter compared to 53.8 μg/g in the gray matter.[31] The white matter of the frontal cortex,[32] temporal cortex, motor cortex, and occipital cortex[33] all have quantitatively more iron than the corresponding gray matter. These latter observations are consistent with our histochemical observations and reports that much of the brain iron is associated with the myelin fraction.[34] More recently, magnetic resonance imaging (MRI) studies contributed support to the concept that considerable levels of iron are found in the white matter.[35]

The reason for the discrepancy between our results for iron in white matter and the established views probably results from tissue processing and handling. Tissue which has been immersed in formalin (especially nonbuffered) for long periods of time will allow iron to leach out of cells, consequently decreasing the stainable iron. Thus, in order to use histochemistry to realistically determine iron presence, tissue must be processed rapidly (within 24 to 48 h). Tissue sections which have been prepared on a Vibratome or microtome provide superior iron staining to those which have been processed through paraffin. Perhaps the most significant advancement for detecting iron in tissue is the intensification of the Perls' reaction with 3,3'diaminobenzidine.[23,24,36] Additional modifications of the Perls' procedure include using low levels of detergents (Triton-X 100) with the reaction.[37] Our protocol for the Perls' reaction used in the studies reported here has been published.[25,38]

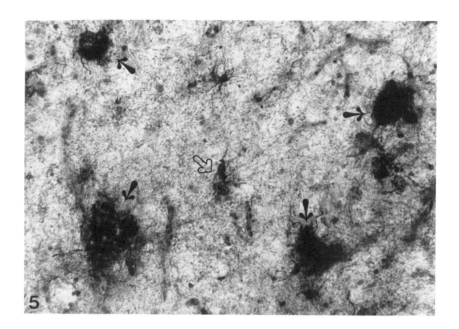

FIGURE 5. Four relatively large (black arrows) senile plaques and one smaller (younger?) plaque (clear arrow) in the cerebral cortical gray matter from an AD brain. Both types of plaques contain both intracellular accumulations of iron as well as a homogeneous apparently extracellular deposition of iron. The plaques were identified previously using either Congo Red or thioflavin-S. (Original magnification × 600.)

B. ALZHEIMER'S DISEASE

In AD, the characteristic hallmark histological changes in the brain are the presence of senile plaques and neurofibrillary tangles.[1-3] The presence of iron in senile plaques was first discussed to our knowledge in 1953.[39] This report also noted increased iron staining in the walls of the vasculature. Our recent study[38] confirmed both of these findings. Iron staining within plaques is both homogeneously distributed within the plaques (Figure 5) and within cells surrounding the plaques (Figure 6). The iron-containing cells adjacent to the plaque are predominantly microglia and astrocytes. Normal appearing iron-containing oligodendrocytes are present throughout the AD brain. A general increase in iron-containing microglia with age or in AD is not apparent.

No alterations in the iron-staining pattern are seen in the AD white matter.

In the rat brain one of the more striking changes in iron distribution with age is the accumulation of iron as a punctate or granular reaction in the soma of pyramidal neurons in the cerebral cortex and hippocampus (Figures 7 and 8). Iron granules are present but infrequent in younger rats.[24] The granular appearance of the reaction product indicates the iron accumulation in these cells is stored in intracellular organelles (lysosomes?). (See also Chapter 8.) Whether this same phenomenon occurs in the human brain and what effect the iron accumulation has on neuronal physiology is under investigation.

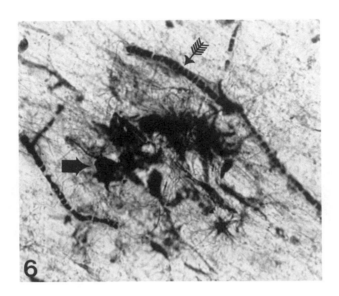

FIGURE 6. A higher power micrograph of iron in a senile plaque. Numerous iron-containing cells are present (e.g., thick arrow) many of which have iron-containing processes which run both into and away from the center of the plaque. Red blood cells containing iron (in hemoglobin) are visible with blood vessels (feathered arrow). (Magnification × 750.)

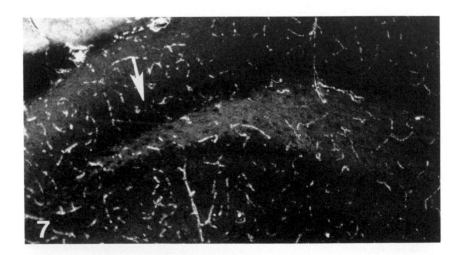

FIGURE 7. A low power darkfield micrograph of the adult rat dentate gyrus. Positive iron-staining appears white. The iron staining in this micrograph is associated mostly with cells within the blood vessels. The band of neurons indicated by the arrow is dark, demonstrating there is no positive reaction. (Photograph supplied by S. A. Benkovic.) (Magnification × 50.)

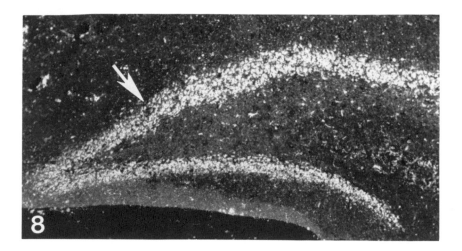

FIGURE 8. In the aged rat dentate gyrus, darkfield microscopy reveals the accumulation of iron in the neurons of the dentate gyrus. The iron-loaded neurons (compare to the dark band in Figure 7) appear as a white band (arrow). (Photograph supplied by S. A. Benkovic.) (Magnification × 50.)

III. FERRITIN

Ferritin is the least studied member of the iron homeostasis system despite reports that one third of the iron in the brain is stored as ferritin.[32,40] Ferritin is a 450,000 mol wt protein involved in iron storage (for general reviews see Chapter 1 and Theil[41]). Oligodendrocytes are the predominant cell type to contain ferritin in the human brain,[25,27] which is consistent with the finding that iron is also found predominantly in oligodendrocytes. In addition to oligodendrocytes, ferritin-positive microglial cells are a frequent finding.[25,42,43] Neuronal cells containing ferritin have not been reported. At present, the distribution of ferritin positive cells has only been reported for the human brain. Recent efforts in our laboratory have demonstrated that ferritin is also present in oligodendrocytes in the rat brain.[43a]

A. NORMAL
Ferritin-positive oligodendrocytes are similar in morphological appearance to those which contain iron. The cells are small and round, and the reaction product is confined to the cell body (Figure 9). Ferritin-containing cells occur in clusters as well as singly. Microglia also immunoreact positively for ferritin and have an elongated cell body and visible processes (Figure 9). Ferritin-positive cells are found in the vicinity of neurons in the gray matter (perineuronal cells) and in association with blood vessels. Unlike with iron, the lining of blood vessels in normal tissue is rarely immunoreactive for ferritin, suggesting the iron (and transferrin) which is present in the endothelial cells is being transported and not stored.

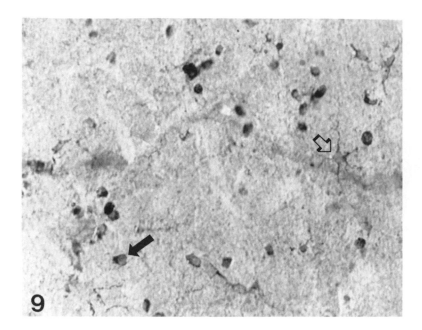

FIGURE 9. Ferritin-containing cells in the human gray matter are of two types. The most abundant is the small, round cell (black arrow) similar to that seen following reactions for iron. The second cell type, which contains ferritin, is more lightly labeled and has thin, ferritin-containing processes (clear arrow). This latter cell type fits the classical description of a microglial cell. (Magnification × 300.)

The distribution of ferritin-containing cells in the white matter is also similar to iron. Patches of ferritin-positive cells are distributed evenly throughout the subcortical white matter. Within the patches the ferritin-positive cells are typical interfascicular oligodendrocytes (Figure 10). Also visible, especially in the white matter, are perivascular ferritin-positive cells which are aligned with blood vessels (Figure 11).

In the gray matter of the basal ganglia, amygdala, and hippocampus, astrocytes containing ferritin can be found in addition to oligodendrocytes.[25] The astrocytic immunostaining with ferritin in these latter regions is age related, increasing in intensity and number of positive cells with age.[25] The number of oligodendrocytes immunolabeling for ferritin is consistent with age in the amygdala and hippocampus, but decreases with age in the basal ganglia.

B. ALZHEIMER'S DISEASE

In the AD brain, ferritin-positive microglia and astrocytes are found within the senile plaques.[38,42,44] In some senile plaques the ferritin reaction product is homogeneously distributed within the plaques in addition to intracellular ferritin immunoreactivity (Figure 12). A striking observation in the AD brain

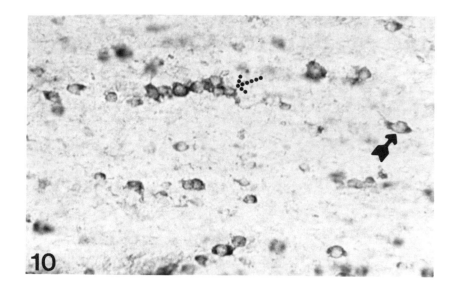

FIGURE 10. Ferritin-positive cells in the white matter are aligned in rows (dotted arrow) but are also frequently found individually (black arrow). (Magnification × 450.)

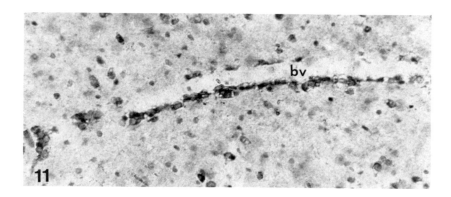

FIGURE 11. Ferritin-positive cells aligned with a blood vessel (bv) from normal human gray matter which is coursing through this micrograph. The cells are small and round and similar to the iron-positive cells. (Original magnification × 300.)

was the altered accumulation of ferritin immunostaining around blood vessels (Figure 13). Unlike the normal appearing perivascular ferritin-positive cells, in the AD brain a robust ferritin reaction in microglia and occasionally astrocytes[38] associated with blood vessels was observed. This observation in conjunction with the observations that iron accumulates abnormally around brain blood vessels in AD strongly suggests that the transport system for iron from plasma to brain has been compromised in AD.

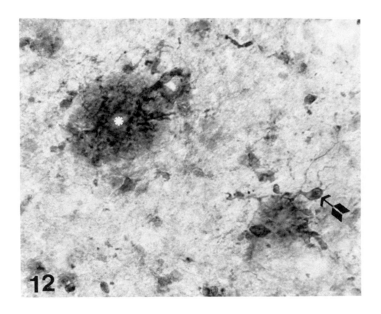

FIGURE 12. Ferritin in senile plaques from gray matter of an AD brain. The core of one of the plaques is indicated with an asterisk (*). The ferritin in the plaques is diffuse and homogeneous as well as intracellular (arrow). (Magnification × 600.)

In support of the concept that transport of nutrients such as iron across endothelial cells in the brain is malfunctioning in AD is the report that a marked decrease in glucose transporter density occurs in AD brains.[45] Furthermore, a decrease in glucose transport occurring across blood vessels in the brain with age[46] has also been reported. Thus, there is evidence that although a complete breakdown in the blood-brain barrier probably does not occur with age, there is a compromise in the uptake of essential nutrients. The uptake and transport of iron through endothelial cells in the brain in AD is another area for study.

IV. TRANSFERRIN

Transferrin is a recognized trophic factor and an essential requirement for growth for almost all cell types.[47] The importance of transferrin (Tf) is presumably its ability to deliver iron. Neurons and glia reportedly receive their iron via a Tf-mediated process.[48,49] Studies by our laboratory[25,50,51] have found Tf normally present predominantly in oligodendrocytes, which is consistent with the observation that the mRNA for Tf is also found in oligodendrocytes.[52] Some neuronal labeling with Tf has been reported in the brain of early postnatal animals[53] and in the adult human brain.[26] However, the majority (>80%) of Tf,[54] Tf mRNA,[55] and the Tf receptor expression[56] in the brain are dependent on a mature population of oligodendrocytes.

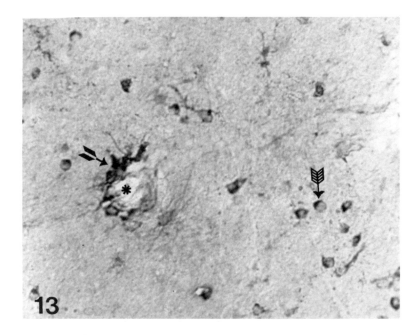

FIGURE 13. Specific to the AD brain is the observation of "reactive" cells in association with blood vessels (*) which contain ferritin (split arrow). Unlike those in the normal brain, these cells contain processes which are strongly labeled with reaction product for ferritin. Normal ferritin-positive cells are also present (feathered arrow). (Magnification × 300.)

A. NORMAL

Tf-positive oligodendrocytes occur in both gray and white matter in the brain. In the gray matter many of the Tf-positive oligodendrocytes are in a perineuronal position (Figure 14) and are found in higher density in the infragranular layers than in the supragranular layers. The distribution and morphological appearance of Tf-containing cells in the gray matter are similar to those reported for iron and ferritin. As mentioned, occasional neuronal immunostaining with Tf is observed in the adult human cerebral cortex,[25,26] but the frequency is low and the labeling is completely inconsistent. It is possible that the neuronal labeling represents fixation artifacts or cells undergoing degenerative or possibly regenerative stages which would allow Tf to be internalized to the point of being detected with immunohistochemistry. Recent interesting reports have been presented in which neurons increase iron uptake (via Tf) following axotomy.[57]

A final immunohistochemical observation in the normal brain for Tf is the appearance of Tf-positive blood vessels. Tf is found within endothelial cells in both human and rat brain tissue.[25,50] The source of Tf in endothelial cells is not clear at present but it is likely hematogenous involved in ferrying iron across the blood-brain barrier.[29,30,58]

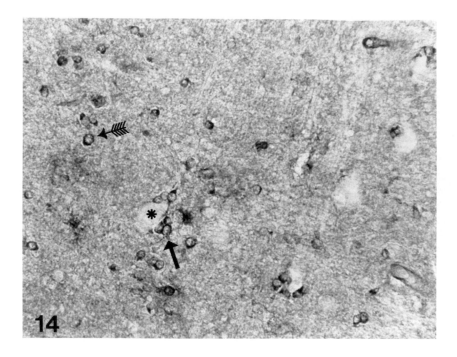

FIGURE 14. Transferrin in the normal human gray matter is contained in cells which are small and round (feathered arrow). Tf-containing processes are rare. The Tf-positive cells in gray matter frequently cluster around neurons (e.g., at *) in groups of 3 to 4 (straight arrow). (Magnification × 300.)

In the white matter, Tf cells have slightly elongated cell bodies which are aligned in rows (Figure 15). Tf immunoreaction product can occasionally be observed in very thin, somewhat beaded processes which run perpendicular to the axonal processes. The presence of Tf-containing processes in the nervous system is particularly noteworthy in the human optic nerve[25] and mouse spinal cord.[25a]

B. ALZHEIMER'S DISEASE

With normal aging, very little change occurs in Tf immunostaining in the human brain (studies on aging rat brain are in progress). In AD, Tf is found in association with senile plaques as iron and ferritin are. The Tf immunostaining is more frequently homogeneous throughout the plaque (Figure 16) than is iron or ferritin and is rarely intracellular.

The most striking observation with Tf immunohistochemistry in AD is the appearance of Tf-positive astrocytes in the cerebral cortical white matter (Figure 17). There is a direct inverse relationship between the number of Tf-labeled oligodendrocytes and Tf-labeled astrocytes in AD white matter. In many AD cases, no Tf-positive oligodendrocytes are present in white matter,

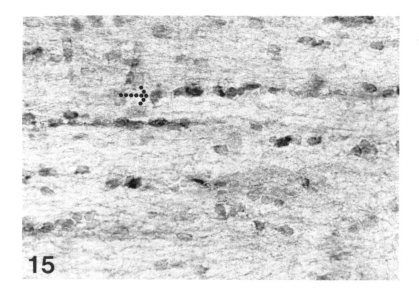

FIGURE 15.   In the normal human white matter, transferrin-positive cells are aligned in rows similar to ferritin- and iron-containing cells (arrow), but do not occur in patches. (Magnification × 400.)

only astrocytes. No other disruptions of Tf cell patterns are noted (except for Tf in senile plaques) in other brain areas in AD tissue. Indeed, the fimbria of the hippocampus was noted for its intense Tf immunostaining in oligo-dendrocytes even in AD cases where Tf-positive astrocytes predominated in cerebral cortical white matter.[38]

In summary, the cellular pattern for ferritin, iron, and Tf shows alterations which are specific to AD. The source of the iron, ferritin, and Tf in the senile plaques is not presently known but we hypothesize that it is hematogenous. Whether the proposed extravasation of iron and the attempt of microglia and astrocytes to sequester the potentially toxic iron are involved in plaque formation and amyloid secretion has not been examined. The developmental sequence of a senile plaque is not known but one hypothesis is that plaques are associated with blood vessels. A speculative scenario for plaque formation could include extravasated iron (as a result of local hypoxia or hypertension, among many possibilities) stimulating microglia and astrocytic synthesis of ferritin (a damage control response). Part of the damage control response by glia and endothelial cells could be the secretion of amyloid precursor protein.

The altered cellular distribution of Tf in AD white matter, especially in the presence of a decreased number of Tf-positive oligodendrocytes, is also indicative of altered iron processing in the AD brain. Future studies are focusing on whether the astrocytes in AD white matter have acquired the Tf by uptake from the blood (suggesting a compromised iron uptake) or whether a previously repressed gene for Tf expression in astrocytes has been dere-

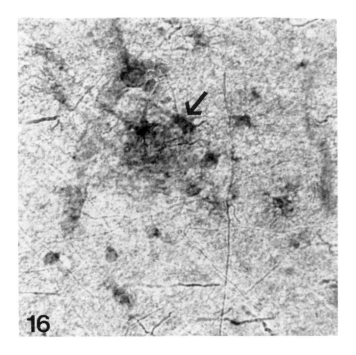

FIGURE 16. Transferrin in a senile plaque in gray matter from an AD brain. Transferrin is normally diffusely distributed throughout the plaque, and transferrin-labeled cells in association with the plaques although present (arrow) are rare. Transferrin cells present within plaques have processes running both within and away from the plaque core. (Magnification × 600.)

pressed. In either event, the histochemical data imply that iron utilization and consequently iron homeostasis in AD white matter are different from normal.

V. QUANTITATIVE STUDIES

Quantitative studies have shown considerable levels of iron in the brain; indeed in the basal ganglia the concentration of iron (per unit weight) is equal to that found in the liver.[32] The latter organ is the major iron storage organ in the body. The amount of iron in the brain is lowest in the neonate and increases during postnatal development with a sharp rise around the time myelination is beginning.[59,60] Iron levels continue to increase in most brain regions with age up to the 30th decade in humans, at which time a plateau is reached[32] and maintained for life.

Comparison of brain iron levels in normal vs. AD has been determined both in bulk brain analyses and in specific nuclei. Analysis of iron in bulk brain samples revealed no difference in iron levels in normal vs. AD. However, when the brain samples were divided into gray and white matter, iron levels were increased 38% in AD gray matter and 27% in AD white matter

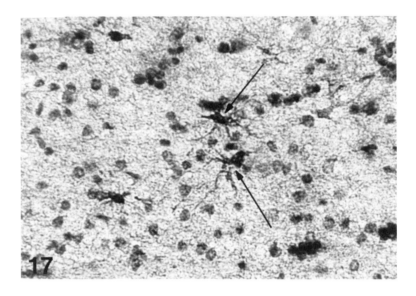

FIGURE 17. Transferrin in the white matter of AD brain tissue is found in astrocytes (arrows). This section has been counterstained with hematoxylin to reveal the presence of other cells in addition to the transferrin-containing astrocytes.

compared to controls.[31] Iron levels in the amygdala, hippocampus, and nucleus basalis reportedly are elevated in AD compared to normal.[61]

Iron, transferrin, and ferritin were recently measured in my laboratory in the same samples from normal, aged, and AD tissue.[33] We chose three cerebral cortical areas for analysis: superior temporal gyrus (an area highly susceptible to change in aging and AD); the motor cortex (area 4, an area reportedly high in iron, and also affected by age and AD); and the occipital cortex (an area relatively high in iron, but in which little change is noted with age or in AD). The samples were separated into gray and white matter. The data are presented in Table 1. The changes of iron, transferrin, and ferritin in aged and AD brains relative to normal are presented in Figure 18.

A. NORMAL

Our results agree with an earlier report[32] that the motor cortex has the highest iron levels followed by the occipital cortex. In the normal brains, iron levels were consistently higher in the white matter than in the gray matter of the corresponding brain region.

Like iron, the iron regulatory proteins are also normally found in greater quantities in the white matter than in the gray matter with the exception of ferritin in the motor cortex. Also similar to iron, the highest levels of both Tf and ferritin are found in the motor cortex. In general, ferritin levels are ten times higher than those found for Tf in each of the cerebral cortical areas examined. Ferritin levels have been determined in brain regions in addition

TABLE 1
Iron, Ferritin, and Transferrin Levels in Brain

		Normal control	Aged control	Alzheimer's disease
Iron (μmol/mg protein)				
Temporal	Gray	7.94 ± 2.79	12.37 ± 1.90	11.42 ± 1.64
cortex	White	12.87 ± 1.02	13.28 ± 1.32	12.56 ± 1.89
Motor	Gray	20.74 ± 4.32	16.00 ± 2.96	25.17 ± 2.32[b]
cortex	White	24.97 ± 3.33	22.39 ± 3.55	27.03 ± 1.87
Occipital	Gray	9.04 ± 1.96	20.85 ± 7.89[a]	6.71 ± 0.95[b]
cortex	White	14.25 ± 2.77	16.16 ± 5.59	7.08 ± 1.36[b]
Ferritin (ng/μg protein)				
Temporal	Gray	25.65 ± 4.75	24.20 ± 4.55	22.65 ± 2.89
cortex	White	44.87 ± 11.16	33.50 ± 6.16	27.44 ± 5.32[a]
Motor	Gray	40.20 ± 9.59	22.13 ± 9.12	50.30 ± 4.08[b]
cortex	White	30.38 ± 7.16	21.51 ± 3.20	29.99 ± 6.08
Occipital	Gray	9.34 ± 2.09	34.27 ± 3.98[a]	24.59 ± 4.19[a]
cortex	White	13.81 ± 2.09	31.38 ± 2.88[a]	30.16 ± 4.27[a]
Transferrin (ng/μg protein)				
Temporal	Gray	1.84 ± 0.15	1.08 ± 0.12	1.22 ± 0.13
cortex	White	3.82 ± 0.59	2.52 ± 0.63[a]	1.82 ± 0.29[a]
Motor	Gray	2.91 ± 0.56	2.93 ± 0.64	1.92 ± 0.28
cortex	White	5.75 ± 1.60	7.34 ± 1.12	4.47 ± 0.51[b]
Occipital	Gray	1.75 ± 0.36	1.67 ± 0.12	1.59 ± 0.14
cortex	White	3.53 ± 0.67[b]	6.07 ± 1.58	2.71 ± 0.32[b]

Note: Human brain material was collected at autopsy. The normal group (n = 9) has a mean age of 55 years (range 44 to 64). The aged control group (n = 11) has a mean age of 71.6 (range 65 to 80). The mean age for the Alzheimer's group (n = 13) is 74.6 years (range 62 to 84). The diagnosis of AD was according to NIH/ADRDA guidelines. Additional details and protocols for immunoassay and iron analysis are presented in Reference 33.

[a] Statistically significant ($p < 0.05$) from normal controls.
[b] Statistically significant ($p < 0.05$) from aged controls.

to those reported here and are considerably higher in basal ganglia structures compared to the cerebral cortex or cerebellum.[62] From these data we conclude that within the cerebral cortex, iron requirements are highest in the motor cortex. In general, we can also conclude that iron requirements in the brain demonstrate regional specificity similar to those already reported for glucose utilization.

Relative Changes of Fe, Frt, and Tf as a function of Brain Area in Normal Control vs. Aged Control and AD Patients

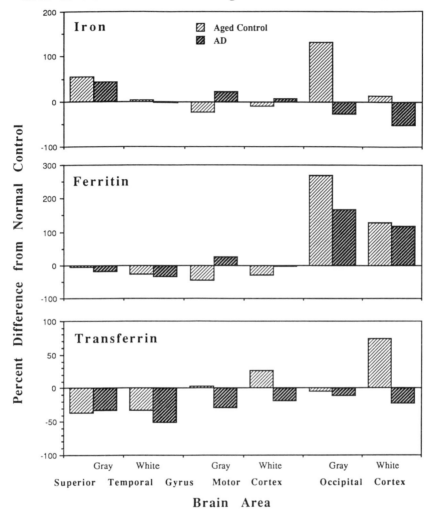

FIGURE 18. This figure summarizes the relative changes (in percent difference) compared to the normal adult in iron (Fe), ferritin (Frt), and transferrin (Tf) in the gray and white matter of each of the brain regions. The zero line represents the value obtained for the normal control brain.

B. AGING/ALZHEIMER'S DISEASE

1. Iron

Both in normal aging and in AD, iron increases in the gray matter of the superior temporal gyrus although the increase in AD gray matter is slightly less than in the normal aged. In the motor cortex gray matter, iron levels decrease by 23% with normal aging, but increase by the same magnitude in AD. Consequently, the levels of iron in AD gray matter are 56% higher than in the age-matched (aged) non-AD group in this brain area.

In the occipital cortex gray matter during normal aging, there is an increase of over 100% in iron levels (the greatest increase seen in any of the regions examined) whereas in AD the iron levels did not increase with age and are decreased by almost 300% compared with normal aging.

In the white matter, iron levels are somewhat more stable relative to the gray matter. Little change is noted in the superior temporal gyrus. In motor cortex white matter, changes in iron levels are only slightly changed from normal, but the changes are in opposite directions resulting in 20% more iron in the AD white matter compared to normal aging. White matter iron levels in the occipital cortex normally increase with age (13%), but with AD the iron levels decrease with age (51%).

The results for iron clearly suggest alterations in iron-related functions in the brain in aging and in AD, and demonstrate that these changes are specific to certain brain regions. Our results for the superior temporal gyrus and motor cortex agree with published results[31] that iron is increased in AD compared to normal aging. However, in the occipital cortex iron is decreased in comparison to both normal and aged controls in both gray and white matter.

2. Ferritin

These results are also summarized in Table 1 and Figure 18.

Ferritin generally has a more consistent pattern of decrease with both age and AD than iron does. Ferritin decreases slightly in gray matter (6%) and more so in white matter (26%) in the superior temporal gyrus with age. In AD brains the decrease in ferritin levels is greater than with normal aging in both the gray (13%) and white (39%) matter.

In the motor cortex gray matter ferritin levels decrease with normal aging (81%), but increase by 25% in AD. Thus, there is over 127% difference in the levels of ferritin in the gray matter between AD and the age-matched, non-AD control group. In motor cortical white matter, ferritin decreases by almost one third with age but remains at normal control levels in the AD group. These data may also be viewed as showing AD motor cortical white matter has one third more ferritin than the age-matched controls.

Ferritin levels in the occipital cortex increase dramatically with age in both gray (three to four times) and white (two times) matter. In the AD occipital cortex, ferritin levels increase as in normal aging in both the gray and white matter, but the increase is slightly less (three times) than in normal aging although still relatively considerable.

Only one other quantitative study on ferritin (using analysis of bulk brain on two cases) changes in the brain in AD exists to our knowledge, and this study reported ferritin increased by more than 50% in the AD brains.[63] This finding would be consistent with our observation in the motor cortex, but is not consistent with our overall observations. Ferritin also has been reported to decrease in the cerebral cortex and basal ganglion structures in Parkinson's disease[62] although there is a discrepancy in the literature.[64]

3. Transferrin

These data are summarized in Table 1 and Figure 18.

Transferrin levels change more consistently in aging and in AD than either iron or ferritin levels do. Tf is decreased in the gray and white matter in each brain region examined in AD. In the superior temporal gyrus, the Tf decrease is similar in the gray matter both with normal aging (38%) and AD (33%). In the white matter Tf also decreases with normal aging and AD but the decrease in the AD brain tissue was greater (34 vs. 52%).

In the motor cortex, the Tf values did not change with normal aging in the gray matter, but decreased compared to normal (and age-matched controls) in the AD brains (34%). In the white matter of the motor cortex the Tf levels increased with normal aging (27%), but decreased in a nearly equal though opposite amount in AD (28%). Thus, the actual difference between AD and age-matched controls in the motor cortical white matter is a 64% decrease in the AD brains.

In the occipital cortex, Tf levels are altered by <10% in the gray matter either with AD or in normal aging. However, in the white matter with normal aging Tf levels in the occipital cortex increased 71% while in the AD tissue Tf levels decreased by 23%. The difference in Tf levels between the normal aged controls and AD for occipital cortical white matter was 56%.

Quantitative comparison of the iron regulatory proteins and iron in normal, aged controls, and AD demonstrates clearly an altered iron homeostasis in the aging brain which is exacerbated by AD. The superior temporal gyrus which undergoes relatively more age- and AD-related atrophy than the other cortical area examined has elevated iron levels in the gray matter in both normal aging and AD while both Tf and ferritin levels decrease. This observation suggests ferritin may have acquired more iron per mole of protein, a concept with support in the literature.[63] The increase in iron per mole of ferritin coupled with the decrease in transferrin in this brain region supports our general hypothesis of a decreased iron mobility in the brain in aging and AD.

In the white matter of the superior temporal gyrus, iron levels are unchanged whereas ferritin and Tf have decreased, again suggesting ferritin may be storing more iron and cells in the white matter have less access to that iron. The superior temporal gyrus loses more Tf with normal aging (in both gray and white matter) than any other brain region examined. Whether this observation reflects the normal degenerative changes with age in the superior temporal gyrus or is a causative factor has yet to be investigated.

In the motor cortex, iron and ferritin decrease in both the gray and white matter with normal aging while Tf levels are either unaffected by age (gray matter) or increase (white matter). In AD, iron and ferritin both increase about the same amount compared to normal in the gray matter with little change in the white matter. Tf levels, on the other hand, decrease considerably in both the gray and white matter in AD, again suggesting diminished capacity of the brain to mobilize iron.

In the occipital cortex, with age and in AD the changes in iron and iron regulatory proteins are less consistent than in the other brain regions. Ferritin and iron increase in both the gray and white matter with normal aging whereas Tf decreases slightly in the gray matter but increases in the white matter. In AD, the changes in ferritin and iron are in opposite directions in both the gray and white matter; iron decreases and ferritin increases. Tf decreases in both gray and white matter in this region in AD.

The increase in ferritin in the occipital cortex without a concomitant increase in iron is enigmatic. However, it is possible from recent reports that ferritin can store other metals in addition to iron could account for a ferritin increase in the absence of an iron increase. Ferritin in the brain has been shown to contain six times more aluminum in AD[63] compared to aged controls. It is interesting but speculative to suggest that some of the sparring of the occipital cortex to changes in AD could be associated with the ability of ferritin in this region to store and thus detoxify aluminum. Why such a phenomenon would occur in one brain region instead of another could be related to iron storage levels, iron utilization requirements, or activity of the microglial population among other possibilities. The ability of metals other than iron to regulate synthesis of ferritin has not been examined but is a field ripe for study.

The histological data which revealed iron in senile plaques and around blood vessels would suggest that the increased iron measured in some of the brain regions we examined comes from the blood. It would follow that iron in brain regions which have a high density of plaques would be "artificially" elevated. In this regard, it is interesting to note that the occipital cortex, which has a low density of senile plaques, does not have an increase in iron in AD brains.

The consistent quantitative decrease in Tf levels in AD white matter in all the brain regions examined becomes even more significant when considered with the altered cellular immunostaining in AD (Tf localized to astrocytes rather than oligodendrocytes) and indicates a dramatic change in iron homeostasis in AD white matter. The data suggest that the iron (stored in ferritin) is present in AD white matter oligodendrocytes but cannot be mobilized. Consequently, a decrease in oxidative metabolism in oligodendrocytes would occur leading to an inability to support normal cell function, in this case production and maintenance of myelin.

AD has generally been considered a "gray matter" disease because of the associated neurodegeneration with the disease. However, recent studies including those using brain-imaging techniques have revealed a much greater involvement with white matter in AD than previously considered.[65-67] It appears that the role of white matter degeneration has been underinvestigated in AD.

VI. RELATIONSHIP OF IRON REGULATORY PROTEINS TO OTHER METALS

The iron regulatory proteins will also bind with reasonable affinity a number of metals other than iron. Tf will specifically bind aluminum, zinc, manganese, and gallium among others.[68] Thus in addition to generating knowledge regarding iron regulation in the brain, the study of Tf and ferritin may lead to information regarding general metal regulation in the brain. This section of the chapter will focus on the relationship of Tf and aluminum because of the interest in aluminum and AD.[69]

Tf will bind aluminum specifically with an affinity which approaches that reported for iron.[70] Indeed some studies indicate that the major aluminum-binding fraction of plasma is Tf.[71] Consequently, the aluminum (and iron) which have been detected in senile plaques in AD could have been transported there via plasma Tf. The hypothesis that aluminum is a pathogenic toxin in AD lacked general scientific support perhaps primarily because aluminum had not been demonstrated to cross the blood-brain barrier under normal circumstances. Our laboratory has recently shown that when complexed to transferrin, aluminum can use the transferrin-transferrin receptor system which exists for uptake of iron into the brain to gain access to cells within the brain. Our study revealed that the Tf-aluminum complex will interact with brain Tf receptors with an affinity similar to Tf iron.[72] Another group has shown the regional distribution of Tf gallium (in which radioactive gallium was used as a substitute for aluminum) into the brain is similar to Tf iron.[73] These latter observations directly attack the long-standing argument against aluminum as a primary pathogenic agent in AD because it shows that aluminum can gain access to neurons under normal physiological conditions and does not require prior damage to cell membranes initiated by some unknown toxic agent.

The relationship between iron, aluminum, and transferrin presents scientists with a focal point from which to pursue aluminum neurotoxicity. The relationship, if any, that aluminum continues to have with iron-requiring activities within cells has yet to be explored. The mechanism of Tf-aluminum uptake and release of aluminum intracellularly is a critical area of research in this field. Aluminum uptake into the brain may actually increase in cases of iron deficiency.[74] The mechanism by which aluminum is involved in cellular toxicity also requires further study in view of the present comments. There is evidence that aluminum may enhance lipid peroxidative damage in the brain possibly through an interaction with iron.[75]

Clinical studies have also examined the relationship between Tf, iron, and aluminum in AD. A recent study reported that Tf iron saturation was higher in groups with AD or Down's syndrome compared to normal and disease controls.[76] This study also reported the iron saturation of Tf was due to a variant form of Tf which bound iron more tightly than normal and is present in higher frequency in AD patients. The investigators suggested that this variant form of Tf would become saturated with iron (normally only 30% of the plasma Tf is bound to iron) leaving aluminum to complex with citrate and thus to have greater access to the brain than normal. The possibilities presented in this latter study are very interesting, but some points require caution in interpretation. For example, Tf may have been saturated with metals other than iron or in addition to iron (such as aluminum). Second, the variant form of Tf may not be a genetic subtype which would suggest a genetic predisposition to AD (or Down's syndrome), but rather an alteration in the number of sialic residues in the carbohydrate moiety of the Tf protein such as occurs in chronic alcoholics.[77] Such a sialovariant form of Tf would indicate a post-translational modification in the glycosylation process rather than a molecular alteration. Nonetheless, the possibility of a variant form of Tf present in AD is exciting and worthy of pursuit.

The relationship between Tf iron and aluminum and the possibility of interventive therapy is in its initial stages of investigation. The use of desferrioxamine, a compound more widely known as an iron chelator, has been utilized to reverse behavioral deficits which followed aluminum ingestion in animals.[78] In a somewhat controversial study,[79] patients with probable AD received desferrioxamine over a 2-year period and the investigators concluded this treatment "may slow the clinical progression of dementia associated with AD". Desferrioxamine has been used successfully to reverse "dialysis dementia" which is presumed to result from aluminum toxicity.[80] Additional clinical and basic scientific experiments are necessary to ascertain both the mechanism of cell disruption by aluminum and the role of chelators such as desferrioxamine in preventing or reversing cell damage. The recent advent of antioxidant compounds which may cross the blood-brain barrier promises to be an area of exciting investigation in the near future in AD.

VII. TRANSFERRIN RECEPTORS

One remaining aspect of iron regulation in the brain which has received little attention to date is the transferrin receptor in the brain. Immunohistochemical studies have shown the receptor is present on endothelial cells in the brain,[58] oligodendrocytes,[81,82] and neurons.[58,82] Autoradiographic studies reveal a heterogeneous distribution of the receptor in the rat brain.[83,84] Neurons in which axons have been severed increase Tf receptor expression and iron uptake.[57] In animals in which the population of oligodendrocytes fails to reach maturity, the receptor density is decreased by approximately two thirds.[56] The only work to our knowledge on the Tf receptor with a potentially direct relationship to AD is a recent study suggesting that areas in the human brain with a high density of Tf receptors are more susceptible to neuropathological changes associated with dialysis encephalopathy.[85] Of particular interest in this latter study is the observation that the nucleus basalis of Meynert has a relatively high density of Tf receptors. This nucleus is a major source of cholinergic cells in the brain. The neurotransmitter acetylcholine is secreted by these cells and is consistently found to be decreased in AD. The reasons for the consistent and specific loss of cholinergic neurons in AD are unknown and have been subjects of intense research activity for some years. As mentioned earlier, the cholinergic system is extremely sensitive to impairments in oxidative metabolism.[4] It is interesting to speculate that disruption in iron metabolism in the nucleus of Meynert could have dramatic effects on the cholinergic system.

VIII. SUMMARY

The data reported in this chapter and the data regarding iron regulation in the brain are mostly at the descriptive level due to the relative immaturity of the field. As would be expected of a new field, many more questions than answers exist at this point. The goal of this chapter was to provide a comprehensive review of the status of iron regulation in the aging brain and present suggestions for additional research pursuits.

So many neurological systems are disrupted in AD that it is difficult to reconcile the loss of one neurotransmitter or the overproduction (for currently unknown reasons) of certain proteins as wreaking the havoc seen in the AD brain. Possibly the most attractive feature of the disruption of iron homeostasis hypothesis in AD is that iron is involved in such a myriad of systems that a general brain iron imbalance could be related to each of the known changes in AD.

ACKNOWLEDGMENTS

I am grateful to my colleagues Drs. Elliott Mufson, Javad Towfighi, and Richard Fine who supplied the brain tissue used in these investigations. Dr. John Beard performed the iron measurements and Brian Snyder performed the quantitative analysis of the proteins. Suzanne St. Martin and Sharon Menzies are responsible for the histological work and Ms. Menzies also prepared the micrographs for this chapter. This work was supported by funds from Alzheimer's Disease Research, a program of the American Health Assistance Foundation, Rockville, MD; American Federation for Aging Research; and United States Public Health Service grants AG09063 and NS22671.

REFERENCES

1. **Katzman, R. and Saitoh, T.**, Advances in Alzheimer's disease, *FASEB J.*, 5, 278, 1991.
2. **Perry, R.**, Recent advances in neuropathology, *Br. Med. Bull.*, 42, 34, 1986.
3. **Gottfries, C. G.**, Alzheimer's disease and senile dementia: biochemical characteristics and aspects of treatment, *Psychopharmacology*, 86, 245, 1985.
4. **Gibson, G. E. and Peterson, C. P.**, Aging decreases oxidative metabolism and the release and synthesis of acetylcholine, *J. Neurochem.*, 37, 978, 1981.
5. **Yehuda, S. and Youdmin, M. B. H.**, Brain iron deficiency: biochemistry and behavior, in *Brain Iron: Neurochemical and Behavioural Aspects*, Yehuda, S. and Youdim, M. B. H., Eds., Taylor & Francis, London, 1988, 89.
6. **Blass, J. P. and Gibson, G. E.**, The role of oxidative abnormalities in the pathophysiology of Alzheimer's disease, *Rev. Neurol.*, 147, 513, 1991.
7. **Crichton, R. R. and Charloteaux-Wauters, M.**, Iron transport and storage, *Eur. J. Biochem.*, 164, 485, 1987.
8. **Youdim, M. B. H., Green, A. R., Bloomfield, M. R., Mitchell, B. D., Heal, D. J., and Grahame-Smith, D. G.**, The effects of iron deficiency on brain biogenic monoamine biochemistry and function in rats, *Neuropharmacology*, 19, 259, 1980.
9. **Hill, J. M.**, Iron concentration reduced in ventral pallidum, globus pallidus, and substantia nigra by GABA-transaminase inhibitor, gamma-vinyl GABA, *Brain Res.*, 342, 18, 1985.
10. **Bourre, J. M., Pascal, G., Durand, G., Masson, M., Dumont, O., and Picotti, M. J.**, Alterations in the fatty acid composition of rat brain cells (neurons, astrocytes and oligodendrocytes) and subcellular fractions (myelin and synaptosomes) induced by a diet devoid of n-3 fatty acids, *J. Neurochem.*, 43, 342, 1984.
11. **Larkin, E. C. and Rao, A.**, Importance of fetal and neonatal iron: adequacy for normal development of central nervous system, in *Brain, Behaviour, and Iron in the Infant Diet*, Dobbing, J., Ed., Springer-Verlag, New York, 1990, chap. 3.
12. **Kabara, J. J.**, A critical review of brain cholesterol metabolism, *Prog. Brain Res.*, 40, 363, 1973.
13. **Mason, R. P., Shajenko, L., Chambers, T. E., Grazioso, H. J., Shoemaker, W. J., and Herbette, L. G.**, Biochemical and structural analysis of lipid membranes from temporal gyrus and cerebellum of Alzheimer's diseased brains, *Biophys. J.*, 59, 592, 1991.
14. **Arai, H., Kogure, K., Sugioka, K., and Nakano, M.**, Importance of two iron-reducing systems in lipid peroxidation of rat brain: implications for oxygen toxicity in the central nervous system, *Biochem. Int.*, 14, 741, 1987.
15. **Subarao, K. V. and Richardson, J. S.**, Iron-dependent peroxidation of rat brain: a regional study, *J. Neurosci. Res.*, 26, 224, 1990.
16. **Jesberger, J. A. and Richardson, J. S.**, Oxygen free radicals and brain dysfunction, *Intern. J. Neurosci.*, 57, 1, 1991.
17. **Zaleska, M. M. and Floyd, R.**, Regional lipid peroxidation in rat brain *in vitro:* possible role of endogenous iron, *Neurochem. Res.*, 10, 397, 1985.
18. **Aschner, M. and Aschner, J. L.**, Manganese transport across the blood brain barrier: relationship to iron homeostasis, *Brain Res. Bull.*, 24, 857, 1990.
19. **Zaleski, S.**, *Arch. Exp. Pathol. Pharmako.*, 23, 77, 1887 (cited in Reference 21).
20. **Spatz, H.**, Uber den Eisennachweis im Gehirn, besonders in Zentren des extrapyramidalmotorischen systems, *Z. Ges. Neruol. Psychiat. Berl.*, 77, 261, 1922.
21. **Diezel, P. B.**, Iron in the brain: a chemical and histochemical examination, in *Biochemistry of the Developing Nervous System*, Waelsch, H., Ed., Academic Press, New York, 1955, 145.
22. **Gans, A.**, Iron in the brain, *Brain*, 46, 128, 1923.
23. **Hill, J.M. and Switzer, R. C.**, The regional distribution and cellular localization of iron in the rat brain, *Neuroscience*, 11, 595, 1984.

24. **Connor, J. R. and Menzies, S. L.**, Altered cellular distribution of iron in the central nervous system of myelin deficient rats, *Neuroscience, 34,* 265, 1990.
25. **Connor, J. R., Menzies, S. L., St. Martin, S., and Mufson, E. J.,** The cellular distribution of transferrin, ferritin and iron in the human brain, *J. Neurosci. Res.,* 27, 595, 1990.
25a. unpublished observations.
26. **Dwork, A. J., Schon, E. A., and Herbert, J.,** Nonidentical distribution of transferrin and ferric iron in human brain, *Neuroscience,* 27, 333, 1988.
27. **Gerber, M. R. and Connor, J. R.,** Do oligodendrocytes mediate iron regulation in the human brain?, *Ann. Neurol.,* 26, 95, 1989.
28. **Craelius, W., Migdal, M. W., Luessenhop, C. P., Sugar, A., and Mihalakis, I.,** Iron deposits surrounding multiple sclerosis plaques, *Arch. Pathol. Lab. Med.,* 106, 397, 1982.
29. **Pardridge, W. M., Eisenber, J., and Yang, J.,** Human blood-brain barrier transferrin receptor, *Metabolism,* 36, 892, 1987.
30. **Fishman, J. B., Rubin, J. B., Handrahan, J. V., Connor, J. R., and Fine, R. E.,** Receptor-mediated transcytosis of transferrin across the blood brain barrier, *J. Neurosci. Res.,* 25, 576, 1987.
31. **Ehmann, W. D., Markesbery, W. R., Alauddin, M., Hossain, T. I. M., and Brubaker, E. H.,** Brain trace elements in Alzheimer's Disease, *Neurotoxicology,* 7, 197, 1986.
32. **Hallgren, B. and Sourander, P.,** The effect of age on the nonhaemin iron in the human brain, *J. Neurochem.,* 3, 41, 1958.
33. **Connor, J. R., Snyder, B. S., Beard, J. L., Fine, R. E., and Mufson, E. J.,** The regional distribution of iron and iron regulatory proteins in the brain in aging and Alzheimer's disease, *J. Neurosci. Res.,* 31, 327, 1992.
34. **Rajan, K. S., Colburn, R. W., and Davis, J. M.,** Distribution of metal ions in the subcellular fractions of several rat brain areas, *Life Sci.,* 18, 423, 1976.
35. **Curnes, J. T., Burger, P. C., Djang, W. T., and Boyko, O. B.,** MR imaging of compact white matter pathways, *AJNR,* 9, 1961, 1988.
36. **Nguyen-Legros, J., Bizot, J., Bolesse, M., and Publicani, J. P.,** Noir de diamino-benzidine: une nouvelle methode histochimique de revelation du fer exogene, *Histochemistry,* 66, 239, 1980.
37. **Levine, S. M. and Macklin, W. B.,** Iron-enriched oligodendrocytes: a reexamination of their spatial distribution, *J. Neurosci. Res.,* 26, 508, 1990.
38. **Connor, J. R., Menzies, S. L., St. Martin, S., Fine, R. E., and Mufson, E. J.,** Altered cellular distribution of transferrin, ferritin and iron Alzheimer's disease brains, *J. Neurosci. Res.,* 31, 75, 1991.
39. **Goodman, L.,** Alzheimer's disease: a clinico-pathologic analysis of twenty-three cases with a theory on pathogenesis, *J. Nerv. Ment. Dis.,* 118, 97, 1953.
40. **Octave, J. N., Schneider, Y. J., Trouet, A., and Crichton, R. R.,** Iron uptake and utilization by mammalian cells. I. Cellular uptake of transferrin and iron, *Trends Biochem. Sci.,* 8, 217, 1983.
41. **Theil, E. C.,** Ferritin: structure, gene regulation, and other cellular function in animals, plants and microorganisms, *Ann. Rev. Biochem.,* 56, 289, 1987.
42. **Kaneko, Y., Kitamoto, T., Tateishi, J., and Yamaguchi, K.,** Ferritin immunohisto-chemistry as a marker for microglia, *Acta Neuropathol. (Berl.),* 79, 129, 1989.
43. **Koeppen, A. H. and Dentinger, M. P.,** Brain hemosiderin and superficial siderosis of the central nervous system, *J. Neuropathol. Exp. Neurol.,* 47, 249, 1988.
43a. **Connor, J. R. and Berkovic, S. A.,** Iron regulation in the brain: histochemical, and molecular considerations. *Ann. Neurol. (Suppl.),* in press.
44. **Grundke-Igbal, I., Fleming, J., Tung, Y.-C., Lassmamm, H., Igbal, K., and Joshi, J. G.,** Ferritin is a component of the neuritic (senile) plaque in Alzheimer dementia, *Acta neuropathol.,* 81, 105, 1990.

45. **Kalria, R. N. and Harik, S. I.,** Reduced glucose transporter at the blood-brain-barrier and in cerebral cortex in Alzheimer's disease, *J. Neurochem.,* 53, 1083, 1989.
46. **Mooradian, A. D., Morin, A. M., Cipp, L. J., and Haspel, H. C.,** Glucose transport is reduced in the blood-brain barrier of aged rats, *Brain Res.,* 551, 145, 1991.
47. **Aisen, R. and Listowsky, I.,** Iron transport and storage proteins, *Ann. Rev. Biochem.,* 49, 357, 1980.
48. **Swaiman, K. F. and Machen, V. L.,** Iron uptake by mammalian cortical neurons, *Ann. Neurol.,* 16, 66, 1984.
49. **Swaiman, K. F. and Machen, V. L.,** Iron uptake by glial cells *Neurochem. Res.,* 10, 1635, 1985.
50. **Connor, J. R. and Fine, R. E.,** The distribution of transferrin immunoreactivity in the rat central nervous system, *Brain Res.,* 368, 319, 1986.
51. **Connor, J. R. and Fine, R. E.,** Development of transferrin-positive oligodendrocytes in the rat central nervous system, *J. Neurosci. Res.,* 17, 51, 1987.
52. **Bloch, B., Popovici, T., Levin, M. J., Tuil, D., and Kahn, A.,** Transferrin gene expression visualized in oligodendrocytes of the rat brain using *in situ* hybridization and immunohistochemistry, *Proc. Natl. Acad. Sci. U.S.A.,* 82, 6706, 1985.
53. **Oh, T. H., Markelonis, G. J., Royal, G. M., and Bregman, B. S.,** Immunocyto-chemical distribution of transferrin and its receptor in the developing chicken nervous system, *Dev. Brain Res.,* 30, 207, 1986.
54. **Connor, J. R., Phillips, T. M., Lakshman, M. R., Barron, K. D., Fine, R. E., and Csiza, C. K.,** Regional variation in the levels of transferrin in the CNS of normal and myelin-deficient rats, *J. Neurochem.,* 49, 1523, 1987.
55. **Bartlett, W. P., Li, X.-S., and Connor, J. R.,** Expression of transferrin mRNA in the CNS of normal and jimpy mice, *J. Neurochem.,* 57, 318, 1991.
56. **Roskams, A. J. and Connor, J. R.,** The transferrin receptor in the myelin deficient (md) rat, *J. Neurosci. Res.,* in press.
57. **Graeber, M. B., Raivich, G., and Kreutzberg, G. W.,** Increase of transferrin receptors and iron uptake in regenerating motor neurons, *J. Neurosci. Res.,* 23, 342, 1989.
58. **Jefferies, W. A., Brandon, M. R., Hunt, S. V., Williams, A. F., Gatter, K. C., and Mason, D. Y.,** Transferrin receptor on endothelium of brain capillaries, *Nature (London),* 312, 162, 1984.
59. **Jackson, A. J., Michael, L. M., and Schumacher, H. J.,** Improved tissue solubilization of iron in the rat brain, *Anal. Chem.,* 44, 595, 1972.
60. **Taylor, E. M. and Morgan, E. H.,** Developmental changes in transferrin and iron uptake by the brain in the rat, *Dev. Brain Res.,* 55, 35, 1990.
61. **Thompson, C. M., Marksberry, W. R., Ehmann, W. D., Mao, Y.-X., and Vance, D. E.,** Regional brain trace-element studies in Alzheimer's disease, *Neurotoxicology,* 9, 1, 1988.
62. **Dexter, D. T., Carayon, A., Vidailhet, M., Ruberg, M., Agid, F., Agid, Y., Lees, A. J., Wells, F. R., Jenner, P., and Marsden, C. D.,** Decreased ferritin levels in brain in Parkinson's disease, *J. Neurochem.,* 55, 16, 1990.
63. **Fleming, J. and Joshi, J. G.,** Ferritin: isolation of aluminum-ferritin complex from brain, *Proc. Natl. Acad. Sci. U.S.A.,* 84, 7866, 1987.
64. **Sofic, E., Riederer, P., Heinsen, H., Beckmann, H., Reynolds, G. P., Hebenstreit, G., and Youdim, M. B. H.,** Increased iron(III) and total iron content in postmortem substantia nigra of Parkinsonian brain, *J. Neural. Trans.,* 74, 199, 1988.
65. **Blennow, K., Wallin, A., Uhlemann, C., and Gottfries, C. G.,** White matter lesion on CT in Alzheimer patients: relation to clinical symptomatology and vascular factors, *Acta Neurol. Scand.,* 83, 187, 1991.
66. **Miller, A. K. H., Alston, R. L., and Corsellis, J. A. N.,** Variation with age in the volumes of grey and white matter in the cerebral hemispheres of man: measurements with an image analyzer, *Neuropathol. Appl. Neurobiol.,* 6, 119, 1980.

67. **Gottfries, C. G.,** Neurochemical aspects on aging and diseases with cognitive impairment, *J. Neurosci. Res.,* 27, 541, 1990.

68. **de Jong, G., van Dijk, J. P., and van Eijk, H. G.,** The biology of transferrin, *Clin. Chimica Acta,* 190, 1, 1990.

69. **Perl, D. P. and Good, P. F.,** The association of aluminum, Alzheimer's disease, and neurofibrillary tangles, *J. Neural. Trans.,* 24, 205, 1987.

70. **Cochran, M., Coates, J., and Neoh, S.,** The competitive equilibrium between aluminum and ferric iron for the binding sites of transferrin, *FEBS Lett.,* 176, 129, 1984.

71. **Martin, R. B.,** The chemistry of aluminum as related to biology and medicine, *Clin. Chem.,* 32, 1797, 1986.

72. **Roskams, A. J. and Connor, J. R.,** Aluminum access to the brain: a possible role for the transferrin receptor, *Proc. Natl. Acad. Sci. U.S.A.,* 87, 9024, 1990.

73. **Pullen, R. G. L., Candy, J. M., Morris, C. M., Taylor, G., Keith, A. B., and Edwardson, J. A.,** Gallium-67 as a potential marker for aluminum transport in rat brain: implication for Alzheimer's disease, *J. Neurochem.,* 55, 251, 1990.

74. **Cannata, J. B., Fernandez-Soto, I., Fernandez-Menendez, M. J., Fernandez-Martin, J. L., McGregor, S. J., Brock, J. H., and Halls, D.,** Role of iron metabolism in absorption and cellular uptake of aluminum, *Kidney Int.,* 39, 799, 1991.

75. **Fraga, C. G., Oteiza, P. I., Golub, M. S., Gershwin, M. E., and Keen, C. L.,** Effects of aluminum on brain lipid peroxidation, *Toxicol. Lett.,* 51, 213, 1990.

76. **Farrar, G., Altmann, P., Welch, S., Wychrij, O., Ghose, B., Lejeune, J., Corbett, J., Proaher, V., and Blair, J. A.,** Defective gallium-transferrin binding in Alzheimer disease and Down syndrome: possible mechanism for accumulation of aluminum in brain, *Lancet,* 335, 747, 1990.

77. **Stibler, H., Sydow, O., and Borg, S.,** Quantitative estimation of abnormal microheterogeneity of serum transferrin in alcoholics, *Pharmacol. Biochem. Behav.,* 13, 47, 1980.

78. **Connor, D. J., Harrel, L. E., and Jope, R. S.,** Reversal of an aluminum-induced behavioral deficit by administration of deferoxamine, *Behav. Neurosci.,* 103, 779, 1989.

79. **Crapper-McLachlan, D. R., Dalton, A. J., Kruck, T. P. A., Bell, M. Y., Smith, W. L., Kalow, W., and Andrews, D. F.,** Intramuscular desferrioxamine in patients with Alzheimer's disease, *Lancet,* 337, 1304, 1991.

80. **Simon, P., Ang, K. S., Cam, G., Allain, P., and Mauras, Y.,** Desferrioxamine, aluminum, and dialysis, *Lancet,* 2, 1489, 1983.

81. **Lin, H. H. and Connor, J. R.,** The development of the transferrin-transferrin receptor system in relation to astrocytes, MBP, and galactosecerebroside in normal and myelin-deficient rat optic nerves, *Dev. Brain Res.,* 49, 281, 1989.

82. **Giometto, B., Bozza, F., Argentiero, V., Gallo, P., Pagni, S., Piccinno, M. G., and Tavolato, B.,** Transferrin receptor in rat central nervous system. An immunohistochemical study, *J. Neurol. Sci.,* 98, 81, 1990.

83. **Hill, J. M., Ruff, M. R., Weber, R. J., and Pert, C. B.,** Transferrin receptors in rat brain: neuropeptide-like pattern and relationship to iron distribution, *Proc. Natl. Acad. Sci. U.S.A.,* 82, 4553, 1985.

84. **Mash, D. C., Pablo, J., Flynn, D. D., Efange, S. M. N., and Weiner, W. J.,** Characterization and distribution of transferrin receptors in the rat brain, *J. Neurochem.,* 55, 1972, 1990.

85. **Morris, C. M., Candy, J. M., Oakley, A. E., Taylor, G. A., Mountfort, S., Bishop, H., Ward, M. K., Bloxham, C. A., and Edwardson, J. A.,** Comparison of the regional distribution of transferrin receptors and aluminum in the forebrain of chronic renal dialysis patients, *J. Neurol. Sci.,* 94, 295, 1989.

16. Iron-Promoted Oxidative Damage in Rheumatic Diseases

C. W. Trenam, Paul G. Winyard, Chris J. Morris, and David R. Blake

The Inflammation Group, The London Hospital Medical College, London, U.K.

I. INTRODUCTION

Iron would appear to be the most important metal in human metabolism. Oxygen, clearly critical to aerobic metabolism, has an unusual electron configuration; two isolated electrons occupy separate orbitals, with magnetic moments which align in similar directions. For oxygen to accept two electrons, it requires an electron from an incoming electron pair to spin invert. This restriction leads oxygen to accept electrons one at a time. Because an iron atom can exist in two valency states, ferrous and ferric, iron became the primordial partner of oxygen in evolution. However, as elegantly expressed by De Sousa[1] "like many other long standing partnerships, this one, to survive, had to use protective devices that would not allow toxicity of either partner to be expressed in the presence of each other." A range of intracellular antioxidant defense systems limits the toxic potential of intermediates formed during the four-electron reduction of oxygen to water. Of particular importance is the enzyme superoxide dismutase (SOD) which, by catalyzing the dismutation of the superoxide anion radical ($O_2^{\cdot-}$) to the reactive oxygen species (ROS) hydrogen peroxide (H_2O_2), maintains intracellular $O_2^{\cdot-}$ levels at approximately 10^{-11} M during normal metabolism. The divalent reduction of oxygen leads to H_2O_2, and once again, the cell is protected from its potential toxicity, either by the heme enzyme catalase or by the selenoenzyme glutathione peroxidase. The most toxic of all the ROS, the hydroxyl radical ($OH^{\cdot}$), lacks a specific enzyme-based defense system. Its production in biological systems is generated by the consequences of the reducing agent $O_2^{\cdot-}$ reacting with ferric or cupric ions

$$Fe^{3+} + O_2^{\cdot-} \rightarrow O_2 + Fe^{2+}$$

Ferrous iron, now reacting with H_2O_2, produces the hydroxyl radical:

$$Fe^{2+} + H_2O_2 \rightarrow OH^{\cdot} + OH^- + Fe^{3+}$$

The hydroxyl radical is highly unstable, reacting within one to five molecular diameters of its site of formation, with a rate constant almost diffusion controlled (10^{-9} mol/s).[2,3] Because of the toxicity of $OH^{\cdot}$, probably the most powerful biological oxidant, iron is compartmentalized intracellularly, thereby limiting its formation. The protein apoferritin serves this purpose. Extracellularly iron is, for the most part, bound to transferrin or lactoferrin, and intravascularly is found in hemoglobin. These proteins not only protect against the toxicity of iron, but also allow for the delivery of oxygen to tissues and the controlled release of iron for a multitude of critical enzymic processes. How may this system break down and promote an inflammatory synovitis?

II. IRON AND JOINT PATHOLOGY

Iron and joint inflammation were first associated by Hochstatter in his description in 1674 of the arthritis associated with excessive bleeding,[4] effectively a description of the synovitis associated with hemophilia. Hemophilic arthropathy is characterized by a florid and proliferative synovitis and associated with erosive bone damage and cartilage destruction.[5] Bleeding into an otherwise normal joint is clearly associated with damage. In patients with an abnormal joint, for instance rheumatoid synovitis, iron may also play a role in perpetuating inflammatory damage.

The peripheral synovial joint is unique in being a mobile organ, subjected to substantial intra-articular pressure (IAP) fluxes once inflamed (*vide infra*). The synovium, though in health a simple structure and relatively acellular, is rapidly populated with cells of the inflammatory response, becoming much thickened and prone to microbleeding, a process leading to intracellular ferritin production and iron deposition (*vide infra*). Iron can also be redirected to the synovium by cytokine-driven uptake as the synovium functions as an extension of the reticuloendothelial (RE) system. Such tissue sequestration of iron leads to the anemia of chronic disease.

III. THE ANEMIA OF CHRONIC DISEASE

Although rheumatoid arthritis (RA) mainly affects peripheral synovial joints, it is also a systemic disease being accompanied by anemia, weight loss, and increase in erythrocyte sedimentation rate. Vascular, cardiac, and pulmonary lesions are also produced. All rheumatoid patients with persistent inflammation develop the anemia of chronic disease (ACD). This is a mild anemia characterized by a disturbance in iron metabolism which results in hypoferremia (low serum iron and hemoglobin levels), despite iron stores that range from adequate to raised. Other features of the ACD include a decrease in both plasma total iron-binding capacity (TIBC) and transferrin (Tf) saturation with iron. There is, however, a marked increase in serum ferritin, and, in RA serum, ferritin levels may reach 250% of initial values.[6,7] (See also Chapter 6.)

The most widely accepted explanation for the low serum iron appears to be that iron deposited in the RE cells is not properly released to Tf in the circulation, i.e., it is poorly reutilized.[8] The RE system plays a central role in iron metabolism, processing hemoglobin from senescent erythrocytes.[9] Under normal circumstances the RE system provides most of the iron required for erythropoiesis, and iron storage and release by the RE system are in equilibrium. After a lag period due to heme catabolism, the RE cells release iron into the plasma by a two-phase process. The first is an early phase (immediate release from heme catabolism), which is completed within a few hours; and the second is a late phase corresponding to iron release from RE stores.[10]

Lee[11] describes two mechanisms for the impaired RE iron release during inflammation. The first is that the iron-binding protein lactoferrin (LF) is liberated from specific granules of leukocytes and competes with the extracellular transport protein transferrin for iron (particularly at the low pH existing at inflammatory sites).[12] The Lf then returns the iron to the macrophage where it is stored as ferritin,[12] but not to erythropoietic cells.[14] In the second mechanism, first proposed by Konijn and Hershko,[15] the hypoferremia of inflammation results from an increase in intracellular synthesis of the iron storage protein, apoferritin. (See also Chapter 2.) Serum apoferritin behaves as an acute phase reactant and is glycosylated within hepatocytes prior to secretion.[18] In acute inflammatory states it tends to parallel changes in another acute phase protein, haptoglobin. The apoferritin provides a storage depot for incoming iron delivered via Lf or from effete erythrocytes. As well as increasing the synthesis of ferritin, interleukin-1 (IL-1) contributes toward the hypoferremia by increasing Lf production from the specific granules of neutrophils.[17] Storage iron is less available to the plasma iron transport system than iron recently derived from destroyed erythrocytes. Therefore, it would be expected that a diversion of iron into stores would result in hypoferremia and an iron supply insufficient for erythropoiesis.[15]

Recently, Fillet and co-workers[18] characterized RE iron kinetics in patients with inflammatory disease and in normal controls. As compared with normal subjects, the patients with inflammation had significantly lower serum iron levels and higher plasma ferritin levels. Early release of radiolabeled iron from the RE cells was significantly reduced and the late release was significantly increased. There was a significant negative correlation between the percentage of early release and plasma ferritin, but no correlation was found between the percentage of early release and biological markers of inflammation (erythrocyte sedimentation rate, fibrinogen, or α_2-globulin). This showed that early release was decreased because RE stores were increased and not because of the intensity of inflammation itself. Ferritin production is enhanced in the inflammatory RE cells,[15] and this precedes the decrease in serum iron levels. Thus, Fillet et al.[18] have supported the hypothesis of increased ferritin synthesis as a mechanism for the reduction in iron output from the RE cells.

These changes are the result of the production of inflammatory mediators from a variety of different cell types. The increased synthesis of acute phase proteins is driven by IL-1,[19] interleukin-6 (IL-6),[20] and tumor necrosis factor (TNF).[21] Specific acute phase proteins are regulated differently by the inflammatory mediators IL-1, IL-6, and TNF.[22] In 1989, Brock and Alvarez-Hernandez[23] demonstrated that TNF is more important than IL-1 in the changes in iron metabolism associated with inflammation. TNF was shown to alter the ability of macrophages to take up, process, and release iron.

IV. THE ROLE OF IRON IN RHEUMATOID ARTHRITIS

There is a strikingly large number of ferritin molecules in rheumatoid synovial lining cells. Muirden[24] was the first to suggest that the large amounts of iron sequestered in the rheumatoid synovial membrane may contribute toward the anemia of the disease. This author found large amounts of iron-loaded ferritin molecules particularly in type A (macrophage-like) synovial lining cells. The ferritin was scattered throughout the cell cytoplasm but was frequently concentrated in lysosomes. All the synovial biopsies which contained iron were removed from patients who were either severely or moderately anemic.

In further studies, Muirden and co-workers[25] demonstrated that synovial cells in culture have the capacity to ingest hemoglobin prepared from hemolyzed red cells, and the subsequent appearance of ferritin in these cells implied that they were able to synthesize apoferritin. The authors suggested that both the synthesis of ferritin and the breakdown of hemoglobin takes place within the same lysosome, and that iron from lysed erythrocytes is likely to be an important source of the iron deposits in the rheumatoid synovium. A light microscopic study of synovia from rheumatoid patients as well as synovia of other joint diseases demonstrated that iron deposits are a constant feature of the pathology of RA.[26] Prussian blue (Perls') positive staining, indicating the presence of ferric iron, was seen in all but one of the 27 synovial biopsies examined. In the exception, material processed for electron microscopy revealed ferritin granules in some of the surface cells. Hemosiderin granules were seen in 15 of the 27 biopsies. The authors suggested that iron deposits in RA arise from continued oozing of blood from the vascular granulation tissue into the synovial cavity. In highly inflamed rheumatoid joints, simple weight bearing or the stress of motion is likely to compress the hyperplastic villi and synovial folds leading to bleeding. These large deposits of iron play a significant contributory role in the anemia and pathogenesis of this disease.

Muirden[27] provided further evidence for the link between synovial iron and pathogenesis of RA. In 28 patients there was a significant relationship between the presence of anemia due to RA and a histological estimate of the extent of iron deposits. There was also a relationship between the duration of the disease, the grade of X-ray change, and the extent of iron deposition. An isotope kinetic method, utilizing ^{59}Fe to label plasma Tf, was employed to study the rate and mechanism of iron deposition in the synovial membrane in 13 rheumatoid knees.[28] Iron accumulation occurred only after incorporation of labeled iron into circulating erythrocytes. This led to the conclusion that intermittent intra-articular hemorrhages were the source of iron deposits in the rheumatoid synovium. This hypothesis has been tested using the rat allergic air pouch model which produces a similar membrane structure to that of human synovium. The addition of autologous whole blood to this naturally remitting allergic model prolongs a low grade inflammatory state[29] as in RA, where microbleeding occurs. The proinflammatory factor in these studies was present in erythrocytes only and would confirm an active role for heme iron, rather than the breakdown products of hemoglobin, such as hemin, which depresses ferritin synthesis *in vitro*.[30] Macrophage ferritin synthesis was much enhanced in this model[31] as in the rheumatoid synovium.

In an extensive study of RA patients, Blake et al.[32] showed that the amount of ferritin within synovial macrophages was significantly associated with the activity of early rheumatoid disease at the time of biopsy. In contrast, the amount of Perls' positive iron was associated with the persistence of the disease. The authors suggested either that ferritin production may fail in a population of synovial macrophages, iron derived from effete erythrocytes becoming available in a form able to induce the synthesis and release of collagenase and prostaglandins (PG), or that ferric iron may be reduced to the ferrous form catalyzing the formation of the $OH^{\cdot}$ radical and subsequent lipid peroxidation (LPO).[33] Hydroxyl radicals and LPO cause extensive disruption of cellular organelle membranes and promote inflammatory tissue damage. Polyunsaturated fatty acids in plasma low density lipoproteins (LDL) can be oxidized by iron, endothelial cells, and macrophages. This oxidized LDL (o-LDL) has chemotactic properties for monocytes and is cytotoxic to endothelial cells and smooth muscle fibers. This group has recently shown the presence of both intra- and extracellular staining for o-LDL in the rheumatoid synovium.[34] Intracellular staining was confined to foamy macrophages. Type A synoviocytes did not form foam cells but did show a surface-staining pattern. The infiltration of the rheumatoid synovium by chronic inflammatory cells may be due to a tendency for these cells, which have receptors for iron-binding proteins, to migrate toward deposits of iron.

Using ultrastructural methods, iron was seen in 25% of the synovial cells from patients with RA.[35] The iron was usually deposited in siderosomes in type B (fibroblast-like) synovial cells, which were the predominant cell type; and no tissue damage was observed in the vicinity of these iron-rich siderosomes. This is in contrast with the findings in type A cells where siderosomes were associated with considerable cytoplasmic damage. The authors suggested that the apparent dominance of the type B cells may be due to type A cell damage and death, reflecting the capacity for reactive oxygen production in these macrophage-like cells in response to iron. Alternatively, there may be a failure of type A cells to produce an apoferritin response with the subsequent precipitation of intracellular proteins by iron. The authors also put forward the idea that the synovial cells may change their function, with a transition from A to B cell morphology as a result of inflammation.[36] This second hypothesis would explain the apparent correlation between the amount of iron in the synovia and the extent of erosive damage,[29] as it is the synovial B cells that have the capacity to cause local bone resorption via the generation of

PGE_2. Another observation is that rheumatoid synovial cells are more sensitive to oxidative stress than normal cells as shown by Rogers et al.[37] They showed that stress induced by H_2O_2 and heat shock cause a collapse of the vimentin intermediary filaments from a transcytoplasmic to a perinuclear position. This is accompanied by a substantial decrease in thiol level in the vimentin protein[38] and a complete loss of intracellular free glutathione.

Low molecular weight iron chelates which are capable of catalyzing OH˙ formation and LPO have been detected in rheumatoid synovial fluid (SF)[39] using the bleomycin method.[40] The concentration of this bleomycin-detectable iron correlated with thiobarbituric acid (TBA)-reactive material in the SF and with indices of disease activity (knee score, leukocyte count, and SF C-reactive protein). Recently, Parkes et al.[41] have confirmed the presence of these low molecular weight iron complexes and characterized them to be predominantly complexes with endogenous citrate.

In rheumatoid SF, the concentration of ferritin is significantly higher than in the serum.[42] This ferritin, however, contains very little iron.[16] Apoferritin has the ability to stimulate O_2^- production from neutrophils which are abundant in rheumatoid SF. The O_2^- is capable of mobilizing iron from ferritin,[43] which may explain the low-iron loading of SF ferritin.

Further work by Blake and Bacon[44] has demonstrated a significant association between SF ferritin concentration, SF immune complexes, and other indices of inflammatory activity in patients with RA. They suggest that this association may be due to excess iron within the synovial RE cell having a direct toxic effect reducing the ability of such cells to clear immune complexes.

These conclusions have recently been supported in studies by Ahmadzadeh and co-workers[45] who measured the iron-binding proteins, "free" iron, and bound iron in the SF of 30 rheumatoid patients and compared them with those of patients with osteoarthritis. They demonstrated a significant increase in SF ferritin and Lf but not Tf. Despite a significant increase in bleomycin-detectable iron, there was a decrease in the saturation index of SF ferritin and Tf. The concentration of both free iron and bound iron in SF correlated with indices of inflammatory activity such as rheumatoid factor and immune complex levels in the SF of RA patients. These data suggest that iron participates in the local inflammatory process and has an important role in the pathogenesis of articular damage in RA patients.

Further evidence for the damaging effects of iron in RA is provided by the exacerbation of synovitis observed when iron is administered to rheumatoid patients. In addition to the ACD, some rheumatoid patients develop true iron deficiency anemia: figures of up to 75% of RA patients have been quoted.[46] In these iron-deficient patients there is a clinical need to provide iron in a safe and nontoxic form. Oral iron supplements in the form of ferrous sulfate have produced a flare of the peripheral synovitis within 48 h of ingestion.[47] This was demonstrated by both clinical and laboratory indices. A large number of RA patients receive multiple drug therapy (including penicillamine, which binds iron) and are intolerant of oral iron supplements. Intramuscular preparations of iron are difficult to administer due to poor muscle bulk and local tenderness. In this population, a total dose infusion of iron dextran is usually given. Reddy and Lewis[48] reported that five of seven rheumatoid patients treated with i.v. iron dextran showed a flare in their arthritis. In each instance the flare took place within 24 h of iron dextran administration, but only in those joints already affected by arthritis. The joints demonstrated increased swelling, heat, and pain. We have attempted to mimic the clinical situation in which anemic rheumatoid patients are given iron supplements in the presence of clinical joint symptoms by employing the adjuvant arthritis model in rats and administering iron in the presence of, rather than prior to, clinical manifestations of joint symptoms. Iron produced an exacerbation of joint inflammation between days 3 to 5 postinjection.[49] This is similar to the findings of Lloyd and Williams[50] who showed that nine patients out of ten had an exacerbation of arthralgia for up to 7 d when given a total dose infusion of iron dextran. The joint symptoms were accompanied by a feeling of general malaise, a low-grade fever, and a definite rise in erythrocyte sedimentation rate.

Two studies by our group[51,52] have provided clear evidence that iron-catalyzed reactions are the causative factors in the exacerbation of synovial inflammation consequent to total dose infusion of iron dextran. In the first study we showed that the exacerbation corresponded with saturation of serum iron-binding capacity. The levels of immune complexes were unaltered, implying a normal RE cell function and hence ruling out the dextran as a causative factor. In one patient, an increase in LPO products (as measured by TBA-reactive material and conjugated dienes) in the SF corresponded with the exacerbation of synovitis. The authors confirmed this by an *in vitro* study which demonstrated that it was the iron component of the iron dextran complex which stimulated LPO. The second study demonstrated that exacerbation of rheumatoid synovitis produced by total dose infusion of iron dextran corresponded with saturation of serum and SF iron-binding capacity, giving rise to low molecular weight iron chelates which are capable of causing oxidative damage. Simultaneously, LPO and the concentration of dehydroascorbate increased in both serum and SF. Hepatic function was transiently disturbed 7 d after the infusion, implying hepatic oxidant stress within the iron-loaded liver.

V. IRON AND HYPOXIC REPERFUSION INJURY

Many of our clinical observations led us to the conclusion that iron may have a relatively specific influence on synovitis as opposed to inflammation generally. Certainly we were and remain unaware of iron dextran flaring other chronic, noninfective, inflammatory conditions in man. The observations that joints needed to be mobile with preexisting inflammation and that the mechanism was essentially via oxidative injury led us to propose that the joint was subject to iron-promoted hypoxic reperfusion injury.[53] This hypothesis we now believe to be proved. The data supporting this view have been extensively published, and are reviewed in Lunec and Blake.[2] Our observations are summarized as follows.

Ischemia-induced tissue injury is recognized as a major factor in the pathogenesis of life-threatening diseases, for example, coronary artery disease. (See Chapter 10 and the Epilogue.) It is now becoming clear that the mechanism of so-called ischemic damage is not simple. It is certainly true that protracted ischemia by itself will ultimately produce tissue death. However, in some clinical situations a substantial part of the injury may be more properly termed reperfusion injury.[54] That is to say, much of the injury may not occur during the period of temporary hypoxia, but rather during the period when oxygen is reintroduced to the tissue by restoration of the blood supply. When this circumstance arises, free radicals may be generated in abundance due to the uncoupling of a variety of intracellular redox systems, and play a major role in producing microvascular and parenchymal damage.

Radical-promoted hypoxic-reperfusion injury was first demonstrated in the cat intestine. Transient ischemia to the small bowel of the cat resulted in an increased intestinal capillary permeability and albumin clearance, which was magnified tenfold on reperfusion. However, the increased intestinal capillary permeability that was observed during reperfusion was blocked by predosing with the radical-scavenging enzymes superoxide dismutase (SOD) or catalase, allopurinol (oxidized to oxypurinol, inhibiting xanthine oxidase), or an iron chelator.[55] Hypoxic-reperfusion injury has been applied to many disease states, including transient coronary or cerebral ischemia, ischemic acute renal failure, and early renal and bone transplant rejection. One source of free radicals, established as a result of multiple investigations into hypoxic-reperfusion injury, is the xanthine oxidase/dehydrogenase enzymatic system.[54] The mechanism for the production of O_2^- in postischemic tissues appears to be affected by changes in purine metabolism within ischemic cells. During temporary ischemia, low oxygen concentrations halt mitochondrial oxidative phosphorylation and cellular ATP production becomes dependent on anaerobic glycolysis. This is an inefficient means of ATP production from glucose and also results in the production of lactate. Increasing levels of lactate, together with an increasing ratio of NADH to oxidized nicotinamide adenine dinucleotide (NAD^+), eventually leads to the inhibition of glycolysis. Moreover, intracellular ATP and adenosine diphosphate (ADP) levels, already reduced, fall further. This leads to raised levels of adenosine and of its breakdown products, including hypoxanthine and xanthine which are the substrates for the cytosolic xanthine oxidase/dehydrogenase enzyme system.

Xanthine oxidase normally catalyzes the oxidation of hypoxanthine and xanthine to uric acid. It is widely distributed among tissues and is predominantly located in the capillary endothelium.[56] The enzyme is synthesized as xanthine dehydrogenase (type D), which transfers electrons to NAD^+. However, in ischemic conditions a Ca^{2+}-dependent protease alters the enzyme critically, converting it to an oxidase (O) form, which no longer transfers electrons to NAD^+ but to O_2-producing $O_2^{\cdot-}$. Upon reperfusion of temporarily ischemic tissue, the O form of the enzyme — supplied with oxygen as an electron acceptor and high levels of hypoxanthine — produces a flux of $O_2^{\cdot-}$ which either may be converted spontaneously or by the enzyme SOD to H_2O_2. In addition, the O form of xanthine oxidase can mobilize iron from ferritin, by a mechanism largely dependent on the generated $O_2^{\cdot-}$. The released iron has the ability to catalyze the formation of $OH^{\cdot}$ from $O_2^{\cdot-}$ and H_2O_2. Iron with this capacity has recently been found bound to citrate in synovial fluid.[57] The complement component C_5a, as well as the monocyte product TNF-α, also cause the conversion of cellular xanthine dehydrogenase to xanthine oxidase in a rapid and irreversible fashion.[58] Activated neutrophils acting on endothelial cells have a similar effect.

Hence, during ischemia important biochemical changes occur within tissue:

1. A new enzyme activity appears, along with one of its two required substrates.
2. The remaining substrate required for type O activity is molecular O_2, which is supplied during the reperfusion of the tissue; with it comes a burst of $O_2^{\cdot-}$ and H_2O_2 production.
3. Iron is decompartmentalized, allowing it to catalyze $OH^{\cdot}$ generation.

VI. XANTHINE OXIDASE AND THE JOINT

From the previous discussion it follows that the presence of xanthine oxidase in human synovium may be central to the proposal of hypoxic-reperfusion injury to the joint. We have demonstrated that both normal and rheumatoid synovia exhibit xanthine oxidase/dehydrogenase activity,[59] located in the capillary endothelium and rapidly converted from a dehydrogenase to an oxidase form.

Electron-spin resonance (ESR) spectroscopy is widely used as a method of identifying and characterizing free radicals in chemical systems. We used ESR spectroscopy coupled with spin-trapping techniques to study free-radical generation in rheumatoid synovium subjected to hypoxic/normoxic cycles *in vitro* and observed radical generation which was suppressed by allopurinol, thereby implicating xanthine oxidase as a source.[60,61]

It can be seen that under appropriate conditions, the human synovium has the biochemical potential to generate oxygen-derived free radicals. Does the joint possess the pathophysiological characteristics to produce a hypoxic-reperfusion event?

VII. HYPOXIC-REPERFUSION INJURY AND INFLAMMATORY SYNOVITIS

Several physiological features present within the inflamed human joint suggest that movement will provide the potential environment for hypoxic-reperfusion injury.

The IAP in the normal knee joint of both humans and animals is at or slightly below atmospheric pressure,[62,63] and it has been shown that quadriceps contraction produces a subatmospheric pressure. In contrast, patients with RA had significantly higher resting pressures than control subjects with a simulated effusion of the same volume. On quadriceps setting RA patients produced IAPs as high as 200 mmHg, well in excess of the synovial capillary perfusion pressure of 30 to 60 mmHg.[63] We fully support these findings, and find a dynamic inverse relationship between SF oxygen tension and IAP in inflammatory synovitis.[64]

The pO_2 in inflamed joints has been measured by several groups, and it is clear that inflammatory effusions have lower oxygen tensions than non-inflammatory effusions. One determinant of synovial fluid oxygen tension is the blood supply to the synovium. This should be related to the IAP, as the synovial membrane and joint capsule form a closed environment in which the IAP is transmitted directly to the synovial membrane vasculature.

We have recently studied microvascular perfusion dynamics within the synovium of the human knee during exercise using laser Doppler flowmetry. In the normal knee there was a negligible reduction of capillary perfusion during exercise. In contrast, exercise of the inflamed knee produced occlusion of the synovial capillary bed for the duration of the exercise period. Reperfusion of the synovial membrane occurred on cessation of exercise.[65]

An interesting clinical observation is that joints with acute synovitis secondary to trauma do not proceed to develop chronic synovitis. We have demonstrated that due to reflex muscle inhibition there is a failure of pathological IAP generation during exercise of joints with acute traumatic synovitis.[66] This provides protection against putative hypoxic-reperfusion injury thereby providing explanation for this clinical conundrum.

Exercise of the inflamed human knee joint provides the potential pathophysiological environment for the promotion of hypoxic-reperfusion injury. We have recently verified this by demonstrating exercise-induced oxidative damage to lipids and immunoglobulin G (IgG) within the knee joint of patients with inflammatory synovitis.[67] We employed proton Hahn spin-echo Fourier transform nuclear magnetic resonance spectroscopy (SEFT-NMR) to investigate the production of low molecular weight oligosaccharides derived from the oxygen radical-mediated depolymerization of SF hyaluronate. A resonance attributable to the *N*-acetyl methyl protons of a molecularly mobile oligosaccharide was detectable, and the signal increased in intensity subsequent to exercise.[68]

VIII. IRON CHELATION THERAPY IN RHEUMATOID ARTHRITIS

The process of hypoxic-reperfusion injury suggests many novel therapeutic approaches. One that we studied previously was the use of an iron chelator, desferrioxamine, in an attempt to suppress iron-promoted oxygen injury. This maneuver had been successful in animal models, significantly reducing the incidence and severity of inflammation and associated soft tissue swelling in rat adjuvant polyarthritis.[69] The approach cannot be recommended in patients, however, as desferrioxamine induced both cerebral and ocular toxicity.[70] In a pilot study, seven patients with rheumatoid disease were treated with desferrioxamine. Two of these patients, who also received the antiemetic prochlorperazine for nausea, lost consciousness for 48 to 72 h and then fully recovered. It is thought that the nausea was induced by the effect of iron chelators on the iron-dependent enzyme ribonucleotide reductase in the gut. Electroencephalographic studies showed abnormalities associated with the metabolic disturbance. Analysis of cerebrospinal fluid from one patient showed a decrease in loosely bound catalytic iron, and an increase in loosely bound (catalytic) copper, total iron, and products of lipid peroxidation with values approaching normal as symptoms resolved. This patient showed abnormal pyramidal features and subsequently developed an optic neuropathy and pigmentary retinopathy. Two other patients not receiving concomitant prochlorperazine developed retinal problems which later improved. Our ongoing investigations suggest a mechanism dependent on the ability of desferrioxamine to mobilize copper, to which it has an appreciable affinity (10^{14} for Cu[II], 10^{32} for Fe[III]).[71] An animal-based model for studying desferrioxamine-induced retinopathy was established in the albino rat.[72,73] The model measured the electroretinogram b wave amplitude. Ocular damage was exacerbated by increased levels of white light and oxygen. Intriguingly, studies in the model showed that darkness, and in particular red light, protected the eye against desferrioxamine toxicity. A family of novel orally active chelators, the hydroxypyridinones, have been tested for anti-inflammatory activity in animal models by our group. The hydroxypyridinones successfully compete for iron with apotransferrin and, under certain conditions, exceed desferrioxamine in their iron-scavenging abilities.[74] Many of these compounds are not ocularly toxic in our model and hold promise for clinical use.

IX. IRON AND DNA DAMAGE

The foregoing discussion has dealt with the mechanisms by which iron-catalyzed oxygen radical reactions may play a role in the pathogenesis of rheumatoid synovitis. We have indicated some pathways by which we believe iron may exacerbate an ongoing inflammatory process, but in this final section we wish to draw attention to the possible role of iron in the etiology of autoimmune inflammatory diseases. In the field of carcinogenesis, there is growing interest in the role of oxygen radical-mediated damage to DNA, a process in which iron is likely to play a critical role. It has now become clear that in mammalian systems, oxygen can become reduced to ROS by a wide variety of both enzymatic and nonenzymatic pathways as a result of normal metabolic processes. For example, up to 5% of the electrons entering the mitochondrial respiratory chain become uncoupled from it at a variety of points and singly "leak out" onto O_2 to form $O_2^{\cdot-}$. Uncoupling of electrons from the endoplasmic reticulum electron transport system can also occur, and is increased following exposure to various environmental agents.

It has been suggested that the endogenous production of oxygen radicals may play a part in carcinogenesis, via DNA damage and mutation.[75] We suggest[76] that oxygen radical-induced somatic mutation may play a role in the etiology of certain inflammatory autoimmune diseases, such as RA and systemic lupus erythematosus (SLE), for example, by producing mutant cells displaying "altered self" antigenic determinants.

Single- and double-strand scissions of DNA, together with hydroxylation of constituent bases, are changes characteristic of oxygen radical attack on DNA. An important mechanism is site-specific hydroxyl radical generation, catalyzed by iron bound to cellular DNA.[77] For example, the reaction of the hydroxyl radical with the DNA nucleoside deoxyguanosine results in the formation of 8-hydroxydeoxyguanosine (8-OHdG).[78] This adduct causes an increase in the frequency of misincorporation of DNA bases both at the damaged base and at the bases adjacent to it,[79] suggesting that it is a mutagen. Intracellular iron also appears to be essential for the induction of DNA strand breaks by H_2O_2 in cultured cells;[80] and it is thought that H_2O_2 diffuses through cell membranes into the nucleus of the cell, where it reacts with DNA-bound iron to generate $OH^{\cdot}$ locally.

Background levels of 8-OHdG are found in normal tissues as a result of normal metabolic production of ROS. However, 8-OHdG may be induced by exposure of target cells to ROS-generating agents or ROS themselves, e.g., X-irradiation[78] and H_2O_2.[80] *In vivo,* 8-OHdG is induced by exposure of rats to the ROS-generating carcinogens γ-irradiation,[78] 2-nitropropane,[81] clofibrate (a peroxisome proliferator),[82] and ferric-nitrilotriacetate.[83] The repair of 8-OHdG in DNA is catalyzed by an endonuclease, 8-OHdG DNA glycosylase, which appears to have identity with the previously isolated protein formamidopyrimidine DNA glycosylase (FPG protein).[84] As well as inducing DNA damage, oxidative stress inhibits the repair of DNA lesions.[85,86]

Gas chromatography-mass spectrometry with selected ion monitoring has been applied to the analysis of the base products produced by exposure of DNA to the hypoxanthine/xanthine oxidase system in the presence of iron ions.[87] The site specificity of $OH^{\cdot}$ generation could be altered by adding unchelated iron ions which bound to the DNA-leading to "site-specific" $OH^{\cdot}$ generation — or by adding Fe^{3+}-EDTA — leading to $OH^{\cdot}$ generation in free solution. They quantitated seven major products, but the relative proportions of these products were dependent on whether the system was set up for site-specific OH˙ generation. For example, for site-specific OH˙ formation, 8-OHdG was the major product with no marked increase in the level of 2,6-diamino-4-hydroxy-5-formamidopyrimidine (FapyGua); for free OH˙ formation FapyGua was the major product, followed by 8-OHdG. Comparative measurement of these products might allow "fingerprinting" of the extent to which site-specific OH˙-induced damage occurs.

High-performance liquid chromatography (HPLC) with electrochemical detection allows the determination of this adduct in femtomole amounts.[88] Using this technique, Ames' group[89] studied the oxidation state of DNA isolated from the nuclear DNA and mitochondrial DNA of rat liver. 8-OHdG was present at a level of 1 per 130,000 bases in nuclear DNA and 1 per 8,000 bases in mitochondrial DNA, and it was therefore proposed that mitochondrial DNA is exposed to greater fluxes of oxygen radicals. Given our recent understanding of uncoupling events in the respiratory chain (*vide supra*), this is a plausible hypothesis.

Levels of 8-OHdG have also been measured in human and rodent urine. Preliminary results indicate a trend toward lower levels in CGD patients than in normal control subjects.[90] It is also reported that urinary 8-OHdG levels are higher in mice than in humans.[91] However, it is not known whether this product in urine is derived exclusively from DNA via repair enzyme processes; oxidation of free guanine, normal purine metabolism, and/or dietary factors might contribute to urinary 8-OHdG.

Isolated human granulocytes produce high levels of ROS after exposure to tumor promoter tetradeconylphorbolacetate (TPA). Floyd et al.[88] showed that TPA-activated cells contained increased levels of 8-OHdG (about 1 8-OHdG per 600 guanine bases in their DNA) compared with nonactivated cells. This increase was prevented by the presence of SOD during exposure of the cells to TPA. This observation suggests that levels of 8-OHdG might be increased in the DNA of inflammatory cells from patients with various inflammatory diseases, making this DNA oxidation product a sensitive marker of cellular activation. Furthermore, our recent preliminary studies[88a] indicate increased levels of 8-OHdG in blood lymphocyte DNA from patients with RA and SLE compared with normal individuals.

Many chemotherapeutic drugs, e.g., adriamycin and bleomycin, appear to exert their cytotoxic actions by virtue of their ability to redox cycle within tumor cells, thus catalyzing DNA damage. Bleomycin forms a ternary complex with iron and DNA. The complex is then activated by the cytochrome P_{450} system to oxidize DNA in an oxygen-dependent reaction, possibly involving OH˙. The resulting DNA damage includes single- and double-strand breaks and release of bases.[92] It has also been shown that bleomycin will catalyze the hydroxylation of deoxyguanosine in DNA to form 8-OHdG.[93] However, we have found that although both bleomycin and γ-irradiation induce 8-OHdG formation in isolated DNA, no increase in 8-OHdG above control levels could be detected in intact human/rat hepatocytes exposed to bleomycin *in vitro* at 4 or 37°C.[94] Bleomycin does, however, induce unscheduled DNA synthesis in isolated, nonpermeabilized hepatocytes ([³H]thymidine incorporation), implying that 8-OHdG formation is not a major determinant of bleomycin-induced DNA repair.[76]

Unfortunately, oxidant-generating chemotherapeutic drugs produce long-term side effects, such as fibrosis, which may be related to extracellular generation of free radicals. Immediately following chemotherapy, patients have high plasma levels of catalytic iron, which might reflect ROS-mediated cell damage.[95] In isolated rat nuclei, SOD inhibits bleomycin-induced membrane peroxidation, but has no effect on bleomycin-catalyzed DNA scission.[92] Thus, it may be possible to use iron chelators to reduce the toxic extracellular side effects of these drugs, while leaving the intracellular therapeutic mode of action unaltered. In fact, it has been demonstrated that the cardiotoxicity of adriamycin can be inhibited by the chelating agent, ICRF-187.[95]

Relatively low levels of oxygen radicals stimulate fibroblast proliferation and collagen production[96] and may also play a role in the connective tissue disease scleroderma, which is characterized by excessive deposition of collagen and vascular damage. Several lines of evidence support this hypothesis: (1) a scleroderma-like condition can be produced in rats after repeated administration of bleomycin;[97] (2) the chromosomal aberrations seen in lymphocytes from scleroderma patients are suggested to be induced by oxygen radical-mediated DNA damage;[98] (3) 97% of scleroderma patients have Raynaud's phenomenon (episodic digital ischemia), a condition in which oxygen radical-mediated reperfusion injury has been implicated;[99] and (4) the plasma concentration of the vascular endothelial cell-derived von Willebrand factor antigen is elevated in scleroderma, but this rise is not paralleled by an increase in von Willebrand factor functional activity.[100] A similar phenomenon has been noted in acute respiratory failure,[101] possibly reflecting the oxidative inactivation of von Willebrand factor during its release from injured endothelial cells, which are putative target cells in both diseases.

Serum anti-DNA antibodies are a feature of several connective tissue diseases, including SLE. Preincubation of isolated DNA with a ROS-generating system resulted in a dose-dependent increase in binding of SLE anti-DNA antibodies.[102] This increased binding was inhibited by the ROS scavenger thiourea and the iron chelator desferrioxamine. It was suggested that oxidatively modified DNA is antigenic, stimulating the release of anti-DNA antibodies. This would be a process analogous to that proposed earlier for free-radical-modified IgG. Anti-IgG antibodies (rheumatoid factor) are present in rheumatoid extracellular fluids and have been shown to react with free-radical-altered IgG produced *in vitro*. As mentioned earlier, oxidatively modified IgG has been detected in rheumatoid synovial fluid from patients who have undergone an exercise program, indicating that this could be the antigenic stimulus for rheumatoid factor production.

DNA damage is an early event in cells killed by oxygen radicals. The capacity of endogenous intracellular antioxidants or the efficiency of repair mechanisms for oxidative DNA damage might determine the susceptibility of different cell populations to either killing or mutation. Lawley et al.[103] have demonstrated that circulating lymphocytes from patients with certain autoimmune diseases, e.g., RA, SLE, and Behcet's syndrome, show increased sensitivity to the toxic effects of the alkylating agent N-methyl-N-nitrosourea compared with normal subjects and patients with other disorders. The autoimmune disease cells are also relatively deficient in the DNA repair of O^6-methylguanine. Furthermore, lymphocytes from patients with a wide variety of autoimmune inflammatory conditions (e.g., RA, SLE) have a higher susceptibility to X-irradiation.[104] Such ionizing radiation can damage DNA by production of OH˙ radicals formed in the aqueous surroundings of the target DNA. In view of these findings, it is noteworthy that there is increasing evidence that oxygen radicals may play a part in mutation induced by a wide variety of agents.[105] Finally, attention should be drawn to the increased incidence of malignancy found at sites of chronic inflammation. It has been suggested that the link may be iron-promoted oxygen radical damage, since oxygen radicals are thought to be involved in both processes.[106]

X. SUMMARY

In conclusion, we have attempted to describe the central role of iron in disease from promotion through to carciongenesis including the persistence and exacerbation of an ongoing inflammatory response in RA and other diseases. Central to this argument is the metabolism and availability of iron in a form able to catalyze the formation of OH˙ (Figure 1). This we believe to be due to an alteration in normal RE iron kinetics leading to an increase in ferritin synthesis and deposition in the synovium and the anemia of chronic disease. Release of iron from ferritin by O_2^- produces hemosiderin and low molecular weight iron chelates. Another source of free iron is heme from intra-articular bleeding. The increase in acute phase reactants such as ferritin and lactoferrin is brought about by inflammatory mediators such as TNF-α, IL-1, and IL-6 as well as the production of ROS themselves. We have also described the production of ROS by hypoxic reperfusion where reflux of O_2 in the synovium activates the O form of xanthine oxidase, itself releasing iron from ferritin via the production of O_2^- leading to OH˙ formation. Evidence exists that there is an inverse relationship between SF pO_2 and IAP in synovium during exercise due to quadriceps contraction providing a suitable environment for ROS production. This leads to a cascade of damaging reactions to proteins (such as altered IgG giving rise to rheumatoid factor), carbohydrates, lipid peroxidation, and DNA damage. These hypotheses have been backed up by various clinical studies including the beneficial effects of iron chelation therapy.

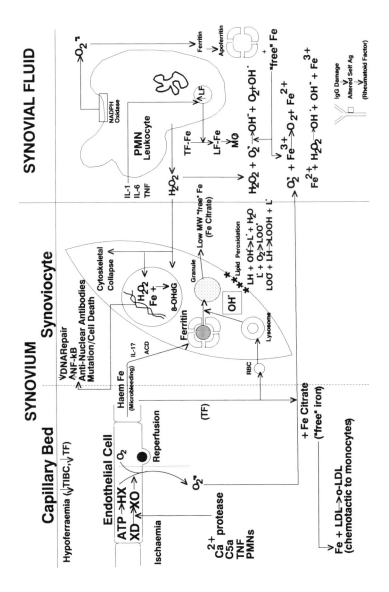

FIGURE 1. Schematic diagram summarizing the sources and interrelating actions of reactive oxygen species within the inflamed joint. The diagram also shows some possible sources of catalytic iron for the production of the hydroxyl radical.

We also describe evidence that iron bound to DNA leads to site-specific production of OH·, leading to DNA strand breaks and formation of 8-OHdG. Elegant evidence of the central role of ROS and iron in the inflammatory response has very recently been described by Schreck et al.[107] They have shown that ROS can act as intracellular second messengers via the activation of the inactive cytoplasmic form of a multisubunit transcription factor, NF-kB, by the release of the inhibitory subunit IkB. NF-kB activates the expression of genes involved in inflammatory, immune, and acute phase responses (including TNF-α, IL-6, interferon-β, granulocyte/macrophage colony-stimulating factor [GM-CSF], and induction of MHC class I antigens and IL-2 receptor). Furthermore, NF-kB has been identified in pre-B, B, and T lymphocytes; macrophages; monocytes; and a murine fibroblast cell line, Ltk⁻. Activation of NF-kB by H_2O_2 is dose dependent from 30 μM up to at least 150 μM (higher doses are cytotoxic). In addition, it appears that a metabolite of H_2O_2 activates NF-kB, as increased levels of thiols (such as glutathione) and the addition of iron chelators (such as desferrioxamine and o-phenanthroline) inhibit its induction. This suggests that it may be the iron-catalyzed production of OH· that is the activating factor.[107] Therefore, endogenous ROS defense mechanisms and ROS-producing enzymes may also be controlling factors of intracellular messengers that at elevated levels are cytotoxic.

REFERENCES

1. **De Sousa, M.,** Iron and the lymphomyeloid system: A growing knowledge, in *Iron in Immunity, Cancer and Inflammation,* de Sousa, M. and Brock, J. H., Eds., John Wiley & Sons, New York, 1989, 3.
2. **Lunec, J. and Blake, D. R.,** Oxidative damage and its relevance to inflammatory joint disease, in *Critical Reviews in Chemistry, Cellular Antioxidant Defense Mechanisms,* Vol. 3, Ching Quang Chow, Ed., CRC Press, Boca Raton, FL, 1988, 143.
3. **Lunec, J. and Blake, D. R.,** Oxygen free radicals: relevance to disease process, in *The Metabolic and Molecular Basis of Acquired Disease,* Cohen, R. D., Alberti, K. G. M. M., Lewis, B., and Denman, A. M., Eds., Bailliere Tindall, London, 1990, 29.
4. **Bullock, W. and Fildes, P.,** Haemophilia, in *A Treasury of Human Inheritance,* Vol. 1, Dulau & Co., London, 1912, section XIVa, 169.
5. **Morris, C. J., Wainwright, A. C., Steven, M. M., and Blake, D. R.,** The nature of iron deposits in haemophilic synovitis. An immunohistochemical, ultrastructural and X-ray microanalytical study, *Virchows Arch. A.,* 404, 75, 1984.
6. **Bentley, D. P. and Williams, P.,** Serum ferritin concentration as an index of storage iron in rheumatoid arthritis, *J. Clin. Pathol.,* 27, 786, 1974.
7. **Hansen, T. M., Hansen, N. E., Birgens, H. S., Holund, B., and Lorenzen, I.,** Serum ferritin and the assessment of iron deficiency in rheumatoid arthritis, *Scand. J. Rheumatol.,* 12, 353, 1983.
8. **Cartwright, G. E. and Lee, G. R.,** The anaemia of chronic disorders, *Br. J. Haematol.,* 21, 147, 1971.
9. **Deiss, A.,** Iron metabolism in reticuloendothelial cells, *Semin. Haematol.,* 20, 81, 1983.

10. **Fillet, G., Cook, J. D., and Finch, C. A.**, Storage iron kinetics VII. A biologic model for reticuloendothelial iron transport, *J. Clin. Invest.*, 53, 1527, 1974.

11. **Lee, G. R.**, The anaemia of chronic disease, *Semin. Haematol.*, 20, 61, 1983.

12. **Van Snick, J. L., Masson, P. L., and Heremans, J. F.**, The involvement of lactoferrin in the hyposideremia of acute inflammation, *J. Exp. Med.*, 140, 1068, 1974.

13. **Markowetz, B., Van Snick, J. L., and Masson, P. L.**, Binding and ingestion of human lactoferrin by mouse alveolar macrophages, *Thorax*, 34, 209, 1977.

14. **Brock, J. H. and Esparza, I.**, Failure of reticulocytes to take up iron from lactoferrin saturated by various methods, *Br. J. Haematol.*, 42, 481, 1979.

15. **Konijn, A. M. and Hershko, C.**, Ferritin synthesis in inflammation. Pathogenesis of impaired iron release, *Br. J. Haematol.*, 37, 7, 1977.

16. **Brailsford, S., Lunec, J., Winyard, P., and Blake, D. R.**, A possible role for ferritin during inflammation, *Free Radical Res. Commun.*, 1, 101, 1985.

17. **Smith, B. J., Speziale, S. C., and Bowman, B. J.**, Properties of interleukin-1 as a complete secretagogue for human neutrophils, *Biochem. Biophys. Res. Commun.*, 130, 1233, 1985.

18. **Fillet, G., Beguin, Y., and Baldelli, L.**, Model of reticuloendothelial iron metabolism in humans: abnormal behaviour in idiopathic haemochromatosis and in inflammation, *Blood*, 74, 844, 1989.

19. **Ramadori, G., Sipe, J. D., Dinarello, C. A., Mizel, S. B., and Colten, H. R.**, Pretranslational modulation of acute phase hepatic protein synthesis by murine recombinant interleukin-1 (IL-1) and purified human IL-1, *J. Exp. Med.*, 162, 930, 1985.

20. **Houssian, F. A., Devogelaer, J.-P., Damme, J. V., Deuxchaisnes, C. N., and Van Snick, J.**, Interleukin-6 in synovial fluid and serum of patients with rheumatoid arthritis and other inflammatory arthritides, *Arthritis Rheum.*, 31, 784, 1988.

21. **Darlington, G. J., Wilson, D. R., and Lachman, L. B.**, Monocyte-conditioned medium, interleukin-1 and tumour necrosis factor stimulate the acute phase response in human hepatoma cells *in vitro*, *J. Cell Biol.*, 103, 787, 1986.

22. **Andus, T., Geigner, T., Hirano, T., Kishimoto, T., and Heinrich, P. C.**, Action of recombinant human interleukin 6, interleukin 1 beta and tumour necrosis factor alpha of the mRNA induction of acute phase proteins, *Eur. J. Immunol.*, 18, 739, 1988.

23. **Brock, J. H. and Alvarez-Hernandez, X.**, Modulation of macrophage iron metabolism by tumour necrosis factor and interleukin 1, *FEMS Microbiol. Immunol.*, 1, 309, 1989.

24. **Muirden, K. D.**, Ferritin in synovial cells in patients with rheumatoid arthritis, *Ann. Rheum. Dis.*, 25, 387, 1966.

25. **Muirden, K. D., Fraser, J. R. G., and Clarris, B.**, Ferritin formation by synovial cells exposed to haemoglobin *in vitro*, *Ann. Rheum. Dis.*, 26, 251, 1969.

26. **Muirden, K. D. and Senator, G. B.**, Iron in the synovial membrane in rheumatoid arthritis and other joint disease, *Ann. Rheum. Dis.*, 27, 38, 1968.

27. **Muirden, K. D.**, The anaemia of RA: the significance of iron deposits in the synovial membrane, *Aust. Ann. Med.*, 2, 97, 1970.

28. **Bennet, R. M., Williams, E. D., Lewis, S. M., and Holt, P. J. L.**, Synovial Iron deposition in RA, *Arthritis Rheum.*, 16, 298, 1973.

29. **Yoshino, S., Blake, D. R., Hewitt, S., Morris, C., and Bacon, P. A.**, Effect of blood on the activity and persistence of antigen induced inflammation in the rat air pouch, *Ann. Rheum. Dis.*, 44, 485, 1985.

30. **Lin, J.-J., Danich-McQueen, S., Patino, M. M., Gaffield, L., Walden, W. E., and Thach, R. E.**, Depression of ferritin messenger RNA-translation by haemin *in vitro*, *Science*, 247, 74, 1990.

31. **Morris, C. J., Blake, D. R., Hewitt, S. D., and Lunec, J.**, Macrophage ferritin and iron deposition in the rat air pouch model of inflammatory synovitis, *Ann. Rheum. Dis.*, 46, 334, 1987.

414

32. **Blake, D. R., Gallagher, P. J., Potter, A. R., Bell, M. J., and Bacon, P. A.,** The effect of synovial iron on the progression of rheumatoid disease, *Arthritis Rheum.,* 27, 495, 1984.

33. **Blake, D. R., Hall, N. D., Bacon, P. A., Dieppe, P. A., Halliwell, B., and Gutteridge, J. M. C.,** The importance of iron in rheumatoid disease, *Lancet,* 8256, 1142, 1981.

34. **Winyard, P. G., Tatzber, F., Esterbauer, H., Blake, D. R., and Morris, C. J.,** Presence of oxidised low density lipoprotein-containing foam cells in the synovial membrane from patients with rheumatoid arthritis, *J. Clin. Invest.,* in press.

35. **Morris, C. J., Blake, D. R., Wainwright, A. C., and Steven, M. M.,** Relationship between iron deposits and tissue damage in the synovium: an ultrastructural study, *Ann. Rheum. Dis.,* 45, 21, 1986.

36. **Hamerman, D.,** Synovial joints. Aspects of structure and function, in *Chemistry and Molecular Biology of the Intercellular Matrix,* Balazs, E. S., Ed., Academic Press, London, 1970, 1259.

37. **Rogers, K. R., Morris, C. J., and Blake, D. R.,** Cytoskeletal rearrangement by oxidative stress, *Int. J. Tissue React.,* 11, 309, 1989.

38. **Rogers, K. R., Morris, C. J., and Blake, D. R.,** Oxidation of thiol in the vimentin cytoskeleton, *Biochem. J.,* 275, 789, 1990.

39. **Rowley, D. A., Gutteridge, J. M. C., Blake, D. R., Farr, M., and Halliwell, B.,** Lipid peroxidation in rheumatoid arthritis: thiobarbituric acid-reactive material and catalytic iron salts in synovial fluid from rheumatoid patients, *Clin. Sci.,* 66, 691, 1984.

40. **Gutteridge, J. M. C., Rowley, D. A., and Halliwell, B.,** Superoxide-dependent formation of hydroxyl radicals in the presence of iron salts. Detection of free iron in biological systems by using bleomycin-dependent degradation of DNA, *Biochem. J.,* 199, 263, 1981.

41. **Parkes, H. G., Allen, R. E., Furst, A., Blake, D. R., and Grootveld, M. C.,** Speciation of non-transferrin bound iron in synovial fluid from patients with rheumatoid arthritis by proton nuclear magnetic resonance spectroscopy, *J. Pharm. Biomed. Anal.,* 9, 29, 1991.

42. **Blake, D. R. and Bacon, P. A.,** Synovial fluid ferritin in rheumatoid arthritis, *Br. Med. J.,* 281, 715, 1980.

43. **Biemond, P., Eijk, H. G. V., Swaak, A. J. G., and Koster, J. F.,** Iron mobilization from ferritin by superoxide derived from stimulated PMN leucocytes, *J. Clin. Invest.,* 73, 1576, 1984.

44. **Blake, D. R. and Bacon, P. A.,** Synovial fluid ferritin in rheumatoid arthritis: an index or cause of inflammation, *Br. Med. J.,* 282, 189, 1981.

45. **Ahmadzadeh, N., Shingu, M., and Nobunaga, M.,** Iron-binding proteins and free iron in synovial fluids of rheumatoid arthritic patients, *Clin. Rheumatol.,* 8, 345, 1989.

46. **Hansen, T. M. and Hansen, N. E.,** Serum ferritin as indicator of iron responsive anaemia in patients with RA, *Ann. Rheum. Dis.,* 45, 596, 1986.

47. **Blake, D. R. and Bacon, P. A.,** Effect of oral iron on rheumatoid patients, *Lancet,* 1, 623, 1982.

48. **Reddy, P. A. and Lewis, M.,** Adverse effect of intravenous iron-dextran in rheumatoid arthritis, *Arthritis Rheum.,* 12, 454, 1969.

49. **Dabbagh, A. J., Morris, C. J., and Blake, D. R.,** Effect of iron complexes on adjuvant arthritis in the rat, *Ann. Rheum. Dis.,* in press, 1992.

50. **Lloyd, K. N. and Williams, P.,** Reactions to total dose infusion of iron dextran in RA, *Br. Med. J.,* 2, 323, 1970.

51. **Blake, D. R., Lunec, J., Ahern, M., Ring, E. F. J., Bradfield, J., and Gutteridge, J. M. C.,** Effect of i.v. iron dextran on rheumatoid synovitis, *Ann. Rheum. Dis.,* 44, 183, 1985.

52. **Winyard, P. G., Blake, D. R., Chirico, S., Gutteridge, J. M. C., and Lunec, J.,** Mechanism of exacerbation of rheumatoid synovitis by total-dose iron-dextran infusion: *in vivo* demonstration of iron promoted oxidant stress, *Lancet,* 1, 69, 1987.

53. **Woodruff, T., Blake, D. R., Freeman, J., Andrews, F. J., Salt, P., and Lunec, J.,** Is chronic synovitis an example of reperfusion injury?, *Ann. Rheum. Dis.,* 45, 608, 1986.

54. **McCord, J. M.,** Oxygen-derived free radicals in post-ischaemic tissue injury, *N. Engl. J. Med.,* 312, 159, 1985.

55. **Granger, D. N., Hollwarth, M. E., and Parks, D. A.,** Ischaemia reperfusion injury: role of oxygen derived free radicals, *Acta Physiol. Scand.,* Suppl. 548, 47, 1986.

56. **Jarasch, E. D., Bruder, G., and Heid, H. W.,** Significance of xanthine oxidase in capillary endothelial cells, *Acta Physiol. Scand.,* Suppl. 548, 39, 1986.

57. **Parkes, H. G., Allen, R. E., Furst, A., Blake, D. R., and Grootveld, M. C.,** Speciation of non-transferrin iron in synovial fluid from patients with rheumatoid arthritis by proton nuclear magnetic resonance spectroscopy, *J. Pharm. Biomed. Anal.,* 9, 29, 1991.

58. **Feidl, H. P., Till, G. O., Ryan, U. S., and Ward, P. A.,** Mediator-induced activation of xanthine oxidase in endothelial cells, *FASEB J.,* 3, 2512, 1989.

59. **Allen, R. E., Outhwaite, J., Morris, C. J., and Blake, D. R.,** Xanthine oxido-reductase is present in human synovium, *Ann. Rheum. Dis.,* 46, 843, 1987.

60. **Allen, R. E., Blake, D. R., Nazhat, N. B., and Jones, P.,** Superoxide radical generation by inflamed human synovium after hypoxia, *Lancet,* 2, 282, 1989.

61. **Nazhat, N. B., Yang, G., Allen, R. E., Blake, D. R., and Jones, P.,** Does 3,5,dibromo-4-nitrosobenzene sulphonate spin trap superoxide radicals, *Biochem. Biophys. Res. Commun.,* 166, 807, 1990.

62. **Dixon, A. and Hawkins, C., Eds.,** *Raised Intra-articular Pressure — Clinical Consequences,* Bath Institute for Rheumatic Diseases, Bath, 1990.

63. **Jayson, M. I. V. and Dixon, A.,** Intra-articular pressure in rheumatoid arthritis of the knee. III. Pressure changes during joint use, *Ann. Rheum. Dis.,* 29, 401, 1970.

64. **Unsworth, J., Outhwaite, J., Blake, D. R., Morris, C. J., Freeman, J., and Lunec, J.,** Dynamic studies of the relationship between intra-articular pressure, synovial fluid oxygen tension and lipid peroxidation in the inflamed knee: an example of reperfusion injury, *Ann. Clin. Biochem.,* 25, 8, 1988.

65. **Blake, D. R., Merry, P., Unsworth, J., Outhwaite, J., Morris, C. J., Gray, L., and Lunec, J.,** Hypoxic-reperfusion injury in the inflamed human joint, *Lancet,* 1, 289, 1989.

66. **Merry, P., Williams, R., Cox, N., King, J. B., and Blake, D. R.,** Comparative study of intra-articular pressure dynamics in acute traumatic and chronic inflammatory joint effusions: potential implications for hypoxic reperfusion injury, *Ann. Rheum. Dis.,* 50, 917, 1991.

67. **Merry, P., Grootveld, M., Lunec, J., and Blake, D. R.,** Oxidative damage to lipids within the inflamed human joint provides evidence of radical-mediated hypoxic-reperfusion injury, *Am. J. Clin. Nutr.,* 53, 362S, 1991.

68. **Henderson, E. B., Grootveld, M., Farrell, A., Smith, E. C., and Blake, D. R.,** A pathological role for damaged hyaluronan in synovitis, *Ann. Rheum. Dis.,* 50, 196, 1991.

69. **Andrews, F. J., Morris, C. J., Kondratowicz, G., and Blake, D. R.,** Effect of iron chelators on inflammatory joint disease, *Ann. Rheum. Dis.,* 46, 327, 1987.

70. **Blake, D. R., Winyard, P., and Lunec, J.,** Cerebral and ocular toxicity induced by desferrioxamine, *Q. J. Med.,* 56, 345, 1985.

71. **Pall, H., Blake, D. R., and Winyard, P.,** Ocular toxicity of desferrioxamine. An example of copper promoted auto-oxidative damage, *Br. J. Opthalmol.,* 73, 29, 1989.

72. **Good, P. A., Blake, D. R., Claxson, A., and Morris, C. J.,** Experimental models for desferrioxamine and oxygen toxicity of the retina, using the albino rat, in *Free Radicals, Diseased States and Anti-Radical Interventions,* Rice Evans, C., Ed., Richelieu Press, London, 1989, 167.

73. **Good, P. A., Claxson, A., Morris, C. J., and Blake, D. R.,** A model for desferrioxamine induced retinopathy using the albino rat, *Opthalmology,* 201, 32, 1990.

416

74. **Hewitt, S. D., Hider, R. C., Sarpong, P., Morris, C. J., and Blake, D. R.,** Investigation of the anti-inflammatory properties of hydroxypyridinones, *Ann. Rheum. Dis.,* 48, 382, 1989.

75. **Ames, B. N. and Saul, R. L.,** in *Theories of Carcinogenesis,* Inverson, O. H., Ed., Hemisphere Publ., Cambridge, 1988, 203.

76. **Winyard, P. G., Perrett, D., Blake, D. R., Harris, G., and Chipman, J. K.,** Measurement of DNA oxidation products, *Anal. Proc. (R. Soc. Chem.),* 27, 224, 1990.

77. **Loeb, L. A., James, E. A., Waltersdorph, A. M., and Klebanoff, S. J.,** Mutagenesis by the autoxidation of iron with isolated DNA, *Proc. Natl. Acad. Sci. U.S.A.,* 85, 3918, 1988.

78. **Kasai, H., Crain, P. F., Kuchino, Y., Nishimura, S., Ootsuyama, A., and Tanooka, H.,** Formation of 8-hydroxyguanine moiety in cellular DNA by agents producing oxygen radicals and evidence for its repair, *Carcinogenesis,* 7, 1849, 1986.

79. **Kuchino, Y., Mori, F., Kasai, H., Inoue, H., Iwai, S., Miura, K., Ohtsuka, E., and Nishimura, S.,** Misreading of DNA templates containing 8-hydroxydeoxyguanosine at the modified base and at adjacent residues, *Nature (London),* 327, 77, 1987.

80. **Schraufstatter, I., Hyslop, P. A., Jackson, J., and Cochrane, C. C.,** Oxidant-induced DNA damage of target cells, *J. Clin. Invest.,* 82, 1040, 1987.

81. **Fiala, E. S., Conaway, C. C., and Mathis, J. F.,** Oxidative DNA and RNA damage in the livers of Sprague-Dawley rats treated with the hepatocarcinogen 2-nitropropane, *Cancer Res.,* 49, 5518, 1989.

82. **Kasai, H., Okada, Y., Nishimura, S., Rao, M. S., and Reddy, J. K.,** Formation of 8-hydroxydeoxyguanosine in liver DNA of rats following long-term exposure to a peroxisome proliferator, *Cancer Res.,* 49, 2603, 1989.

83. **Unemura, T., Sai, K., Takagi, A., Hasegawa, R., and Kurokawa, Y.,** Formation of 8-hydroxyguanosine (8-OHdG) in rat kidney DNA after intraperitoneal administration of ferric nitrilotriacetate (Fe-NTA), *Carcinogenesis,* 11, 345, 1990.

84. **Tchou, J., Kasai, H., Shibutani, S., Chung, M.-H., Laval, J., Grollman, A. P., and Nishimura, S.,** 8-oxoguanine (8-hydroxyguanine) DNA glycosylase and its substrate specificity, *Proc. Natl. Acad. Sci. U.S.A.,* 88, 4690, 1991.

85. **Krokan, H., Grafstrom, R. C., Sundqvist, K., Esterbauer, H., and Harris, C. C.,** Cytotoxicity, thiol depletion and inhibition of O^6-methylguanine-DNA methyltransferase by various aldehydes in cultured human bronchial fibroblasts, *Carcinogenesis,* 6, 1755, 1985.

86. **Pero, R. W., Anderson, M. W., Doyle, G. A., Anna, C. H., Romagna, F., Markowitz, M., and Byrngelsson, C.,** Oxidative stress induces DNA damage and inhibits the repair of DNA lesions induced by N-acetoxy-2-acetylaminofluorene in human peripheral monomuclear leukocytes, *Cancer Res.,* 50, 4619, 1990.

87. **Aruoma, O. I., Halliwell, B., and Dizdaroglu, M.,** Iron ion-dependent modification of bases in DNA by the superoxide radical-generating system hypoxanthine/xanthine oxidase, *J. Biol. Chem.,* 264, 13024, 1989.

88. **Floyd, R. A., Watson, J. J., Harris, J., West, M., and Wong, P. K.,** Formation of 8-hydroxydeoxyguanosine, hydroxyl free radical adduct of DNA in granulocytes exposed to the tumour promoter, tetradeconylphorbolacetate, *Biochem. Biophys. Res. Commun.,* 137, 841, 1986.

88a. **Bashir, S., Harris, G., Blake, D. R., Dunman, A. M., Black, C. M., and Winyard, P. G.,** Oxidative DNA damage in human autoimmune disease, *Int. J. Radiat. Biol.,* in press.

89. **Richter, C., Park, J.-W., and Ames, B. N.,** Normal oxidative damage to mitochondrial and nuclear DNA is extensive, *Proc. Natl. Acad. Sci. U.S.A.,* 85, 6465, 1988.

90. **Cundy, K. C., Kohen, R., and Ames, B. N.,** Determination of 8-hydroxydeoxyguanosine in human urine: a possible assay for *in vivo* oxidative DNA damage, in *Oxygen Radicals in Biology and Medicine,* Simic, M. G., Taylor, K. A., Ward, J. F., and von Sonntag, C., Eds., Plenum Press, New York, 1988, 479.

91. **Bergtold, D. S., Simic, M. G., Alessio, H., and Cutler, R. G.,** Urine biomarkers for oxidative DNA damage, in *Oxygen Radicals in Biology and Medicine,* Simic, M. G., Taylor, K. A., Ward, J. F., and von Sonntag, C., Eds., Plenum Press, New York, 1988, 483.

92. **Ciriolo, M. R., Peisach, J., and Magliozzo, R. S.,** A comparative study of the interactions of bleomycin with nuclei and purified DNA, *J. Biol. Chem.,* 264, 1443, 1989.

93. **Kohda, K., Kasai, H., Ogawa, T., Suzuki, T., and Kawazoe, Y.,** Deoxyribonucleic acid (DNA) damage induced by bleomycin-Fe(II) *in vitro*: formation of 8-hydroxyguanine residues in DNA, *Chem. Pharm. Bull.,* 37, 1028, 1989.

94. **Smith, A. J., Winyard, P. G., and Chipman, J. K.,** Bleomycin and gamma-radiation induced hydroxylation of deoxyguanosine *in vitro,* in *Int. Symp. Biol. React. Intermediates,* Abstract of the Fourth International Symposion of Biological Reactive Intermediates, Tuscon, January 1990.

95. **Halliwell, B. and Bomford, A.,** ICRF-187 and doxorubicin-induced cardiac toxicity, *N. Engl. J. Med.,* 320, 399, 1989.

96. **Murrell, G. A. C., Francis, M. J. O., and Bromley, L.,** Free radicals and Dupuytren's contracture, *Br. Med. J.,* 295, 1373, 1987.

97. **Mountz, J. D., Downs Minor, M. B., Turner, R., Thomas, M. B., Richards, F., and Pisko, E.,** Bleomycin-induced cutaneous toxicity in the rat: analysis of histopathology and ultrastructure compared with progressive systemic sclerosis (scleroderma), *Br. J. Dermatol.,* 108, 679, 1983.

98. **Emerit, I., Keck, M., Levy, A., Feingold, J., and Michelson, A. M.,** Activated oxygen species at the origin of chromosome breakage and sister-chromatid exchanges, *Mutat. Res.,* 103, 165, 1982.

99. **Chopra, M., Smith, W. E., Ansell, D., and Belch, J. J. F.,** Free radical pathology in Raynaud's phenomenon, *Acta Chir. Scand.,* 546 (Suppl.), 51a, 1988.

100. **Greaves, M., Malia, R. G., Ward, A. M., Moult, J., Holt, C. M., Lindsey, N., Hughes, P., Goodfield, M., and Rowell, N. R.,** Elevated von Willebrand factor antigen in systemic sclerosis: relationship to visceral disease, *Br. J. Rheumatol.,* 27, 281, 1988.

101. **Carvalho, A. C. A., Bellman, S. M., Saullo, V. J., Quinn, D., and Zapol, W. M.,** Altered factor VIII in acute respiratory failure, *N. Engl. J. Med.,* 307, 1113, 1982.

102. **Blount, S., Griffiths, H. R., and Lunec, J.,** Reactive oxygen species induce antigenic changes in DNA, *FEBS Lett.,* 245, 100, 1989.

103. **Lawley, P. D., Topper, R., Denman, A. M., Hylton, W., Hill, I. D., and Harris, G.,** Increased sensitivity of lymphocytes from patients with systemic autoimmune diseases to DNA alkylation by the methylating carcinogen *N*-methyl-*N*-nitrosourea, *Ann. Rheum. Dis.,* 47, 445, 1988.

104. **Harris, G., Cramp, W. A., Edwards, J. C., George, A. M., Sabovljev, S. A., Hart, L., Hughes, G. R. V., Denman, A. M., and Yatvin, M. B.,** Radiosensitivity of peripheral blood lymphocytes in autoimmune disease, *Int. J. Radiat. Biol.,* 47, 689, 1985.

105. **Hsie, A. W., Recio, L., Katz, D. S., Lee, C. Q., Wagner, M., and Schenley, R. L.,** Evidence for reactive oxygen species inducing mutations in mammalian cells, *Proc. Soc. Acad. Sci. U.S.A.,* 83, 9616, 1986.

106. **Trush, M. A., Seed, J. L., and Kensler, T. W.,** Oxidant-dependent metabolic activation of polycyclic aromatic hydrocarbons by phorbol ester-stimulated human polymorphonuclear leukocytes: possible link between inflammation and cancer, *Proc. Natl. Acad. Sci. U.S.A.,* 82, 5194, 1985.

107. **Schreck, R., Rieber, P., and Baeuerle, P. A.,** Reactive oxygen intermediates as apparently widely used messengers in the activation of the NF-kB transcription factor and HIV-1, *EMBO J.,* 10, 2247, 1991.

17. Iron and Ethanol-Induced Tissue Damage: Generation of Reactive Oxygen Intermediates and Possible Mechanisms for Their Role in Alcohol Liver Toxicity

ARTHUR I. CEDERBAUM

Department of Biochemistry, The Mount Sinai School of Medicine, New York, New York

I. INTRODUCTION

There is growing interest in the role that reactive oxygen intermediates play in a variety of diseases, in the reaction systems which generate these radicals, and in the antioxidative systems which protect against the toxic actions of these radicals. Reactive oxygen intermediates have been implicated in the toxicity associated with ionizing radiation, ozone, and cigarette smoke; deficiency of essential metals such as selenium or vitamins such as α-tocopherol (vitamin E); iron overload; halogenated solvents such as carbon tetrachloride; a variety of xenobiotics including acetaminophen, polycyclic aromatic hydrocarbons, and nitrosamines; and redox cycling antitumor agents such as adriamycin, halothane, etc. Oxygen radicals have also been implicated in cancer, ischemia-reperfusion injury, and aging and alcohol toxicity. The purpose of this chapter is to review some of the chemistry of oxygen radicals, especially the critical role of iron, and to describe possible mechanisms by which alcohol can result in increased production of reactive oxygen intermediates. Special significance will be attached to the interaction of iron with biological organelles such as microsomes and the effects of alcohol on these interactions.

A free radical is a species which contains an unpaired electron in an outer orbital. Such radicals may be neutral, e.g., quinone, vitamin E, glutathione radical; or positively (cation) charged, e.g., paraquat radical; or negatively (anion) charged, e.g., superoxide radical. Free radicals are very reactive because of the tendency of the unpaired electron to pair with another electron. Because aerobic metabolism yields considerably more energy than anaerobic metabolism, most species utilize molecular oxygen as a final electron acceptor in the ultimate degradation of the food stuff which they ingest. Under certain conditions, oxygen can be toxic, inactivating enzymes, destroying membranes, mutating DNA, and producing cell death. It is now clear that the toxicity of molecular oxygen is not due to oxygen per se, which by itself possesses weak reactivity, but is due to the production of reactive oxygen intermediates such as superoxide radical, hydrogen peroxide, singlet oxygen, and the hydroxyl radical ($OH^{\cdot}$).

In the ground state, oxygen is paramagnetic since it contains two unpaired electrons in its outer orbitals. These electrons have parallel spins which make oxygen poorly reactive, since direct addition of a pair of electrons from a substrate to oxygen is spin-forbidden, i.e., one of the electrons in the outer orbital of oxygen would have to be inverted in order to avoid having two electrons with the same spin in one orbital. Inversion of electronic spin is relatively slow as compared to the lifetime of a collisional complex, therefore ground-state oxygen (triplet oxygen) is relatively inert toward direct two-electron reduction. By contrast, singlet oxygen, in which one of the outer electrons has been inverted, is very reactive, especially with high electron-dense species, e.g., unsaturated substrates. Because of this spin restriction, molecular oxygen is more amenable to univalent reduction, which yields the superoxide anion radical.

A scheme for the tetravalent reduction of oxygen follows:

$$\text{Triplet oxygen } {}^3O_2 \longrightarrow {}^1O_2 \text{ (singlet)}$$
$$\downarrow e^-$$

$$\text{Superoxide} \quad O_2^{\cdot -} \xrightarrow{\text{pK 4.8}} HO_2^{\cdot}$$
$$\downarrow e^-$$

$$\text{Peroxide} \quad O_2^{=} \xrightarrow{\text{pK 14}} HO_2^{-} \xrightarrow{\text{pK 12}} H_2O_2$$
$$\downarrow e^-$$

$$[O_2^{3-}] \xrightarrow{2H^+} H_2O$$

$$\downarrow$$

$$\text{Hydroxyl} \quad O^- \xrightarrow{\text{pK 12}} OH^{\cdot}$$
$$\downarrow e^-$$

$$O^{=} \xrightarrow{2H^+} H_2O$$

II. REACTIVE OXYGEN INTERMEDIATES

A. SUPEROXIDE RADICAL

There is considerable evidence for the production of superoxide in biological systems.[1-7] This radical is produced by a variety of oxidative enzymes such as xanthine oxidase, aldehyde oxidase, and dihydroorotic acid dehydrogenase; by organelles which possess electron-transfer systems such as mitochondria, chloroplasts, microsomes, and nuclei; by autoxidation of substrates such as flavins, quinones, and catecholamines; by autoxidation of proteins such as hemoglobin or ferredoxin; by radiation; and even by intact cells, e.g., the respiratory burst of activated phagocytes. Superoxide is the conjugate base of a weak acid, the perhydroxyl radical ($HO_2^{\cdot}$) with a pK of 4.8; although $HO_2^{\cdot}$ is much more reactive than superoxide radical at physiological pH, more than 99% of univalent-reduced oxygen is in the superoxide form. Superoxide is a good reductant with a redox potential of about -0.30 V ($O_2^{\cdot -} \rightarrow O_2$) and a good oxidant with a redox potential of about $+1.7$ V ($O_2^{\cdot -} \rightarrow O_2^{2-}$). An important reaction which superoxide undergoes is reaction with itself. In this dismutation, one superoxide is oxidized, while the other is reduced:

$$O_2^{\cdot -} + O_2^{\cdot -} + 2H^+ \rightarrow O_2 + H_2O_2 \quad K < 100/M/s \quad (1)$$

$$HO_2^{\cdot} + O_2^{\cdot-} + H^+ \rightarrow O_2 + H_2O_2 \quad K = 8.5 \times 10^7 \quad (2)$$

$$HO_2^{\cdot} + HO_2^{\cdot} \rightarrow O_2 + H_2O_2 \quad K = 7.6 \times 10^5 \quad (3)$$

At physiological pH, the dismutation is quite slow because of charge repulsion; however, the reaction is markedly accelerated to a rate constant of about $2 \times 10^9/M/s$ by the enzyme superoxide dismutase (SOD). Indeed, the discovery of SOD by McCord and Fridovich,[8] which ascribed an enzymatic function for proteins such as erythrocuprein, hepatocuprein, and cerebrocuprein, led to the rapid growth and development of the role of free radicals in biology and medicine, since it provided a tool for the biochemist to evaluate these reactions.

There are three types of SOD: an iron-containing enzyme found in bacteria, a manganese-containing enzyme found in mitochondria, and a copper/zinc enzyme found in the cytosol of eukaryotes. The mechanism, at least for the Cu/Zn SOD, is fairly well understood, with the Cu^{2+} being reduced by one superoxide, and the resulting Cu^+ being oxidized by the second superoxide:

$$Cu^{2+} + O_2^{\cdot-} \rightarrow Cu^+ + O_2 \quad (4)$$

$$Cu^+ + O_2^{\cdot-} \rightarrow Cu^{2+} + O_2^{2-} \quad (5)$$

SOD possesses one of the highest turnover numbers known. To date, its only known function is to catalyze the dismutation of superoxide.

The literature is replete with studies which demonstrate that superoxide reacts with cellular molecules such as cytochrome c and epinephrine; inactivates various enzymes; depolymerizes macromolecules such as hyaluronic acid and collagen; oxidizes polyunsaturated fatty acids; nicks DNA; causes membrane lysis; promotes inflammation; and kills viruses, bacteria, and mammalian cells. The superoxide theory of oxygen toxicity essentially proposes that oxygen is toxic because of the production of the superoxide radical, and that SOD is an important antioxidative defense against oxygen toxicity because it catalyzes the rapid removal of superoxide. There appears to be a positive correlation between the content of SOD or its inducibility and the tolerance to oxygen and to agents that are toxic because of the production of oxygen radicals (e.g., paraquat). While not all investigators have accepted the superoxide theory of oxygen toxicity (see following), it still remains an attractive theory which accommodates much of the data in the literature. With respect to the protective role of SOD, increased production of H_2O_2 caused by catalysis of superoxide dismutation can at times lead to toxicity,[9] since H_2O_2 is also reactive. Hence, SOD must function in conjunction with other enzymes which can remove H_2O_2.

B. HYDROGEN PEROXIDE

H_2O_2 is the most stable of the reactive oxygen intermediates and is produced from the dismutation of superoxide and from the divalent reduction of oxygen by oxidases found primarily in the peroxisomes, as well as decay of the peroxy-cytochrome P-450 intermediate. H_2O_2 is an oxidizing agent, and is especially reactive with thiol residues of proteins and enzymes. H_2O_2 may also be toxic because it is a precursor of OH· (see following). Similar to studies with superoxide, there are numerous reports that H_2O_2 inactivates enzymes, causes membrane lysis, and is cytotoxic. The major two peroxidases in most mammalian cells which remove H_2O_2 are catalase and glutathione (GSH) peroxidase. Catalase is a heme-containing enzyme found primarily in the peroxisomes; it can remove H_2O_2 via a catalatic or peroxidatic mode of action.

$$H_2O_2 + H_2O_2 \rightarrow 2H_2O + O_2 \tag{6}$$

$$H_2O_2 + AH_2 \rightarrow 2H_2O + A \tag{7}$$

AH_2 can be substrates such as methanol, ethanol, formate, or formaldehyde. Catalase has been of interest in the alcohol field as being a possible pathway of ethanol oxidation, as playing a role in the microsomal ethanol oxidizing system, and in generating acetaldehyde in the central nervous system.

In view of the cellular localization of catalase, the rather higher K_m for H_2O_2 coupled to second order kinetics for catalatic activity, and the fact that acatalasemics which lack catalase survive rather well, the need and presence of a second enzyme system to detoxify H_2O_2 is apparent. GSH peroxidase is found in the cytosolic and mitochondrial fractions of the cell and catalyzes the following reaction:

$$2GSH + H_2O_2 \rightarrow GSSG + 2H_2O \tag{8}$$

The GSH peroxidase functions together with another enzyme, GSH reductase, to regenerate GSH and remove GSSG, which can be toxic because of the formation of mixed disulfides:

$$GSSG + 2NADPH \rightarrow 2GSH + 2NADP^+ \tag{9}$$

GSH peroxidase contains selenocysteine at the active site and can also remove lipid and organic hydroperoxides besides H_2O_2. Conditions which promote oxidative stress result in depletion of NADPH and accumulation of GSSG. It would appear that the GSH peroxidase system is important for removal of H_2O_2 produced in the mitochondria, microsomes, and cytosol, whereas catalase removes H_2O_2 produced in the peroxisomes.

C. HYDROXYL RADICAL

The hydroxyl radical is the most reactive of the various oxygen intermediates, reacting with almost anything it comes in contact with. While this radical can be directly produced from radiation of aqueous solutions ($H_2O \rightarrow H^{\cdot} + OH^{\cdot}$), in most biological systems, $OH^{\cdot}$ is derived from H_2O_2 by a metal-catalyzed reaction. Early studies found that $OH^{\cdot}$ was produced by systems in which superoxide was generated, and it was proposed that the $OH^{\cdot}$ was produced by a Haber-Weiss type of reaction:[10-12]

$$O_2^{\cdot-} + H_2O_2 \rightarrow OH^{\cdot} + OH^- + O_2 \qquad (10)$$

Although thermodynamically feasible, this reaction was kinetically too slow to reasonably account for the production of $OH^{\cdot}$ in most reaction systems. Reaction 10 can be catalyzed by metals such as iron or copper, and it was therefore proposed that $OH^{\cdot}$ was produced by a metal-catalyzed Haber-Weiss reaction in which superoxide functions to reduce the metal, followed by a Fenton reaction between the reduced metal and H_2O_2 to yield $OH^{\cdot}$:

$$Fe^{3+}(Cu^{2+}) + O_2^{\cdot-} \rightarrow Fe^{2+}(Cu^+) + O_2 \qquad (11)$$

$$Fe^{2+}(Cu^+) + H_2O_2 \rightarrow Fe^{3+}(Cu^{2+}) + OH^- + OH^{\cdot} \qquad (12)$$

The net result of these two reactions is the Haber-Weiss reaction in which the metal continues to redox cycle between the reduced and oxidized forms. Since superoxide itself is poorly reactive with most biochemical intermediates and macromolecules (whereas $OH^{\cdot}$ is extremely reactive), formation of $OH^{\cdot}$ from O_2 was proposed to account for the toxicity of $O_2^{\cdot-}$. An important role for superoxide in this superoxide theory of oxygen toxicity was to promote the reduction of oxidized metals to the reduced redox state, and thereby promote the generation of $OH^{\cdot}$ from H_2O_2. SOD, by scavenging superoxide, should prevent this reaction and thus be protective. Consistent with this suggestion are the many observations that the toxicity of oxygen and superoxide is not only prevented by SOD, catalase, and GSH peroxidase, but also by scavengers of $OH^{\cdot}$ as well as by metal-chelating agents.

Immediate controversy concerning the previous reaction pathway revolved around the fact that metals are generally not found in high amounts in the "free" state, e.g., most iron is complexed as ferritin which is inert in generating $OH^{\cdot}$; and that if available, metals such as iron and copper can be reduced by cellular reductants, such as GSH or ascorbate, which are found in much higher concentrations than superoxide. While clear resolution has not been obtained, numerous studies appear to support a role for $OH^{\cdot}$ (and metal catalysis) in superoxide toxicity.

D. LIPID PEROXIDATION

One important mechanism by which reactive oxygen intermediates damage cells appears to be via peroxidation of membrane lipids.[6,13-16] The allylic divinyl methane groups of polyunsaturated fatty acids are very sensitive to hydrogen abstraction by $OH^{\cdot}$ and other oxidants to yield the lipid radical, $L^{\cdot}$. Propagation of $L^{\cdot}$ via interaction with oxygen and with other lipids readily occurs, with the subsequent breakdown of membrane lipids before termination finally occurs. Metals such as iron often play a central role in the lipid peroxidation process:[17]

$$LH + OH^{\cdot}(\text{or other oxidant}) \rightarrow L^{\cdot} + H_2O \quad \text{Initiation} \quad (13)$$

$$L^{\cdot} + O_2 \rightarrow LOO^{\cdot} \quad (14)$$

$$LOO^{\cdot} + L^1H \rightarrow LOOH + L^{1\cdot} \quad \text{Propagation} \quad (15)$$

$$LOOH + Fe^{2+} \rightarrow LO^{\cdot} + Fe^{3+} + OH^- \quad (16)$$

$$LOOH + Fe^{3+} \rightarrow LOO^{\cdot} + H^+ + Fe^{2+} \quad (17)$$

$$LOO^{\cdot} + L^{1\cdot} \rightarrow LOOL^1 \quad \text{Termination} \quad (18)$$

$$L^{\cdot} + \text{vitamin E} \rightarrow LH + \text{vitamin E}^{\cdot} \quad (19)$$

Major defense against lipid peroxidation is via the GSH peroxidase system to remove lipid hydroperoxides (LOOH), and most importantly, vitamin E, which is present in most biological membranes and readily reacts with lipid radicals to cause chain termination. The vitamin E radical so produced is reoxidized back to vitamin E at the expense of ascorbate (vitamin C). Glutathione also helps to regenerate and maintain vitamin E levels.

A variety of analytical methods are available to assay for the occurrence of lipid peroxidation. These include direct assay of the lipid hydroperoxide; the decrease in content of polyunsaturated fatty acids from membrane phospholipids; the production of fragmented products from the breakdown of the lipid peroxide, e.g., malondialdehyde, alkanes such as ethane and pentane, and aldehydic products such as 8-hydroxy-2-nonenal; and the occurrence of conjugated dienes. All methods suffer a variety of weaknesses including lack of specificity and sensitivity, further metabolism and artifactual formation.[13,15,17] Despite these considerable problems, lipid peroxidation has been found to occur under conditions in which generation of reactive oxygen intermediates is increased, e.g., metabolism of halogenated hydrocarbons such as carbon tetrachloride; in the presence of redox cycling agents such as adriamycin; during iron overload; and during ischemia-reperfusion injury. It is, however, not clear whether the peroxidation is a cause of, or a consequence of, the cell toxicity which is occurring. Diluzio[18-20] was among the first to report that ethanol could produce an increase in lipid peroxidation in the liver, and that antioxidants could prevent the ethanol-induced fatty liver. The ability of ethanol to cause lipid peroxidation remains controversial (reviewed by Dianzani[21]), which may not be surprising in view of the numerous variables that exist in the reaction conditions employed by investigators; these have been briefly reviewed elsewhere.[22]; Although considerable more research is required, there is a growing amount of literature that ethanol administered acutely or chronically can increase the production of reactive oxygen species in the liver, at least under certain conditions.

III. SUGGESTED POSSIBILITIES WHEREBY ETHANOL MAY INCREASE OXIDATIVE STRESS IN THE LIVER

The background previously discussed serves to suggest a multitude of ways by which acute and chronic ethanol administration can induce oxidative stress to the liver. Aspects of these possibilities have been reviewed elsewhere.[21-25] A brief summary of some of these potential mechanisms follows. Particular emphasis will be placed on the latter possibilities, since in keeping with the theme of this volume, they involve critical roles for iron.

A. ALTERED ANTIOXIDANT ACTIVITIES

Sufficient levels of antioxidative enzymes and biochemicals are required to remove reactive oxygen intermediates or prevent their formation. Although some controversy exists, in general, ethanol does not appear to significantly alter the activities of catalase, SOD, GSH peroxidase, or GSH reductase.[26,27] Perhaps more significantly, there are many reports that ethanol decreases the content of vitamin E, the most important chain terminator of the lipid peroxidation process.[28-30].

GSH levels in the liver are decreased by acute ethanol administration.[23] GSH is an important antioxidant by itself and as a component of the GSH-peroxidase system. However, the fall in GSH levels are rather modest, typically being in the order of 25 to 40%. In general, GSH levels must be markedly lowered (>90%) before elevation of lipid peroxidation is found.[31] The fall in GSH appears to be due to decreased synthesis and increased turnover rather than an oxidative-related reaction.[32,33] Although acute ethanol lowers GSH, chronic ethanol does not appear to have any significant effect. The finding that mitochondrial GSH may be more sensitive to ethanol than cytosolic GSH[34] could be important because mitochondrial damage is frequently observed after chronic ethanol treatment.[35-37]

B. DAMAGE TO MITOCHONDRIA

Reduction of oxygen by the mitochondrial respiratory chain is normally tightly coupled via cytochrome oxidase to four-electron reduction to water. Inhibition of the respiratory chain and uncoupled respiration increases production of superoxide and peroxide.[38] Damage to the mitochondrial respiratory chain as a consequence of chronic alcohol treatment[36-38] can promote auto-oxidation of reduced electron carriers to yield reactive oxygen species. Increased superoxide production by liver submitochondrial particles after *in vivo* ethanol administration has been reported.[39]

C. CONVERSION OF XANTHINE DEHYDROGENASE TO XANTHINE OXIDASE

Considerable attention has been focused on the role of xanthine oxidase in generating oxidative stress during ischemia reperfusion. Normally this enzyme exists primarily in a dehydrogenase form, but can be converted by proteolysis and/or thiol oxidation to the oxidase form, which yields superoxide and H_2O_2. Ethanol has been shown to convert xanthine dehydrogenase to the oxidase form.[40,41] In addition, redox inhibition of the dehydrogenase form by ethanol-derived NADH can promote the oxidase reaction.[42] Acetaldehyde can serve as a substrate for the enzyme; however, the K_m is very high, and therefore generation of oxygen radicals during acetaldehyde oxidation by xanthine oxidase may not be physiologically significant.

D. ACETALDEHYDE OXIDATION

Acetaldehyde can be oxidized by aldehyde oxidase, yielding superoxide, although the K_m for acetaldehyde is still rather high; a recent study suggested this pathway as a mechanism for acetaldehyde-induced lipid peroxidation.[43] Muller and Sies[44,45] have shown that acetaldehyde oxidation by liver cells results in increased lipid peroxidation; Kera et al.[46] indicated that acetaldehyde metabolism played a role in the lipid peroxidation caused by ethanol. How acetaldehyde oxidation by the low-K_m mitochondrial aldehyde dehydrogenase causes production of oxygen radicals is not clear because direct reaction between GSH and acetaldehyde is weak.[47] Acetaldehyde may react with superoxide or OH˙ to produce excited carbonyl species or acetaldehyde radicals with a more defined cellular lifetime.[48,49]

E. FORMATION OF HYDROXYETHYL RADICAL

Production of ethanol radicals, primarily the hydroxyethyl radical (CH_3 CHOH˙), is receiving increasing interest. This radical will be produced when ethanol is oxidized by potent oxidizing species such as OH˙ or peroxy cytochrome P-450. Albano et al.[50,51] and Reinke et al.[52,53] have observed production of this radical when microsomes were incubated with ethanol and NADPH; suggested mechanisms for its production involved both oxygen radical-dependent and -independent pathways. The latter appeared to be via direct oxidation by P-450; the alcohol-inducible cytochrome P-450 isozyme appeared to be especially reactive in oxidizing ethanol to the hydroxyethyl radical, and it was suggested that the capacity for the alcohol-inducible P-450 isozyme (cytochrome P-4502E1) to reduce oxygen is related to its ability to generate alcohol-free radicals and that the ferric-P-450-oxygen complex might act as an oxidizing species toward alcohols.[54] Concerning the oxygen radical-dependent pathway, a critical role for iron was implicated based on the inhibition by desferrioxamine and the augmentation of the electron-spin resonance (ESR) signal by the addition of iron chelates such as iron EDTA or iron ADP.[50,51,53] Production of the hydroxyethyl radical by this iron-dependent pathway was suggested to involve OH· or a similar oxidant produced via a Fenton-type reaction from microsomal-generated H_2O_2 and iron.[50-52] Direct evidence for *in vivo* formation of free radicals following the acute or chronic administration of ethanol was obtained by a spin-trapping, ESR study.[51] Carbon-centered radicals were found in liver extracts of rats that had been fed an ethanol-containing diet for 2 weeks, whereas no such signals were observed in controls fed a similar diet, but lacking ethanol. The carbon-centered radicals were presumed to be lipid radicals. It was suggested that the carbon-centered radicals might have arisen from the interaction of microsomal lipids with the hydroxyethyl radical, produced from the oxidation of ethanol by the microsomal mixed function oxidase system.[51] Knecht et al.[55] have observed the hydroxyethyl radical in the bile of deer mice that are lacking alcohol dehydrogenase, the major enzyme responsible for oxidation of ethanol, suggesting other alcohol-oxidizing pathways (e.g., microsomal) may be responsible for generating the hydroxyethyl radical. The physiological and toxicological significance of this radical awaits further study. An interesting possibility may be that formation of long-lived hydroxyethyl free radicals may be more toxic to biological systems than short-lived primary radicals.[56]

F. MICROSOMAL INTERACTION WITH IRON AND THE PRODUCTION OF REACTIVE OXYGEN INTERMEDIATES

Isolated microsomes generate O_2^- and H_2O_2 during NADPH-dependent electron transfer.[57-60] It appears that production of these oxidizing species occurs primarily via decay of oxy- or peroxy-cytochrome P-450.[61,62] Microsomes isolated from rats chronically fed alcohol have been shown to produce O_2^- and H_2O_2 at elevated rates compared to pair-fed controls.[63-65] These increases may be due, in part, to increased activity of NADPH-cytochrome P-450 reductase,[64] to the increased content of total cytochrome P-450 produced by the alcohol treatment,[66] or to inefficient coupling between the reductase and P-450. Indeed, the alcohol-inducible cytochrome P-450 isozyme, cytochrome P-4502E1, displays elevated NADPH oxidase activity associated with this inefficient coupling.[67,68] A recent interesting mechanism proposed to explain the fact that alcohol liver injury occurs primarily in the perivenous zone of the liver acinus, the zone where cytochrome P-4502E1 is primarily located, was that the elevated NADPH oxidase activity causes depletion of the lower concentrations of oxygen diffusing into this region of the liver lobule, thereby promoting hypoxia.[69]

As discussed earlier, superoxide and H_2O_2 in the presence of iron may serve as precursors of OH· via Fenton-type or modified Haber-Weiss types

TABLE 1
Reduction of Ferric Chelates by Rat Liver Microsomes

	Rate of production of ferrous (nmol/min/mg protein)	
Ferric chelate	NADPH	NADH
Ferric desferrioxamine	4 ± 2	6 ± 4
Ferric ATP	52 ± 8	61 ± 14
Ferric citrate	28 ± 8	22 ± 5
Ferric EDTA	37 ± 3	40 ± 9
Ferric DTPA	16 ± 2	26 ± 4

Note: Ferric chelates at a final concentration of iron of 25 μM were incubated with microsomes, a NADPH- or NADH-generating system, and 2,2′-dipyridyl. The production of ferrous dipyridyl was monitored by the absorbance changes at 520 nm.

of reaction. Microsomes also undergo active peroxidation in the presence of iron. In biological systems, iron is present in various chelated forms when not stored in ferritin. It, therefore, was considered that an understanding of the structure-function relationship of various ferric chelates as it concerns interaction with liver microsomes to promote production of potent oxidants capable of initiating lipid peroxidation, causing light emission (chemiluminescence) and generating OH·-like species, would be important, especially with respect to how alcohol treatment influences these reactions. For these studies, ferric ATP and ferric citrate were chosen as representatives of possible physiologically relevant iron complexes, ferric desferrioxamine as a relatively inert iron complex, and ferric EDTA and ferric diethylene-triamine pentaacetic acid (DTPA) as interesting toxicologically significant ferric complexes.

Initial experiments were carried out using liver microsomes from chow-fed rats and NADPH as the microsomal reductant.[70,71] Rat liver microsomes effectively catalyzed the reduction of ferric complexes with ATP, citrate, EDTA, and DTPA; whereas ferric-desferrioxamine was slowly reduced (Table 1). The nature of the ferric complex profoundly influenced microsomal production of potent reactive oxygen intermediates. As shown in Table 2, microsomal lipid peroxidation, as assessed by chemiluminescence or production of thiobarbituric acid reactive components, was strikingly increased by the addition of ferric chloride, ferric ATP, and ferric citrate; whereas ferric EDTA, ferric DTPA, and ferric desferrioxamine were strongly inhibitory. Microsomal production of OH·-like species showed the opposite catalytic effectiveness because ferric EDTA and ferric DTPA were potent stimulators, whereas the

TABLE 2
Effect of Ferric Chelates, Chelating Agents, and Antioxidants on Microsomal Lipid Peroxidation and OH˙ Generation

Addition	Effect on		
	MDA production	Light emission	OH˙ production
A) Ferric chloride	+ 368	+ 328	+ 59
Ferric ATP	+ 343	+ 229	+ 66
Ferric citrate	+ 479	+ 286	+ 52
Ferric EDTA	− 67	− 57	+ 490
Ferric DTPA	− 85	− 86	+ 301
Ferric desferrioxamine	− 89	− 77	− 87
B) EDTA	− 79		+ 243
DTPA	− 87		+ 115
ADP	+ 70		+ 24
Desferrioxamine	− 91		− 70
C) Catalase	+ 17	+ 9	− 76
SOD	+ 18	− 4	− 15
DMSO	− 4	− 8	− 69
Trolox	− 95	− 87	− 7

Note: Lipid peroxidation was measured as malondialdehyde equivalents as determined by production of thiobarbituric acid reactive components or by chemiluminescence, while generation of ethylene gas from 2-keto-4-thiomethylbutyric acid (KMB) was used as an index of the production of OH˙-like species.

other ferric compounds were much less effective. Ferric desferrioxamine remained essentially inert in catalyzing production of reactive oxygen intermediates by microsomes. Experiment B of Table 2 shows that addition of the chelating agent itself influences microsomal lipid peroxidation or OH˙ production in much the same manner (although to a lesser extent) as did the ferric chelate, suggesting the presence of small amounts of nonheme iron in the isolated microsomes.[72]

The opposite pattern of catalytic effectiveness of different ferric complexes toward microsomal lipid peroxidation and the oxidant responsible for oxidizing chemical scavengers such as 2-keto-4-thiomethylbutyric acid (KMB) suggests that different oxidants are responsible for these two activities. Experiment C of Table 2 shows that microsomal lipid peroxidation is insensitive to catalase, superoxide dismutase, and DMSO, indicating little or no role for H_2O_2, O_2^-, and OH˙ in this process. Oxidation of KMB is sensitive to catalase and to a competitive OH˙ scavenger but not to superoxide dismutase. The lack of effect of superoxide dismutase most likely is a consequence of the direct reduction of ferric EDTA or ferric DTPA by the microsomal electron transfer chain.[73]

In other experiments, the ability of the purified NADPH cytochrome P-450 reductase to interact with ferric complexes and catalyze the production of OH˙-like species was determined (Table 3). In the absence of added iron,

TABLE 3
NADPH-Cytochrome P-450 Reductase-Dependent Production of OH˙ in the Absence or Presence of Iron and Paraquat

Ferric complex	Rate of OH˙ production (pmol/min)		Observed rate/ additive rate
	− Paraquat	+ Paraquat	
None	0	19	—
Ferric desferrioxamine	0	34	1.8
Ferric ammonium sulfate	0	84	4.4
Ferric ATP	4	160	7.0
Ferric citrate	7	169	6.5
Ferric EDTA	117	499	3.7
Ferric DTPA	40	327	5.5

Note: Ferric chelates were used at a final concentration of iron of 25 μM. When present, the concentration of paraquat was 1 mM. The production of ethylene gas from KMB was determined as a reflection of the generation of OH˙-like compounds.

the purified reductase did not catalyze production of OH˙ at significant rates. Low rates of OH˙ production were found in the presence of ferric ammonium sulfate, ferric ATP, or ferric citrate, while ferric EDTA or ferric DTPA were very reactive in promoting OH˙ production from the reductase.[74,75] Thus, the pattern of catalytic effectiveness of varying ferric complexes in promoting microsomal production of OH˙-like species was identical to that of the reductase itself. It is important to note that contrary to earlier reports,[76,77] cytochrome P-450 itself does not function as a Fenton or Haber-Weiss catalyst. Under certain conditions, e.g., very low concentrations of ferric EDTA, cytochrome P-450 may be required to generate sufficient amounts of H_2O_2, the precursor of OH˙. Nevertheless, nonheme iron is required to generate OH˙ from H_2O_2.

Also shown in Table 3 is the effect of the redox cycling agent, paraquat, on the reductase-dependent production of OH˙. Redox cycling agents such as paraquat or quinones are toxic in biological systems because of the production of reactive oxygen intermediates. The addition of paraquat produced a small increase in the generation of OH˙ by the reductase, perhaps a reflection of the presence of small amounts of residual iron in the reaction system. In the presence of various ferric complexes, paraquat was a potent catalyst of the production of OH˙-like species (Table 3). Rates of OH˙ production in the presence of paraquat plus an iron complex were more than additive, suggesting synergistic interactions between the redox cycling agent and iron in catalyzing the generation of OH˙-like species by the reductase. Perhaps of toxicological significance is the fact that physiologically relevant iron complexes such as ferric ATP or ferric citrate, which were poor catalysts of OH˙ production by the reductase, were much more reactive catalysts in the presence of paraquat.[78]

TABLE 4
Effect of Chronic Ethanol Consumption on Microsomal Production of Reactive Oxygen Species

Reaction	Addition	Rate	
		Pair-fed	Chronic ethanol
Lipid peroxidation[a]	—	0.27 ± 0.12	0.64 ± 0.19
	Fe ATP	0.44 ± 0.02	1.18 ± 0.20
Chemiluminescence[b]	—	0.188 ± 0.07	0.652 ± 0.13
	Fe citrate	0.255 ± 0.08	0.895 ± 0.17
KMB oxidation[a]	—	0.13 ± 0.01	0.29 ± 0.03
	FeCl$_3$	0.25 ± 0.05	0.46 ± 0.09
	FeADP	0.30 ± 0.03	0.47 ± 0.11
	FeEDTA	4.48 ± 0.09	7.93 ± 0.47

Note: Lipid peroxidation was determined by the production of TBA-reactive material. Light emission over time was plotted and the area under the curve was calculated by weighing the curve. The indicated ferric chelate was used at a final concentration of iron of 25 μM.

[a] nmol/min/mg Microsomal protein.
[b] Area in arbitrary units/mg microsomal protein.

These results suggest the possibility that the toxicity of redox cycling agents such as paraquat in biological systems may be due to synergistic interactions with ferric complexes to promote the production of potent oxidants by organelles such as the microsomes.

To study the effect of chronic ethanol treatment on microsomal interaction with iron and the subsequent production of reactive oxygen species, rats were fed a total liquid diet in which ethanol comprised 36% of total calories, fat 35%, protein 18%, and carbohydrate 11%.[79] Pair-fed controls consumed the same diet except that ethanol calories were replaced by carbohydrate calories. A brief summary of these results[80-84] is shown in Table 4. Microsomal lipid peroxidation and chemiluminescence, in the absence or presence of added iron, were elevated in microsomes isolated from the ethanol-treated rats. The response of the control microsomal preparations and microsomes from the ethanol-treated rats to different iron complexes were identical, e.g., effective iron catalysts were ferric ATP, ferric citrate, or ferric ammonium sulfate; whereas ferric EDTA, ferric DTPA, or ferric desferrioxamine were inhibitory. Lipid peroxidation by both preparations was insensitive to catalase, superoxide dismutase, and OH$^{\cdot}$ scavengers, but inhibited in a similar manner by trolox, propylgallate, and glutathione. A role for cytochrome P-450 in the elevated rates of light emission was determined from the inhibitory effects of carbon monoxide on the increase produced by the ethanol treatment, whereas this inhibitor of cytochrome P-450 function had no effect on the control rates of light emission.[83] Importantly, in studies employing polyclonal antibodies which inhibit catalytic function of P-4502E1, Ekstrom and Ingelman-Sundberg[68] demonstrated that the elevated rates of superoxide and H_2O_2 production and lipid peroxidation found in microsomes after chronic ethanol treatment correlated with the content of the alcohol-inducible cytochrome P-4502E1. This isozyme has also been shown to be very effective in catalyzing reactive β-scission of hydroperoxides,[85] which would propagate the lipid peroxidation process.

Microsomes from the ethanol-fed rats catalyzed the oxidation of OH˙ chemical scavenging agents at elevated rates compared to the pair-fed controls (Table 4). These elevated rates were observed in the presence of various ferric complexes (Table 4) and in the presence of redox cycling agents such as menadione and paraquat.[84] Rates of oxidation of KMB by both microsomal preparations displayed similar sensitivities to desferrioxamine, catalase, and competitive OH˙ scavengers. Increased oxidation of chemical scavengers such as KMB and DMSO after chronic ethanol treatment has also been observed by others.[86,87]

Microsomes and other mixed-function oxidase systems have been shown to produce an oxidant which catalyzes the inactivation of a variety of metabolic enzymes.[88-90] This inactivation process is believed to be an initial step in marking the enzyme for eventual degradation by cellular proteases and plays an important role in protein turnover. The inactivation process requires iron, oxygen, and reducing equivalents; inhibition by catalase suggests that an H_2O_2 iron-derived oxidant is responsible for interacting with the added enzyme.[88-90] Since elevated rates of lipid peroxidation and chemiluminescence could be due, in part, to different lipid compositions of the microsomal membranes of the control and the ethanol-treated rats, the ability of these microsomes to catalyze the inactivation of lactic dehydrogenase added *in vitro* to the isolated microsomes was determined.[91] Microsomes from the ethanol-treated rats were twice as reactive as the pair-fed controls in catalyzing inactivation of lactic dehydrogenase (Table 5). Similar results were observed with other added enzymes such as pyruvate kinase and alcohol dehydrogenase.[91] Redox cycling agents increased the percent of inactivation presumably by increasing microsomal rates of production of reactive oxygen species. Nevertheless, rates of inactivation remained highest with the microsomes from the ethanol-treated rats (Table 5). Rates of inactivation were prevented by catalase and glutathione, but not by superoxide dismutase or OH˙ scavengers. Rates of inactivation were also prevented by EDTA, DTPA, and desferrioxamine, indicating that iron was required for the generation of the oxidant by the microsomes.

In summary, in the presence of iron and NADPH, microsomes catalyze the production of potent oxidizing agents which are capable of initiating lipid peroxidation, causing light emission, and oxidizing OH˙ scavengers. The role of iron in these reactions is complex and depends on the chelated form of iron utilized, the concentration used, and the oxygen radical reaction being investigated. Xenobiotics which are toxic because of their redox cycling

TABLE 5
Inactivation of Lactic Dehydrogenase by Oxidants Produced by Microsomes

| | Percent inactivation per 15 min incubation | |
Addition	Pair-fed	Chronic ethanol
Control	22 ± 6	42 ± 7^a
0.02 mM Menadione	41 ± 11	65 ± 10^a
0.10 mM Menadione	65 ± 11	84 ± 5^b
0.10 mM Paraquat	43 ± 17	77 ± 11^a
0.50 mM Paraquat	65 ± 2	84 ± 7^b

Note: 3000 units of lactic dehydrogenase (type I, Sigma Chem. Co.) were incubated for 15 min with microsomes from pair-fed controls or rats chronically fed ethanol, a NADPH-generating system and 25 μM ferric chloride. The microsomes were removed by rapid centrifugation, and the residual activity of lactic dehydrogenase remaining in the supernatant was assayed. The control (0% inactivation) reflects samples incubated in the absence of NADPH and iron. The loss in activity of lactic dehydrogenase is the percent inactivation.

[a] $p < 0.01$.
[b] $p < 0.05$.

capability synergistically interact with iron to increase the catalytic effectiveness of iron in generating reactive oxygen intermediates. Microsomes isolated from rats chronically fed ethanol display elevated rates of production of superoxide and H_2O_2; and in the presence of iron, they increased production of reactive oxygen intermediates which can cause lipid peroxidation, chemiluminescence, oxidation of $OH^{\cdot}$ chemical scavengers, and inactivation of metabolic enzymes. Increased oxygen radical production by microsomes after ethanol feeding may be due to inefficient coupling between the reductase and cytochrome P-450, increased content of enzymes which comprise the mixed-function oxidase system, and increased oxidase activity of the alcohol-inducible cytochrome P-450 isoenzyme. Increased generation of reactive oxygen intermediates by microsomes after chronic ethanol treatment may contribute to the hepatotoxic actions of ethanol, as well as play a role in the perivenous toxicity associated with ethanol consumption.

G. NADH REDUCTION OF IRON

Several of the toxic metabolic actions of ethanol on the liver, e.g., inhibition of fatty acid oxidation, or of gluconeogenesis or of activity of the citric acid cycle appear to be due to the production of NADH when ethanol is oxidized by hepatic alcohol dehydrogenase (ADH).[92-94] The NAD$^+$/NADH redox state of the cytosol is normally in a highly oxidized state, and decreases from a NAD$^+$/NADH ratio of about 700 to a ratio of about 200 when ethanol is oxidized.[95,96] It is interesting to speculate that the increased availability of NADH as a consequence of ethanol oxidation by ADH could promote microsomal generation of reactive oxygen species. Ozols[97] found that a reconstituted system containing ethanol plus NAD$^+$ plus ADH caused reduction of microsomal cytochrome b$_5$ suggesting that NADH-cytochrome b$_5$ reductase can, to some extent, directly reoxidize the NADH arising from ethanol oxidation. As described in the preceding section, in the presence of transition metals such as iron, rat liver microsomes catalyze the production of reactive oxygen species which can initiate lipid peroxidation, produce chemiluminescence, or promote the oxidation of OH$^{\cdot}$ chemical scavenging agents. Most studies on the generation of reactive oxygen intermediates by microsomes have utilized NADPH because this is the required co-factor for the reduction of NADPH-cytochrome P-450 reductase, and subsequently, cytochrome P-450. The interaction of NADH with various ferric complexes and microsomes to catalyze the generation of reactive oxygen intermediates has not been as well defined as the NADPH-dependent reactions. NADH provides electrons to NADH-cytochrome b$_5$ reductase, and subsequently, cytochrome b$_5$. This electron transfer system is important for fatty acid desaturation and elongation[98] and also for the ability of NADH to synergistically enhance NADPH-dependent mixed-function oxidase activity.[99] Therefore, we initiated a series of studies to determine the ability of NADH to interact with various ferric complexes to promote microsomal lipid peroxidation and generation of OH$^{\cdot}$-like species.[100,101]

As shown in Table 1, NADH could catalyze the reduction of various ferric chelates by rat liver microsomes. Indeed, the NADH-dependent rates were as high as the NADPH-dependent rates. The oxidation of DMSO to formaldehyde was determined as a measure of OH$^{\cdot}$ production. In the absence of added iron or in the presence of desferrioxamine, very low or neglible rates of DMSO oxidation were observed. As had been described earlier for the NADPH-dependent reactions, ferric EDTA and ferric DTPA were very reactive in catalyzing NADH-dependent OH$^{\cdot}$ production; while ferric ammonium sulfate, ferric ATP, or ferric citrate were less reactive (Table 6). Similar results were observed for other OH$^{\cdot}$ scavengers, e.g., *t*-butylalcohol[100] and KMB.[101] The oxidation of DMSO was sensitive to catalase and competitive OH$^{\cdot}$ scavengers, but not to superoxide dismutase (Table 6, Experiment B). NAD$^+$ could not replace NADH in catalyzing these reactions. The NADH-dependent rates were 50 to 75% as high as the NADPH-dependent rates of OH$^{\cdot}$ generation. Carbon monoxide had litttle effect on the NADH plus ferric EDTA catalyzed production of OH$^{\cdot}$, indicating little or no role for cytochrome P-450 in the reaction. Rates of H$_2$O$_2$ production in the presence of NADH were about 30 to 40% of the NADPH-dependent rates in the absence of added

TABLE 6
NADH-Dependent Microsomal Oxidation of OH˙-Scavenging Agents and Lipid Peroxidation

	Ferric complex	Addition	Rate of DMSO oxidation (nmol/min/mg protein)	Rate of MDA production
A)	Ferric ammonium sulfate		0.22 ± 0.05	0.76
	Ferric ATP		0.41 ± 0.02	1.22 ± 0.36
	Ferric citrate		0.12 ± 0.06	0.78 ± 0.10
	Ferric EDTA		3.10 ± 0.46	0
	Ferric DTPA		2.37 ± 0.69	0
B)	Ferric EDTA	—	3.76 ± 0.19	
		Catalase	1.00 ± 0.85	
		SOD	2.98 ± 0.08	
		Ethanol	2.81 ± 0.41	
		KMB	1.44 ± 0.04	
C)	Ferric ATP	—		1.22 ± 0.36
		Catalase		0.88 ± 0.18
		SOD		0.90 ± 0.22
		DMSO		0.84 ± 0.20

Note: Control microsomes were incubated with a NADH-generating system, and OH˙ production was evaluated by the production of formaldehyde from DMSO, while lipid peroxidation was measured by the production of malondialdehyde.

iron, and about 70% of the NADPH-dependent rates in the presence of ferric EDTA. NADH also catalyzed a time- and protein-dependent production of TBA-reactive components by microsomes (Table 6). Ferric ATP, ferric citrate, and ferric ammonium sulfate were effective catalysts of microsomal lipid peroxidation, whereas ferric EDTA or ferric DTPA did not promote NADH-dependent lipid peroxidation (Table 6). Microsomal lipid peroxidation in the presence of NADH was only slightly sensitive to catalase, superoxide dismutase, or DMSO (Table 6, Experiment C). The NADH-dependent rates of microsomal lipid peroxidation were about 20% that of the NADH-dependent rates. Essentially similar results were obtained when NADH was added directly to catalyze microsomal interaction with iron to produce reactive oxygen species or when NADH was generated at a constant level in a reconstituted system containing ethanol, NAD^+, and alcohol dehydrogenase.

The effect of chronic ethanol treatment on NADH-dependent microsomal production of reactive oxygen intermediates was determined, and the results are summarized in Table 7. Oxidation of KMB or of DMSO, production of H_2O_2, and generation of TBA-reactive material in the presence of NADH were increased by about 50% after chronic ethanol feeding. The sensitivities of the control microsomal preparations and those from ethanol-fed rats to antioxidants and the catalytic effectiveness of various iron complexes were identical, and were also similar to those previously described for the NADPH-

TABLE 7
Effect of Chronic Ethanol Consumption on NADH-Dependent Microsomal Production of Reactive Oxygen Intermediates

Reaction	Rate of product formation (nmol/min/mg)	
	Pair-fed	Chronic ethanol
OH· production	5.86 ± 0.06	8.91 ± 0.41[a]
H_2O_2 production	13.16 ± 1.36	19.40 ± 2.92[a]
Lipid peroxidation	0.84 ± 0.08	1.30 ± 0.21[a]

[a] $p < 0.02$.

dependent reactions in these preparations. However, the increase in production of reactive oxygen species by microsomes after treatment with ethanol was greater when NADPH (about twofold) was the microsomal reductant than with NADH (about 50%). This probably reflects the fact that NADPH is the preferred reductant for cytochrome P-450.

In summary, NADH was found to be active in catalyzing the reduction of various iron complexes by microsomes and to promote the production of reactive oxygen intermediates. The NADH-dependent reactions with microsomes are about 20 to 70% as reactive as the NADPH-dependent reactions. Since the oxidation of ethanol by alcohol dehydrogenase results in an elevated production of NADH, interaction of NADH and iron with hepatic microsomes to promote the production of potent oxidants may contribute to the overall mechanisms by which alcohol is toxic to the liver. These acute metabolic interactions produced from ethanol-derived NADH are increased, not attenuated, in microsomes from ethanol-fed rats. Although the increases with NADH are less robust than with NADPH, it is interesting to speculate that the combination of the acute metabolic effects of ethanol (increased availability of NADH, which may also lead to increases in NADPH availability) added to the increases produced by chronic ethanol treatment may place an increasing oxidative burden on the liver.

H. EFFECTS OF ETHANOL ON IRON HOMEOSTASIS

In view of the critical role played by iron in the production of reactive oxygen intermediates by microsomes and other cellular organelles, the effect of acute and chronic ethanol treatment on hepatic iron levels and iron homeostasis is of major significance. There are numerous reports that alcoholic liver disease is associated with disorders of iron metabolism and homeostasis. Examples include the decrease in serum levels of the major iron transporter protein, transferrin;[102] the altered plasma iron turnover and iron incorporation into hemoglobin;[103,104] and a variety of other hematological disorders.[105] Chronic alcohol feeding has been shown to increase hepatic iron stores;[106-108] if this iron is available to interact with reducing equivalents and cellular organelles, production of reactive oxygen intermediates would be elevated. The combination of ethanol and iron was especially more toxic to rats than either agent was alone.[109,110] Nordmann and co-workers[111] have shown that ethanol may mobilize iron and increase content of the low molecular weight cytosolic iron pool.[111] Sinaceur et al.[112] observed that desferrioxamine and DTPA produced a small inhibition of the *in vivo* rate of ethanol oxidation, suggesting some contribution by an iron-dependent reaction (OH·?) toward the overall metabolism of ethanol. Shaw and co-workers[113,114] have suggested that ethanol may mobilize iron from its ferritin storage site, perhaps via superoxide generated from xanthine oxidase.

A variety of mechanisms have been suggested to explain the elevated liver iron levels but most are controversial and require further study. Iron is present in certain alcoholic beverages, especially red wine, and consumption of these beverages may therefore cause elevated liver content of iron;[115] others find no relationship between the amount of iron consumed and the extent of liver siderosis.[116] The effects of alcohol on iron absorption are complex with reports ranging from increases[117] to decreases.[118] Elevated iron levels in the liver may arise from decreases in erythropoiesis following chronic intake of alcohol.[119] It is unclear whether some of the effects of ethanol on iron metabolism are due to ethanol itself or to other dietary constituents in the alcoholic beverages, or to the nutritional complications and malnutrition which often accompany alcohol abuse. For example, the presence of liver disease may affect liver deposition of iron because there is increased iron absorption in cirrhosis[120] and increased iron uptake in patients with liver damage.[121] In general, while some correlations between the quantity of iron and alcohol ingested and liver siderosis in alcoholics have been found by some,[122] others find no correlations between liver siderosis and the length of drinking history.[123,124] The elevated iron levels in the liver found in alcoholics are much less than those found in patients with idiopathic hemochromatosis.

Synthesis of transferrin by hepatocytes may be decreased by ethanol, as has been found with several other plasma proteins synthesized and secreted by the liver.[125,126] Ethanol added *in vitro* was found to decrease the uptake of transferrin-bound iron by rat liver hepatocytes.[127] This effect could be prevented by increased buffering capacity of the medium and was suggested to be due to the decrease in pH apparently preventing efficient recycling of the transferrin receptor.[127] Iron uptake from transferrin by isolated rat hepatocytes from chronic ethanol-fed rats was reported to be lower than control values,[128] presumably due to this reduced receptor recycling.[129] There is considerable interest in the effects of alcohol on transferrin, since an abnormal microheterogeneity of transferrin has been observed in the serum of alcoholics.[130,131] This microheterogeneity involves the carbohydrate moiety of the transferrin glycoprotein,[132,133] and it has been suggested that carbohydrate-deficient transferrin may be a marker for alcohol abuse, especially in conjunction with other diagnostic markers.[134,135]

It is apparent that the toxicity of many xenobiotics and of certain metabolic conditions (hyperoxia, reperfusion, vitamin E deficiency) is magnified by metals such as iron which catalyzes Haber-Weiss and Fenton reactions; initiates and propagates lipid peroxidation; and, in general, promotes oxidative stress. The effects of acute and chronic ethanol treatment on cellular iron levels and iron mobilization will likely be an important area of continuing research into mechanisms by which ethanol may promote hepatic injury.

IV. CONCLUSIONS

In addition to the previously mentioned mechanisms, several other possibilities exist whereby ethanol can produce increased oxidative stress to the liver, e.g., direct solvent actions on membranes, increased oxygen uptake due to a hypermetabolic state of the liver, and release of chemoattractants. These various possibilities are not mutually exclusive of one another, and several may occur simultaneously. Ethanol-induced oxidative stress is not relegated only to the liver, e.g., chronic ethanol has been suggested to produce oxidative stress in the heart, testes, and the central nervous system.[136-138] Inasmuch as ethanol is not significantly oxidized in these tissues, many of these possible mechanisms (redox state, acetaldehyde, P-4502E1) can probably be eliminated as explaining the oxidative stress produced by ethanol. It is interesting that the toxic effects of ethanol originate in the pericentral zone of the liver acinus. Reactive oxygen intermediates could play a role in this pericentral hepatotoxicity, e.g., GSH levels are lower in the pericentral zone,[139] P-4502E1 levels are higher,[69,140] and the redox state change (increased NADH) produced by ethanol is more pronounced in this zone.[141] Studies on iron levels, distribution, availability, and mobilization in different zones of the liver may be of importance. Alcohol abuse and hepatotoxicity are more prevalent in the West; the typical Western diet contains greater amounts of iron than the typical Eastern diet. Can elevated iron levels contribute to the toxic actions of alcohol and predispose individuals to alcohol toxicity? Additional research will be needed to clarify the role of iron and reactive oxygen intermediates in the hepatotoxic actions of ethanol. It will be important to overcome the numerous variables and to clearly define the model, the reaction system, and the parameter being measured. Additional studies with intact cells and *in vivo* will also be required. It is likely that advances in the free-radical field (e.g., development of stable spin-trapping agents, more specific quantitative methods to assay oxygen radicals, and lipid peroxidation) and identification of the low molecular weight iron (or other metal) pool which catalyzes production of potent oxidizing species both will be of great value in helping to further assess the role of oxygen radicals in the toxic actions of ethanol.

ACKNOWLEDGMENTS

Experiments by the author were supported by USPHS Grants AA-03312 and AA-03508 (Alcohol Research Center) from the National Institute on Alcohol Abuse and Alcoholism. I thank Ms. Lucy Martinez for typing the manuscript.

REFERENCES

1. **Fridovich, I.**, Superoxide dismutases, *Adv. Enzymol.*, 41, 35, 1974.
2. **Fridovich, I.**, The biology of oxygen radicals, *Science*, 201, 875, 1978.
3. **Halliwell, B.**, Free radicals and metal ions in health and disease, *Proc. Nutr. Soc.*, 46, 13, 1987.
4. **Halliwell, B. and Gutteridge, J. M. C.**, Oxygen toxicity, oxygen radical, transition metals and disease, *Biochem. J.*, 219, 1, 1984.
5. **Oberley, L. W.**, *Superoxide Dismutase*, Vol. 1 and 2, CRC Press, Boca Raton, FL, 1982.
6. **Farber, J. L., Kyle, M. E., and Coleman, J. B.**, Biology of disease; mechanism of cell injury by activated oxygen species, *Lab. Invest.*, 62, 670, 1990.
7. **Freeman, B. A. and Crapo, J. D.**, Biology of disease; free radicals and tissue injury, *Lab. Invest.*, 47, 412, 1982.
8. **McCord, J. M. and Fridovich, I.**, Superoxide dismutase: an enzymatic function for erythrocuprein, *J. Biol. Chem.*, 244, 6049, 1969.
9. **Scott, M. D., Meschnick, S. R., and Eaton, J. W.**, Superoxide dismutase-rich bacteria, paradoxical increase in oxidant toxicity, *J. Biol. Chem.*, 262, 3640, 1987.
10. **Beauchamp, C. and Fridovich, I.**, A mechanism for the production of ethylene from methional. The generation of the hydroxyl radical by xanthine oxidase, *J. Biol. Chem.*, 245, 4641, 1970.
11. **McCord, J. M. and Day, E. D.**, Superoxide-dependent production of hydroxyl radical catalyzed by iron-EDTA complex, *FEBS Lett.*, 86, 139, 1978.
12. **Halliwell, B.**, Superoxide dependent formation of hydroxyl radicals in the presence of iron chelates, *FEBS Lett.*, 92, 321, 1978.
13. **Horton, A. A. and Fairhurst, S.**, Lipid peroxidation and mechanisms of toxicity, *CRC Crit. Rev. Toxicol.*, 18, 27, 1987.
14. **Comporti, M.**, Biology of disease: lipid peroxidation and cellular damage in toxic liver injury, *Lab. Invest.*, 53, 599, 1985.
15. **Kappus, H.**, Lipid peroxidation: mechanisms, analysis, enzymology and biological relevance, in *Oxidative Stress*, Sies, H., Ed., Academic Press, London, 1985, 273.
16. **Tribble, D. L., Aw, T. Y., and Jones, D. P.**, The pathophysiological significance of lipid peroxidation in oxidative cell injury, *Hepatology*, 7, 377, 1987.
17. **Aust, S. D., Morehouse, L. A., and Thomas, C. E.**, Role of metals in oxygen radical reactions, *Free Radical Biol. Med.*, 1, 3, 1985.
18. **Diluzio, N. R.**, Prevention of the acute ethanol-induced fatty liver by the simultaneous administration of anti-oxidants, *Life Sci.*, 3, 113, 1964.
19. **Diluzio, N. R.**, The role of lipid peroxidation and antioxidants in ethanol-induced lipid alterations, *Exp. Mol. Pathol.*, 8, 394, 1968.
20. **Diluzio, N. R. and Hartman, A. D.**, Role of lipid peroxidation in the pathogenesis of ethanol-induced fatty liver, *Fed. Proc.*, 26, 1436, 1967.

21. **Dianzani, M. U.**, Lipid peroxidation in ethanol poisoning: a critical reconsideration, *Alcohol Alcoholism,* 20, 161, 1985.
22. **Cederbaum, A. I.**, Introduction: role of lipid peroxidation and oxidative stress in alcohol toxicity, *Free Radical Biol. Med.,* 7, 537, 1989.
23. **Videla, L. A. and Valenzuela, A.**, Alcohol ingestion, liver glutathione and lipoperoxidation, *Life Sci.,* 32, 2395, 1982.
24. **Nordmann, R., Ribiere, C., and Rouach, H.**, Involvement of iron and iron catalyzed free radical production in ethanol metabolism and toxicity, *Enzyme,* 37, 57, 1987.
25. **Reitz, R. C.**, A possible mechanism for the peroxidation of lipids due to chronic ethanol ingestion, *Biochim. Biophys. Acta,* 380, 145, 1975.
26. **Antonenkov, V. D. and Panchenko, L. F.**, Effect of chronic ethanol treatment under partial catalase inhibition on the activity of enzymes related to peroxide metabolism in rat liver and heart, *Int. J. Biochem.,* 20, 823, 1988.
27. **Harata, J., Nagata, M., Sasaki, E., Ishiguro, I., Ohta, Y., and Murakami, Y.**, Effect of prolonged alcohol administration on activities of various enzymes scavenging activated oxygen radicals and lipid peroxide level in the liver of rats, *Biochem. Pharmacol.,* 32, 1795, 1983.
28. **Bjorneboe, G. A., Bjorneboe, A., Hagen, B. F., Moreland, J., and Drevon, C.**, Reduced hepatic α-tocopherol content after long term administration of ethanol to rats, *Biochim. Biophys. Acta,* 918, 236, 1987.
29. **Kawase, T., Kato, S., and Lieber, C. S.**, Lipid peroxidation and antioxidant defense systems in rat liver after chronic ethanol feeding, *Hepatology,* 10, 815, 1989.
30. **Tanner, A. R., Bantock, I., Hintes, L., Lloyd, B., Turner, N. R., and Wright, R.**, Depressed selenium and vitamin E levels in an alcoholic population, *Digest Dis. Sci.,* 31, 1307, 1986.
31. **Strubelt, O., Younes, M., and Pentz, R.**, Enhancement by GSH depletion of ethanol-induced acute hepatotoxicity *in vitro* and *in vivo, Toxicology,* 45, 213, 1987.
32. **Lauterberg, B. H., Davies, S., and Mitchell, J. R.**, Ethanol suppresses hepatic GSH synthesis in rats, *in vivo, J. Pharmacol. Exp. Ther.,* 230, 7, 1984.
33. **Morton, S. and Mitchell, M. C.**, Effects of chronic ethanol feeding on GSH turnover in the rat, *Biochem. Pharmacol.,* 34, 1559, 1985.
34. **Fernandez-Checa, J. G., Ookhtens, M., and Kaplowitz, N.**, Effect of chronic ethanol feeding on rat hepatocyte glutathione, *J. Clin. Invest.,* 80, 57, 1987.
35. **Cederbaum, A. I. and Rubin, E.**, Molecular injury to mitochondria produced by ethanol and acetaldehyde, *Fed. Proc.,* 34, 2045, 1975.
36. **Cunningham, C. C., Coleman, W. B., and Spach, P. I.**, The effects of chronic ethanol consumption on hepatic mitochondrial energy metabolism, *Alcohol Alcoholism,* 25, 127, 1990.
37. **Thayer, W. S. and Rubin, E.**, Effects of chronic ethanol intoxication on oxidative phosphorylation in rat liver submitochondrial particles, *J. Biol. Chem.,* 254, 7717, 1979.
38. **Forman, H. J. and Boveris, A.**, Superoxide radical and hydrogen peroxide in mitochondria, in *Free Radicals in Biology,* Vol. 5, Pryor, W., Ed., Academic Press, New York, 1982, 65.
39. **Ribiere, C., Sabourault, D., Saffar, I., and Nordmann, R.**, Mitochondrial generation of superoxide free radicals during acute ethanol intoxication in the rat, *Alcohol Alcoholism,* Suppl. 1, 241, 1987.
40. **Oei, H. H. H., Stroo, E., Burton, K. P., and Schaffer, S. W.**, A possible role of xanthine oxidase in producing oxidative stress in the heart of chronically ethanol-treated rats, *Res. Commun. Chem. Pathol. Pharmacol.,* 38, 453, 1982.
41. **Sultatos, L. G.**, Effect of acute ethanol administration on the hepatic xanthine dehydrogenase/oxidase system in the rat, *J. Pharmacol. Exp. Ther.,* 246, 946, 1988.
42. **Kato, S., Kawase, T., Alderman, J., Inatomi, N., and Lieber, C. S.**, Role of xanthine oxidase in ethanol-induced lipid peroxidation in rats, *Gastroenterology,* 98, 203, 1990.

442

43. **Shaw, S. and Jayatilleke, E.,** The role of aldehyde oxidase in ethanol-induced hepatic lipid peroxidation in the rat, *Biochem. J.,* 268, 579, 1990.
44. **Muller, A. and Sies, H.,** Role of alcohol dehydrogenase activity and acetaldehyde in ethanol-induced ethane and pentane production by isolated perfused liver, *Biochem. J.,* 206, 153, 1982.
45. **Muller, A. and Sies, H.,** Ethane release during metabolism of aldehydes and monomines in perfused rat liver, *Eur. J. Biochem.,* 134, 599, 1983.
46. **Kera, Y., Ohbora, Y., and Kumura, S.,** The metabolism of acetaldehyde and not acetaldehyde itself is responsible for *in vivo* ethanol induced lipid peroxidation in rats, *Biochem. Pharmacol.,* 37, 3633, 1988.
47. **Speisky, H., MacDonald, A., Giles, G., Orrego, H., and Israel, Y.,** Increased loss and decreased synthesis of hepatic glutathione after acute ethanol administration, *Biochem. J.,* 225, 565, 1985.
48. **Boh, E. E., Baricos, W. H., Bernofsky, C., and Steele, R. H.,** Mitochondrial chemiluminescence elicited by acetaldehyde, *J. Bioenerg. Biomembrane,* 14, 115, 1982.
49. **Puntarulo, S. P. and Cederbaum, A. I.,** Chemiluminescence from acetaldehyde oxidation by xanthine oxidase involves generation of and interactions with hydroxyl radical, *Alcoholism: Clin. Exp. Res.,* 13, 84, 1989.
50. **Albano, E., Tomasi, A., Goria-Gatti, L., Poli, G., Vannini, V., and Dianzani, M. U.,** Free radical metabolism of alcohols by rat microsomes, *Free Radicals Res. Commun.,* 3, 243, 1987.
51. **Albano, E., Tomasi, A., Goria-Gatti, L, and Dianzani, M. U.,** Spin trapping of free radical species produced during the microsomal metabolism of ethanol, *Chem. Biol. Interact,* 65, 223, 1988.
52. **Reinke, L. A., Lai, E. K., DuBose, C. M., and McCay, P. B.,** Reactive free radical generation *in vivo* in heart and liver of ethanol fed rats, *Proc. Natl. Acad. Sci. U.S.A.,* 84, 9223, 1987.
53. **Reinke, L. A., Rau, J. M., and McCay, P. B.,** Possible roles of free radicals in alcoholic tissue damage, *Free Radical Res. Commun.,* 9, 205, 1990.
54. **Albano, K. E., Tomasi, A., Persson, J. O., Terelius, Y., Goria-Gatti, L., Ingelman-Sundberg, M., and Dianzani, M. U.,** Role of ethanol-inducible cytochrome P-450 in catalyzing free radical activation of aliphatic alcohols, *Biochem. Pharmacol.,* 41, 1895, 1991.
55. **Knecht, K. T., Bradford, B. U., Mason, R. P., and Thurman, R. G.,** *In vivo* formation of a free radical metabolite of ethanol, *Mol. Pharmacol.,* 38, 26, 1990.
56. **Ahmad, F. F., Cowan, D. L., and Sun, A. Y.,** Potentiation of ethanol induced lipid peroxidation of biological membranes by vitamin C, *Life Sci.,* 43, 1169, 1988.
57. **Aust, S. D., Roerig, D. L., and Pederson, T. C.,** Evidence for superoxide generation by NADPH-cytochrome c reductase of rat liver microsomes, *Biochem. Biophys. Res. Commun.,* 47, 1133, 1972.
58. **Prough, R. A. and Masters, B. S. S.,** Studies of the NADPH oxidase reaction of NADPH-cytochrome c reductase. The role of superoxide anion, *Ann. N.Y. Acad. Sci.,* 212, 89, 1973.
59. **Dybing, E., Nelson, S. D., Mitchell, J. R., Sasame, H. A., and Gillette, J. R.,** Oxidation of α-methyldopa and other catechols by cytochrome P-450-generated O_2^-: possible mechanism of methyldopa hepatitis, *Mol. Pharmacol.,* 12, 911, 1976.
60. **Strobel, H. W. and Coon, M. J.,** Effect of superoxide generation and dismutation on hydroxylation reactions catalyzed by liver microsomal cytochrome P-450, *J. Biol. Chem.,* 246, 7826, 1971.
61. **Kuthan, H. and Ullrich, V.,** Oxidase and oxygenase function of the microsomal cytochrome P-450 monooxygenase system, *Eur. J. Biochem.,* 126, 583, 1982.
62. **Kuthan, H., Tsuji, H., Graf, H., Ullrich, V., Werringloer, J., and Estabrook, R. W.,** Generation of superoxide anion as a source of hydrogen peroxide in a reconstituted monooxygenase system, *FEBS Lett.,* 91, 343, 1978.

63. **Boveris, A., Fraga, C. G., Varsavsky, A. I., and Kock, O. R.,** Increased chemiluminescence and superoxide production in the liver of chronically ethanol-treated rats, *Arch. Biochem. Biophys.,* 227, 534, 1983.

64. **Lieber, C. S. and DeCarli, L. M.,** Reduced NADP oxidase: activity enhanced by ethanol consumption, *Science,* 170, 78, 1970.

65. **Thurman, R. G.,** Induction of hepatic microsomal NADPH-dependent production of hydrogen peroxide by chronic prior treatment with ethanol, *Mol. Pharmacol.,* 9, 670, 1973.

66. **Lieber, C. S.,** Microsomal ethanol oxidizing system, *Enzyme,* 37, 45, 1987.

67. **Gorsky, L. D., Koop, D. R., and Coon, M. J.,** On the stoichiometry of the oxidase and monooxygenase reactions catalyzed by liver microsomal cytochrome P-450, *J. Biol. Chem.,* 259, 6812, 1984.

68. **Ekstrom, G. and Ingelman-Sundberg, M.,** Rat liver microsomal NADPH-supported oxidase activity and lipid peroxidation dependent on ethanol inducible cytochrome P-450, *Biochem. Pharmacol.,* 38, 1313, 1989.

69. **Ingelman-Sundberg, M., Johansson, I., Penttila, K. E., Glaumann, H., and Lindros, K. O.,** Centrilobular expression of ethanol inducible cytochrome P-450 (IIE1) in rat liver, *Biochem. Biophys. Res. Commun.,* 157, 55, 1988.

70. **Winston, G. W., Feierman, D. E., and Cederbaum, A. I.,** The role of iron chelates in OH production by rat liver microsomes, NADPH cytochrome P-450 reductase and xanthine oxidase, *Arch. Biochem. Biophys.,* 232, 378, 1984.

71. **Puntarulo, S. and Cederbaum, A. I.,** Comparison of the ability of ferric complexes to catalyze microsomal chemiluminescence, lipid peroxidation and OH generation, *Arch. Biochem. Biophys.* 264, 482, 1988.

72. **Minotti, G.,** NADPH- and adriamycin-dependent microsomal release of iron and lipid peroxidation, *Arch. Biochem. Biophys.,* 277, 268, 1990.

73. **Morehouse, L. A. and Aust, S. D.,** Reconstituted microsomal lipid peroxidation: ADP-Fe^{3+} dependent peroxidation of phospholipid vesicles containing NADPH-cytochrome P-450 reductase and cytochrome P-450, *Free Radical Biol. Med.,* 4, 269, 1988.

74. **Winston, G. W. and Cederbaum, A. I.,** NADPH-dependent production of oxy-radicals by purified components of the rat-liver mixed-function oxidase system, I-oxidation of ˙OH scavenging agents, *J. Biol. Chem.,* 258, 1508, 1983.

75. **Winston, G. W. and Cederbaum, A. I.,** NADPH-dependent production of oxy-radicals by purified components of the rat liver mixed-function oxidase system, II-role in microsomal oxidation of ethanol, *J. Biol. Chem.,* 258, 1514, 1983.

76. **Ingelman-Sundberg, M. and Johansson, I.,** Mechanisms of hydroxyl radical formation and ethanol oxidation by ethanol-inducible and other forms of rabbit liver microsomal cytochrome P-450, *J. Biol. Chem.,* 259, 6447, 1984.

77. **Terelius, Y. and Ingelman-Sundberg, M.,** Cytochrome P-450 dependent oxidase activity and hydroxyl radical production in micellar and membranes types of reconstituted systems, *Biochem. Pharmacol.,* 37, 1383, 1988.

78. **Clejan, L. A. and Cederbaum, A. I.,** Synergistic interactions between NADPH cytochrome P-450 reductase, paraquat and iron in the generation of active oxygen radicals, *Biochem. Pharmacol.,* 38, 1779, 1989.

79. **Lieber, C. S. and DeCarli, L. M.,** The feeding of alcohol in liquid diets: two decades of applications and 1982 update, *Alcoholism: Clin. Exp. Res.,* 6, 523, 1982.

80. **Klein, S. M., Cohen, G., Lieber, C. S., and Cederbaum, A. I.,** Increased microsomal oxidation of hydroxyl radical scavenging agents and ethanol after chronic consumption of ethanol, *Arch. Biochem. Biophys.,* 223, 425, 1983.

81. **Krikun, G., Lieber, C. S., and Cederbaum, A. L.,** Increased microsomal oxidation of ethanol by cytochrome P-450 and ˙OH dependent pathways after chronic ethanol consumption, *Biochem. Pharmacol.,* 33, 3306, 1984.

82. **Krikun, G. and Cederbaum, A. I.,** Effect of chronic ethanol consumption on microsomal lipid peroxidation: role of iron and comparison between controls, *FEBS Lett.,* 208, 292, 1986.

83. **Puntarulo, S. P. and Cederbaum, A. I.,** Increased NADPH-dependent chemiluminescence by microsomes after chronic ethanol consumption, *Arch. Biochem. Biophys.,* 266, 435, 1988.

84. **Dicker, E. and Cederbaum, A. I.,** Hydroxyl radical generation by microsomes after chronic ethanol consumption, *Alcoholism: Clin. Exp. Res.,* 11, 309, 1987.

85. **Vaz, A. D. N., Roberts, E. S., and Coon, M. J.,** Reductive β-scission of the hydroperoxides of fatty acids and xenobiotics: role of alcohol-inducible cytochrome P-450, *Proc. Natl. Acad. Sci. U.S.A.,* 87, 5499, 1990.

86. **Shaw, S., Jayatilleke, E., and Lieber, C. S.,** The effect of chronic alcohol feeding on lipid peroxidation in microsomes: lack of relationship to hydroxyl radical generation, *Biochem. Biophys. Res. Commun.,* 118, 233, 1984.

87. **Ekstrom, G., Cronholm, T., and Ingelman-Sundberg, M.,** Hydroxyl radical production and ethanol oxidation by liver microsomes isolated from ethanol-treated rats, *Biochem. J.,* 233, 755, 1986.

88. **Fucci, L., Oliver, C. N., Coon, M. J., and Stadtman, E. R.,** Inactivation of key metabolic enzymes by mixed function oxidation reactions: possible implications in protein turnover and aging, *Proc. Natl. Acad. Sci. U.S.A.,* 80, 1521, 1983.

89. **Nakamura, K., Oliver, C. N., and Stadtman, E. R.,** Inactivation of glutamine synthetase by a purified rabbit liver microsomal cytochrome P-450 system, *Arch. Biochem. Biophys.,* 240, 319, 1985.

90. **Stadtman, E. R.,** Oxidation of proteins by mixed-function oxidation systems, *Trends Biol. Sci.,* 11, 11, 1986.

91. **Dicker, E. and Cederbaum, A. I.,** Increased oxygen radical dependent inactivation of metabolic enzymes by liver microsomes after chronic ethanol consumption, *FASEB J.,* 2, 2901, 1988.

92. **Lieber, C. S.,** Metabolism of ethanol, in *Medical Disorders of Alcohol,* Lieber, C. S., Ed., W. B. Saunders, Philadelphia, 1982, 1.

93. **Krebs, H. A.,** The effects of ethanol on the metabolic activities of the liver, *Adv. Enzyme Regul.,* 6, 467, 1968.

94. **Williamson, J. R., Scholz, R., Browning, E. T., Thurman, R. G., and Fukami, M. H.,** Metabolic effects of ethanol in perfused rat liver, *J. Biol. Chem.,* 244, 5044, 1969.

95. **Stubbs, M., Veech, R., and Krebs, H. A.,** Control of the redox state of the NAD couple in rat liver cytoplasm, *Biochem. J.,* 126, 59, 1972.

96. **Veech, R. L., Guynn, R., and Veloso, D.,** The time course of the effects of ethanol on the redox and phosphorylation states of rat liver, *Biochem. J.,* 127, 387, 1972.

97. **Ozols, J.,** The role of microsomal cytochrome b_5 in the metabolism of ethanol, drugs and the desaturation of fatty acids, *Ann. Clin. Res.,* 8, 182, 1976.

98. **Strittmater, P., Spatz, L., Cocoran, D., Rogers, M. J., Setlow, B., and Redline, R.,** Purification and properties of rat liver microsomal stearyl coenzyme A desaturase, *Proc. Natl. Acad. Sci. U.S.A.,* 71, 4565, 1974.

99. **Hildebrandt, A. and Estabrook, R. W.,** Evidence for the participation of cytochrome b_5 in hepatic microsomal mixed function oxidation reaction, *Arch. Biochem. Biophys.,* 143, 66, 1971.

100. **Kukielka, E. and Cederbaum, A. I.,** NADH-dependent microsomal interaction with ferric complexes and production of reactive oxygen intermediates, *Arch. Biochem. Biophys.,* 275, 540, 1989.

101. **Dicker, E. and Cederbaum, A. I.,** NADH-dependent generation of reactive oxygen species by microsomes in the presence of iron and redox cycling agents, *Biochem. Pharmacol.,* 42, 529, 1991.

102. **Valberg, L. S., Ghent, C. N., Lloyd, D. A., Frei, J. V., and Chamberlain, N. J.,** Diagnostic efficacy of tests for the detection of iron overload, *Can. Med. Assoc. J.,* 119, 229, 1978.

103. **Beaumier, D. L., Caldwell, M. A. and Holdbein, B. E.,** Inflammation triggers hypoferremia and ceruloplasmia in mice, *Infect. Immunol.,* 46, 489, 1984.

104. **Eichner, E. R. and Hillman, J.,** The evolution of anemia in alcoholic patients, *Am. J. Med.,* 50, 218, 1971.

105. **Colman, N. and Herbert, V.,** Hematologic complications of alcoholism: overview, *Semin. Hematol.,* 17, 164, 1980.

106. **Chapman, R. W., Morgan, M. Y., Laulicht, M., Hoffbrand, D., and Sherlock, S.,** Hepatic iron stores and markers of iron overload in alcoholics and patients with idiopathic hemochromatosis, *Dig. Dis. Sci.,* 27, 909, 1982.

107. **Powell, L. W.,** The relationship between alcohol consumption and hepatic iron metabolism, *Hepatology: Rapid Lit. Rev.,* 2(1), 9, 1981.

108. **Sanchez, J., Casas, M., and Rama, R.,** Effect of chronic ethanol administration on iron metabolism in the rat, *Eur. J. Haematol.,* 41, 321, 1988.

109. **Valenzuela, A., Fernandez, V., and Videla, L. A.,** Hepatic and biliary levels of glutathione and lipid peroxides following iron overload in the rat: effect of simultaneous ethanol administration, *Toxicol. Appl. Pharmacol.,* 70, 87, 1983.

110. **Mazzanti, R., Srai, K. S., Debnam, E. S., Boss, A. M., and Gentilini, P.,** The effect of chronic consumption on iron absorption in rats, *Alcohol Alcoholism,* 22, 47, 1987.

111. **Rouach, H., Mouze, P., Orfanelli, M. T., Gentil, M., Bourdon, R., and Nordmann, R.,** Effect of acute ethanol administration on the subcellular distribution of iron in rat liver and cerebellum, *Biochem. Pharmacol.,* 39, 1095, 1990.

112. **Sinaceur, J., Ribiere, C., Abu-Murad, C., Nordman, J., and Nordman, R.,** Reduction in the rate of ethanol elimination *in vivo* by desferrioxamine and diethylenetriamine pentaacetic acid: suggestion for involvement of hydroxyl radicals in ethanol oxidation, *Biochem. Pharmacol.,* 32, 2371, 1983.

113. **Shaw, S., Jayatilleke, E., and Lieber, C. S.,** Lipid peroxidation as a mechanism of alcoholic liver injury; role of iron mobilization and microsomal induction, *Alcohol,* 5, 135, 1988.

114. **Shaw, S.,** Lipid peroxidation, iron mobilization and radical generation induced by alcohol, *Free Radical Biol. Med.,* 7, 541, 1989.

115. **Barry, M.,** Iron and chronic liver disease, *J. R. Coll. Physicians Lond.,* 8, 52, 1973.

116. **Jakobovits, A. W., Morgan, M. Y., and Sherlock, S.,** Hepatic siderosis in alcoholics, *Dig. Dis. Sci.,* 24, 305, 1979.

117. **Charlton, R. W., Jacobs, P., Seftel, H., and Bothwell, T. H.,** Effects of alcohol on iron absorption, *Br. Med. J.,* 2, 1427, 1964.

118. **Celeda, A., Rudolf, H., and Donath, A.,** Effect of a single ingestion of alcohol on iron absorption, *Am. J. Hematol.,* 5, 225, 1978.

119. **Hourihane, D. O. B. and Weir, D. G.,** Suppression of erythropoiesis by alcohol, *Br. Med. J.,* 1, 86, 1970.

120. **Hoenig, V., Brodanova, M., and Kordac, C.,** Effect of ethanol on iron tolerance and endogenous serum iron in liver cirrhosis, *Scand. J. Gastroenterol.,* 3, 334, 1968.

121. **Heilmeyer, L.,** Pathogenesis of hemochromatosis, *Medicine (Baltimore),* 46, 209, 1967.

122. **Powell, L. W.,** Normal human iron storage and its relation to ethanol consumption, *Aust. Ann. Med.,* 15, 110, 1966.

123. **Powell, L. W.,** The role of alcoholism in hepatic iron storage disease, *Ann. N.Y. Acad. Sci.,* 252, 124, 1975.

124. **Lundvall, O., Weinfeld, A., and Lundin, P.,** Iron stores in alcohol abusers. I. Liver iron, *Acta Med. Scand.,* 185, 259, 1969.

125. **Rothschild, M. A., Oratz, N., Morland, J., Schreiber, S. S., Burks, A., and Martin, B.,** Effects of ethanol on protein synthesis and secretion, *Pharmacol. Biochem. Behav.,* 13 (Suppl. 1), 31, 1980.

126. **Jeejeebhoy, K. N., Phillips, M. J., Bruce-Robertson, A., Ho, J., and Sodtke, U.,** The acute effects of ethanol on albumin, fibrinogen and transferrin synthesis in the rat, *Biochem. J.,* 126, 1111, 1972.

127. **Nunes, R. M., Beloqui, O., Potter, B. J., and Berk, P. D.,** Iron uptake from transferrin by isolated hepatocytes: effect of ethanol, *Biochem. Biophys. Res. Commun.,* 125, 824, 1984.

128. **Beloqui, O., Nunes, R. M., Blades, B., Berk, P. D., and Potter, B. J.,** Depression of iron uptake from transferrin by isolated hepatocytes in the presence of ethanol is a pH dependent consequence of ethanol metabolism, *Alcoholism: Clin. Exp. Res.,* 10, 463, 1986.

129. **Casey, C. A., Kragskow, S. L., Sorrell, M. F., and Tuma, D.,** Effect of chronic ethanol administration on total asialoglycoprotein receptor content and intracellular processing of asialoorosomucoid in isolated rat hepatocyte, *Biochim. Biophys. Acta.,* 1052, 1, 1990.

130. **Stibler, H., Borg, S., and Allgulander, C.,** Clinical significance of abnormal heterogeneity of transferrin in relation to alcohol consumption, *Acta Med. Scand.,* 206, 275, 1979.

131. **Storey, E. L., Mack, U., Powell, L. W., and Halliday, J. W.,** Use of chromatofocusing to detect a transferrin variant in serum of alcoholic subjects, *Clin. Chem.,* 31, 1543, 1985.

132. **Stibler, H. and Borg, S.,** Evidence of a reduced sialic acid content in serum transferrin in male alcoholics, *Alcoholism: Clin. Exp. Res.,* 5, 545, 1981.

133. **Stibler, H. and Borg, S.,** Carbohydrate composition of serum transferrin in alcoholic patients, *Alcoholism: Clin. Exp. Res.,* 10, 61, 1986.

134. **Stibler, H., Borg, S., and Joustra, M.,** Micro anion exchange chromatography of carbohydrate-deficient transferrin in relation to alcohol consumption, *Alcoholism: Clin. Exp. Res.,* 10, 535, 1986.

135. **Behrens, U. J., Worner, T. M., Braly, L. F., Schaffner, F., and Lieber, C. S.,** Carbohydrate-deficient transferrin, a marker for chronic alcohol consumption in different ethnic populations, *Alcoholism: Clin. Exp. Res.,* 12, 427, 1988.

136. **Nordmann, R., Ribiere, C., and Rouach, H.,** Ethanol induced lipid peroxidation and oxidative stress in extrahepatic tissues, *Alcohol Alcoholism,* 25, 231, 1990.

137. **Edes, I., Toszegi, A., Csanady, M., and Bozoky, B.,** Myocardial lipid peroxidation in rats after chronic alcohol ingestion and the effects of different antioxidants, *Cardiovasc. Res.,* 20, 542, 1986.

138. **Rosenblum, E. R., Gavaler, J. S., and Van-Thiel, D. M.,** Lipid peroxidation: a mechanism for alcohol-induced testicular injury, *Free Radical Biol. Med.,* 7, 569, 1989.

139. **Kera, Y., Pentilla, K. E., and Lindros, K. O.,** Glutathione replenishment capacity is lower in isolated perivenous than in periportal hepatocytes, *Biochem. J.,* 254, 411, 1988.

140. **Tsutsumi, M., Lasker, J., Shimizu, M., Rosman, A. S., and Lieber, C. S.,** The intralobular distribution of ethanol-inducible P-450IIE1 in rat and human liver, *Hepatology,* 10, 437, 1989.

141. **Jauhonen, V. P., Baraona, E., Miyakawa, H., and Lieber, C. S.,** Mechanism for selective perivenular hepatotoxicity of ethanol, *Alcoholism: Clin. Exp. Res.,* 6, 350, 1982.

18. Iron Metabolism and Oxygen Radical Injury in Premature Infants

Jerome L. Sullivan

*Veterans Affairs Medical Center, Charleston, South Carolina, and
Department of Pathology and Laboratory Medicine,
Medical University of South Carolina, Charleston*

I. INTRODUCTION

Iron overload is traditionally defined by the presence of large amounts of histologically stainable iron in tissue. Iron overload thus defined occurs only rarely in neonates.[1] Fewer than 50 cases have been reported. In "neonatal hemochromatosis" there is parenchymal deposition of iron in the liver and other organs. These infants are often premature and suffer from hypotension, hyperbilirubinemia, hypoglycemia, hypoxia, and coagulopathy. There is no association with adult hemochromatosis. With histologically demonstrable iron in liver parenchyma there is no disagreement that iron overload exists.

In this chapter, a case will be made for broadening the definition of iron overload in the neonatal period. Several developmental factors conspire to guarantee that many premature infants will have no unsaturated iron-binding capacity for a period of days following birth. Unavailability of iron-binding capacity, combined with ferritin levels in the hundreds or thousands of micrograms per liter and a developmental lack of ferroxidase (ceruloplasmin) activity, in my view, represents a state of clinically significant iron overload. These conditions are commonly encountered in preterm infants, more so in very low birth weight preterm infants. Absence of stainable iron in liver storage compartments and parenchyma in these infants does not exclude the possibility that excess iron is available to promote oxygen radical injury. The relationship of neonatal iron overload, as defined here, to neonatal hemochromatosis is unclear.

The consequences of iron overload in premature infants may be a greatly increased susceptibility to oxygen radical injury.[2-4] Iron overload thus defined may predispose the premature infant to serious injury by critically compromising antioxidant defenses. Many premature infants have essentially no capacity for decreasing the reactivity of endogenous iron in plasma. Deficiency in free iron-binding capacity (i.e., iron overload) can theoretically be corrected by administration of human apotransferrin. Infusing apotransferrin in premature infants with evidence of iron overload may correct the deficiency and protect them from oxygen radical injury. This experiment should help to determine the importance of antioxidants that decrease the reactivity of iron in comparison with other proposed antioxidant deficiencies in the neonatal period. If shown to be protective, exogenous apotransferrin could be used clinically as prophylaxis against a range of neonatal disorders associated with oxygen radical injury. Apotransferrin infusion is a feasible short-term therapy in iron-overloaded preterm infants, since their iron overload is a transient phenomenon, if they survive. Neonatal iron overload may also predispose infants to certain infectious diseases (see Chapter 8).

II. OXYGEN RADICAL DISEASE IN PREMATURITY

Oxygen radical injury has been implicated as a pathogenic mechanism in several neonatal diseases including retinopathy of prematurity, bronchopulmonary dysplasia, subependymal and intraventricular hemorrhage, and necrotizing enterocolitis.[5] The greater incidence of these in preterm infants suggests that some aspect of prematurity increases susceptibility to toxic oxygen species. A possible explanation for increased susceptibility to these disorders in prematurity is that premature infants may have defects in one or more of the antioxidant systems that protect more mature infants and older children. It is not surprising that preterm infants have less effective antioxidant systems. Lower oxygen tensions in the intrauterine environment may allow survival with less potent antioxidant systems.

Hypotheses based on possible antioxidant deficiencies are potentially verifiable. Administration of the deficient antioxidant may allow both verification of the hypothesis and preventive treatment, if the hypothesis is confirmed. Many proteins and other endogenous substances have antioxidant activity *in vitro*. These include superoxide dismutase, catalase, glutathione peroxidase, vitamin E, ascorbic acid, ceruloplasmin, and apotransferrin. The relative importance of each component *in vivo* in health and disease remains unclear. Results of *in vitro* assays are of limited value in addressing this question.[6] Studies with vitamin E in retinopathy of prematurity illustrate this point. *In vitro* vitamin E is a potent, lipophilic, chain-breaking antioxidant. Vitamin E is also known to be at a relatively low concentration in preterm plasma. These findings appear to be strong circumstantial evidence that low vitamin E levels predispose premature infants to retinopathy of prematurity. However, administration of vitamin E to preterm infants does not reliably protect them from retinopathy of prematurity.[7,8] On the other hand, vitamin E may confer some protection against brain hemorrhage in neonates.[9]

III. ANTIOXIDANT DEFICIENCIES IN PRETERM IRON OVERLOAD

Iron overload as defined here has a negative impact on endogenous antioxidants that decrease the reactivity of iron. Much of the preventive antioxidant activity of plasma is associated with apotransferrin and ceruloplasmin.[10-12] As preventive antioxidants, these proteins are at least two orders of magnitude more potent than vitamin E, compared on a molar basis.[10,11] The antioxidant activities of both proteins depend on decreasing the reactivity of iron in oxygen radical reactions. Ceruloplasmin is a ferroxidase catalyzing the oxidation of ferrous to ferric iron.[12] Inhibition of its ferroxidase activity blocks antioxidant activity. Oxidation to the ferric state may facilitate binding of iron to transferrin. Transferrin in the unsaturated, apo- form acts as an antioxidant by binding iron.[10,11] The antioxidant activity of uric acid may also depend on interactions with iron.[13]

The plasma concentrations of both transferrin[14-16] and ceruloplasmin[17,18] are low by adult standards in term neonates and are even lower in premature infants. Such a pattern would be expected for antioxidants of importance in the pathogenesis of oxygen radical injury in premature infants. Also, shortly after birth, in both term and preterm infants, there are major changes in iron metabolism that substantially increase transferrin saturation and thus diminish its antioxidant activity.[14-16,19-22] The preterm infant is especially at risk of high transferrin saturation because of developmentally low levels of transferrin.

IV. NEONATAL IRON METABOLISM

Birth is a transition from a relatively iron-rich environment in utero to the nutritionally iron-poor extrauterine environment. In utero, iron is available from the mother in excess of needs. At birth, normal neonates have excess iron in storage.[20] After birth, acquisition of adequate iron to support maximal growth is not always assured.

Birth also marks a transition to an environment with higher oxygen concentration. This is associated with a virtual cessation of red cell formation that persists for 6 to 8 weeks after birth.[21,22] The adjustment has major effects on neonatal iron metabolism. Red cell senescence and lysis continue despite the cessation of erythropoiesis. If there is a hemolytic process, the rate of iron release from lysed red cells increases over basal levels. Thus, there is a large increase in the amount of iron to be stored. The usual postnatal pause in erythropoiesis is undoubtedly a large part of the explanation for the major increases in transferrin saturation and plasma ferritin levels seen in term and preterm infants shortly after birth. In the study of Siimes et al.,[19] the median serum ferritin level in normal infants rose to a peak of 356 µg/l at 1 month of age and fell to 30 µg/l by 6 months of age.

In preterm infants, much higher levels of serum ferritin can be seen, particularly in those who receive iron supplements or blood transfusions. These small patients have a very limited capacity to assimilate exogenous iron. Premature infants are also at risk of iron overload because their absorption of iron is unregulated.[21] Iron absorption is proportional to dietary iron regardless of need. In those given supplemental iron or blood transfusions, Shaw[21] reported some very high values for serum ferritin (1000 to 2000 µg/l). In an adult, such numbers would suggest the diagnosis of homozygous hemochromatosis.

At birth, preterm infants have less total body iron than term infants. Premature birth interrupts iron acquisition from the mother during the period of maximal iron absorption by the fetus. The lower total body iron pool does not protect the preterm infant from very high transferrin saturations. Transferrin saturations of 100% often occur. The developmentally low levels of transferrin put the premature infant at great risk of having totally saturated transferrin. Transferrin concentration increases with gestational age and correlates closely with gestational age. Developmental factors appear to be much more important than iron status in regulating transferrin level at birth.[14,22]

V. CERULOPLASMIN IN PRETERM INFANTS

Ceruloplasmin is another plasma protein whose antioxidant activity depends on interactions with iron. As a ferroxidase it may exert some of its antioxidant activity by facilitating the binding of iron to transferrin. Even in the absence of transferrin, however, ceruloplasmin is a potent antioxidant.[12] Iron appears to be most effective in promoting lipid peroxidation when ferric and ferrous ions are present in equal concentrations. Ferric iron alone is much less effective than a 1:1 mixture of ferric and ferrous iron.[23] Ceruloplasmin may have an antioxidant effect by increasing the ferric/ferrous ratio.

Preterm infants have a lower plasma concentration of ceruloplasmin than term infants.[12,17,18] Even fully mature infants have only about a third as much ceruloplasmin per volume of plasma as do older children and adults. There is evidence that preterm infants with respiratory distress syndrome have lower cord serum ceruloplasmin than unaffected preterm infants.[24]

VI. HYPOTHESIS

The following hypothesis is proposed: preterm infants are abnormally susceptible to oxygen radical injury because of a clinically significant state of iron overload. Iron overload in premature infants is characterized by developmentally low levels of transferrin and ceruloplasmin/ferroxidase activity, combined with postnatal changes in iron metabolism that increase transferrin saturation. This is not to say that the iron present is excessive in terms of the amount required for erythropoiesis and growth. Rather, the available iron overloads the infant's limited iron-handling capacity. Because of the limited amount of iron present, the strategy for correcting this form of iron overload must involve increasing the available iron-binding capacity, and not removing excess iron.

The hypothesis does not exclude an important role for other factors in the pathogenesis of oxygen radical diseases of prematurity. It does not explain why injury is more prominent in the retina of one infant and in the lungs of another. Additional factors must be acting to determine which site of injury predominates in each case. The hypothesis does suggest that correction of a deficiency in iron-binding capacity may decrease the incidence of a broad range of serious neonatal disorders.

VII. VERIFICATION

Several testable predictions arise from the hypothesis, the most significant of which involve possible modes of preventive therapy. Existing data on iron metabolism, ceruloplasmin, and transferrin in the neonatal period generally support the proposed hypothesis.[14-22] There is indirect evidence of an inverse association between the mean transferrin level and disease incidence. Verification of the hypothesis will require demonstration of such an association in individual patients. Disease should occur more frequently in those infants with high transferrin saturation, high ferritin, and/or low ceruloplasmin levels. Verification will require studies of transferrin saturation, ferritin, and ceruloplasmin levels in relation to the occurrence of disease in a series of preterm infants. Positive findings in such studies should be followed by attempts to prevent disease by pharmacological augmentation of apotransferrin and/or ceruloplasmin levels in premature infants.

VIII. ANTIOXIDANT ACTIVITY AND PLASMA TRANSFUSION

Infusion of purified apotransferrin should increase the antioxidant activity of an infant's plasma. Apotransferrin is often routinely given to sick newborns in the form of donor plasma. Since adult plasma has greater concentrations of apotransferrin than term, and especially preterm infant plasma, transfusion of donor plasma can also potentially boost the infant's plasma levels of apotransferrin. The established safety of plasma transfusion in neonates gives some assurance that purified apotransferrin would at least do no harm.

How much of an increase can be achieved? If the plasma donor were also a frequent blood donor, he could be iron depleted or marginally iron deficient.[25] Uncomplicated iron deficiency is associated with a substantial increase in plasma free transferrin.[26] A preterm infant can have essentially no free transferrin, i.e., in cases with a transferrin saturation of 100%. Thus, even a normal adult level of plasma apotransferrin can exceed that of a preterm infant's level by several orders of magnitude.

Serologically compatible plasma is regarded as a fairly uniform commodity. However, there are large differences from unit to unit in the amounts of apotransferrin. Its concentration can be measured by widely available assays. Donor plasma could be selected to assure maximal augmentation of the infant's free iron-binding capacity. Transfusions of plasma rich in apotransferrin may be an effective preventive therapy against oxygen radical injury in premature infants.

IX. ANTIOXIDANT ACTIVITY AND BLOOD TRANSFUSION

Excess blood transfusions may enhance oxygen radical injury by increasing a preterm infant's iron load.[2,4] Packed red blood cell transfusions contain hundreds of times more hemoglobin iron than plasma iron-binding capacity. The small amount of plasma in the blood transfusion contributes only a negligible amount of free transferrin. The amounts of blood transfused in neonates are small by adult standards, but large in relation to the infant's total body iron. A single 10 ml transfusion of packed red blood cells contains about one fifth of the total body iron of a typical 1000 g premature infant. An increase in total body iron from excess transfusions may partially explain the reported positive association between blood transfusions and retinopathy of prematurity.[27]

X. DEFEROXAMINE AS AN ANTIOXIDANT

In principle, deferoxamine should be clinically useful for augmenting iron-binding capacity in premature infants with 100% transferrin saturation.[2,4] However, as has been pointed out previously, deferoxamine treatment imposes a potentially serious hazard.[4] Deferoxamine-bound iron is not retained by the kidneys. Premature infants have only a very small amount of total body iron. Administration of deferoxamine may quickly deplete the tiny iron storage compartment and perhaps iron from other sites as well. Deferoxamine treatment in premature baboon infants with hyaline membrane disease has been shown to be rapidly fatal.[28] There may be other modes of toxicity in addition to sudden iron depletion. In the baboon model, deferoxamine may have cardiovascular toxicity through an unknown mechanism. High molecular weight forms of deferoxamine may not deplete iron stores so quickly and should be tested in the premature baboon model. Exogenous purified apotransferrin may be superior to deferoxamine because it does not cause iron loss. Exogenous apotransferrin could be given intravenously or directly into the lung in aerosolized form.

The apparent cardiovascular toxicity of deferoxamine in premature baboon infants may be a species-specific effect. In a necrotizing enterocolitis model using weanling rats, deferoxamine showed significant protective effects.[29] Both survival and mucosal histology were superior in deferoxamine-treated animals.

XI. MILK AND THE ANTIOXIDANT ACTIVITY OF APOLACTOFERRIN

Both human milk and purified apolactoferrin have substantial antioxidant activity *in vitro*.[29a] Human apolactoferrin given intravenously to rats protects them in a dose-dependent manner against acute lung injury *in vivo* in a complement- and neutrophil-dependent model system.[30] Human milk, especially colostrum, is rich in apolactoferrin.[31,32] Premature infants absorb large amounts of intact macromolecules from milk into their plasma.[33] Maternal lactoferrin is found in the urine of premature infants.[34] Milk apolactoferrin may be absorbed in amounts sufficient to increase the infant's plasma antioxidant activity and partially correct the iron overload. Enhanced neonatal antioxidant protection may be another of the many benefits of breast feeding.[4] Absorbed apolactoferrin may be a partial explanation for the reported lower incidence of retinopathy of prematurity in breast-fed infants.[35]

XII. TRANSFERRIN IN THE LUNG

Transferrin may have a special antioxidant role in the lung. Studies of antioxidant activity in adult lung epithelial lining fluid (ELF) suggest that transferrin is the predominant antioxidant.[36] Vitamin E, vitamin C, and albumin do not function as antioxidants in ELF, and ceruloplasmin makes only a minimal contribution.[36] In other studies, Skinner and co-workers[37] found that transferrin gene expression occurs in the fibroblasts of fetal rat lung. These experiments suggest that transferrin synthesis in the lung follows a strict developmental schedule, peaking in the last few days before birth. Immunohistochemical staining for transferrin showed intense staining alveolar and capillary basement membranes. The sharp increase in transferrin gene expression in the lung shortly before term is consistent with the idea that transferrin is a crucially important antioxidant at the lung/air boundary at birth.

XIII. IRON OVERLOAD AND HEMOLYTIC DISEASE IN THE NEWBORN

Recent work on iron and rhesus hemolytic disease (RHD) lends support to the concept of iron overload in the neonatal period. Berger and co-workers[38] found increased serum ferritin and decreased apotransferrin in infants with severe RHD. The reported associations do not demonstrate conclusively that iron overload was the cause of the reported increase in lipid peroxidation products,[38] but the findings are consistent with the present hypothesis.

XIV. CONCLUDING REMARKS

Postnatal increases in serum ferritin and transferrin saturation have been known for some time. Until recently these patterns were apparently regarded as benign phenomena. For example, one investigator recently commented on ferritins up to 2000 $\mu g/l$ in premature infants[21] stating, ''I am not aware of any harmful sequelae, and the levels tend to fall spontaneously.'' However, these perturbations in ferritin and transferrin are large even by adult standards. The changes clearly increase, rather than decrease, the potential for free iron occurring *in vivo*. They are seen during a narrow temporal window of increased susceptibility to oxygen radical injury. The scale, direction, and timing of these changes suggest that iron overload, i.e., deficiency in iron-binding capacity, has an important role in promoting oxygen radical injury in premature infants.

ACKNOWLEDGMENT

This chapter is an updated and revised version of a paper originally published in the *American Journal of Diseases of Children*, 142, 1341, (De-

REFERENCES

1. **Halliday, J. W.**, Inherited iron overload, *Acta Paediatr. Scand.*, Supp. 361, 86, 1989.
2. **Sullivan, J. L.**, Retinopathy of prematurity and iron: a modification of the oxygen hypothesis, *Pediatrics,* 78, 1171, 1986.
3. **Sullivan, J. L. and Newton, R. B.**, Serum antioxidant activity in neonates, *Arch. Dis. Child.*, 63, 748, 1988.
4. **Sullivan, J. L.**, Iron, plasma antioxidants, and the 'oxygen radical disease of prematurity', *Am. J. Dis. Child.*, 142, 1341, 1988.
5. **Saugstad, O. D.**, Oxygen toxicity in the neonatal period, *Acta Paediatr. Scand.*, 79, 881, 1990.
6. **Dormandy, T. L.**, Free-radical oxidation and antioxidants, *Lancet,* 1, 647, 1978.
7. **Phelps, D. L., Rosenbaum, A. L., Isenberg, S. J., Leake, R. D., and Dorey, F. J.**, Tocopherol efficacy and safety for preventing retinopathy of prematurity: a randomized, controlled, double-masked trial, *Pediatrics,* 79, 489, 1987.
8. **Hittner, H. M., Speer, M. E., Rudolph, A. J., Blifeld, C., Chadda, P., Holbein, M. E. B., Godio, L. B., and Kretzer, F. L.**, Retrolental fibroplasia and vitamin E in the preterm infant: comparison of oral versus intramuscular:oral administration, *Pediatrics,* 73, 238, 1984.
9. **Chiswick, M., Gladman, G., Sinha, S., Toner, N., and Davies, J.**, Vitamin E supplementation and periventricular hemorrhage in the newborn, *Am. J. Clin. Nutr.,* 53, 370S, 1991.
10. **Stocks, J., Gutteridge, J. M. C., Sharpe, R. J., and Dormandy, T. L.**, Assay using brain homogenate for measuring the antioxidant activity of biological fluids, *Clin. Sci.,* 47, 215, 1974.
11. **Stocks, J., Gutteridge, J. M. C., Sharp, R. J., and Dormandy, T. L.**, The inhibition of lipid autoxidation by human serum and its relation to serum proteins and alpha-tocopherol, *Clin. Sci.,* 47, 223, 1974.
12. **Gutteridge, J. M. C. and Stocks, J.**, Caeruloplasmin: physiological and pathological perspectives, *CRC Crit. Rev. Clin. Lab. Sci.,* 14, 257, 1981.
13. **Davies, K. J. A., Sevanian, A., Muakkassah-Kelly, S. F., and Hochstein, P.**, Uric acid-iron ion complexes: a new aspect of the antioxidant functions of uric acid, *Biochem. J.,* 235, 747, 1986.
14. **Scott, P. H., Berger, H. M., Kenward, C., Scott, P., and Wharton, B. A.**, Effect of gestational age and intrauterine nutrition on plasma transferrin and iron in the newborn, *Arch. Dis. Child.*, 50, 796, 1975.
15. **Galet, S., Schulman, H. M., and Bard, H.**, The postnatal hypotransferrinemia of early preterm newborn infants, *Pediatr. Res.*, 10, 118, 1976.
16. **Saarinen, U. M. and Siimes, M. A.**, Developmental changes in serum iron, total iron-binding capacity, and transferrin saturation in infancy, *J. Pediatr.*, 91, 875, 1977.
17. **Hilderbrand, D. C., Fahim, Z., James, E., and Fahim, M.**, Ceruloplasmin and alkaline phosphatase levels in cord serum of term, preterm, and physiologically jaundiced neonates, *Am. J. Obstet. Gynecol.*, 118, 950, 1974.
18. **Buffone, G. I., Brett, E. M., Lewis, S. A., Iosefsohn, M., and Hicks, J. M.**, Limitations of immunochemical measurements of ceruloplasmin, *Clin. Chem.*, 25, 749, 1979.

19. **Siimes, M. A., Addiego, J. F., and Dallman, P. R.,** Ferritin in serum: diagnosis of iron deficiency and iron overload in infants and children, *Blood,* 43, 581, 1974.

20. **Brittenham, G. M., Danish, E. H., and Harris, J. W.,** Assessment of bone marrow and body iron stores: old techniques and new technologies, *Semin. Hematol.,* 18, 194, 1981.

21. **Shaw, J. C. L.,** Iron absorption by the premature infant: the effect of transfusion and iron supplements on the serum ferritin levels, *Acta Paediatr. Scand.,* Suppl. 299, 83, 1982.

22. **Lukens, J. N.,** Iron metabolism and iron deficiency anemia, in *Blood Diseases of Infancy and Childhood,* Miller, D. R., Baehner, R. L., McMillan, C. W., and Miller, L. P., Eds., St. Louis, C. V. Mosby, 1984, 115.

23. **Braughler, J. M., Duncan, L. A., and Chase, R. L.,** The involvement of iron in lipid peroxidation: importance of ferric to ferrous ratios in initiation, *J. Biol. Chem.,* 261, 10282, 1986.

24. **Omene, J. A., Longe, A. C., Ihongbe, J. C., Glew, R. H., and Holzman, I. R.,** Decreased umbilical cord serum ceruloplasmin concentrations in infants with hyaline membrane disease, *J. Pediatr.,* 99, 136, 1981.

25. **Finch, C. A., Cook, J. D., Labbe, R. F., and Culala, M.,** Effect of blood donation on iron stores as evaluated by serum ferritin, *Blood,* 50, 441, 1977.

26. **Herbert, V.,** Recommended dietary intakes (RDI) of iron in humans, *Am. J. Clin. Nutr.,* 45, 679, 1987.

27. **Sacks, I. M., Schaffer, D. B., Anday, E. K., Peckham, G. J., and Delivoria-Papadopoulos, M.,** Retrolental fibroplasia and blood transfusion in very low birth weight infants, *Pediatrics,* 68, 770, 1981.

28. **deLemos, R. A., Roberts, R. J., Coalson, J. J., deLemos, J. A., Null, D. M., and Gertsmann, D. R.,** Toxic effects associated with the administration of deferoxamine in the premature baboon with hyaline membrane disease, *Am. J. Dis. Child.,* 144, 915, 1990.

29. **Lelli, J. L., Pradhan, S., and Cobb, I. M.,** Blockade of reperfusion injury of the bowel in a necrotizing enterocolitis model, *Pediatr. Res.,* 20, 353A, 1986.

29a. **Sullivan, J. L. and Newton, R. B.,** unpublished observations, 1987.

30. **Ward, P. A., Till, G. O., Kunkel, R., and Beauchamp, C.,** Evidence for role of hydroxyl radical in complement and neutrophil-injury, *J. Clin. Invest.,* 72, 789, 1983.

31. **Siimes, M. A., Vuori, E., and Kuitunen, P.,** Breast milk iron — a declining concentration during the course of lactation, *Acta Paediatr. Scand.,* 68, 29, 1979.

32. **Fransson, G. B. and Lonnerdal, B.,** Iron in human milk, *J. Pediatr.,* 96, 380, 1980.

33. **Jakobsson, I., Lindberg, T., Lothe, L., Axelsson, I., and Benedktsson, B.,** Human alpha-lactalbumin as a marker for macromolecular absorption, *Gut,* 27, 1029, 1986.

34. **Hutchens, T. W., Henry, J. F., Yip, T.-T., Hachey, D. L., Schanler, R. J., Motil, K. J., and Garza, C.,** Origin of intact lactoferrin and its DNA-binding fragments found in the urine of human milk-fed preterm infants. Evaluation by stable isotopic enrichment, *Pediatr. Res.,* 29, 243, 1991.

35. **Cunningham, A. S.,** Breast-feeding, antioxidants, and retinopathy of prematurity, *Am. J. Obstet. Gynecol.,* 156, 1040, 1987.

36. **Pacht, E. R. and Davis, W. B.,** Role of transferrin and ceruloplasmin in antioxidant activity of lung epithelial lining fluid, *J. Appl. Physiol.,* 64(5), 2092, 1988.

37. **Skinner, S. J. M., Somervell, C. E., Buch, S., and Post, M.,** Transferrin gene expression and transferrin immunolocalisation in developing fetal rat lung, *J. Cell Sci.,* in press, 1991.

38. **Berger, H. M., Lindeman, J. H. N., van Zoernen-Grobben, D., Houdkamp, E., Schrijver, J., and Kanhai, H. H.,** Iron overload, free radical damage, and rhesus haemolytic disease, *Lancet,* 335, 933, 1990.

Part VI
Implications for Prevention and Therapy

19. Preventive Measures for the Maintenance of Low but Adequate Iron Stores

RANDALL B. LAUFFER

NMR Center, Massachusetts General Hospital and Harvard Medical School, Boston, Massachusetts

I. INTRODUCTION

The evidence in this book has important implications for preventive health care in Western societies where high iron levels are commonplace. As an oxidative catalyst and a limiting nutrient for tumor cells and pathogenic organisms, iron appears to contribute to an enormous number of diseases which afflict the Western world including cardiovascular disease and cancer, the leading killers. Whether the role of iron in these many conditions is confirmed in subsequent research and whether reductions in iron levels will be palliative or even lifesaving are two of the many questions for future research. Nonetheless, the evidence to date is persuasive enough to begin to discuss various preventive approaches based on this new information on iron.

Many investigators and physicians understandably consider the epidemiological and animal data in a stage too early to issue public health recommendations. It is true that the "iron story" is lagging some 40 to 50 years behind that of the "cholesterol story". A well-publicized Framingham-type study that includes detailed iron balance profiles is desperately needed. There are, however, a number of other considerations that make public health recommendations justified today.

One of the most important considerations is whether the new recommendations would be safe and whether they would be consistent with existing guidelines. If preliminary but provocative evidence indicates that high iron stores can make a heart attack more deadly or promote tumor growth, then why not inform the public that their new low-fat diet — with its lower meat content — is also likely to lower their iron levels? This information cannot do harm to people, and it gives them new ways to think about eating healthy foods.

This disagreement among investigators as to whether to give the public this preliminary information is understandable and common in the nutrition and preventive health fields. Considerable acrimony still exists in the debate over whether lowering cholesterol levels actually saves lives. Complete agreement is indeed rare, and this is never a good reason *not* to inform the public. In addition, it is unlikely that the natural level of confusion on the part of the public with regard to nutrition and health advice can be alleviated by waiting years for the results of large clinical trials before informing them. The public is constantly bombarded by good and bad advice, and one can only hope that they can begin to receive more of the former. Cultural factors, unrelated to science, also have undue influence, especially in the case of iron.[1] Furthermore, people have a right to make their own choices based on whatever information set they deem reasonable and meaningful for their own lives. Ours is increasingly a sophisticated public, at least the subset of the public that pays close attention to health matters, and individual choice has as much relevance in the arena of health as it does in other areas of life.

A final reason for increasing the public's awareness of the potential harm from excess iron is to facilitate the early diagnosis and treatment of homo-

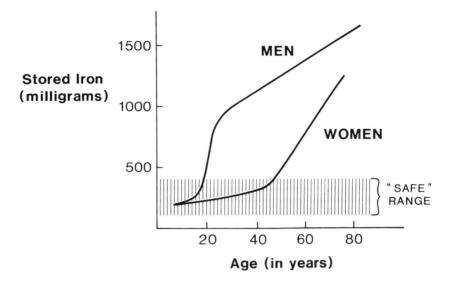

FIGURE 1. Iron stores in men and women as a function of age. Total iron stores were estimated as ten times the average serum ferritin values found in the study of Cook et al.[2] An adequate but not excessive level of iron (100 to 400 mg), roughly equal to the range exhibited by premenopausal women, is shown as a theoretical "safe range". (From Lauffer, R. B., *Iron Balance*, St. Martin's Press, New York, 1991. With permission.)

zygous hemochromatosis. Only a fraction of the estimated 3 to 5 per 1000 individuals are ever diagnosed. This is changing as doctors are becoming aware that the prevalence estimates in many textbooks are erroneously low. Blood chemistry testing services are beginning to include serum ferritin and transferrin saturation in standard screens, leading to many new diagnoses. The layman, too, can contribute to increased awareness. I am aware of several instances where a person informed about iron overload and its symptoms offered a preliminary diagnosis to a friend and encouraged him or her to get tested.

The following sections outline the basic preventive measures to maintain low but adequate iron stores. In a recently published book for the lay public I proposed that, based on the preliminary information to date, the best estimate for optimal iron stores would be in the range of roughly 100 to 400 mg, the general range exhibited by premenopausal women.[1] This theoretical "safe range" is shown in Figure 1 along with the iron stores for American men and women as estimated from serum ferritin measurements.[2] One can begin to establish this level of iron stores through one or more of the following measures: dietary changes, occasional blood donation, or possibly exercise. A new approach to iron nutrition also requires that physicians change their views concerning routine iron supplementation for mild anemia and pregnancy. This is discussed in Section II.

II. EXERCISING CAUTION IN IRON SUPPLEMENTATION FOR ANEMIA AND PREGNANCY

An important public health goal with regard to iron is to convince physicians to approach the diagnosis and treatment of iron deficiency and iron deficiency anemia with extreme caution. Pharmacological iron supplementation is probably the most rapid means by which to build iron stores to unnecessarily high levels. In addition, one unjustified recommendation of iron supplements to a patient can begin a habit that the person carries throughout life. There are several reports in the literature of secondary hemochromatosis in women who had taken iron supplements for many years.[3-6] In addition, one study reported that only 12 weeks of iron supplementation can cause mild liver damage as evidenced by transient elevations in the concentration of liver enzymes in serum.[7] There are, of course, a wide range of mild side effects of iron supplements, such as constipation, nausea, heartburn, upper gastric discomfort, and diarrhea.

All evidence points to iron deficiency anemia as being one of the most overdiagnosed and overtreated diseases. In a recent survey of 265 general practitioners in England, half of the respondents admitted that they often treated patients with iron without even requesting a laboratory blood test.[8] Up to 40% of the doctors admitted prescribing iron when patients had nonspecific complaints such as fatigue or even when the patients themselves requested iron.

The prevalence of iron deficiency in developed countries has been constantly exaggerated.[1] This is largely due to early population studies of hemoglobin levels or other nonspecific indices where artificial and inappropriate cutoffs between normal and iron-deficient subjects were applied. Iron, hemoglobin, and hematocrit levels in populations span a large range with no clear cutoffs for deficiency. Some evidence of harm or function in each individual is required to be confident that treatment is justified.[9]

The 1976 to 1980 National Health and Nutrition Examination Survey (NHANES II) has been the bench mark for recent discussions of iron deficiency anemia.[10] Subjects were judged to have "impaired iron status" if at least two of the following tests results were in the ranges shown:

Serum ferritin: <12 μg/l
Transferrin saturation: $<16\%$
Erythrocyte protoporphyrin: >70 μg/l of red blood cells
(Cutoffs applicable to both men and women, ages 15 to 74)

The prevalence of iron deficiency anemia among men was found to be very low: 0.6% of men aged 20 to 44 and 1.9% aged 45 to 64 had "impaired iron status". Women, as expected, were more likely to have abnormal results: 9.6% of those aged 20 to 44 and 4.8% of age 45 to 64. Thus, physicians should not expect to find true iron deficiency anemia in more than one of ten women seen in general practice.

Although NHANES II is the best study to date, its data on iron are still open to debate. There is considerable overlap between the values obtained for abnormal subjects and those judged normal. For example, 31% of those women with low hemoglobin readings (less than 11.9 g/100 ml) had *not one* abnormal reading, whereas 22% of those women with hemoglobin values in the normal range had at least one abnormal reading. In addition, true evidence of harm to health or function was not obtained in this large study.

The most prudent approach seems to be to treat only those patients with lab tests at least as abnormal as that defined by the NHANES II study. General screening must include, at the minimum, the serum ferritin test in addition to the other common tests such as hemoglobin. A low serum ferritin (<10 μg/l for ages 3 to 4 years and <12 μg/l for ages >15 years) justifies obtaining transferrin saturation, erythrocyte protoporphyrin, and perhaps other tests. Cautious iron supplementation (as described by Crosby[11,12]) seems justified if two of three tests are abnormal, but iron levels should be closed monitored with serum ferritin measurements. In addition, the original cause of the iron deficiency should be sought.

Even greater care should be applied to the monitoring and treatment of pregnant women. While the iron demands of pregnancy appear high (300 mg for the fetus and 500 mg for the expanded blood supply), the fetus is rarely deficient and much of the iron required is recovered after birth. The current U.S. Recommended Dietary Allowance (RDA) for pregnant women is 15 mg of iron plus a 30 mg supplement.[13] Despite this, women are commonly prescribed prenatal supplements containing 65 mg of iron or more. A more cautious approach has been recommended wherein iron is given only to those patients with low serum ferritin or other readings.[14] This approach is supported by a recent study which showed that a group of women who were routinely supplemented with iron experienced prolonged pregnancies and higher infant mortality than a group who were supplemented selectively.[15] In addition to prenatal death, prolonged pregnancy can lead to increased incidence of placental lesions, fetal hypoxia and asphyxia, intrauterine growth retardation, macrosomia, and meconium staining and aspiration.[16] It is thought that excess iron might prolong pregnancy by inhibiting the absorption of zinc which is required for labor.

III. PREVENTIVE MEASURES FOR MAINTAINING LOW IRON STORES

A. DIET

Dietary changes may, over time, reduce iron levels. If the absolute amount of iron lost through bodily fluids, cells that slough off, gastrointestinal bleeding, etc. exceeds that absorbed from the diet, gradual reduction in iron stores can be expected. Though blood donation is the most efficient measure, dietary recommendations regarding iron are probably the most efficacious public health step that could be taken at the present time. (The relative value of each method to reduce iron stores is discussed further in Section IV.)

There are three basic dietary strategies to reduce iron uptake: (1) minimizing intake of heme iron in meat; (2) minimizing nonheme iron intake; and (3) minimizing nonheme iron absorption. Little is known of practical methods to decrease heme iron absorption (the fourth possible strategy).

1. Minimizing Intake of Heme Iron in Meat

The high consumption of meat in the developed Western world is thought to contribute to the prevalence of heart disease, obesity, certain forms of cancer, and other diseases. The lower prevalence of these conditions in Asian countries is often ascribed, in part, to the lower intake of meat. One of the latest findings, by Willett et al.[17] (part of the Nurses Health Study), is that meat consumption, particularly of red meat (beef, pork, or lamb), is associated with increased risk of colon cancer.

While most investigators point to the high saturated fat content of the meat-containing diet, it is also entirely possible that the high iron availability from meat is also an important factor, at least in regard to diseases in which iron is a catalyst for oxygen free-radical tissue damage or a vital nutrient for the growth of tumor or infectious cells. Past, present, and future epidemiological studies of diet and health should be scrutinized in an attempt to discern the relative contributions of fat and iron.[18]

The high consumption of meat, linked directly to improved socioeconomic conditions and developments in food production and preservation, is a relatively recent occurrence in human history. It is a legitimate question whether the human body, which evolved in leaner times, can withstand the high iron content of this modern diet.

Meat intake is the single most important dietary factor in determining iron status. A number of studies have shown that meat intake increases total iron stores or decreases the prevalence of "iron deficiency".[19-23]

There are several reasons for the importance of meat intake in determining total iron stores. While heme iron may only contribute about 10 to 15% of the total iron in the diet, the percentage absorption of heme iron is some 5 to 10 times greater than for nonheme iron. Except for unreasonably large doses, the percentage of heme iron absorbed does not appear to decrease with increasing meat content in the diet.[24] Also, while nonheme iron absorption decreases drastically in individuals with high-iron stores, the absorption of heme iron does not appear to be as sensitive to a person's iron status.[25] An additional reason why meat content in the diet leads to higher iron stores is that some unique factors in meat, not yet firmly identified, result in a roughly 50% increase in the absorption of nonheme iron.[24]

In offering advice to hemochromatosis patients or others who would like to minimize iron uptake from their diets, one can suggest reducing either the

RANKING MEATS FOR THE LOW-FAT, LOW-IRON LIFESTYLE

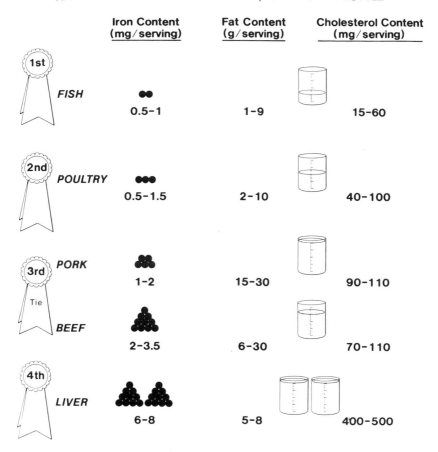

FIGURE 2. A chart for the lay reader to show that low-iron meats are generally lower in fat and/or cholesterol. Iron content is portrayed using stacked cannonballs, and the general fat/cholesterol level is crudely denoted by a graduated beaker containing fluid (i.e., oil). (From Lauffer, R. B., *Iron Balance,* St. Martin's Press, New York, 1991. With permission.)

frequency of meat intake or the size of the portions consumed. Also, a good rule of thumb is that the meats lowest in fat and cholesterol — fish and poultry — are also generally lower in iron.[1] Figure 2 shows for the lay reader a simple ranking of various meats in terms of iron, fat, and cholesterol content. While the percentage absorption of heme iron from each of these meats is what is most important (and not fully cataloged), the iron contents can serve as a rough guide for the consumer. The crude correspondence between fat/cholesterol and iron contents makes it easy for the consumer to remember which meats are healthiest.

2. Minimizing Nonheme Iron Intake

Because of the importance of the percentage absorption of nonheme iron rather than its total intake, attempting to minimize total nonheme iron intake is not a good means to control iron stores. Furthermore, foods naturally rich in iron, such as certain vegetables, are also good sources of other nutrients and thus should not be avoided. One can, of course, avoid food products with exogenously added iron, such as enriched white flour (which should be replaced with whole wheat) or highly supplemented breakfast cereals. In fact, the growing awareness of hemochromatosis and the role of iron in other diseases should renew the debate over the safety of such foods.[1] Cooking in iron pots, which can increase the content of some foods (particularly those that are acidic), can also be avoided.

3. Minimizing Nonheme Iron Absorption

Since the amount of nonheme iron absorbed is very sensitive to the contents of the meal, the inclusion of inhibiting substances such as phytate and polyphenols and the avoidance of enhancing factors such as excessive alcohol or vitamin C can be an effective way to control iron absorption.

a. Phytate

In recommending the reduction of meat content in the diet, it is implied that the consumption of other protein sources such as grains and legumes must increase. Many of these foods are rich in phytic acid, the highly negatively charged hexaorthophosphate ester of myo-inositol which avidly binds metal ions including iron.[26] Widdowson and McCance[27] showed in 1942 that the total amount of iron absorbed from phytate-rich brown bread was less than that from white bread even though the former had 50% more iron. Many studies since have revealed the importance of phytic acid in determining nonheme iron absorption. Hallberg and co-workers[28] showed that phytate-rich bran could reduce the absorption of iron by more than 90%, regardless of whether the subject was a long-term vegetarian or omnivore. In 1985, Graf and Eaton[29] proposed that the iron-chelating ability of phytic acid in the gut could be important in preventing colon cancer; unfortunately, despite the attractiveness of this proposal, it does not appear to have been tested in large clinical or epidemiological studies.

Table 1 lists the phytic acid content of selected foods. Many of these can be recommended as part of a healthy, low-meat diet. An easy-to-remember recommendation for the layman is to include whole grain products at every meal. Also, it is helpful to emphasize heavier breads made with little or no yeast to raise the dough; yeast contains a phytase enzyme that degrades the phytic acid in a time- and dose-dependent manner.[30]

b. Polyphenols

Iron-binding phenolic substances, such as tannins and chlorogenic acid, in tea and coffee decrease nonheme iron absorption almost as efficiently as

TABLE 1
Phytic Acid Content in Selected Foods

Food item	Phytic acid[26,30,31] (% Dry wt)
Sesame seeds	5.3
Wheat bran cereals	3.0—5.0
Pumpkin seeds	4.3
Lima beans	0.9—2.5
Oatmeal	2.4
Wild rice	2.2
Red kidney beans	1.2—2.1
Pinto beans	0.6—2.0
Sunflower seeds	1.9
Peanuts	1.9
Navy beans	1.8
Shredded wheat	1.5
Rye bread	0.8—1.5
Corn bread	1.4
Soybeans	1.4
Peas	0.9—1.2
Whole wheat bread	0.6—1.0
Barley	1.0
Brown rice	0.9
Corn	0.9
Pumpernickel bread	0.16
White bread or French bread	0.03—0.13
Cornflakes	0.05

phytic acid. Percentage decreases in iron absorption of 35 to 83%, depending on the brand of tea or coffee, were found in several studies; the beverage must be consumed during or within 1 hour after meals for greatest effect.[32,33] The growing interest in the potential health benefits of plant-based polyphenols, especially as documented in Asian populations,[34] should eventually shed some light on whether a simple mechanism such as iron binding might have broad explanatory power.

In recommending tea or coffee consumption to consumers, one has to add a caution about excess caffeine consumption. It is thought that one should limit caffeine intake to 300 mg/d, the equivalent of roughly two cups of coffee or four cups of tea. Also, herb teas and decaffeinated tea and coffee can be recommended; preliminary indications are that these beverages contain polyphenols, though in variable quantities.

c. Alcohol

Alcohol enhances nonheme iron absorption, and in addition alcohol abusers exhibit profound changes in iron metabolism. Alcohol increases the acidity of the gastrointestinal tract, which may solubilize more iron for absorption. It also slows erythropoiesis, freeing up some iron which adds to existing stores. In abusers, liver damage leads to increased hepatic iron storage. Several studies have revealed elevated iron levels in alcohol users.[35-37]

Recent studies, summarized by Cederbaum in Chapter 17, indicate that iron is intimately involved in the tissue damage caused by alcohol. The metabolism of alcohol results in the production of NADH-reducing equivalents which may convert storage ferric iron to a more labile pool of ferrous iron. This may be a critical factor in governing the severity of the oxidative stress caused by alcohol.[38-40]

Current U.S. government dietary guidelines recommend no more than two drinks a day for men and only one for women.[41] The consistent protective effect of alcohol observed in studies of coronary artery disease, presumably due to either an elevation of high-density lipoprotein levels or a decrease in platelet aggregation, is often used to justify these guidelines. While it has not been shown that one or two drinks a day can lead to organ damage, close scrutiny of alcohol-iron interactions may soon expose new health risks for even moderate drinking.

For hemochromatosis patients and others concerned with maintaining low but adequate iron stores, it appears that alcohol should be used quite sparingly, perhaps no more than two or three drinks per week.

d. Vitamin C

Ascorbate is a strong enhancing factor in nonheme iron absorption. Although it is not known whether chronic vitamin C supplementation leads to greater iron stores, numerous studies consistently reveal significantly increased absorption from individual meals containing added vitamin C.[42] This is presumably due to either the reduction or chelation of iron in the gut which increases its bioavailability.

Ascorbate and other antioxidants are best viewed from the context of oxidative balance (see the Epilogue). As reducing agents, antioxidants can inhibit damage to lipids, etc., but they can also stimulate iron-catalyzed reactions. It is well known, for example, that vitamin C supplementation in iron overload victims can exacerbate cardiac damage, sometimes leading to severe heart failure and death.[43-45] It is also possible that supplementation could be harmful, though over a period of time, to people with high-iron stores but lacking overt iron overload.

It seems justified to recommend caution in regard to vitamin C supplementation. The public can also be advised that proper timing if their intake of vitamin C-rich foods can minimize the enhancing effects on iron absorption while still allowing for adequate vitamin uptake. For example, one could recommend that citrus juices be consumed at snack time rather than during meals. Due to this added complexity of timing intake, however, it is unlikely that all but the most avid, health-conscious individuals would adopt this measure.

B. BLOOD DONATION

Blood donation is the only method by which to reduce iron stores significantly over a short period of time. Each pint of hemoglobin-rich whole blood contains approximately 240 mg of iron in men and 210 mg, in women. A review of four studies showed that regular blood donation reduced the average iron stores, as estimated by serum ferritin measurements, from 1240 to 470 mg for men and from 460 to 250 mg for women.[46] Although lower iron stores lead to an enhancement in the absorption of iron from the diet, the dietary measures discussed in the previous section may counter this to some extent.

While bloodletting was greatly misused in medieval medicine and soon fell into disfavor, it is a well-recognized, lifesaving treatment for hereditary hemochromatosis, polycythemia vera, and porphyria cutanea tarda.[47] Reduction of excess iron by bloodletting in hemochromatosis patients without liver cirrhosis restores their natural life expectancy.[48]

Sullivan[49] was the first to propose that reduction of iron levels via blood donation might have health benefits. Sullivan's interests were in the area of coronary artery disease (see Chapter 11), but his theory could be extended to infection, cancer, and diseases involving oxygen free-radical chemistry.[1,50] A series of adequately designed clinical trials are desperately needed to test this provocative idea.[51]

For now, the public at least shoud be aware of the effect of blood donation on their iron levels. They, of course, should be encouraged to donate to the precious national blood supply primarily for altruistic reasons. They also should be informed of the potential health benefits with the normal caveats that further study is still needed.

Blood donation appears to be safe enough to serve as a preventive health measure. Mild reactions such as fainting occur in less than 1% of blood donors. More serious reactions, such as convulsions, vomiting, or myocardial infarction, are exceedingly rare. The donor must be informed not to donate more frequently than once every 8 weeks to allow restoration of normal hematocrit.[52,53] It might be preferable for the donor to visit primarily one clinic so that accurate records can be kept. (It should also be noted that people over the age of 65 are eligible for blood donation at the discretion of the medical director of the donor center. One study showed that the elderly are excellent and willing donors.[54])

If the donor desires to reduce his total iron stores to roughly 100 to 400 mg, a serum ferritin measurement is required at the beginning of the program. Using the rough relationship that total iron stores in milligrams are equal to ten times the serum ferritin result (expressed in nanograms per milliliter or micrograms per liter), the donor can calculate how many donations would be required assuming roughly 200 mg of iron lost per donation.[1] The donor is protected from developing iron deficiency anemia to a great extent by the rather high hemoglobin and hematocrit minimums required for donation. After completing the schedule of donations over 1 to 2 years, one donation per year should be adequate to prevent excessive iron accumulation. This is difficult to predict since the percentage absorption of iron from the diet will be enhanced. Periodic serum ferritin measurements, perhaps every 5 years would be helpful in monitoring any residual iron buildup.

C. EXERCISE

A number of studies have shown that exercise reduces both heart disease and cancer mortality rates.[55-57] The proposed mechanisms for the beneficial effects of exercise, while intriguing and no doubt operative to some extent, lack generality, particularly in regard to these two very different diseases.[58] How, for example, could the stimulation of macrophage activity by exercise, which may lead to enhanced scavenging of tumor cells, be good for heart disease? Would this not accelerate atherogenesis by stimulating the uptake of oxidized low-density lipoprotein by macrophages in the coronary artery wall?[59] While the improved circulation from exercise might be good for the heart, would it not also increase the vascularity and viability of tumor cells?

I have proposed[58,60,61] that part of the beneficial effects from exercise may stem from either reductions in total iron stores or reductions in the concentration of "free" (chelatable) iron in the body. As discussed in other chapters of this book, iron is a possible risk factor for both heart disease and cancer. Thus, alterations in iron metabolism would be a general mechanism that might account for the preventive effects.

Figure 3 shows two pathways by which exercise may confer health benefits via changes in iron homeostasis. The first is overt iron loss through gastrointestinal bleeding, sweat, or hemolysis. Long-distance running, for example, has been noted to lead to iron losses from gastrointestinal bleeding up to 1 mg or more per session.[62] More mild aerobics/fitness-type exercise was also found to lead to a 20% drop in serum ferritin values in women after 6 weeks, although no further change was noted after 7 additional weeks.[63]

The second, more speculative pathway involves enhanced iron storage in cells via increased synthesis of ferritin as part of a mild acute phase response triggered by exercise (see Chapter 2). One might expect the more frequent replenishment of apoferritin levels to restrict the size of the potentially damaging "free iron pool".

Although the second pathway deserves further study, it appears that the iron losses from the first mechanism, while significant, are not sufficient to recommend exercise as a way to reduce iron levels. Exercise, of course, should be recommended to increase the general fitness level and well-being of the individual.

IV. RECOMMENDATIONS FOR SCREENING AND PREVENTIVE HEALTH GUIDELINES

The identification of patients at greatest risk for iron-induced adverse health effects is easily performed by serum tests such as serum ferritin and

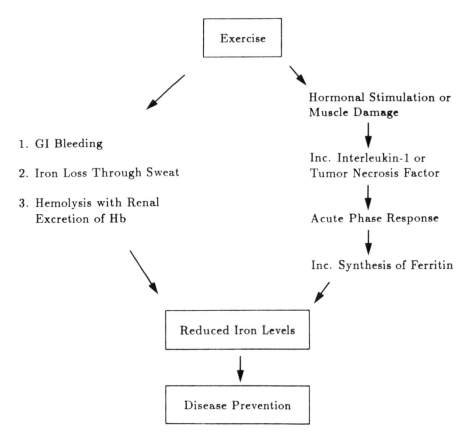

FIGURE 3. Possible pathways for exercise-induced disease prevention via alterations in iron homeostasis. Inc. = increased, GI = gastrointestinal, Hb = hemoglobin. (From Lauffer, R. B., *Med. Hypotheses,* 35, 103, 1991. With permission.)

transferrin saturation. Although there is increasing interest in including such tests on standard blood chemistry profiles, the tests do add cost to preventive health screening. The cost-effectiveness of screening for homozygous hereditary hemochromatosis has been shown by a recent analysis.[64] If it is a reasonable assumption that at least 50% of homozygotes develop disease symptoms, then mass transferrin saturation screening is estimated to save both lives and money.

A strong case can also be made for the cost-effectiveness of screening for patients with high iron stores who lack the genetic defect characteristic of homozygous hemochromatosis. The prevalence of "Western" diseases in which iron may play a role is so enormous that, even if iron is shown to be only one of many risk factors for only one of these conditions, it is likely that screening will be well justified.

TABLE 2
Comparison of Three Methods to Reduce Iron Stores

	Diet	Blood donation	Exercise
Effectiveness in reducing iron stores	+	+ + +	?
Safety	+ + +	+	+ +
Consistency with other health recommendations	+ + +	−	+ + +
Likelihood that the public will respond	+ + +	+	+ +

The following recommendations for routine screening seem warranted today. They can be modified as new insights on iron-related diseases are gained.

All adults over 30 years of age should be periodically screened (e.g., once every 5 years) for hemochromatosis or high iron stores using transferrin saturation and serum ferritin measurements.

1. If the transferrin saturation is 62% or greater in men or 50% or greater in women and the serum ferritin is abnormally high (e.g., greater than 300 μg/l [or ng/ml], although the normal range will vary with laboratories), hemochromatosis is likely, and a definitive diagnosis should be made with a liver biopsy. If the diagnosis is confirmed, phlebotomy therapy should begin immediately.

2. If the transferrin saturation is 62% or greater in men or 50% or greater in women but the serum ferritin appears normal, the individual should undergo periodic phlebotomies (perhaps every 2 to 3 months) and the tests should be repeated at least every 5 years.[65,66]

3. Those adults with either transferrin saturation values greater than, for example, 40% or serum ferritin values greater than 200 μg/l should be advised of their high iron status just as high-cholesterol patients are advised today.

What preventive health recommendations should be offered to people without homozygous hemochromatosis but with high-iron stores? This large fraction of the population in developed societies may include part of the estimated 13.4% of the population who are heterozygous for hemochromatosis[65] and may exhibit some tendency toward excess iron absorption. This is likely to be an area of heated debate for some time due to the paucity of good epidemiological studies on this topic. Table 2 grades the possible remedies for high iron stores from four perspectives: effectiveness in lowering iron stores, safety, consistency with other health recommendations, and likelihood that people will adopt the recommendation.

Dietary measures to reduce iron absorption have the advantage of: safety (there is no known harm from well-balanced, low- or no-meat diets); consistency with other health recommendations ("low-fat" roughly equals "low-iron"); and likelihood that the public will understand the link between diet and high iron stores and realize that they now have a second reason, in addition to improving their lipid profile, to eat a healthier diet. The only disadvantage is that, while long-term vegetarians have been noted to have lower iron levels than omnivores, we do not know how long it would take by dietary measures alone for a person to reduce his or her relatively high iron stores or whether it would be effective at all. However, it seems reasonable that the dietary measures would, at the very least, inhibit additional accumulation of iron. Furthermore, the low-fat, low-iron, low-meat diet could have other important benefits such as reducing the risk of colon cancer, which may be independent of iron stores or could depend on the free iron or heme concentration in the lumen of the gut or other factors provided by this type of diet.

Despite its unparalleled effectiveness in reducing iron stores, blood donation may be too controversial a preventive health measure for many physicians. Bloodletting has a distinctly antiquated and negative connotation despite its present-day acceptance in many specialities. The safety of repeated blood donations to individuals is thought to be high, but certainly the occasional bruises and mild reactions place this potential preventive health measure below a low-fat diet in terms of safety from potential adverse effects. In addition, the public is likely to be puzzled by this new recommendation, so unlike any others; and, because many fear the needle, they may be unlikely to give blood donation a try. (It has been estimated that only 6% of the American population have ever donated blood.[1]) Nonetheless, the public should be informed of the potential health benefits, and they should be encouraged to help others by donating.

Exercise, the third possible way to reduce iron levels, is already part of the standard preventive health message. However, its effectiveness in actually reducing iron stores in high-iron individuals has yet to be shown. Again, however, the public needs to be informed of the possible effects of exercise on iron metabolism, although they should be encouraged to exercise for traditional reasons.

With these observations and limitations in mind, I propose the following as a first draft of possible preventive health recommendations for the public in response to our growing understanding of iron as a double-edged nutrient.

A. HOW YOU CAN PREVENT IRON OVERLOAD

1. If you are 30 years of age or older, ask your doctor to perform two simple blood tests (serum ferritin and transferrin saturation) to see if you have iron overload.
2. Eat a low-fat, low-iron diet.

a. Include plenty of whole grains (at each meal), fruits, and vegetables. If you eat meat, choose, low-fat, low-iron selections such as fish, chicken, or turkey. Try to eat smaller portions of meat, perhaps using it as a condiment rather than the centerpiece of the meal.

b. Avoid iron-containing vitamin/mineral supplements and breakfast cereals or other foods which have been fortified with iron to more than 25% of the U.S. RDA.

c. Avoid excessive intake of alcoholic beverages, no more than two drinks per day for men and one for women.

d. If you like tea or coffee, drink some with your meals or within 1 hour after you eat.

3. Donate blood occasionally to aid others and reduce your iron levels, but do not donate more frequently than once every 8 weeks.

4. Get plenty of exercise.

REFERENCES

1. **Lauffer, R. B.**, *Iron Balance*, St. Martin's Press, New York, 1991.
2. **Cook, J. D., Finch, C. A., and Smith, N. J.,** Evaluation of the iron status of a population, *Blood*, 48, 449, 1976.
3. **Anon.,** Case records of the Massachusetts General Hospital, *N. Engl. J. Med.*, 247, 992, 1952.
4. **Turnberg, L. A.,** Excessive oral iron therapy causing hemochromatosis, *Br. Med. J.*, 1, 1360, 1965.
5. **Johnson, B. F.,** Hemochromatosis resulting from prolonged oral iron therapy, *N. Engl. J. Med.*, 278, 1100, 1968.
6. **Green, P., Eviatar, J. M., Sirota, P., and Avidor, I.,** Secondary hemochromatosis due to prolonged iron ingestion, *Isr. J. Med. Sci.*, 25, 199, 1989.
7. **Sas, F., Nemesanszky, E., Brauer, H., and Scheffer, K.,** On the therapeutic effects of trivalent and divalent iron in iron deficiency anemia, *Arzneim.-Forsch.*, 34, 1575, 1984.
8. **Waller, D. G. and Smith, A. G.,** Attitudes to prescribing iron supplements in general practice, *Br. Med. J.*, 294, 94, 1987.
9. **Beaton, G. H.,** Epidemiology of iron deficiency, in *Iron in Biochemistry and Medicine*, Jacobs, A. and Worwood, M., Eds., Academic Press, London, 1974, chap. 13.
10. Expert Scientific Working Group, Summary of a Report on Assessment of the Iron Nutritional Status of the United States Population, *Am. J. Clin. Nutr.*, 42, 1318, 1985.
11. **Crosby, W. H.,** The rationale for treating iron deficiency anemia, *Arch. Intern. Med.*, 144, 471, 1984.
12. **Crosby, W. H.,** Overtreating the deficiency anemias, *Arch. Intern. Med.*, 146, 779, 1986.
13. **Herbert, V.,** Recommended dietary intakes (RDI) of iron in humans, *Am. J. Clin. Nutr.*, 45, 679, 1987.
14. **Hibbard, B. M.,** Iron and folate supplements during pregnancy: supplementation is valuable only in selected patients, *Br. Med. J.*, 297, 1324, 1988.

15. **Hemminki, E. and Rimpela, U.,** A randomized comparison of routine versus selective iron supplementation during pregnancy, *J. Am. Coll. Nutr.,* 10, 3, 1991.

16. **Jovanovic-Peterson, L.,** Guest editorial: what is so bad about a prolonged pregnancy?, *J. Am. Coll. Nutr.,* 10, 1, 1991.

17. **Willett, W. C., Stampfer, M. J., Colditz, G. A., Rosner, B. A., and Speizer, F. E.,** Relation of meat, fat, and fiber intake to the risk of colon cancer in a prospective study among women, *N. Engl. J. Med.,* 323, 1664, 1990.

18. **Sullivan, J. L.,** Vegetarianism, ischemic heart disease, and iron, *Am. J. Clin. Nutr.,* 37, 882, 1983.

19. **Takkunen, H. and Seppanen, R.,** Iron deficiency and dietary factors in Finland, *Am. J. Clin. Nutr.,* 28, 1141, 1975.

20. **Faber, J., Gouws, E., Spinnler Benade, A. J., and Labadarios, D.,** Anthropometric measurements, dietary intake and biochemical data of South African lacto-ovovegetarians, *S. Afr. Med. J.,* 69, 733, 1986.

21. **Bindra, G. S. and Gibson, R. S.,** Iron status of predominantly lacto-ovo vegetarian East Indian immigrants to Canada: a model approach, *Am. J. Clin. Nutr.,* 44, 643, 1986.

22. **Worthington-Roberts, B. S., Breskin, M., and Monsen, E. R.,** Iron status of premenopausal women in a university community and its relationship to habitual dietary sources of protein, *Am. J. Clin. Nutr.,* 47, 275, 1988.

23. **Leggett, B. A., Brown, N. N., Bryant, S. J., Powell, L. W., and Halliday, J. W.,** Factors affecting the concentrations of ferritin in serum in a healthy Australian population, *Clin. Chem.,* 36, 1350, 1990.

24. **Cook, J. D.,** Adaptation in iron metabolism, *Am. J. Clin. Nutr.,* 51, 301, 1990.

25. **Lynch, S. R., Skikne, B. S., and Cook, J. D.,** Food iron absorption in idiopathic hemochromatosis, *Blood,* 74, 2187, 1989.

26. **Graf, E. and Eaton, J. W.,** Antioxidant functions of phytic acid, *Free Radical Biol. Med.,* 8, 61, 1990.

27. **Widdowson, E. M. and McCance, R. A.,** Iron exchanges of adults on white and brown bread, *Lancet,* 1, 588, 1942.

28. **Brune, M., Rossander, L., and Hallberg, L.,** Iron absorption: no intestinal adaptation to a high-phytate diet, *Am. J. Clin. Nutr.,* 49, 542, 1989.

29. **Graf, E. and Eaton, J. W.,** Dietary suppression of colonic cancer: fiber or phytate?, *Cancer,* 56, 717, 1985.

30. **Harland, B. F. and Harland, J.,** Fermentive reduction of phytate in rye, wheat, and whole wheat breads, *Cereal Chem.,* 57, 226, 1980.

31. **Harland, B. F. and Prosky, L.,** Development of dietary fiber values for foods, *Cereal Foods World,* 24, 387, 1979.

32. **Morck, T. A., Lynch, S. R., and Cook, J. D.,** Inhibition of food iron absorption by coffee, *Am. J. Clin. Nutr.,* 37, 416, 1983.

33. **Brune, M., Rossander, L., and Hallberg, L.,** Iron absorption and phenolic compounds: importance of different phenolic structures, *Eur. J. Clin. Nutr.,* 43, 547, 1989.

34. **Worthy, W.,** Fruits, vegetables, green tea may cut cancer risk, *Chem. Eng. News,* September 16, 27, 1991.

35. **Chapman, R. W., Morgan, M. Y., Bell, R., and Sherlock, S.,** Hepatic iron uptake in alcoholic liver disease, *Gastroenterology,* 84, 143, 1983.

36. **Chapman, R. W., Morgan, M. Y., Laulicht, M., Hoffbrand, A. V., and Sherlock, S.,** Hepatic iron stores and markers of iron overload in alcoholics and patients with idiopathic hemochromatosis, *Dig. Dis. Sci.,* 27, 909, 1982.

37. **Friedman, I. M., Kraemer, H. C., Mendoza, F. S., and Hammer, L. D.,** Elevated serum iron concentration in adolescent alcohol users, *Am. J. Dis. Child.,* 142, 156, 1988.

38. **Nordmann, R., Ribiere, C., and Rouach, H.,** Ethanol-induced lipid peroxidation and oxidative stress in extrahepatic tissues, *Alcohol Alcoholism,* 25, 231, 1990.

39. **Rouach, H., Houze, P., Orfanelli, M.-T., Gentil, M., Bourdon, R., and Nordmann, R.,** Effect of acute ethanol administration on the subcellular distribution of iron in rat liver and cerebellum, *Biochem. Pharmacol.,* 39, 1095, 1990.

476

40. **Cederbaum, A. I.**, Oxygen radical generation by microsomes: role of iron and implications for alcohol metabolism and toxicity, *Free Radical Biol. Med.*, 7, 559, 1989.
41. **Hilts, P. J.**, U.S. Dietary Guide Sets Fat and Alcohol Limits, *New York Times*, November 6, 1990.
42. **Hallberg, L.**, in *Nutrition Reviews' Present Knowledge in Nutrition*, The Nutrition Foundation, Washington, D.C., 1984, chap. 32.
43. **Nienhuis, A. W.**, Vitamin C and iron, *N. Engl. J. Med.*, 304, 170, 1981.
44. **McLaran, C. J., Bett, J. H. N., Nye, J. A., and Halliday, J. W.**, Congestive cardiomyopathy and haemochromatosis — rapid progression possibly accelerated by excessive ingestion of ascorbic acid, *Aust. N.Z. J. Med.*, 12, 187, 1982.
45. **Olson, J. A. and Hodges, R. E.**, Recommended dietary intakes (RDI) of vitamin C in humans, *Am. J. Clin. Nutr.*, 45, 693, 1987.
46. **Skikne, B., Lynch, S., Borek, D., and Cook, J.**, Iron and blood donation, *Clin. Haematol.*, 13, 271, 1984.
47. **Weintraub, L. R.**, Current uses of phelobotomy therapy, *Hosp. Pract.*, 22, 251, (June 15) 1987.
48. **Niederau, C., Fischer, R., Sonnenberg, A., Stremmel, W., Trampisch, H. J., and Strohmeyer, G.**, Survival and causes of death in cirrhotic and noncirrhotic patients with primary hemochromatosis, *N. Engl. J. Med.*, 313, 1256, 1985.
49. **Sullivan, J. L.**, Iron and the sex difference in heart disease risk, *Lancet*, 1, 1293, 1981.
50. **Weinberg, R. J., Ell, S. R., and Weinberg, E. D.**, Blood-letting, iron homeostasis, and human health, *Med. Hypotheses*, 21, 441, 1986.
51. **Sullivan, J. L.**, Is blood donation good for the donor? Iron, heart disease, and donor recruitment, *Vox. Sang.*, 61, 161, 1991.
52. American Red Cross, Blood Donor Information, Form No. 05-007B, Rev. 12/86-100M.
53. **Huestis, D. W.**, *Practical Blood Transfusion*, 4th ed., Little, Brown, Boston, 1988.
54. **Pindyck, J., Avorn, J., Kuriyan, M. et al.**, Blood donation by the elderly. Clinical and policy considerations, *J. Am. Med. Assoc.*, 257, 1186, 1987.
55. **Vena, J. E., Graham, S., Zielezny, M., Swanson, M. K., Barnes, R. E., and Nolan, J.**, Lifetime occupational exercise and colon cancer, *Am. J. Epidemiol.*, 122, 357, 1985.
56. **Ekelund, L.-G., Haskell, W. L., Johnson, J. L., Whaley, F. S., Criqui, M. H., and Sheps, D. S.**, Physical fitness as a predictor of cardiovascular mortality in asymptomatic North American men. The Lipid Research Clinics Mortality Follow-up Study, *N. Engl. J. Med.*, 319, 1379, 1988.
57. **Blair, S. N., Kohl, H. W., III, Paffenbarger, R. S., Clark, D. G., Cooper, K. H., and Gibbons, L. W.**, Physical fitness and all-cause mortality: a prospective study of healthy men and women, *JAMA*, 262, 2395, 1989.
58. **Lauffer, R. B.**, Exercise as prevention: do the health benefits derive in part from lower iron levels?, *Med. Hypotheses*, 35, 103, 1991.
59. **Steinberg, D., Parthasarathy, S., Carew, T. E., Khoo, J. C., and Witztum, J. L.**, Beyond cholesterol: modifications of low-density lipoprotein that increases its atherogenicity, *N. Engl. J. Med.*, 320, 915, 1989.
60. **Lauffer, R. B.**, Exercise, fitness, and mortality, *JAMA*, 263, 2047, 1990.
61. **Lauffer, R. B.**, Iron depletion and coronary disease, *Am. Heart J.*, 119, 1448, 1990.
62. **Newhouse, I. J. and Clement, D. B.**, Iron status atheletes. An update, *Sports Med.*, 5, 337, 1988.
63. **Blum, S. M., Sherman, A. R., and Boileau, R. A.**, The effects of fitness-type exercise on iron status in adult women, *Am. J. Clin. Nutr.*, 43, 456, 1986.
64. **Guzman, G., Phatak, P. D., Woll, J., and Phelps, C. E.**, Cost-effectiveness of screening for hemochromatosis, *Clin. Res.*, 39, 348A, 1991.
65. **Edwards, C. Q., Griffen, L. M., Goldgar, D., Drummond, C., Skolnick, M. H., and Kushner, J. P.**, Prevalence of hemochromatosis among 11,065 presumably healthy blood donors, *N. Engl. J. Med.*, 318, 1355, 1988.
66. Hemochromatosis Research Foundation, Hereditary (genetic or idiopathic) hemochromatosis, Albany, New York, 1984 pamphlet.

20. Therapeutic Strategies to Inhibit Iron-Catalyzed Tissue Damage

Philip E. Hallaway and Bo E. Hedlund

Biomedical Frontiers, Inc., Minneapolis, Minnesota

478

I. BACKGROUND

Iron is a ubiquitous metal present in various forms in all mammalian cells. However, in spite of the abundance of iron in the body, very little is present in a free or "reactive" form.[1] Instead, iron is found associated with heme-containing proteins (such as a hemoglobin or myoglobin); in the active sites of a variety of redox active enzymes; in ferritin and hemosiderin, or in the iron-binding and transport proteins, transferrin and lactoferrin. In normal human plasma, only about 30% of the total iron-binding sites on transferrin are occupied, thereby making it an effective buffer against free iron in the vascular compartment.

In this review we will discuss the mechanistic and therapeutic aspects of two separate types of iron-mediated pathophysiologies. In the first of these, the adverse effects are directly related to an excessive intake of iron which overwhelms the body's normal iron-processing and defense mechanisms. Acute iron intoxication, occurring through the accidental or deliberate ingestion of iron-containing medicaments, can be a life-threatening situation requiring immediate medical attention. Likewise, the toxicity of chronic iron accumulation and the need for its removal is well recognized in iron overload states occurring secondary to chronic transfusion therapy or in individuals suffering from diseases associated with abnormal iron absorption, such as homozygous hereditary hemochromatosis.

In addition to the syndromes associated with acute and chronic iron intoxication, there is increasing evidence that, under appropriate conditions, reactive iron can be liberated from otherwise safe body stores. The concept of endogenously derived iron as an important contributor to tissue injury in individuals with normal iron status is becoming increasingly accepted, particularly in conditions associated with "reperfusion injury".

Iron has also been implicated in such diverse disease states as rheumatoid arthritis,[2,3] autoimmune disease,[4] inflammation,[5-7] central nervous system trauma,[8] diabetes,[9,10] Parkinson's and Alzheimer's diseases,[11,12] cancer,[13,14] alcohol-mediated hepatotoxicity,[15] and toxicity of drugs such as adriamycin[16] and paraquat.[17-19] An excellent review of general aspects of the role of the oxygen radical and iron in biology and medicine has been provided by Halliwell and Gutteridge.[20]

II. IRON-DEPENDENT MOLECULAR DAMAGE AND ITS PREVENTION

A. INTRODUCTION

The toxicity of iron is closely linked to its ability to transfer electrons and to catalyze the formation of other reactive species, specifically oxygen and lipid derived reactive compounds, leading to the subsequent destruction of biomolecules. Suggested mechanisms for this biological damage include the formation hydroxyl radicals via Fenton chemistry, the direct oxidation by ferryl and perferryl iron complexes, or the catalytic decomposition of lipid hydroperoxides leading to the formation of alkoxy and peroxy radicals. (See also Chapter 7.)

Much of the recent interest in iron-mediated tissue damage has centered on the formation of the extremely reactive hydroxyl radical via an iron-catalyzed Haber-Weiss reaction between superoxide and hydrogen peroxide.[3] In this scheme, the hydroxyl radical is produced by the Fenton reaction[2] and the superoxide provides not only the reducing equivalents necessary for cycling of ferric iron back to the ferrous state[1] but also a constant source of hydrogen peroxide via the dismutation of superoxide:

$$Fe^{3+} + O_2^{\cdot -} \rightarrow Fe^{2+} + O_2 \tag{1}$$

$$Fe^{2+} + H_2O_2 \rightarrow Fe^{3+} + OH^{\cdot} + OH^{-} \tag{2}$$

$$O_2^{\cdot -} + H_2O_2 \rightarrow O_2 + OH^{\cdot} + OH^{-} \tag{3}$$

Prevention of hydroxyl radical formation by Fenton chemistry can be achieved by elimination of hydrogen peroxide, superoxide, or the catalyst of the reaction, iron. Prevention of superoxide production by enzyme inhibitors or antineutrophil agents or scavenging of superoxide and its by-product, hydrogen peroxide, will effectively interrupt the Fenton reaction. Hydroxyl radical-mediated injury can also be limited by low molecular weight compounds, so-called radical scavengers, which react with hydroxyl radicals with rate constants higher than most biomolecules.

Removal of the catalytic component of the reaction can be achieved by rendering iron nonreactive with appropriate chelators or by interrupting the redox cycling of iron. In addition to the hydroxyl radical, it has been proposed that ferryl and perferryl complexes between iron and oxygen are important oxidants capable of promoting lipid peroxidation and destruction of other biomolecules.[21]

Iron-dependent stimulation of lipid peroxidation can also occur independently of hydroxyl radicals or iron-oxygen complexes via the iron catalyzed decomposition of lipid hydroperoxides and the formation of alkoxy and peroxy radicals,[4] which can then propagate further lipid peroxidation by hydrogen abstraction from other lipid molecules.[5,6]

$$2 \text{ LOOH} \xrightarrow{\text{Iron catalyst}} \text{LO}^\cdot + \text{LOO}^\cdot + \text{H}_2\text{O} \qquad (4)$$

$$\text{LH} + \text{LOO}^\cdot \longrightarrow \text{L}^\cdot + \text{LOOH} \qquad (5)$$

$$\text{L}^\cdot + \text{O}_2 \longrightarrow \text{LOO}^\cdot \qquad (6)$$

As a means of protecting the lipid membrane against iron-catalyzed lipid peroxidation, lipid soluble chelators and radical chain breakers can be introduced. Iron-catalyzed tissue damage involves a series of physiological events, and therefore many therapeutic interventions have been proposed to interrupt the process at various steps in the cascade. In general, these approaches are of two types, primary or secondary. Primary interventions are aimed at limiting the availability and reactivity of iron, whereas secondary interventions focus on protection of biological molecules subject to potential iron-mediated destruction. Figure 1 illustrates the important steps in iron-mediated tissue damage and possible points for therapeutic interdiction. However, because this area of research is newly emerging and because many of the concepts are controversial in nature, Figure 1 is intended only as a working model. In addition, more than one mechanism can often be invoked for the protective effect of a given therapeutic entity. Undoubtedly, this scheme will have to be modified as more data is accumulated from both basic and clinical studies.

B. PRIMARY INTERVENTION METHODS
1. Iron Chelation and Neutralization

Limiting the availability of free iron can be accomplished either by chelation therapy or by inhibiting its release from endogenous iron-containing compounds. In cases of acute iron poisoning or transfusion-dependent iron overload, chelation is the most appropriate therapy because of the grossly elevated iron levels and lack of residual transferrin iron-binding capacity. Currently, the drug of choice for these two clinical indications is deferoxamine (deferoxamine mesylate; Desferal®; CIBA-Geigy), a bacterial siderophore isolated from *Streptomyces pilosus*. Since its introduction in the 1960s, deferoxamine has proven to be a relatively safe and efficacious iron chelator, and has clearly decreased the mortality rate associated with acute and chronic iron poisoning.[22-24] Deferoxamine binds iron with a high affinity ($K_d \sim 10^{-31}$ M) and specificity,[25] and because it is a hexadentate ligand it prevents the iron-catalyzed formation of hydroxyl radicals.[26] However, deferoxamine has several shortcomings which limit its potential usefulness, and this has spurred interest in finding alternative iron chelators. Specifically, deferoxamine is not absorbed when given orally,[25] it has a plasma half-life of only 5 to 10 min,[27] and has both acute and chronic side effects.[28] Most prominent of these effects are the tendency to produce severe hypotension at high doses,[29-33] and neurotoxicity associated with auditory and ocular dysfunction.[34]

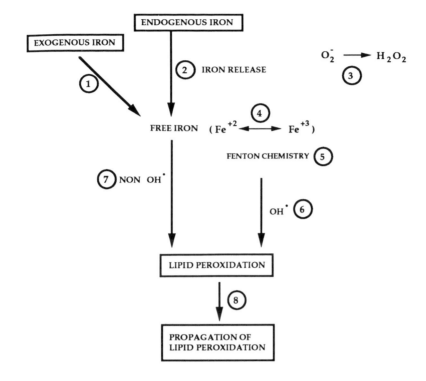

POSSIBLE THERAPEUTIC INTERVENTIONS AT THE NUMBERED AREAS:

1. IRON CHELATORS

2. IRON CHELATORS, SOD, SOD-MIMICS, ANTI-NEUTROPHIL
   AGENTS, XANTHINE OXIDASE INHIBITORS, CERULOPLASMIN,

3. CATALASE, GLUTATHIONE PEROXIDASE

4. IRON CHELATORS, SOD, CERULOPLASMIN

5. IRON CHELATORS, SOD, CATALASE

6. RADICAL SCAVENGERS

7. IRON CHELATORS, 21-AMINOSTEROIDS

8. VITAMIN E, 21-AMINOSTEROIDS

FIGURE 1. Potential therapeutic interventions in the prevention of iron-mediated tissue injury.

The two naturally occurring iron-binding proteins, transferrin and lactoferrin, are effective chelators of iron and may act as endogenous buffers against the deleterious consequences of free iron.[35] Lactoferrin, with its ability to bind iron at low pH, may provide protection against iron-catalyzed damage to host endothelial cells during the respiratory burst of activated granulocytes.[2,36,37] However, the use of these two proteins for therapeutic purposes is probably not feasible because of the large quantity required for adequate chelation (apotransferrin has only two iron-binding sites on a protein of 80,000 mol wt) and because of the inherent high cost of production.

2. Removal of Superoxide

Superoxide can be an important participant in the series of events leading to iron-mediated tissue injury for three reasons. First, it can provide reducing equivalents necessary for the reductive liberation of iron from otherwise nonreactive forms. Second, it provides reducing equivalents for the redox-cycling of iron in Fenton-type reactions. Third, it provides a constant source of hydrogen peroxide via the superoxide dismutation reaction.

Several mechanisms may exist for the delocalization of iron from otherwise safe storage proteins and hemeproteins. Iron can be reductively displaced from ferritin by superoxide anion,[38-41] by xanthine oxidase independently of superoxide;[41-43] or by radicals of compounds such as paraquat,[44] adriamycin,[45] and alloxan.[46] Superoxide-mediated release of iron is much slower from hemosiderin than from ferritin[47] and does not occur with transferrin or lactoferrin, except at pH values of 5 or less.[48] Low levels of superoxide are continuously produced during normal cellular activities, for example, by "leakage" from the mitochondrial cytochrome oxidase system[49] or from the intraerythrocytic oxidation of hemoglobin.[50] This constant flux of superoxide is detoxified sequentially by the initial conversion of superoxide to hydrogen peroxide by superoxide dismutase, followed by removal of hydrogen peroxide by catalase or glutathione peroxidase. In addition to this continuous generation, high localized concentrations of superoxide may occur in a variety of clinical situations via xanthine oxidase,[51] the NADPH oxidase system of activated neutrophils,[52] or by redox cycling of certain xenobiotics and quinones.[53]

The prevention of superoxide formation or its accumulation can be accomplished by several methods and may be beneficial not only in preventing iron delocalization but also in limiting its reactivity. Following ischemia/reperfusion, increases in superoxide formation are hypothesized to be a result of the proteolytic conversion of xanthine dehydrogenase to xanthine oxidase in an environment containing an abundant supply of purine substrates resulting from the breakdown of ATP.[51] Suppression of xanthine oxidase-mediated production of superoxide is easily achieved by administration of the enzyme-specific inhibitors allopurinol or oxypurinol. Superoxide production by activated neutrophils can be inhibited with adenosine,[54] with monoclonal antibodies to the neutrophil NADPH oxidase,[55] or by monoclonal antibodies to several of the neutrophil adhesion molecules.[56,57]

Superoxide, if formed, can be effectively scavenged by superoxide dismutase (SOD) or mimics thereof. Although many investigators have reported efficacy of superoxide dismutase in preclinical models, an equally large number have reported negative results, particularly in the cardiology literature.[58,59] In addition, the initial enthusiasm for the therapeutic use of SOD has been tempered by the lack of successful clinical studies. Superoxide dismutase for preclinical and clinical use either of bovine origin or has been manufactured by recombinant technology. Proponents of the recombinant form of the protein point to potential adverse immunogenic responses as the main reason for not using the bovine-derived enzyme. Regardless of the source, the potential therapeutic use of SOD is limited by its rapid excretion by the kidneys, the inability to traverse cell membranes, and a possible exacerbation of tissue injury at high doses of SOD. The efficient filtration of native SOD by the kidney may account for demonstrated efficacy of this protein in a model of renal ischemia[60] and in a human trial of renal transplantation.[61] The short circulatory half-life of superoxide dismutase, approximately 5 to 10 min,[62,63] can be prolonged by modification of the native molecule or by entrapment in liposomes. Covalent attachment of SOD to polyethylene glycol yields a much larger but still enzymatically active molecule, having a circulatory half-life of 18 to 40 h, a reduced immunogenicity, and an increased ability to enter cells and cross the blood-brain barrier.[64-66] A hybrid molecule has been produced by coupling two Cu/Zn SOD subunits to human IgA, resulting in 750-kDa polymers which exhibit superoxide dismutase activity.[63] Encapsulation of SOD into liposomes results in an effective plasma half-life of about 4 h and about one order of magnitude enhancement of intracellular SOD activity.[62,67]

General aspects of the use of superoxide dismutase in human medicine have been reviewed recently by Greenwald.[68] The large number of preclinical studies involving SOD will not be reviewed unless there is specific relevance to the involvement of iron in the disease being investigated. Reviews by Ward et al.[69] and Reilly and co-workers[70] describe general aspects of the pharmacology of oxygen radical-mediated tissue injury without the emphasis on iron that is the focus of this review.

Despite many reports indicating therapeutic efficacy of superoxide dismutase in experimental protocols intended to model free-radical-mediated tissue injury, it appears that elevated levels of SOD are not always protective, but may be actually harmful.[71-73] These deleterious effects of SOD may be due to the biological toxicity of hydrogen peroxide, the dismutation product of superoxide;[71,74] and to the increased activity of endothelial-derived relaxing factor (nitric oxide) normally inactivated by superoxide, leading to extravasation and edema or to excessive removal of superoxide which may be important in the termination of lipid peroxidation.[73]

Other than SOD, several low molecular weight compounds exhibit superoxide dismutase activity and have been proposed as potential therapeutics for use in limiting superoxide-mediated cytotoxicity. Many of these SOD mimics are transition metal chelates of copper, iron, or manganese.[75-78] Although capable of entering cells, several of these compounds tend to dissociate *in vivo,* thereby losing their activity and posing a potential metal-dependent toxicity.[77,79] More recently, a class of metal-independent cyclic nitroxide radicals have been identified as synthetic superoxide dismutases having greater *in vivo* stability and less toxicity than the metal chelates.[79,80] Because of their small size the SOD mimics probably will be able to penetrate cell membranes, be nonimmunogenic, and be relatively inexpensive to manufacture. However, in spite of these apparent advantages these compounds may suffer from the same shortcomings described earlier for SOD, in addition to unknown long-term toxicity. Although protection against superoxide-mediated toxicity has been documented with several of these compounds in cell culture,[78,79,81,82] their efficacy has not yet been documented in animal studies.

3. Removal of Hydrogen Peroxide

Hydrogen peroxide poses a biological threat not only as a direct oxidant, but also because of the potential for release of free iron through the destruction of heme compounds, for reaction with ferrous iron leading to the formation of hydroxyl radicals via the Fenton reaction, or for production of reactive hypochlorous acid by the neutrophil myeloperoxidase system. The major source of this hydrogen peroxide is predominantly from the spontaneous or enzymatic-mediated dismutation of previously formed superoxide. Therefore, any of the therapeutic interventions which reduce the formation of superoxide, e.g., inhibition of xanthine oxidase or inhibition of the phagocytic respiratory burst, will lessen the potential for subsequent hydrogen peroxide formation. Parental administration of catalase can be used to scavenge hydrogen peroxide, but its inability to enter cells and its rapid vascular clearance diminish its utility. Like superoxide dismutase, these two problems can be overcome, while retaining enzymatic activity, either by entrapment in liposomes[62] or by conjugation with polyethylene glycol.[64]

In addition to its intrinsic toxicity, hydrogen peroxide can be involved in liberation of iron from heme-containing compounds such as myoglobin and hemoglobin.[83-85] These hemeproteins may provide a source of potentially available iron, especially when they escape from their usual milieu and the intracellular protection afforded by the detoxifying enzymes, superoxide dismutase, catalase, and glutathione peroxidase. Plasma myoglobin levels can be increased following myocardial infarction[86] or muscle trauma;[87] and the appearance of free hemoglobin in the plasma, due to intravascular hemolysis, can occur following exposure to oxidant drugs[88] or thermal injury.[89,90] Increased levels of oxidant species capable of destroying the heme ring would be expected in situations involving the activation of granulocytes or xanthine oxidase leading to the production of superoxide and its dismutation product, hydrogen peroxide; or in instances of inadequate activity of hydrogen peroxide-catabolizing enzymes. The extracellular compartment has an almost total lack of catalase, and therefore provides poor enzymatic protection against hydrogen peroxide. The inactivation of glutathione peroxidase can often be the consequence of an oxidant stress leading to the consumption of its substrate, reduced glutathione.

C. SECONDARY INTERVENTION METHODS

1. Direct Radical Scavenging

Any organic compound can, in principle, compete with biomolecules for the highly reactive hydroxyl radical. Certain compounds, such as dimethylsulfoxide and dimethyltiourea react with the hydroxyl radical with very high rate constants, thereby protecting neighboring biomolecules. Unlike the enzymatic scavengers which are restricted to the vascular compartment, the low molecular weight scavengers can either localize in the cell membrane or enter the cell to react with intracellularly generated radicals.

The choice of a nonenzymatic scavenger for use in a preclinical, and potentially clinical, situation is based on two primary criteria, namely, its rate of reaction with various radical species and its inherent toxicity. The use of radical scavengers started with relatively nontoxic compounds, such as dimethyl sulfoxide and mannitol. More recent studies have provided evidence that other, often chemically related, compounds offer better combinations of efficacy and low toxicity. Thus, thiourea, and more recently, dimethylthiourea (DMTU), and 2-mercapto-propionyl-glycine (MPG) have proven highly efficacious in reducing radical-mediated cellular injury in both *in vitro* and *in vivo* models. However, since this therapeutic approach falls outside the main focus of this review, it will not be discussed in detail.

It should be noted that the protective mode of action of both enzymatic and nonenzymatic oxygen radical scavengers is, in many instances, not entirely clear and that the observed effect may be due to more than one mechanism.

2. Interruption of Lipid Peroxidation

Once initiated, a chain reaction of lipid peroxidation can be propagated by alkoxy and peroxy lipid radicals via hydrogen abstraction from other lipid molecules leading to the continuous formation of more lipid radicals via Reactions 3 and 4 shown earlier. This reaction can be interrupted, however, by the reaction of "chain-terminating" compounds such as vitamin E (α-tocopherol) with peroxy lipid radicals to form a lipid hydroperoxide and a vitamin E radical:[5]

$$LOO^{\cdot} + \text{vitamin E} \rightarrow LOOH + \text{vitamin E radical} \qquad (7)$$

The resulting vitamin E radical does not have sufficient energy to abstract a hydrogen from other membrane lipids, thereby interrupting the peroxidative chain reaction. Because of its hydrophobicity, vitamin E accumulates in cell membranes and will provide some defense against lipid peroxidation. This protection, however, will last only as long as there is a source of reduced vitamin E. A recently published review[91] dealing with vitamin E and oxidant stress will provide the reader with ample background.

Recently a group of antioxidant compounds, collectively known as 21-aminosteroids or "lazaroids", have been developed which localize in cell membranes and inhibit iron-mediated lipid peroxidation. Several of these compounds show promise for the treatment of ischemia and traumatic injury, particularly in models involving the central nervous system.[92] The 21-aminosteroids all lack glucocorticoid activity,[93,94] but they vary in their antioxidant capacity and apparently in their mode of action. Inhibition of lipid peroxidation is probably through the scavenging of lipid peroxy radicals, in a manner similar to vitamin E, or through an interaction with ferrous iron.[92,93] It was initially suggested that some of the 21-aminosteroids, such as compound U74006F, functioned simply by scavenging lipid peroxy radicals while others, such as compound U74500A, functioned by both mechanisms. However, it has been reported that although both of these compounds can scavenge LOO$^\cdot$ and that this may contribute to their antioxidant activity, they are much less effective in this regard than vitamin E.[95] Apparently other mechanisms, such as iron binding or sparing of endogenous vitamin E, are involved in the protection afforded by these compounds. Although the action of the 21-aminosteroids is not fully understood mechanistically, efficacy has been demonstrated in several *in vivo* models of shock, trauma, and ischemia.

III. THERAPEUTIC INTERVENTION IN PATHOPHYSIOLOGICAL STATES ASSOCIATED WITH EXCESS TISSUE IRON LEVELS

A. ACUTE IRON POISONING

In cases of acute iron intoxication, much of the damage to the gastrointestinal tract and the liver may be a result of high, localized, iron concentrations and concomitant free-radical generation[96] leading to hepatotoxicity via lipid peroxidation and destruction of the hepatic mitochondria.[97,98] Therefore, rapid removal of iron from the gut as well as from the circulatory system must be achieved to prevent tissue damage. Gastric decontamination with orally administered deferoxamine (DFO) has been advocated by several clinicians[99,100] but this therapeutic approach is not supported by most toxicologists.[101] Unlike deferoxamine, the iron-saturated form of the drug, ferrioxamine, is absorbed in the gut[29,30,102] and has been shown to be toxic.[30] Systemic chelation with deferoxamine is the therapy of choice for acute iron intoxication, but presents a problem to the clinician because the dose and route of administration are limited by the hypotensive effect of the drug.[101,103]

Recently, macromolecular forms of deferoxamine prepared by the covalent attachment of deferoxamine to large, biocompatible polymers such as dextran and hydroxyethyl starch[32] have been shown to be highly effective in a murine model of acute iron poisoning.[104] These high molecular weight chelators retain the iron-binding characteristics of native deferoxamine but they have, in contrast, circulatory half-lives of many hours and a much lower acute toxicity, as evidenced by a murine LD_{50} of 4000 mg DFO equivalents per kilogram of body weight as compared to an LD_{50} of 250 mg/kg for native deferoxamine.[32]

Mahoney et al.[104] demonstrated that intravenous administration of these conjugated forms of deferoxamine, but not the native drug, prevented mortality after otherwise lethal oral or intraperitoneal doses of iron sulfate, even when the conjugate was given 1 h after administration of the iron. It was assumed that the superiority of these high molecular weight chelators was due to their low toxicity, thereby permitting administration of very high doses of chelator without any associated hypotension. In addition to their potential use for the intravenous therapy of systemic iron toxicity, the polymer deferoxamine conjugates may be excellent candidates for gastric decontamination following iron poisoning. Presently, there do not appear to be additional compounds offering advantages over deferoxamine for the removal of reactive iron for the prevention of iron-mediated tissue damage following acute iron poisoning.

B. CHRONIC IRON OVERLOAD

Unlike acute iron intoxication, iron overload secondary to chronic transfusion therapy is an area in which alterative chelators are being actively researched with the aim of developing a safe and orally active chelator. Despite the obvious improvement in life expectancy and minimal iatrogenic complications in iron-overload patients treated with deferoxamine, some of the drug's undesirable properties, as mentioned previously, have stimulated the search for improved chelators. Because of poor absorption when given orally and rapid circulatory excretion, deferoxamine must be given by chronic subcutaneous infusion to obtain net negative iron balance.[105-107] Unfortunately, this method of administration is expensive and cumbersome, resulting in a high incidence of noncompliance in much of the patient population.[108] Intravenous therapy appears to provide more effective iron removal, but is not widely available.[109] Finally, increasing evidence of long-term toxicity suggests that careful monitoring of patients and dosages are required.[28,34]

Ferric iron chelators, in general, are of the following types: hydroxamic acids, catecholates, amino carboxylates, aryl hydrazones, and hydroxypyridones. In order to limit iron-catalyzed tissue damage via the removal of reactive iron, these compounds should be preferably high affinity, hexadentate ligands. Bidentate or tridentate ligands can form partially coordinated iron complexes at low ligand concentrations, and therefore actually promote hydroxyl radical formation.[26,110] The toxicity of the iron-free and iron-bound form of the chelator should be low to allow for the administration and maintanance of high-circulating concentrations of the active ingredient. Also, the iron-bound form of the chelator should be stable *in vivo,* easily excretable, and incapable of translocating and later releasing iron to other parts of the body.[110] For the treatment of iron overload, the chelator should be orally active to increase patient compliance. The physicochemical properties and *in vivo* toxicity and efficacy of various iron chelators, especially in the context of iron overload, are amply reviewed in several recent publications.[110,111]

IV. IRON-MEDIATED PATHOPHYSIOLOGY IN CONDITIONS ASSOCIATED WITH NORMAL LEVELS OF IRON

Other than a consequence of excess intake, free iron may be the result of decompartmentalization of endogenous stores following some form of "oxidant stress." Early evidence for this type of iron release was provided by Mazur and co-workers,[112] who demonstrated that iron, in quantities sufficient to completely saturate the available transferrin-binding capacity, was released during a prolonged period of hypovolemic shock. Similar results were obtained by Janoff et al.[113] Paller and Hedlund[114] have reported a tenfold increase in the urinary iron concentration during reperfusion following a 60-min period of renal ischemia; Robinson and Hedlund[115] noted a significant increase in the plasma iron concentration in rats exposed to 90 min of total intestinal ischemia. In addition, localized iron mobilization has been documented in the brain after a period of global ischemia induced by cardiac arrest[116,117] and in myocardial tissue following 2 h of *in vivo* ischemia.[118]

A. ISCHEMIA AND REPERFUSION
1. Introduction
Extended ischemic insults to mammalian cells will eventually lead to cell death. Shorter periods of ischemia lead to metabolic depletion due to lack of oxygen, and such biochemical imbalance can be restored when oxygen becomes available. The definition of the extent of injury caused by an ischemic insult to a whole organ is often less well-defined. As a first approximation it is often convenient to classify ischemic organ injury into two general categories: vascular, usually microvascular, or parenchymal. Endothelial cell swelling is an example of a morphologically defined vascular injury, while microvascular leakage of macromolecules represents a physiological measure of vascular integrity. An example of modest, reversible organ injury is the "stunned" myocardium,[119] observed after a relatively brief occlusion of the blood supply to a region of the heart. At the other extreme is cell death and subsequent infarction.

Until recently it was assumed that most, if not all, cellular injury observed after an ischemic insult was caused by a lack of oxygen, i.e., metabolic depletion within the cell. However, our increased knowledge of the biochemical and physiological events occurring at reflow suggest that much of the cellular injury sustained during ischemia and subsequent reoxygenation takes place within minutes of reflow. Based on studies with a variety of novel detection techniques, it is now generally accepted that a burst of reactive oxygen-derived radicals are formed at reoxygenation.[120-125] The injury caused by these toxic compounds at the time of reflow, beyond that caused by the ischemic insult alone, is referred to as "reperfusion injury". In an experimental setting it is often difficult to determine how much of the observed molecular, cellular, or whole organ injury is caused by reperfusion as opposed to that caused by the ischemic insult itself. In an attempt to separate these two components of the observed injury, a therapeutic agent can be given either prior to ischemia or immediately prior to reoxygenation. A number of studies of this type will be briefly reviewed in the following section.

Since this volume deals primarily with the role of iron in human disease, the following discussion of ischemia and reperfusion will emphasize those studies implicating iron in the observed pathophysiology. Similarly, studies using agents aimed at reducing the oxidant role of iron have been selected over those dealing with more general antioxidant approaches. As noted earlier, a broader based review by Reilly and co-workers[70] deals with general aspects of pharmacological intervention aimed at attenuating radical-mediated injury.

2. Myocardial Ischemia

The ischemic and reperfused heart has received considerable attention since studies dealing with reperfusion injury were initiated nearly 10 years ago. (See also Chapter 10.) Several recent reviews have been dedicated to the present status of preclinical research pertaining to radical-mediated reperfusion injury of the myocardium.[59,126-130] This section will focus on *in vivo* as opposed to *ex vivo* studies. Only selected articles, dealing primarily with iron-mediated injury and its prevention, will be discussed.

In general, preclincal studies of myocardial ischemia can be classified not only in terms of severity but also in timing of the therapeutic intervention. Depending on the length of the ischemic insult a reversible or irreversible injury will result. Studies of reversible injury, i.e., the "stunned" myocardium,[119] usually utilize functional end points as the index of therapeutic efficacy. In more severe models involving myocardial infarction, assessment of efficacy is based on infarct size in treated and untreated animals. The time at which a protective agent is given in the experimental protocol not only can determine its efficacy, but also can provide valuable information on the time course of injury caused by ischemia and reperfusion.

Deferoxamine pretreatment has been shown to limit infarct size in several studies. In a canine model involving 120-min left anterior descending (LAD) coronary artery occlusion and 240-min reperfusion, Reddy et al.[131] documented a decrease in myocardial infarct size in dogs given deferoxamine intravenously 30 min prior to occlusion as compared to saline controls. However, no protective benefit was afforded when the deferoxamine was given only 5 min prior to reperfusion. In both cases the deferoxamine dose was 10 mg/kg for the first hour followed by a maintenance dose of 1.5 mg/kg/h until the end of reperfusion.

Likewise, Lesnefsky et al.[132] using a 90-min canine LAD occlusion model with 240 min of reperfusion, showed that deferoxamine treatment (15 mg/kg) initiated 30 min prior to occlusion significantly reduced infarct size. Iron-loaded deferoxamine administered preocclusion or deferoxamine given only 15 min prior to reperfusion afforded no protection compared to normal saline. In addition, pretreatment with deferoxamine was the only regimen which decreased the release of oxidized glutathione into the coronary sinus, presumably indicating a decrease in oxidative reactions. The same group[133] subsequently demonstrated that high dose, hydroxyethyl starch-conjugated deferoxamine (75-mg deferoxamine equivalents per kilogram) failed to reduce infarct size when administered late during the ischemic insult.

A recent study suggests that targeting deferoxamine directly into the high risk microcirculation increases the therapeutic efficacy. Kobayashi et al.[134] demonstrated that the iron chelator is effective in reducing myocardial infarct size following coronary occlusion only when given directly to the area at risk via the coronary vein. In this porcine, open-chest myocardial infarct model the LAD was occluded for 60 min and deferoxamine (10 mg/kg) administered for 5 min, beginning 15 min prior to reperfusion, either by retrograde infusion into the anterior interventricular vein or systemically by intravenous infusion. The infarct size expressed as percent of area at risk was 73.9 ± 13.5 for saline treated controls, 70.6 ± 16.4 for systemically treated animals, and 48.5 ± 21.4 for animals treated by retrograde infusion. The observed decrease in the latter group was statistically significant.

Thus, in two of the studies discussed previously deferoxamine reduced infarct size when administered prior to the ischemic insult. These results suggest that the chelator protects against injury occurring during the ischemic phase as well as during the subsequent reperfusion. However, when administered late during ischemia the chelator failed to influence infarct size in three of four studies. In the only report documenting reduction of infarct size, the therapeutic agent was given late in the ischemic period directly into the coronary venous circulation by means of retrograde perfusion.

Deferoxamine has also been used in several preclinical studies of the stunned myocardium. In a pretreatment model, Bolli et al.[135] demonstrated that recovery of contractile function following 15 min of occlusion of the LAD and 4 h of reperfusion was significantly better in animals treated with deferoxamine compared to normal saline. Deferoxamine was given intravenously for 45 min, beginning 30 min before occlusion at a dose of 10 mg/kg and then given at a dose of 1.7 mg/kg throughout the reperfusion period for a total dose of 17 mg/kg.

In a similar canine model, also using 15 min of LAD occlusion, Farber et al.[136] documented significant improvement in functional recovery in animals pretreated with deferoxamine at a total dose of 500 mg administered intra-atrially over a 30-min period, beginning 15 min before occlusion. In addition, these investigators noted improved normalization of endocardial ATP levels, suppression of the reperfusion-induced rebound increase in phosphocreatine, and prevention of tissue edema in the deferoxamine-treated animals.

Bolli and co-workers[124] utilized the thiol-containing radical scavenger 2-mercapto-propionyl-glycine (MPG) to assess the time course of reperfusion injury in the canine stunned myocardium model (15 min of LAD occlusion followed by 4 h of reperfusion). Although this study does not deal directly with the role of iron, it is important because it provides mechanistic data pertaining to reperfusion injury. The scavenger was given by intracoronary infusion at a dose of 8 mg/kg/h. Four different groups of animals were used. Group one received the scavenger prior to, during occlusion, and for 2 h following reperfusion. A second group received the drug 2 min prior to reperfusion and for another 2 h thereafter. The third group received MPG at 1 min after reperfusion and for another 2 h of reperfusion. A fourth group received vehicle. Both groups that received the scavenger prior to reperfusion had a highly significant recovery of systolic function, while the group receiving the protective agent 1 min after reperfusion was indistinguishable from the control group.

Free-radical production during the reperfusion phase was assessed by intracoronary infusion of the spin trap α-phenyl *N-tert*-butyl nitrone (PBN). In separate control animals, radical adducts to this spin trap were detected in the coronary venous effluent within seconds of reflow and peaked after 4 min of reperfusion. The release of PBN adducts continued for at least 2 h. In animals receiving MPG 1 min after reperfusion, there was modest diminution of PBN adducts, while in the group receiving the scavenger immediately prior to reperfusion there was a dramatic decrease in the amount of these radical adducts.

MPG is a highly efficient scavenger of the hydroxyl radical, but reacts only slowly with superoxide anion and hydrogen peroxide. MPG is reported to easily enter cells, although the rate of cell permeation is not well documented.[124,137] Therefore, it is believed to interact with hydroxyl radicals generated within cells as well as in the vascular compartment. A rather remarkable conclusion that can be drawn from Bolli's study is that the protective effect of a therapeutic agent is largely lost if it is introduced into the previously ischemic organ as little as 1 min following reperfusion.

The question of involvement of iron in the pathophysiology of the stunned myocardium was addressed by Bolli and co-workers[138] in a subsequent study. Using protocols very similar to those employed in the MPG study discussed earlier, these investigators have provided direct evidence for the involvement of iron-catalyzed free-radical reactions in the stunned myocardium. In these experiments, the effects of intracoronary administration of deferoxamine 2 min before reperfusion, 1 min after reperfusion, or as the iron-saturated form of the drug were compared. The only group which had improved recovery of contractile function as compared to saline controls was the group receiving deferoxamine prior to reperfusion.

Again, free-radical production during the reperfusion phase was assessed by intracoronary infusion of PBN. Deferoxamine, given 2 min prior to reperfusion, significantly decreased the production of PBN-radical adducts. These results clearly indicate that antioxidant intervention can be administered late during ischemia and still attenuate functional injury. Furthermore, it appears that a compound, such as deferoxamine, that does not significantly penetrate membranes[139,140] can limit reperfusion injury, suggesting that a significant component of this damage occurs in the extracellular compartment.

In another study using the canine model of the stunned myocardium, Maruyama et al.[141] provide information about the site of reperfusion injury. These investigators compared the effect of conventional DFO with that of polymer-conjugated DFO.[32] Both compounds were administered intravenously in a pretreatment mode beginning 30 min before occlusion and continuing throughout the ischemic period at a dose of 50-mg deferoxamine equivalents per kilogram. Significant improvements in recovery of cardiac function, as measured by segmental shortening, were noted in animals treated intravenously with the high molecular weight form of the drug. Animals treated with free deferoxamine and iron-saturated DFO conjugate were not significantly different from saline-treated animals.

The lack of protective effect of free deferoxamine observed by Maruyama et al.[141] differs from an earlier study from the same laboratory[136] and also conflicts with the first reported use of DFO in the same model.[135] However, in the study by Farber et al.,[136] the drug was administered intra-atrially, which is likely to provide higher concentrations of the protective agent in the coronary circulation. It should also be noted that, unlike the polymer-DFO conjugates, the dose of free DFO used by Maruyama et al.[141] caused modest, but statistically significant, hypotension. This may have compromised the potential efficacy of the drug. The effectiveness of the polymer-DFO conjugates in this model also suggests that the ability of an agent to diffuse into the intracellular space is not a requirement for therapeutic efficacy.

In summary, the therapeutic efficacy of antioxidant treatment of the ischemic and reperfused myocardium is dependent on several variables. The timing of the administration (prior to, during, or at reperfusion); the site of infusion (intracardiac, intrasinus, or systemic), and the distribution of the therapeutic agent (vascular, interstitial, or intracellular) will profoundly influence the observed efficacy. All these variables must be carefully considered when one or more antioxidants are to be considered for introduction in human medicine. It should be noted that deferoxamine has been incorporated into human cardiac surgery in at least one center.[142,143]

3. Brain Injury and Ischemia

There are a large number of studies pertaining to antioxidant intervention following ischemic injury to the brain. However, relatively few deal directly with the role of iron in promoting injury occurring secondary to cerebral ischemia and reperfusion. (See also Chapter 12.)

Using a rat model of cardiac arrest and resuscitation, Babbs[144] showed a doubling of the probability of long-term survival, following 7 min of total circulatory arrest, by administration of deferoxamine (50 mg/kg) within the first few minutes after cardiopulmonary resuscitation (CPR). In addition, the surviving animals did not show any overt neurological deficit. Similar improvements in survival and neurological outcome have been achieved with administration of deferoxamine and the calcium entry blocker, lidoflazine, after 7 min of cardiorespiratory arrest in the rat[145] and 15 min of cardiac arrest in the dog.[146]

Patt et al.[147] demonstrated that an iron-deficient diet decreased the magnitude of brain edema observed following brain ischemia in the gerbil. Administration of deferoxamine prior to reperfusion also afforded protection in this model. Promising results with polymer-conjugated DFO[32] have also been obtained in a cardiac arrest/brain resuscitation model in which rats were subjected to 6.5 min of cardiopulmonary arrest.[148] Following arrest, successfully resuscitated animals received either normal saline or polymer-conjugated DFO (100-mg deferoxamine equivalents per kilogram) and were monitored for survival and neurological impairment for 10 d. Mortality was not different between the two groups in the first 24 h, but delayed mortality among 24-h survivors was only 13% in chelator-treated animals, compared to 42% in saline controls. In addition, neurological deficit scores were also significantly improved in the animals treated with polymer-conjugated DFO.

The 21-aminosteroid, U74006F, has also shown promise in models of global and focal ischemia. Natale et al.[149] examined the effect of U74006F on morbidity and mortality in a 10-min canine model of cardiopulmonary arrest. A 15-min bolus injection of 25 mM citrate vehicle or U74006F (1.5 mg/kg) was administered as soon as spontaneous circulation was established after the ischemic period and a maintenance dose of 0.125 mg/kg was continued for the next 12 h. At 24 h after arrest, survival in the vehicle-treated group was only 2 of 12, while in the group that received aminosteroid the survival was 8 of 12. In addition, neurological function was significantly improved in the U74006F group at 1, 2, and 24 h postarrest. These authors also documented that the aminosteroid-treated animals had significantly lower concentrations of lipid hydroperoxides in the plasma at 12 h postarrest and higher plasma vitamin E levels at 1, 2, and 6 h postarrest. Based on the hydroperoxide levels and the vitamin E data, the authors speculate that the protective effects of U74006F may be due to an antioxidant mechanism.

In a concussive head injury model in the mouse, Hall et al.[150] documented that administration of a single intravenous dose of U74006F (1 mg/kg) 5 min after injury improved long-term survival to 78.6% as compared to only 27.3% in vehicle-treated controls. Neurological function, as measured by a simple grip test, was also significantly improved at both 1 and 4 h in treated animals.

Additional evidence of efficacy of the 21-aminosteroids in traumatic CNS injury comes from the feline spinal cord injury work of Anderson and co-workers.[151] Thirty minutes after compression trauma of the upper lumbar spinal cord, animals received intravenous bolus injections of either vehicle or U74006F, followed by a constant intravenous infusion for 42 h. Total treatment doses ranged from 0.048 to 160 mg/kg. Neurological recovery, 4 weeks after injury, was approximately 75% of normal in animals receiving doses between 1.6 and 160 mg/kg and approximately 50% for animals receiving doses between 0.16 and 0.48 mg/kg as compared to 20% for vehicle-treated controls.

4. Intestine, Stomach, and Liver

Several pioneering studies dealing with the role of oxygen radicals and the injury sustained seconary to ischemia and reperfusion were performed using the feline intestinal model. The study by Granger and colleagues,[51] using capillary permeability as an indicator of capillary integrity, was one of the earliest studies clearly illustrating the protective effect of superoxide dismutase following an ischemic insult.

Evidence pointing to the importance of iron in the genesis of intestinal ischemia/reperfusion-induced injury was provided by Hernandez et al.[152] using the feline intestine. In this model, 1 h of ischemia and 30 min of reperfusion increased the intestinal vascular permeability from 0.08 to 0.40 in controls. However, in animals given deferoxamine intravenously during the last 5 min of ischemia and the first 15 min of reperfusion, the vascular permeability increased only to 0.15. Iron-loaded deferoxamine afforded no protection, with the vascular permeability increasing to 0.44. These investigators also provided support for the concept of *in vivo* protection by iron-binding proteins, by demonstrating that apotransferrin was as effective as deferoxamine in limiting the increase in vascular permeability caused by ischemia/reperfusion.

Several studies published in recent years indicate that the ability of antioxidants and oxygen radical scavengers to protect the intestine is strongly dependent on the severity of ischemic injury.[153] Park et al.[154] demonstrated that in a rat model of intestinal venous occlusion varied from 1 to 90 min, there was no evidence of exacerbation of mucosal injury by reperfusion over that caused by the ischemic insult.

The role of oxygen radicals in the pathophysiology of gastric mucosal injury following ischemia and reperfusion has been clearly demonstrated.[155,156] The importance of iron in this context was subsequently investigated by Smith et al.[157] Using clearance of radiolabeled red cells as a measure of mucosal integrity following reperfusion, it was noted that animals receiving 50 mg/kg of deferoxamine had dramatically decreased permeability to red cells. Likewise, superoxide dismutase and xanthine oxidase deficiency, achieved by feeding animals a tungsten diet, provided partial protection against reperfusion injury.

In a rat model of hepatic ischemia/reperfusion, Drugas et al.[158] demonstrated that polymer-conjugated DFO provides significant protection to the microcirculation. In these *in vivo* experiments, hepatic ischemia was maintained for 120 min followed by 90 min of reperfusion. Animals were treated 5 min before initiation of reperfusion with a 2-ml bolus of polymer-conjugated DFO (100-mg deferoxamine equivalents per kilogram), hydroxyethyl starch vehicle, or saline. The extent of hepatic injury at the end of reperfusion was determined by measuring serum alanine aminotransaminase (ALT), tissue edema, and sinusoidal perfusion, using a flourescein-albumin infusion technique followed by examination of frozen sections. These results were compared against sham-operated animals not subjected to ischemia. The reperfusion-induced rises in ALT and edema seen in the untreated animals were each suppressed 50% in animals receiving polymer-conjugated DFO. More importantly, the number of perfused microvessels in the chelator-treated group was not different from nonischemic controls, as compared to a 30% loss of microcirculatory perfusion in the untreated ischemic groups.

5. Lung

The adult respiratory distress syndrome and its association with oxygen radicals, complement, and neutrophils has been well established.[159,160] The involvement of iron in this syndrome is, in part, based on observed protection against pulmonary injury by the iron-binding protein lactoferrin, and deferoxamine.[36,37] Using systemic activation of the complement system with cobra venom factor (CVF), these investigators demonstrated that both apolactoferrin and deferoxamine significantly decreased plasma levels of conjugated dienes following treatment with CVF, while the iron-saturated forms of these compounds failed to reduce lipid peroxidation.

More recently, Kennedy et al.[161] have proposed that phosgene pulmonary injury is partially mediated by iron. These authors proposed that the observed protective effect afforded by ibuprofen may be due to iron chelation, although the structure of this drug does not suggest such a property.

6. Kidney

There are a limited number of studies indicating that iron chelators are effective in reducing renal injury following an ischemic insult and subsequent reperfusion. Paller et al.[60] first demonstrated that antioxidants, including superoxide dismutase and dimethylthiourea, were effective in an *in vivo* model of renal ischemia. Paller[162] also noted that renal tubular injury induced by hemeproteins is mediated by iron and, therefore, presumably by oxygen radicals. More recently, Paller and Hedlund[114] demonstrated that deferoxamine and inulin-conjugated DFO, but not dextran-conjugated DFO, protected against injury sustained during 60 min of warm ischemia and subsequent reperfusion. The iron chelator was administered immediately prior to reperfusion, indicating that a significant fraction of overall injury is sustained during reperfusion. The results clearly implicate iron as a mediator of renal reperfusion injury and suggest that the therapeutic agent must be efficiently filtered in order to afford protection.

In a study of relevance to renal transplantation, Fuller and co-workers[163] documented that DFO at a dose of 15 mg/kg provided protection against oxidant injury following 24 h of cold storage prior to autotransfusion. The same group[164] has also shown that a low molecular weight, chelatable pool of iron is formed during cold ischemia in rabbit kidneys.

7. Hemorrhagic Shock and Burn Injury

A role for delocalized iron in the etiology of hypovolemic shock, possibly through a free-radical-mediated mechanism, is suggested by the observations that serum iron increases during hemorrhagic shock in animals.[112,113] Sanan et al.[165] have examined this possibility and the potential therapeutic benefit of systemic iron chelation in a canine model of hypovolemic shock. The shock state, produced by rapid arterial bleeding to a mean arterial blood pressure of 35 mmHg, was maintained for 4 h at which time the animals were resuscitated by return of the shed blood. Deferoxamine was administered intramuscularly at 2, 3, and 4 h after blood loss at a dose of 25 mg/kg, and return of consciousness and survival were monitored for 72 h postresuscitation. Histopathological liver examinations were performed in a separate group of animals subjected to the same protocol, but sacrificed at 2 h after return of blood. Animals receiving deferoxamine had a more rapid return of consciousness, improved survival, and less histopathological change than untreated animals. Outcomes were dependent on the time of administration of the deferoxamine, with the best results obtained when the chelator was given just before resuscitation (4 h postbleed), presumably because of the greater availability of the chelator during the resuscitation phase. Survival was 100% (10/10) in those animals receiving deferoxamine at 4 h compared to only 50% (5/10) for the untreated group. In addition, the treated animals did not have the magnitude of liver histopathology seen in the untreated group.

In a recent study, Jacobs and co-workers[166] demonstrated that a conjugate between deferoxamine (DFO) and hydroxyethyl starch, as well as the colloid itself, greatly improved survival in a porcine hemorrhagic shock model. Animals were bled to a mean arterial blood pressure of 45 mmHg, maintained at this pressure for 1 h, and then resuscitated with one volume of colloid or colloid-DFO conjugate (one volume equals the shed blood volume) or three volumes of lactated Ringer's solution. All animals treated with crystalloid died within 24 h, while 100% survival was noted in both colloid-treated groups. However, hepatocellular injury appeared to be less severe in animals receiving the chelator because of decreased plasma levels of alanine aminotransferase and reduced hepatic lipid peroxidation compared to animals receiving the colloid control.

In a feline model of hemorrhagic shock, Hall and associates[167] have shown that animals treated with the 21-aminosteroid, U74006F, had improved hemodynamic recovery in comparison to animals treated with vehicle and gluco-corticoid. A dose of 10 mg/kg of the lazaroid was compared with a dose of 30 mg/kg of the glucocorticoid, methylprednisolone. Both agents were administered prior to reinfusion of shed blood following a 2-h period of hypotension (45 to 50 mmHg mean arterial blood pressure).

Burn injury is not associated with an ischemic insult followed by reperfusion, but is probably best characterized as a global inflammatory response to an initial trauma, usually involving the skin. However, there is abundant evidence that the damage to secondary organs, particularly the liver and the lung, observed following burn are, in part, caused by oxygen-derived radicals.[168-171] Recent studies by Demling and associates[172] suggest that this inflammatory response can be modulated by systemic iron chelation. In an ovine model involving 40% of total body surface area third-degree burn, animals treated with the hydroxyethyl starch-deferoxamine conjugate had significantly improved overall hemodynamics and significantly decreased lipid peroxidation compared with animals receiving either the colloid or lactated Ringer's solution.

B. IRON-MEDIATED INFLAMMATION AND AUTOIMMUNE DISEASE

The involvement of activated phagocytic cells, including activated neutrophils and macrophages, is one of the hallmarks of inflammatory processes. It is often the inappropriate effects of these cells on the host that cause many of the syndromes associated with inflammation, including microvascular leakage leading to edema, and the inflammatory responses associated with skin and joint diseases.[6,7]

Rheumatoid arthritis has been associated with altered iron homeostasis in the joint since early studies by Muirden and associates.[173,174] Deferoxamine has been tried as a therapeutic agent for the treatment of rheumatoid arthritis,[3,5,175] but results were confounded by drug-induced toxicity. The radical scavenger, tiopronin (2-mercapto-propionyl-glycine or MPG), has been used in the treatment of this disease, but promising results were also complicated by drug-induced toxicity.[176] The observed protective effect of tiopronin has been proposed to be related to the scavenging of hypochlorous acid released by activated neutrophils.[177]

In a model of experimental allergic encephalomyelitis (EAE) in rats manifested by hind leg paralysis, Bowern et al.[4] demonstrated that deferoxamine, given at various times before onset of symptoms, dramatically suppressed the severity and duration of the disease. EAE is considered an animal model of multiple sclerosis. The authors suggest that the protective effect of the chelator was related to its suppression of T cell responsiveness and therefore a decreased invasiveness of these cells into the inflammatory lesions. As an example of the beneficial effect of iron chelators other than deferoxamine,

Hewitt et al.[178] have demonstrated an anti-inflammatory effect of the hydroxypyridin-4-one and hydroxypyrone-type chelators in a pleural inflammation model.

C. ROLE OF IRON IN DRUG TOXICITY
1. Paraquat

The human toxicity manifested by the commonly used herbicide, paraquat, is thought to be associated with an enzymatic univalent reduction to a free-radical species, leading to the formation of activated oxygen species through redox cycling.[179] In addition, paraquat is efficient at liberating iron from ferritin,[45] and transition metals may be necessary for paraquat toxicity.[17-19,180,181] For these reasons, several investigators have examined the effect of deferoxamine on the toxicity of paraquat. Kohen and Chevion[17] and Van Asbeck et al.[19] have demonstrated protection against paraquat toxicity by deferoxamine, while Osheroff et al.[180] have documented a lack of protection by the chelator. Kohen and Chevion administered 5-mg injections of deferoxamine intraperitoneally 24 h prior to a single intraperitoneal injection of paraquat (17 mg/kg) followed by additional injections of deferoxamine twice daily following the paraquat injection. Animals receiving paraquat alone began dying at 24 h postinjection, 50% had died by 32 h and none survived past 3 d. In contrast, those animals receiving deferoxamine in addition to the paraquat did not begin dying until 40 h postparaquat, with 50% surviving to 90 h and 20 to 30% surviving more than 3 months. Because of the lung damage seen clinically in patients suffering from paraquat poisoning, these investigators also measured the activity of lung acetylcholine esterase and water content as an index of lung damage following injection of paraquat, with or without deferoxamine. Deferoxamine therapy eliminated the loss of acetylcholine esterase activity and prevented the increase in lung edema seen in untreated animals.

Van Asbeck et al.[19] have also shown protection against paraquat-induced mortality and lung damage by continuous intravenous administration of deferoxamine in a vitamin E-deficient model in the rat. In this model, deferoxamine therapy was initiated immediately, 6 or 16 h after injection of paraquat (20 mg/kg) and continued for 14 d. Survival to 35 d was significantly improved in animals receiving deferoxamine (100 mg/kg/24 h) either immediately or 6 h after, but not at 16 h after paraquat administration. Histological examinations of treated and untreated nonsurvivors revealed severe lung damage including edema, necrosis, phagocyte infiltration, and fibrosis. In contrast, deferoxamine-treated animals surviving 14 or 35 d had no apparent lung lesions.

2. Adriamycin

Animal studies,[182-185] as well as an initial clinical trial in women with advanced breast cancer,[186] have shown that the EDTA-like metal chelator,

ICRF-187 ([+]-1,2-bis[3,5-dioxopiperazinyl-1-yl]propane) provides significant protection against the dose-dependent cardiotoxicity induced by the antineoplastic drug, adriamycin (doxorubicin). A proposed mechanism for adriamycin toxicity is through the interaction of the drug and iron, thereby catalyzing free-radical formation and the promotion of lipid peroxidation.[16,187-192]

The protective effect of ICRF-187 has not been elucidated, but may reside in its ability to render iron unavailable for formation of a reactive adriamycin-iron complex. The ring-opened hydrolysis product of ICRF-187 has a structure similar to EDTA and is a strong iron chelator.[193] In addition, ICRF-187 removes iron from preformed adriamycin-iron complexes and can form mixed ligand complexes with adriamycin-iron which are poorly reactive.[194] *In vitro* studies have shown that adriamycin-dependent lipid peroxidation and microsomal Ca ATPase inactivation are inhibited by ICRF-187.[191] Using an isolated rat heart preparation, Rajagopalan et al.[190] demonstrated that the adriamycin-stimulated production of hydroxyl radicals is abrogated by clinically achievable levels of ICRF-187. Other iron-specific chelators such as deferoxamine have not been protective against adriamycin toxicity, possibly because of poor cellular uptake.[195]

V. SUMMARY

This discussion of the role of iron in human disease is divided into two parts. The first part deals with the toxic effects of iron caused either by excess intake of some form of iron, or by genetic disorders leading to the continuous buildup of tissue iron levels. In these situations therapeutic intervention is aimed at achieving reduction of systemic iron levels by chelation therapy. Primary research efforts in the treatment of chronic iron overload are centered on the development of orally active chelators. The second part pertains to situations where, despite normal tissue iron levels, the metal ion can be released from normally sequestered sites and catalyze reactions leading to the formation of highly reactive, oxygen- and lipid-derived radicals. These reactive molecules are mediators in the pathophysiology of a variety of disease states. Although many different approaches have been proposed for limiting iron-mediated tissue injury, it seems clear that a primary intervention based on systemic and/or targeted iron chelation affords the most practical and efficient means of achieving this therapeutic goal.

REFERENCES

1. **Gutteridge, J. M. C., Rowley, D. A., and Halliwell, B.,** Superoxide dependent formation of hydroxyl radicals in the presence of iron salts, *Biochem. J.,* 199, 263, 1981.
2. **Halliwell, B., Gutteridge, J. M. C., and Blake, D.,** Metal ions and oxygen radical reactions in human inflammatory joint disease, *Philos. Trans. R. Soc. London, Ser. B,* 311, 659, 1985.
3. **Andrews, F. J., Morris, C. J., Kondratowicz, G., and Blake, D. R.,** Effect of iron chelation on inflammatory disease, *Ann. Rheum. Dis.,* 46, 327, 1987.
4. **Bowern, N., Ramshaw, I. A., Clark, I. A., and Doherty, P. C.,** Inhibition of autoimmune neuropathological process by treatment with an iron-chelating agent, *J. Exp. Med.,* 160, 1532, 1984.
5. **Blake, D. R., Hall, N. D., Bacon, P. A., et al.,** Effect of a specific iron chelating agent on animal models of inflammation, *Ann. Rheum. Dis.,* 42, 89, 1983.
6. **Halliwell, B., Hoult, J. R., and Blake, D. R.,** Oxidants, inflammation, and anti-inflammatory drugs, *FASEB J.,* 2, 2867, 1988.
7. **Ward, P. A., Warren J. S., and Johnson, K. J.,** Oxygen radicals, inflammation, and tissue injury, *Free Radical Biol. Med.,* 5, 403, 1988.
8. **Braughler, J. M. and Hall, E. D.,** Central nervous system trauma and stroke. I. Biochemical considerations for oxygen radical formation and lipid peroxidation, *Free Radical Biol. Med.,* 6, 289, 1989.
9. **Oberley, L. W.,** Free radicals and diabetes, *Free Radical. Biol. Med.,* 5, 113, 1988.
10. **Cutler, P.,** Deferoxamine therapy in high-ferritin diabetes, *Diabetes,* 38, 1207, 1989.
11. **Halliwell, B.,** Oxidants and the central nervous system: some fundamental questions. Is oxidant damage relevant to Parkinson's disease, Alzheimer's disease, traumatic injury or stroke?, *Acta Neurol. Scand.,* Suppl. 126, 23, 1989.
12. **Adams, J. D. and Odunze, I. N.,** Oxygen free radicals and Parkinson's disease, *Free Radical Biol. Med.,* 10, 161, 1991.
13. **Weinberg, E. D.,** Iron and neoplasia, *Biol. Trace Elem.,* 3, 55, 1981.
14. **Stevens, R. G., Jones, D. Y., Micozzi, M. S., and Taylor, P. R.,** Body iron stores and the risk of cancer, *N. Engl. J. Med.,* 319, 1047, 1988.
15. **Nordmann, R., Ribière, C., and Rouach, H.,** Involvement of iron and iron-catalyzed free radical production in ethanol metabolism and toxicity, *Enzyme,* 37, 57, 1987.
16. **Sinha, B. K. and Politi, P. M.,** Anthracyclines, *Cancer Chem. Biol. Resp. Mod.,* 11, 45, 1990.
17. **Kohen, R. and Chevion, M.,** Paraquat toxicity is enhanced by iron and reduced by desferrioxamine in laboratory mice, *Biochem. Pharmacol.,* 34, 1841, 1985.
18. **Korbashi, P., Kohen, R., Katzhendler, J., and Chevion, M.,** Iron mediated paraquat toxicity in *Escherichia coli, J. Biol. Chem.,* 261, 12472, 1986.
19. **Van Asbeck, B. S., Hillen, F. C., Boonen, H. C. N., et al.,** Continuous intravenous infusion of deferoxamine reduces mortality by paraquat in vitamin E-deficient rats, *Am. Rev. Respir. Dis.,* 139, 769, 1989.
20. **Halliwell, B. and Gutteridge, J. M. C.,** Oxygen free radicals and iron in relation to biology and medicine: some problems and concepts, *Arch. Biochem. Biophys.,* 246, 501, 1986.
21. **Minotti, G. and Aust, S. D.,** The role of iron in oxygen radical mediated lipid peroxidation, *Chem. Biol. Interact.,* 71, 1, 1989.
22. **Westlin, W. F.,** Deferoxamine as a chelating agent, *Clin. Toxicol.,* 4, 587, 1971.
23. **Zurlo, M., Destefano, P., Borgna-Pignatti, C., et al.,** Survival and causes of death in thalassemia major, *Lancet,* 1, 27, 1989.
24. **Giardina, P. J., Grady, R. W., Ehlers, K. H., et al.,** Current therapy of Cooley's anemia. A decade of experience with subcutaneous desferrioxamine, *Ann. N.Y. Acad. Sci.,* 612, 275, 1990.

25. **Keberle, H.,** The biochemistry of desferrioxamine and its relation to iron metabolism, *Ann. N.Y. Acad. Sci.,* 119, 758, 1964.
26. **Graf, E., Mahoney, J. R., Bryant, R. G., and Eaton, J. W.,** Iron-catalyzed hydroxyl radical formation. Stringent requirement for free iron coordination site, *J. Biol. Chem.,* 259, 3620, 1984.
27. **Summers, M. R., Jacobs, A., Tudway, D., et al.,** Studies in desferrioxamine and ferrioxamine metabolism in normal and iron-loaded subjects, *Br. J. Haematol.,* 42, 547, 1979.
28. **Bentur, Y., McGuigan, M., and Koren, G.,** Deferoxamine (desferrioxamine). New toxicities for an old drug, *Drug Safety,* 6, 37, 1991.
29. **Whitten, C. F., Gibson, G. W., Good, M. H., et al.,** Studies in acute iron poisoning. I. Desferrioxamine in the treatment of acute iron poisoning: clinical observations, experimental studies, and theoretical considerations, *Pediatrics,* 36, 322, 1965.
30. **Whitten, C. F., Chen, Y., and Gibson, G. W.,** Studies in acute iron poisoning. II. Further observations on desferrioxamine in the treatment of acute experimental iron poisoning, *Pediatrics,* 38, 102, 1966.
31. **Westlin, W. F.,** Deferoxamine in the treatment of acute iron poisoning. Clinical experiences with 172 children, *Clin. Ped.,* 5, 531, 1966.
32. **Hallaway, P. E., Eaton, J. W., Panter, S. S., and Hedlund, B. E.,** Modulation of deferoxamine toxicity and clearance by covalent attachment to biocompatible polymers, *Proc. Nat. Acad. Sci. U.S.A.,* 86, 10108, 1989.
33. **Forder, J. R., McClanahan, T. B., Gallagher, K. P., et al.,** Hemodynamic effects of intaatrial administration of deferoxamine or deferoxamine-pentafraction conjugate to conscious dogs, *J. Cardiovasc. Pharmacol.,* 16, 742, 1990.
34. **Olivieri, N. F., Buncic, J. R., Chew, W., et al.,** Visual and auditory neurotoxicity in patients receiving subcutaneous desferrioxamine infusions, *N. Engl. J. Med.,* 314, 869, 1986.
35. **Halliwell, B. and Gutteridge, J. M. C.,** Iron toxicity and oxygen radicals, *Baillières Clin. Haematol.,* 2, 195, 1989.
36. **Ward, P. A., Till, G. O., Hatherill, J. R., et al.,** Systemic complement activation, lung injury, and products of lipid peroxidation, *J. Clin. Invest.,* 76, 517, 1985.
37. **Johnson, K. J. and Ward, P. A.,** Role of oxygen metabolites in immune complex injury of lung, *J. Immunol.,* 126, 2365, 1981.
38. **Thomas, C. E., Morehouse, L. A., and Aust, S. D.,** Ferritin and superoxide-dependent lipid peroxidation, *J. Biol. Chem.,* 260, 3275, 1985.
39. **Biemond, P., Swaak, A. J. G., van Eijk, H. G., and Koster, J. F.,** Superoxide dependent iron release from ferritin in inflammatory diseases, *Free Radical Biol. Med.,* 4, 185, 1988.
40. **Reif, D. W., Schubert, J., and Aust, S. D.,** Iron release from ferritin and lipid peroxidation by radiolytially generated reducing radicals, *Arch. Biochem. Biophys.,* 264, 238, 1988.
41. **Bolann, B. J. and Ulvik, R. J.,** Release of iron from ferritin by xanthine oxidase. Role of the superoxide radical, *Biochem. J.,* 243, 55, 1987.
42. **Mazur, A., Green, S., Saha, A., and Carleton, A.,** Mechanism of release of ferritin iron *in vivo* by xanthine oxidase, *J. Clin. Invest.,* 37, 1809, 1958.
43. **Duggan, D. E. and Streeter, K. B.,** Inhibition of ferritin reduction by pyrazolo (3,4d) pyrimidines, *Arch. Biochem. Biophys.,* 156, 66, 1973.
44. **Thomas, C. E. and Aust, S. D.,** Reductive release of iron from ferritin by cation free radicals of paraquat and other bipyridyls, *J. Biol. Chem.,* 261, 13064, 1986.
45. **Thomas, C. E. and Aust, S. D.,** Free radicals and environmental toxins, *Ann. Emerg. Med.,* 15, 1075, 1986.
46. **Reif, D. W., Samokyszyn, V. M., Miller, D. M., and Aust, S. D.,** Alloxan- and glutathione-dependent ferritin iron release and lipid peroxidation, *Arch. Biochem. Biophys.,* 269, 407, 1989.

502

47. **Gutteridge, J. M. C. and Hou, Y.,** Iron complexes and their reactivity in the bleomycin assay for radical promoting loosely-bound iron, *Free Radical Res. Commun.,* 2, 143, 1986.

48. **Arouma, O. I. and Halliwell, B.,** Superoxide-dependent and ascorbate-dependent formation of hydroxyl radicals from hydrogen peroxide in the presence of iron, *Biochem. J.,* 241, 273, 1987.

49. **Turrens, J. F. and Boveris, A.,** Generation of superoxide anion by the NADH dehydrogenase of bovine heart mitochondria, *Biochem. J.,* 191, 421, 1980.

50. **Misra, H. P. and Fridovich, I. J.,** Generation of superoxide radical during autooxidation of hemoglobin, *J. Biol. Chem.,* 247, 6960, 1972.

51. **Granger, D. N., Ruttili, G., and McCord, J. M.,** Superoxide radicals in feline intestinal ischemia, *Gastroenterology,* 81, 22, 1981.

52. **Babior, B. M. and Peters, W. A.,** The O_2^- producing enzyme of human neutrophils: further properties, *J. Biol Chem.,* 256, 2321, 1981.

53. **Kappus, H. and Sies, H.,** Toxic drug effects associated with oxygen metabolism: redox cycling and lipid peroxidation, *Experientia,* 37, 1233, 1981.

54. **Cronstein, B. N., Rosenstein, E. D., Kramer, S. B., et al.,** Adenosine: a physiologic modulator of superoxide anion generation by human neutrophils, adenosine acts via an A2 receptor on human neutrophils, *J. Immunol.,* 135, 1366, 1985.

55. **Berton, G., Dusi, S., Serra, M. C., et al.,** Studies on the NADPH oxidase of phagocytes: production of a monoclonal antibody which blocks the enzymatic activity of pig neutrophil NADPH oxidase, *J. Biol. Chem.,* 254, 5564, 1989.

56. **Arfors, K. E., Lundberg, C., Lindbom, L., et al.,** A monoclonal antibody to the membrane glycoprotein complex CD18 inhibits polymorphonuclear leucocyte accumulation and plasma leakage *in vivo, Blood,* 69, 338, 1987.

57. **Vedder, N. B., Winn, R. K., Rice, C. L., et al.,** A monoclonal antibody to the adherence-producing leukocyte glycoprotein, CD18, reduces organ injury and improves survival from hemorrhagic shock and resuscitation in rabbits, *J. Clin. Invest.,* 81, 939, 1988.

58. **Engler, R. and Gilpin, E.,** Can superoxide dismutase alter myocardial infarct size?, *Circulation,* 79, 1137, 1989.

59. **Bolli, R.,** Superoxide dismutase 10 years later: a drug in search of a use, *J. Am. Coll. Cardiol.,* 18, 231, 1991.

60. **Paller, M. S., Hoidal, J. R., and Ferris, T. F.,** Oxygen free radicals in ischemic acute renal failure in the rat, *J. Clin. Invest.,* 74, 1156, 1984.

61. **Schneeberger, H., Illner, W. D., Abendroth, D., et al.,** First clinical experience with superoxide dismutase in kidney transplantation — results of a double-blind randomized study, *Transplant. Proc.,* 21, 1245, 1989.

62. **Turrens, J. F., Crapo, J. D., and Freeman, B. A.,** Protection against oxygen toxicity by intravenous injection of liposome-entrapped catalase and superoxide dismutase, *J. Clin. Invest.,* 73, 87, 1984.

63. **Hallewell, R. A., Laria, I., Tabrizi, A., et al.,** Genetically engineered polymers of human CuZn superoxide dismutase, *J. Biol. Chem.,* 264, 5260, 1989.

64. **Liu, T. H., Beckman, J. S., Freeman, B. A., et al.,** Polyethylene glycol-conjugated superoxide dismutase and catalase reduce ischemic brain injury, *Am. J. Physiol.,* 256, H589, 1989.

65. **White, C. W., Jackson, J. H., Abuchowski, A., et al.,** Polyethylene glycol-attached antioxidant enzymes decrease pulmonary oxygen toxicity in rats, *J. Appl. Physiol.,* 66, 584, 1989.

66. **Somack, R., Saifer, M. G. P., and Williams, L. D.,** Preparation of long-acting superoxide dismutase using high molecular weight polyehylene glycol (41,000-72,000 Daltons), *Free Rad. Res. Commun.,* 12(13), 553, 1991.

67. **Freeman, B. A., Young, S. I., and Crapo, J. D.,** Liposome-mediated augmentation of superoxide dismutase in endothelial cells prevents oxygen injury, *J. Biol. Chem.*, 258, 12534, 1983.

68. **Greenwald, R. A.,** Superoxide dismutase and catalase as therapeutic agents for human diseases. A critical review, *Free Radical Biol. Med.*, 8, 201, 1990.

69. **Ward, P. A., Warren, J. S., Till, G. O., et al.,** Modification of disease by preventing free radical formation: a new concept in pharmacological intervention, *Baillière's Clin. Haematol.*, 2, 391, 1989.

70. **Reilly, P. M., Schiller, H. J., and Bulkley, G. B.,** Pharmacologic approach to tissue injury mediated by free radicals and other reactive oxygen metabolites, *Am. J. Surg.*, 161, 488, 1991.

71. **Scott, M. D., Meshnick, S. R., and Eaton, J. W.,** SOD rich bacteria: paradoxical increase in oxidant toxicity, *J. Biol. Chem.*, 262, 3640, 1987.

72. **Omar, B. A., Gad, N. M., Jordan, M. C., et al.,** Cardioprotection by Cu,Zn-superoxide dismutase is lost at high doses in the reoxygenated heart, *Free Radical Biol. Med.*, 9, 465, 1990.

73. **Omar, B. A. and McCord, J. M.,** The cardioprotective effect of Mn-superoxide dismutase is lost at high doses in the postischemic isolated rabbit heart, *Free Radical Biol. Med.*, 9, 473, 1990.

74. **Kedziora, J. and Bartosz, G.,** Down's syndrome: a pathology involving the lack of balance of reactive oxygen species, *Free Radical Biol. Med.*, 4, 317, 1988.

75. **Younes, M. and Weser, U.,** Superoxide dismutase activity of copper-penicillamine: possible involvement of Cu(I) stabilized sulphur radical, *Biochem. Biophys. Res. Commun.*, 78, 1247, 1977.

76. **Kimura, E., Sakonaka, A., and Nakamoto, M.,** Superoxide dismutase activity of macrocyclic polyamine complexes, *Biochim. Biophys. Acta*, 678, 172, 1981.

77. **Darr, D., Zarilla, K., and Fridovich, I.,** A mimic of superoxide dismutase activity based on desferrioxamine B and manganese, *Arch. Biochem. Biophys.*, 258, 351, 1987.

78. **Nagano, T., Tomohisa, H., and Hirobe, M.,** Novel iron complexes behave like superoxide dismutase in vivo, *Free Radical Res. Commun.*, 12(13), 221, 1991.

79. **Mitchell, J. B., Samuni, A., Krishna, M. C., et al.,** Biologically active metal-independent superoxide dismutase mimics, *Biochemistry*, 29, 2802, 1990.

80. **Samuni, A., Mitchell, J. B., DeGraff, W., et al.,** Nitroxide SOD-mimics: modes of action, *Free Radical Res. Commun.*, 12(13), 187, 1991.

81. **Darr, D. J., Yanni, S., and Pinnell, S. R.,** Protection of chinese hamster ovary cells from paraquat-mediated cytotoxicity by a low molecular weight mimic of superoxide dismutase (DF-Mn), *Free Radical Biol. Med.*, 4, 357, 1988.

82. **Rabinowich, H. D., Privalle, C. T., and Fridovich, I.,** Effects of paraquat on the green alga *Dunaliella salina:* protection by the mimic of superoxide dismutase, desferal-Mn(IV), *Free Radical Biol. Med.*, 3, 125, 1987.

83. **Puppo, A. and Halliwell, B.,** Formation of hydroxyl radicals in biological systems. Does myoglobin stimulate hydroxyl radical formation from hydrogen peroxide?, *Free Radical Res. Commun.*, 4, 415, 1988.

84. **Puppo, A. and Halliwell, B.,** Oxidation of dimethylsulphoxide to formaldehyde by oxyhaemoglobin in the presence of hydrogen peroxide is not mediated "free" hydroxyl radicals, *Free Radical Res. Commun.*, 5, 277, 1989.

85. **Rice-Evans, C., Okunade, G., and Khan, R.,** The suppression of iron release from activated myoglobin by physiological electron donors and by desferrioxamine, *Free Radical Res. Commun.*, 7, 45, 1989.

86. **Drexel, H., Dworzak, E., Kirchmair, W., et al.,** Myoglobinemia in the early phase of acute myocardial infarction, *Am. Heart J.*, 105, 642, 1983.

87. **Odeh, M.,** The role of reperfusion injury in the pathogenesis of crush syndrome, *N. Engl. J. Med.*, 324, 1417, 1991.

88. **Luzzatto, L. and Mehta, A.,** Glucose-6-phosphate dehydrogenase deficiency, in *Metabolic Basis of Inherited Disease,* 6th ed., Scriver, C. R., Beaudet, A. L., Sly, W. S., et al., Eds., McGraw-Hill, New York, 1989, 2237.

89. **Baar, S. and Arrowsmith, D. J.,** Thermal damage to red cells, *J. Clin. Pathol.,* 23, 572, 1970.

90. **Loebl, E. C., Marvin, J.-A., Curreri, P. W., and Baxter, C. R.,** Erythrocyte survival following thermal injury, *J. Surg. Res.,* 16, 96, 1974.

91. **Chow, C. K.,** Vitamin E and oxidative stress, *Free Radical Biol. Med.,* 11, 215, 1991.

92. **Braughler, J. M., Hall, E. D., Jacobsen, E. J., et al.,** The 21-aminosteroids: potent inhibitors of lipid peroxidation for the treatment of central nervous system trauma and ischemia, *Drugs Future,* 14, 143, 1989.

93. **Braughler, J. M., Pregenzer, J. F., Chase, R. L., et al.,** Novel 21-aminosteroids as potent inhibitors of iron-dependent lipid peroxidation, *J. Biol. Chem.,* 262, 10438, 1987.

94. **Jacobsen, E. J., McCall, J. M., Ayer, D. E., et al.,** Novel 21-aminosteroids that inhibit iron-dependent lipid peroxidation and protect against central nervous system trauma, *J. Med. Chem.,* 33, 1145, 1990.

95. **Braughler, J. M. and Pregenzer, J. F.,** The 21-aminosteroid inhibitors of lipid peroxidation: reactions with lipid peroxyl and phenoxy radicals, *Free Radical Biol. Med.,* 7, 125, 1989.

96. **Kang, J. O., Slivka, A., Slater, G., and Cohen, G.,** *In vivo* formation of hydroxyl radicals following intragastric administration of ferrous salt in rats, *J. Inorg. Biochem.,* 35, 55, 1989.

97. **Witzleben, C. L.,** An electron microscopic study of ferrous sulfate induced liver damage, *Am. J. Pathol.,* 49, 1053, 1966.

98. **Ganote, C. E. and Nahara, G.,** Acute ferrous sulfate hepatotoxicity in rats: an electron microscopic and biochemical study, *Lab. Invest.,* 28, 426, 1973.

99. **Robotham, J. L. and Lietman, P. S.,** Acute iron poisoning: a review, *Am. J. Dis. Child.,* 34, 875, 1980.

100. **Henretig, F. M., Karl, S. R., and Weintraub, W. H.,** Severe iron poisoning treated with enteral and intravenous deferoxamine, *Ann. Emerg. Med.,* 12, 306, 1983.

101. **Tenenbein, M.,** Iron poisoning, in *Intensive Care Medicine,* 2nd ed., Rippe, J. M., Irwin, R. S., Alpert, J. S., et al., Eds., Little, Brown, Boston, 1991, 1290.

102. **Banner, W. and Tong, T. G.,** Iron poisoning, *Pediatr. Clin. North Am.,* 33, 393, 1986.

103. *Physicians' Desk Reference,* 44th ed., Medical Economics, Oradell, NJ, 1990, 850.

104. **Mahoney, J. R., Hallaway, P. E., Hedlund, B. E., and Eaton, J. W.,** Acute iron poisoning: rescue with macromolecular chelators, *J. Clin. Invest.,* 85, 1362, 1989.

105. **Propper, R., Cooper, B., Rufo, R., et al.,** Continuous subcutaneous administration of desferrioxamine in patients with iron overload, *N. Engl. J. Med.,* 297, 418, 1977.

106. **Pippard, M. J.,** Desferrioxamine-induced iron secretion in humans, *Baillière's Clin. Haematol.,* 2, 323, 1989.

107. **Hoffbrand, A. V. and Wonke, B.,** Results of long-term subcutaneous desferrioxamine therapy, *Baillière's Clin. Haematol.,* 2, 335, 1989.

108. **Fosburg, M. T. and Nathan, D. G.,** Treatment of Cooley's anemia, *Blood,* 76, 435, 1990.

109. **Cohen, A.,** Current status of iron chelation therapy with deferoxamine, *Semin. Hematol.,* 27, 86, 1990.

110. **Porter, J. B., Huehns, E. R., and Hider, R. C.,** The development of iron chelating drugs, *Baillière's Clin. Haematol.,* 2, 257, 1989.

111. **Hershko, C. and Weatherall, D. J.,** Iron-chelating therapy, *Crit. Rev. Clin. Lab. Sci.,* 26, 303, 1988.

112. **Mazur, A., Baez, S., and Shorr, E.,** The mechanism of iron release from ferritin as related to its biological properties, *J. Biol. Chem.,* 213, 147, 1955.

113. **Janoff, A., Zweifach, B. W., and Shapiro, L. R.,** Levels of plasma-bound iron in experimental shock in the rabbit and dog, *Am. J. Phisol.,* 198, 1161, 1960.

114. **Paller, M. S. and Hedlund, B. E.**, Role of iron in post-ischemic renal injury in the rat, *Kidney Int.*, 34, 474, 1988.

115. **Robinson, E. and Hedlund, B.**, Role of iron in ischemia and reperfusion, *Circ. Shock*, 27, 367, 1989.

116. **Krause, G. S., Joyce, K. M., Nayini, N. R., et al.**, Cardiac arrest and resuscitation. Brain iron delocalization during reperfusion, *Ann. Emerg. Med.*, 14, 1037, 1985.

117. **Krause, G. S., Nayini, N. R., White, B. C., et al.**, Natural course of iron delocalization and lipid peroxidation during the first eight hours following a 15-minute cardiac arrest in dogs, *Ann. Emerg. Med.*, 16, 1200, 1987.

118. **Holt, S., Gunderson, M., Joyce, K., et al.**, Myocardial tissue iron delocalization and evidence for lipid peroxidation after two hours of ischemia, *Ann. Emerg. Med.*, 15, 1155, 1987.

119. **Braunwald, E. and Kloner, R. A.**, The stunned myocardium: prolonged, postischemic ventricular dysfunction, *Circulation*, 66, 1146, 1982.

120. **Zweier, J. L., Flaherty, J. T., and Weisfeldt, M. L.**, Direct measurement of free radical generation following reperfusion of ischemic myocardium, *Proc. Natl. Acad. Sci. U.S.A.*, 84, 1404, 1987.

121. **Zweier, J. L., Kuppusamy, P., Williams, R., et al.**, Measurement and characterization of postischemic free radical generation in the isolated perfused heart, *J. Biol. Chem.*, 264, 18890, 1989.

122. **Arroyo, C. M., Kramer, J. H., Leiboff, G. W., et al.**, Spin trapping of oxygen and carbon-centered free radicals in ischemic canine myocardium, *Free Radical Biol. Med.*, 3, 313, 1987.

123. **Davies, M. J.**, Direct detection of radical production in the ischaemic and reperfused myocardium: current status, *Free Radical Biol. Med.*, 7, 275, 1989.

124. **Bolli, R., Jeroudi, M. O., Patel, B. S., et al.**, Marked reduction of free radical generation and contractile dysfunction by antioxidant therapy begun at the time of reperfusion, *Circ. Res.*, 65, 607, 1989.

125. **Tsao, P. S. and Lefer, A. M.**, Time course and mechanism of endothelial dysfunction in isolated ischemic- and hypoxic-perfused rat hearts, *Am. J. Physiol.*, 259, H1660, 1990.

126. **Gauduel, Y. and Duvelleroy, M. A.**, Role of oxygen radicals in cardiac injury due to reoxygenation, *J. Mol. Cell Cardiol.*, 16, 459, 1984.

127. **Hess, M. L. and Manson, N. H.**, Molecular oxygen: friend and foe, *J. Mol. Cell Cardiol.*, 16, 969, 1984.

128. **Kloner, R. A., Przyklenk, K., and Whittaker, P.**, Deleterious effects of oxygen radicals in ischemia/reperfusion: resolved and unresolved issues, *Circulation*, 80, 1115, 1989.

129. **Opie, L. H.**, Reperfusion injury and its pharmacologic modification, *Circulation*, 80, 1049, 1989.

130. **Lucchesi, B. R.**, Myocardial ischemia, reperfusion, and free radical injury, *Am. J. Cardiol.*, 65, 141, 1990.

131. **Reddy, B. R., Kloner, R. A., and Przyklenk, K.**, Early treatment with deferoxamine limits myocardial ischemic/reperfusion injury, *Free Radical Biol. Med.*, 7, 45, 1989.

132. **Lesnefsky, E. J., Repine, J. E., and Horwitz, L. D.**, Deferoxamine pretreatment reduces canine infarct size and oxidative injury, *J. Pharmacol. Exp. Therap.*, 253, 1103, 1990.

133. **Lesnefsky, E. J., Hedlund, B. E., Hallaway, P. E., and Horwitz, L. D.**, High-dose iron-chelator therapy during reperfusion with deferoxamine-hydroxyethyl starch conjugate fails to reduce canine infarct size, *J. Cardiovasc. Pharmacol.*, 16, 523, 1990.

134. **Kobayashi, S., Tadokoro, H., Yasushi, W., et al.**, Coronary venous retroinfusion of deferoxamine reduces infarct size in pigs, *J. Am. Coll. Cardiol.*, 18, 621, 1991.

135. **Bolli, R., Patel, B. S., Zhu, W. Y., et al.**, The iron chelator deferoxamine attenuates post-ischemic dysfunction, *Am. J. Physiol.*, 253, H1372, 1987.

506

136. **Farber, N. E., Vercellotti, G. M., Jacob, H. S., et al.,** Evidence for a role of iron-catalyzed oxidants in functional and metabolic stunning in the canine heart, *Circ. Res.,* 63, 351, 1988.

137. **Devi, P. U.,** Chemical radiation protection by alpha-mercaptopropionylglycine, *J. Nucl. Med. Allied Sci.,* 27, 327, 1983.

138. **Bolli, R., Patel, B. S., Jeroudi, M. O., et al.,** Iron mediated radical reactions upon reperfusion contribute to myocardial "stunning", *Am. J. Physiol.,* 259, H1901, 1990.

139. **Rice-Evans, C., Baysal, E., Singh, S., et al.,** The interactions of desferrioxamine and hydroxypyridone compounds with haemoglobin and erythrocytes, *FEBS Lett.,* 256, 17, 1989.

140. **Lloyd, J. B., Cable, H., and Rice-Evans, C.,** Evidence that desferrioxamine cannot enter cells by passive diffusion, *Biochem. Pharmacol.,* 41, 1361, 1991.

141. **Maruyama, M., Pieper, G. M., Kalyanaraman, B., et al.,** Effects of hydroxyethyl starch conjugated deferoxamine on myocardial functional recovery following coronary occlusion and reperfusion in dogs, *J. Cardiovasc. Pharmacol.,* 17, 166, 1991.

142. **Menasché, P., Pasquier, C., Bellucci, S., et al.,** Deferoxamine reduces neutrophil-mediated free radical production during cardiopulmonary bypass in man, *J. Thorac. Cardiovasc. Surg.,* 96, 582, 1988.

143. **Menasché, P., Grousset, C., Mouas, C., and Piwnica, A.,** A promising approach for improving the recovery of heart transplants. Prevention of free radical injury through iron chelation by deferoxamine, *J. Thorac. Cardiovasc. Surg.,* 100, 13, 1990.

144. **Babbs, C. F.,** Role of iron ions in the genesis of reperfusion injury following successful cardiopulmonary resuscitation: preliminary data and a biochemical hypothesis, *Ann. Emerg. Med.,* 14, 777, 1985.

145. **Badylak, S. F. and Babbs, C. F.,** The effect of carbon dioxide, lidoflazine and deferoxamine upon long term survival following cardiopulmonary arrest in rats, *Resuscitation,* 13, 165, 1985.

146. **Aust, S. D. and White, B. C.,** Iron chelation prevents tissue injury following ischemia, *Adv. Free Radical Biol. Med.,* 1, 1, 1985.

147. **Patt, A., Horesh, I. R., Berger, E. M., et al.,** Iron depletion or chelation reduces ischemia/reperfusion-induced edema in gerbil brains, *J. Ped. Surg.,* 25, 224, 1990.

148. **Rosenthal, R. E., Chanderbhan, R., Granville, M., and Fiskum, G.,** Prevention of post-ischemic brain lipid conjugated diene production and neurological injury by hydroxyethyl starch-conjugated deferoxamine, *Free Radical Biol. Med.,* 12, 29, 1991.

149. **Natale, J. E., Schott, R. J., Hall, E. D., et al.,** Effect of the aminosteroid U74006F after cardiopulmonary arrest in dogs, *Stroke,* 19, 1371, 1988.

150. **Hall, E. D., Yonkers, P. A., McCall, J. M., and Braughler, J. M.,** Effects of the 21-aminosteroid U74006F on experimental head injury in mice, *J. Neurosurg.,* 68, 456, 1988.

151. **Anderson, D. K., Braughler, J. M., Hall, E. D., et al.,** Effects of treatment with U74006F on neurological outcome following experimental spinal cord injury, *J. Neurosurg.,* 69, 562, 1988.

152. **Hernandez, L. A., Grisham, M. B., and Granger, D. N.,** A role for iron in oxidant-mediated ischemic injury to intestinal microvasculature, *Am. J. Physiol.,* 253, G49, 1987.

153. **Haglund, U., Bulkley, G. B., and Granger, D. N.,** On the pathophysiology of intestinal ischemic injury, *Acta Chir. Scand.,* 153, 321, 1987.

154. **Park, P. O., Haglund, U., Bulkley, G. B., and Fält, K.,** The sequence of development of intestinal tissue injury after strangulation ischemia and reperfusion, *Surgery,* 107, 574, 1990.

155. **Itoh, M. and Guth, P. H.,** Role of oxygen-derived free radicals in hemorrhagic shock-induced gastric lesions in the rat, *Gastroenterology,* 88, 1162, 1985.

156. **Perry, M. A., Wadhwa, S., Parks, D. A., et al.,** Role of oxygen radicals in ischemia-induced lesions in the cat stomach, *Gastroenterology,* 90, 362, 1986.

157. **Smith, S. M., Grisham, M. B., Manci, E. A., et al.,** Gastric mucosal injury in the rat: role of iron and xanthine oxidase, *Gastroenterology,* 91, 950, 1987.

158. **Drugas, G. T., Paidas, C. N., Yahanda, A. M., et al.,** Conjugated deferoxamine attenuates hepatic microvascular injury following ischemia-reperfusion, *Circ. Shock,* 34, 278, 1991.

159. **Johnson, K. J. and Ward, P. A.,** Role of oxygen metabolites in immune complex injury of lung, *J. Immunol.,* 126, 2365, 1981.

160. **Till, G. and Ward, P. A.,** Oxygen radicals in complement and neutrophil-mediated acute lung injury, *J. Free Radical. Biol. Med.,* 1, 163, 1985.

161. **Kennedy, T. P., Rao, N. V., Noah, W., et al.,** Ibuprofen prevents oxidant lung injury and *in vitro* lipid peroxidation by chelating iron, *J. Clin. Invest.,* 86, 1565, 1990.

162. **Paller, M. S.,** Hemoglobin- and myoglobin-induced acute renal failure in rats: role of iron in nephrotoxicity, *Am. J. Physiol.,* 255, F539, 1988.

163. **Fuller, B. J., Lunec, J., Healing, G., et al.,** Reduction of susceptibility to lipid peroxidation in rabbit kidneys subjected to 24-hour cold ischemia and reperfusion, *Transplantation,* 43, 604, 1987.

164. **Healing, G., Gower, J., Fuller, B., and Green, C.,** Intracellular iron redistribution. An important determinant of reperfusion damage to rabbit kidneys, *Biochem. Pharmacol.,* 39, 1239, 1990.

165. **Sanan, S., Sharma, G., Malhotra, R., et al.,** Protection by desferrioxamine against histopathological changes of the liver in the post-oligaemic phase of clinical hemorrhagic shock in dogs: correlation with improved survival rate and recovery, *Free Radical Res. Commun.,* 6, 29, 1989.

166. **Jacobs, D. M., Julsrud, J. M., and Bubrick, M. P.,** Iron chelation with a deferoxamine conjugate in hemorrhagic shock, *J. Surg. Res.,* 51, 484, 1991.

167. **Hall, E. D., Yonkers, P. A., and McCall, J. M.,** Attenuation of hemorrhagic shock by the nongluccorticoid 21-aminosteroid U74006F, *Eur. J. Pharmacol.,* 147, 299, 1988.

168. **Jin, L. J., LaLonde, C., and Demling, R. H.,** Lung dysfunction after thermal injury in relation to prostanoid and oxygen radical release, *J. Appl. Physiol.,* 61, 103, 1986.

169. **Oldham, K., Guice, K., Till, G., et al.,** Activation of complement by hydroxyl radical in thermal injury, *Surgery,* 104, 272, 1988.

170. **Demling, R. H. and LaLonde, C.,** Early postburn lipid peroxidation: effect of ibuprofen and allopurinol, *Surgery,* 107, 85, 1990.

171. **Ward, P. A. and Till, G. O.,** Pathophysiologic events related to thermal injury of skin, *J. Trauma,* 30, S75, 1990.

172. **Demling, R. H., LaLonde, C., Knox, J., et al.,** Fluid resuscitation with deferoxamine prevents systemic burn induced oxidant injury, *J. Trauma,* 31, 538, 1991.

173. **Muirden, K. D.,** Ferritin in synovial cells in patients with rheumatoid arthritis, *Ann. Rheum. Dis.,* 25, 387, 1966.

174. **Senator, G. B. and Muirden, K. D.,** Concentration of iron in synovial membrane, synovial fluid and serum in rheumatoid arthritis and other joint diseases, *Ann. Rheum. Dis.,* 27, 49, 1968.

175. **Polson, R. J., Jawad, A. S. M., Bomford, A., et al.,** Treatment of rheumatoid arthritis with desferrioxamine, *Q. J. Med.,* 61, 1153, 1986.

176. **Amor, B., Mery, C., and De Gery, A.,** Tiopronin (*N*-[2-mercaptopropionyl] glycine) in rheumatoid arthritis, *Arthritis Rheum.,* 25, 698, 1982.

177. **Cuperus, R. A., Muijsers, A. O., and Wever, R.,** Antiarthritic drugs containing thiol groups scavenge hypochlorite and inhibit its formation by myeloperoxidase from human leukocytes, *Arthritis Rheum.,* 28, 1228, 1985.

178. **Hewitt, S. D., Hider, R. C., Sarpong, P., et al.,** Investigation of the anti-inflammatory properties of hydroxypyridones, *Ann. Rheum. Dis.,* 48, 382, 1989.

179. **Bus, J. S., Aust, S. D., and Gibson, J. E.,** Paraquat toxicity: proposed mechanism of action involving lipid peroxidation, *Environ. Health Prospect.,* 16, 139, 1976.

508

180. **Osheroff, M. R., Schaich, K. M., Drew, R. T., and Borg, D. C.,** Failure of desferrioxamine to modify the toxicity of paraquat in rats, *Free Radical Biol. Med.,* 1, 71, 1985.

181. **Korbashi, P., Katzhendler, J., Saltman, P., and Chevion, M.,** Zinc protects *Escherichia coli* against copper-mediated paraquat-induced damage, *J. BIol. Chem.,* 264, 8479, 1989.

182. **Perkins, W. E., Schroeder, R. L., Carrano, R. A., and Imondi, A. R.,** Effect of ICRF-187 on doxorubicin-induced myocardial effects in the mouse and guinea pig, *Br. J. Cancer,* 46, 662, 1982.

183. **Herman, E. H., Ferrans, V. J., Jordan, W., et al.,** Reduction of chronic daunorubicin cardiotoxicity by ICRF-187 in rabbits, *Res. Commun. Chem. Pathol. Pharmacol.,* 31, 85, 1981.

184. **Herman, E. H. and Ferrans, V. J.,** Influence of vitamin E and ICRF-187 on chronic doxorubicin cardiotoxicity in miniature swine, *Lab. Invest.,* 49, 69, 1983.

185. **Herman, E. H., El-Hage, A., and Ferrans, V. J.,** Reduction of chronic doxorubicin cardiotoxicity in dogs by pretreatment with (+ / −)1,2-bis(3,5-dioxopiperazinyl-1-yl)propane (ICRF-187), *Cancer Res.,* 41, 3436, 1988.

186. **Speyer, J. L., Green, M. D., Kramer, E., et al.,** Protective effect of the bispiperazinedione ICRF-187 against doxorubicin-induced cardiac toxicity in women with advanced breast cancer, *N. Engl. J. Med.,* 319, 745, 1988.

187. **Myers, C. E., Gianni, L., Simone, C. B., et al.,** Oxidative destruction of erythrocyte ghost membranes catalyzed by the doxorubicin-iron complex, *Biochemistry,* 21, 1707, 1982.

188. **Eliot, H., Gianni, L., and Myers, C. E.,** Oxidative destruction of DNA by the adriamycin-iron complex, *Biochemistry,* 23, 928, 1984.

189. **Gianni, L., Zweier, J., Levy, A., and Meyers, C. E.,** Characterization of the cycle of iron-mediated electron transfer from adriamycin to molecular oxygen, *J. Biol. Chem.,* 260, 6820, 1985.

190. **Rajagopalan, S., Politi, P. M., Sinha, B. K., and Myers, C. E.,** Adriamycin-induced free radical formation in the perfused rat heart: implications for cardiotoxicity, *Cancer Res.,* 4, 84766, 1988.

191. **Vile, G. F. and Winterbourn, C. C.,** Inhibition of adriamycin-promoted microsomal lipid peroxidation by α-carotene, α-tocopherol and retinol at high and low oxygen partial pressures, *FEBS Lett.,* 238, 353, 1988.

192. **Winterbourn, C. C., Vile, G. F., and Monteiro, H. P.,** Ferritin, lipid peroxidation and redox-cycling xenobiotics, *Free Radical Res. Comm.,* 2(13), 107, 1991.

193. **Hasinoff, B. B., Reinders, F. X., and Clark, V.,** The enzymatic hydrolysis-activation of the adriamycin cardioprotective agent (+)-1,2-bis(3,5-dioxopiperazinyl-1-yl)propane, *Drug. Metab. Disp.,* 19, 74, 1991.

194. **Hasinoff, B. B.,** The iron(III) and copper(II) complexes of adriamycin promote the hydrolysis of the cardioprotective agent ICRF-187 ((+)-1,2-bis(3,5-dioxopiperazinyl-1-yl)propane), *Agents Actions,* 29, 374, 1990.

195. **Dorr, R. T.,** Chemoprotectants for cancer chemotherapy, *Semin. Oncol.,* 18, 48, 1991.

Epilogue

Iron and Oxidative Balance

Joe M. McCord

Webb-Waring Lung Institute, University of Colorado Health Sciences Center, Denver, Colorado

I. INTRODUCTION

From the time it was first realized that iron is a necessary nutrient, essential for strong bodies and healthy blood, there was a natural tendency to assume that more must be better. Physicians and scientists were no more immune from this line of reasoning than the rest of society. Accordingly, for several decades we were bombarded with "iron-supplemented" this and "iron-fortified" that, possibly to our eventual detriment, as documented by many of the chapters in this book.

When it was realized that biological systems are capable of producing free radicals and other potent oxidants, the natural tendency of conventional wisdom was to view the oxidants as "bad" and the antioxidants as "good". Things are rarely that simple. Now, after two decades of contemplation and experimentation, there is a growing recognition that a balance between oxidants and antioxidants is a more realistic depiction of the relationship. There were many early clues, most of which were ignored or otherwise dismissed due to their circumstantial nature, or, more probably, due to the fact that they flew in the face of conventional wisdom. With the recognition that life must carefully juggle oxidants against antioxidants has come the recognition that iron, as the most common redox-active transition element present in biological systems, is an active participant in this precarious balancing act.

II. IRON AND FREE-RADICAL-MEDIATED INJURY

The discovery of superoxide dismutase[1] provided a highly specific probe for the implication of the superoxide free radical ($O_2^{\cdot -}$) in numerous biological processes. From the beginning, though, there were those who were disquieted by the rather robust nature of the damage which was apparently inflicted by this relatively mild-mannered radical. Soon, evidence suggested that the superoxide radical was not acting alone but was, in fact, collaborating with hydrogen peroxide (the product of its dismutation) to produce a species with much greater oxidizing potential than either of the co-conspirators.[2] This new species was presumed to be the hydroxyl radical ($OH^{\cdot}$), generated via a reaction first proposed in 1934 by Haber and Weiss.[3]

$$O_2^{\cdot -} + H_2O_2 \rightarrow O_2 + OH^- + OH^{\cdot} \tag{1}$$

This suggestion, too, left some uneasy. Weinstein and Bielski[4] reported the rate constant for this reaction to be so slow as to preclude biological relevance. Iron, however, was found to catalyze the reaction:[5,6]

$$O_2^{\cdot -} + Fe^{3+} \rightarrow O_2 + Fe^{2+} \tag{2}$$

$$Fe^{2+} + H_2O_2 \rightarrow Fe^{3+} + OH^- + OH^{\cdot} \tag{3}$$

$$O_2^{\cdot -} + H_2O_2 \rightarrow O_2 + OH^- + OH^{\cdot} \tag{1}$$

This combination of reactions is now commonly referred to as the iron-catalyzed Haber-Weiss reaction, or as superoxide-driven Fenton chemistry, as Reaction 3 had been proposed much earlier by Fenton.[7] It would seem proper as well to refer to it simply as Haber-Weiss chemistry, since these authors postulated all three reactions.[3]

The question of mechanism does not end there. While nearly everyone agrees that the interaction of superoxide, iron, and hydrogen peroxide generates a potent oxidant, not everyone agrees that the species is the hydroxyl radical. In some systems, the reactivity of the oxidant differs from that of the radiolytically generated hydroxyl radical.[8,9] Koppenol[8] has suggested that Reaction 3 might be written alternatively as follows:

$$Fe^{2+} + H_2O_2 \rightarrow FeO^{2+} + H_2O \tag{4}$$

The ferryl ion (FeO^{+2}) has oxidant properties similar to but somewhat less potent than the hydroxyl radical.

From a physiological or clinical perspective, the important point to appreciate is that iron may seriously exacerbate any oxidative stress. It is interesting to note that higher organisms are particularly careful about how iron is handled. There is little "free" or loosely chelated iron in the healthy state. It is transported in the ferric state, bound to transferrin, in a complex that is especially difficult to reduce. Likewise, it is stored in the ferric state by ferritin, a protein found in virtually all tissues and in plasma. Importantly, the superoxide radical is capable of reducing ferritin-bound iron to the ferrous state, whereupon it is released.[10,11] It is this iron, liberated by the pathological production of superoxide, that is now free to catalyze Haber-Weiss chemistry and to wreak additional cellular havoc.

III. THE CONCEPT OF OXIDANT/ANTIOXIDANT BALANCE

Very early in the history of superoxide dismutase (SOD) it was recognized that the protein might be therapeutic in certain pathological situations,[12] again bolstering the concept that "more is better". Yet, if this were the case, why was the activity distributed within such narrow limits? If more were truly better, surely some organism would have discovered the advantage of boosting its SOD production to preempt the pathology; however, this has not occurred. SOD is distributed with remarkable constancy of activity across virtually all aerobic organisms.[13]

In 1973 it was discovered that activated phagocytes put radical production to a constructive use: the killing of bacteria.[14] That might explain the advantage of having relatively little SOD in the extracellular fluids, where phagocytes roam.

The human condition known as Down's syndrome, or trisomy 21, has provided some provocative clues regarding the concept of balance between oxidants and antioxidants. The human cytosolic Cu/Zn SOD gene is located on chromosome 21,[15] and persons with trisomy 21 exhibit a gene-dosage effect;[16] i.e., their cells contain 50% more than the normal amount of Cu/Zn SOD due to the presence of a third copy of the gene. Their platelets, however, contain one third less Mn SOD.[17] This suggests a regulatory mechanism which attempts to control SOD concentration within the cell or, conversely, to regulate the superoxide concentration at low, but nonzero value. Down's syndrome patients display numerous metabolic and physiological aberrations, including an abnormal neuromuscular junction in the tongue,[18] increased lipid peroxidation in brain homogenates,[19] and decreased uptake of serotonin by platelets.[20] Because of the many genes present on the extra chromosome, there was no reason to attribute any of these abnormalities to the extra SOD until recently. The development of animal and cultured cell models which allow examination of specific gene-dosage effects has shed new light on the subject.

With the advent of molecular biology, it has become possible to manipulate levels of gene expression. Bacteria can be induced to produce huge quantities of recombinant SOD, accounting for >10% of their total cellular protein.[21] Cultured mammalian cells[22] and even intact transgenic rodents[23] can be induced to produce several times the normal amount of SOD. These overproducing cells are not the "supercells" some expected they would be; instead, they exhibit some interesting and unexpected deficits and frailties. In so doing, they have provided new understanding of the pathological mechanisms of Down's syndrome and suggest that some of the symptoms of the syndrome are, in fact, a reflection of the gene dosage of SOD per se. The tendency for lipid peroxidation seen in tissues from Down's syndrome[19] is also seen in transfected human HeLa cells and mouse L cells which overexpress the Cu/Zn SOD by about sixfold.[22] The diminished serotonin uptake by platelets seen in Down's syndrome is also seen in platelets from transgenic mice with increased Cu/Zn SOD activity.[20] Finally, and most amazingly, the abnormal neuromuscular junction seen in the tongue in Down's syndrome is reproduced in mice transgenic for the human Cu/Zn SOD.[24] These observations make a strong case for the importance of the concept of balance between oxidants and antioxidants.

The mechanism whereby too much SOD may become toxic to cells is not at all clear. At least one superoxide-utilizing enzyme, indoleamine-2,3-dioxygenase, has been described.[25] This enzyme, and possibly others like it, is in competition with SOD for the available superoxide. Interestingly, the indoleamine-2,3-dioxygenase degrades serotonin, a neurotransmitter, and dimethyltryptamine, a normal metabolite which is hallucinogenic. Michelson and co-workers surveyed a large variety of populations (old, young, rural, urban, sick, healthy, etc.), finding significantly higher levels of erythrocyte SOD in a population of mentally ill adult patients[26] and among infants with developmental psychoses.[27]

Some believe that more SOD results in more formation of H_2O_2, the product of the dismutation. This can be true only under special conditions, namely, if much of the intracellular superoxide were serving to reduce another species:

$$O_2^{\cdot-} + X \rightarrow O_2 + X^{\cdot-} \tag{5}$$

Excess SOD would, in this case, force half the $O_2^{\cdot-}$ into H_2O_2 production. However, if nearly all the superoxide were undergoing spontaneous dismutation, excess SOD would serve only to lower the steady-state concentration of $O_2^{\cdot-}$, but would have no effect on the rate of H_2O_2 formation.[1] If, on the other hand, much of the intracellular superoxide were serving to oxidize another species:

$$O_2^{\cdot-} + HX + H^+ \rightarrow H_2O_2 + X^{\cdot} \tag{6}$$

then excess SOD would force half the $O_2^{\cdot-}$ into O_2 production, decreasing the rate of H_2O_2 production. Hence, in the absence of data showing that the first condition holds, the argument that excess SOD causes increased cellular production of H_2O_2 is not a convincing one.

We have recently suggested a mechanism whereby the low concentrations of superoxide (or its conjugate acid, the hydroperoxyl radical, $HO_2^{\cdot}$) produced by normal metabolism and buffered by normal concentrations of SOD may serve a useful role to the cell by scavenging the lipid peroxyl radicals ($LOO^{\cdot}$) which propagate lipid peroxidation.[28] The only way a radical may be eliminated, after all, is by an annihilation reaction with another radical. The superoxide radical is constantly supplied by normal metabolism and is, as radicals go, a mild-mannered and relatively nonreactive free radical. These qualities would seem to make it an ideal candidate for use in the annihilation of other more noxious radicals. In this scheme $R^{\cdot}$ represents any free radical capable of abstracting a hydrogen atom from an unsaturated lipid, LH, to initiate lipid peroxidation:

$$OH^{\cdot} + LH \rightarrow H_2O + L^{\cdot} \qquad \text{Initiation} \tag{7}$$

$$\begin{aligned} L^{\cdot} + O_2 &\rightarrow LOO^{\cdot} \\ LOO^{\cdot} + LH &\rightarrow LOOH + L^{\cdot} \end{aligned} \qquad \text{Propagation} \tag{8}$$

$$LOO^{\cdot} + HO_2^{\cdot} \rightarrow LOOH + O_2 \qquad \text{Termination} \tag{9}$$

Alternatively, if the lipid peroxidation is iron dependent, ferrous iron may cause the reductive lysis of the oxygen-oxygen bond in a preexisting lipid hydroperoxide molecule, giving rise to a lipid alkoxyl radical (LO·) which may then serve as an initiating radical in the previous scheme. If this lipid alkoxyl radical were scavenged by O_2^-, then an entire chain of reactions would be prevented:

$$Fe^{2+} + LOOH \rightarrow Fe^{3+} + LO· + OH^- \qquad \text{Preinitiation} \qquad (10)$$

$$LO· + HO_2^- \rightarrow LOH + O_2 \qquad \text{Termination} \qquad (11)$$

Therefore, overscavenging of superoxide by increased amounts of SOD would eliminate important termination steps of lipid peroxidation, thereby amplifying cellular damage.

In support of this hypothesis, Thom and Elbuken[29] recently reported that increasing oxygen concentrations (and the resulting increases in superoxide production) slow the propagation of lipid peroxidation initiated by xanthine oxidase/hypoxanthine, while having no effect on the efficiency of initiation. They, too, proposed termination reactions between hydroperoxyl radical and lipid peroxyl or alkoxyl radicals, although they speculate that the products may be oxidized to carbonyl compounds rather than the alcohols or hydroperoxides we proposed earlier in this chapter.

IV. THERAPEUTIC IMPLICATIONS

A few chelating agents are known, notably desferrioxamine (deferoxamine or Desferal®) and diethylenetriamine pentaacetic acid (DTPA or DETAPAC), which are capable of binding ferric iron extremely tightly, and with such a shift in redox potential that the iron is not easily reduced.[30] Like superoxide dismutase, desferrioxamine has become a useful probe for detection of the involvement of iron in any circumstance producing biological injury.

Williams et al.[31] found that desferrioxamine treatment significantly improves functional and metabolic recovery of isolated perfused rabbit hearts subjected to 30 min of global ischemia. Studies by Reddy et al.[32] and Lesnefsky et al.[33] found a significant decrease in infarct size in animals pretreated with the drug. Yet another study by Maxwell et al.[34] using an in vivo rabbit model failed to find any effect on infarct size, even with preischemic administration. Thus, as with virtually all interventions aimed at reducing myocardial reperfusion injury, this one is also controversial.

In 1985, Babbs[35] reported that desferrioxamine treatment doubled the probability of survival (from 31 to 62%) of rats subjected to 6 to 10 min of total circulatory arrest, followed by resuscitation. Myers et al.[36] found desferrioxamine protective in the isolated rabbit heart subjected to hypoxia and reoxygenation as evidenced by decreased release of creatine kinase. Subsequent studies in isolated perfused rat hearts confirmed suppression of postischemic creatine kinase release[37] and of reperfusion-induced arrhythmias.[38] Bolli et al.[39] found substantially improved recovery from myocardial "stunning" in desferrioxamine-treated open-chest dogs, as did Farber et al.[40] Desferrioxamine improved postischemic recovery of high-energy phosphate content as measured by ^{31}P nuclear magnetic resonance spectroscopy.[41]

The potential use of desferrioxamine to improve recovery of transplanted organs has not escaped notice. A recent study by Menasché et al.[42] found that the addition of the drug to cardioplegic solution improved postreperfusion ventricular pressure development, maximal rate of rise of ventricular pressure, left ventricular compliance, and coronary flow. Green et al.[43] found that desferrioxamine reduced the susceptibility to lipid peroxidation in cold ischemic rabbit kidneys. Liver subjected to warm ischemia and reperfusion *in vivo* is protected substantially from lipid peroxidation and by histopathological evidence if desferrioxamine is administered at any point prior to reperfusion.[44]

If "liberated" iron can seriously exacerbate the component of reperfusion injury due to free radical production, the question arises as to whether iron status from a nutritional standpoint might be a predisposing factor in ischemic heart disease (see Chapter 11). A study by van der Kraaij et al.[45] has addressed the question by comparing hearts from normal vs. iron-supplemented rats. Langendorff hearts were subjected to 45 min of anoxic perfusion, followed by reoxygenation. Under normoxia, the groups behaved identically. Following a period of anoxia, however, the iron-loaded hearts displayed ventricular fibrillation and significantly lower recovery of contractility, both of which were returned to control values by perfusion with desferrioxamine.

V. CONCLUSION

In controlled moderation, both free-radical formation and ingestion of iron appear to be biological necessities. In excess, both may contribute to serious damage. Furthermore, they are interactive: superoxide is capable of releasing iron and reducing free iron to the more reactive ferrous state; ferrous iron is capable of reducing hydroperoxides, giving rise to alkoxyl or hydroxyl free radicals. Recognition of the interactions between free-radical metabolism and iron metabolism seems crucial to the development of effective therapeutic interventions.

516

REFERENCES

1. **McCord, J. M. and Fridovich, I.**, Superoxide dismutase: an enzymic function for erythrocuprein (hemocuprein), *J. Biol. Chem.*, 244, 6049, 1969.
2. **Beauchamp, C. and Fridovich, I.**, A mechanism for the production of ethylene from methional. The generation of the hydroxyl radical by xanthine oxidase, *J. Biol. Chem.*, 245, 4641, 1970.
3. **Haber, F. and Weiss, J.**, The catalytic decomposition of hydrogen peroxide by iron salts, *Proc. R. Soc. Ser. A*, 147, 332, 1934.
4. **Weinstein, J. and Bielski, B. H. J.**, Kinetics of the interaction of HO_2 and O_2^- radicals with hydrogen peroxide. The Haber-Weiss reaction, *J. Am. Chem. Soc.*, 101, 58, 1979.
5. **McCord, J. M. and Day, E. D., Jr.**, Superoxide-dependent production of hydroxyl radical catalyzed by iron-EDTA complex, *FEBS Lett.*, 86, 139, 1978.
6. **Halliwell, B.**, Superoxide-dependent formation of hydroxyl radicals in the presence of iron chelates, *FEBS Lett.*, 92, 321, 1978.
7. **Fenton, H. J. H.**, Oxidation of tartaric acid in the presence of iron, *J. Chem. Soc.*, 65, 899, 1894.
8. **Koppenol, W. H.**, The reaction of ferrous EDTA with hydrogen peroxide: evidence against hydroxyl radical formation, *J. Free Radical Biol. Med.*, 1, 281, 1985.
9. **Winterbourn, C. C. and Sutton, H. C.**, Iron and xanthine oxidase catalyze formation of an oxidant species distinguishable from OH˙: comparison with the Haber-Weiss reaction, *Arch. Biochem. Biophys.*, 244, 27, 1986.
10. **Biemond, P., van Eijk, H. G., Swaak, A. J. G., and Koster, J. F.**, Iron mobilization from ferritin by superoxide derived from stimulated polymorphonuclear leukocytes. Possible mechanism in inflammation diseases, *J. Clin. Invest.*, 73, 1576, 1984.
11. **Biemond, P., Swaak, A. J., Biendorff, C. M., and Koster, J. F.**, Superoxide-dependent and -independent mechanisms of iron mobilization from ferritin by xanthine oxidase. Implications for oxygen free-radical-induced tissue destruction during ischaemia and inflammation, *Biochem. J.*, 239, 169, 1986.
12. **Huber, W., Schulte, T. L., Carson, S., Goldhamer, R. E., and Vogin, E. E.**, Some chemical and pharmacologic properties of a novel anti-inflammatory protein, *Toxicol. Appl. Pharmacol.*, 12, 308, 1968.
13. **McCord, J. M., Keele, B. B., Jr., and Fridovich, I.**, An enzyme-based theory of obligate anaerobiosis: the physiological function of superoxide dismutase, *Proc. Natl. Acad. Sci. U.S.A.*, 68, 1024, 1971.
14. **Babior, B. M., Kipnes, R. S., and Curnutte, J. T.**, Biological defense mechanisms. The production by leukocytes of superoxide, a potential bactericidal agent, *J. Clin. Invest.*, 52, 741, 1973.
15. **Tan, Y. H., Tischfield, J., and Ruddle, F. H.**, The linkage of genes for the human interferon induced anti-viral protein and indophenol oxidase-B traits to chromosome G-21, *J. Exp. Med.*, 137, 317, 1973.
16. **Sinet, P. M., Allard, D., Lejeune, J., and Jerome, H.**, Augmentation d'activite de la superoxyde dismutase erythrocytaire dans la trisomie pour le chromosome 21, *C. R. Acad. Sci. Paris*, 278, 3267, 1974.
17. **Sinet, P. M., Lavelle, F., Michelson, A. M., and Jerome, H.**, Superoxide dismutase activities of blood platelets in trisomy 21, *Biochem. Biophys. Res. Commun.*, 67, 904, 1975.
18. **Yarom, R., Sherman, Y., Sagher, U., Peled, I. J., and Wexler, M. R.**, Elevated concentrations of elements and abnormalities of neuromuscular junctions in tongue muscles of Down's syndrome, *J. Neurol. Sci.*, 79, 315, 1987.
19. **Brooksbank, B. and Balazs, R.**, Superoxide dismutase, glutathione peroxidase, and lipoperoxidation in Down's syndrome fetal brain, *Dev. Brain Res.*, 16, 37, 1984.

20. **Schickler, M., Knobler, H., Avraham, K. B., Elroy-Stein, O., and Groner, Y.,** Diminished serotonin uptake in platelets of transgenic mice with increased Cu/Zn-superoxide dismutase activity, *EMBO J.,* 8, 1385, 1989.

21. **Hartman, J. R., Geller, T., Yavin, Z., et al.,** High-level expression of enzymatically active human Cu/Zn superoxide dismutase in *Escherichia coli, Proc. Natl. Acad. Sci. U.S.A.,* 83, 7142, 1986.

22. **Elroy-Stein, O., Bernstein, Y., and Groner, Y.,** Overproduction of human Cu/Zn-superoxide dismutase in transfected cells: extenuation of paraquat-mediated cytotoxicity and enhancement of lipid peroxidation, *EMBO J.,* 5, 615, 1986.

23. **Epstein, C. J., Avraham, K. B., Lovett, M., et al.,** Transgenic mice with increased Cu/Zn-super-oxide dismutase activity: animal model of dosage effects in Down syndrome, *Proc. Natl. Acad. Sci. U.S.A.,* 84, 8044, 1987.

24. **Avraham, K. B., Schickler, M., Sapoznikov, D., Yarom, R., and Groner, Y.,** Down's syndrome: abnormal neuromuscular junction in tongue of transgenic mice with elevated levels of human Cu/Zn-superoxide dismutase, *Cell,* 54, 823, 1988.

25. **Taniguchi, T., Hirata, F., and Hayaishi, O.,** Intracellular utilization of superoxide by indoleamine 2,3-dioxygenase of rabbit enterocytes, *J. Biol. Chem.,* 252, 2774, 1977.

26. **Michelson, A. M., Puget, K., Durosay, P., and Bonneau, J. C.,** Clinical aspects of the dosage of erythrocuprein, in *Superoxide and Superoxide Dismutases,* Michelson, A. M., McCord, J. M., and Fridovich, I., Eds., Academic Press, London, 1977, 487.

27. **Glos, B., Debray-Ritzen, P., Puget, K., and Michelson, A. M.,** Dosage de la superoxyde dismutase 1 plaquettaire dans les pyschoses infantile de développment, *Nouv. Presse Med.,* 6, 2449, 1977.

28. **Omar, B. A., Gad, N. M., Jordan, M. C., et al.,** Cardioprotection by Cu,Zn-superoxide dismutase is lost at high doses in the reoxygenated heart, *Free Radical Biol. Med.,* 9, 465, 1990.

29. **Thom, S. R. and Elbuken, M. E.,** Oxygen-dependent antagonism of lipid peroxidation, *Free Radical Biol. Med.,* 10, 413, 1991.

30. **Gutteridge, J. M. C., Richmond, R., and Halliwell, B.,** Inhibition of the iron-catalysed formation of hydroxyl radicals from superoxide and of lipid peroxidation by desferrioxamine, *Biochem. J.,* 184, 469, 1979.

31. **Williams, R. E., Zweier, J. L., and Flaherty, J. T.,** Treatment with deferoxamine during ischemia improves functional and metabolic recovery and reduces reperfusion-induced oxygen radical generation in rabbit hearts, *Circulation,* 83, 1006, 1991.

32. **Reddy, B. R., Kloner, R. A., and Przyklenk, K.,** Early treatment with deferoxamine limits myocardial ischemic/reperfusion injury, *Free Radical. Biol. Med.,* 7, 45, 1989.

33. **Lesnefsky, E. J., Repine, J. E., and Horwitz, L. D.,** Deferoxamine pretreatment reduces canine infarct size and oxidative injury, *J. Pharmacol. Exp. Ther.,* 253, 1103, 1990.

34. **Maxwell, M. P., Hearse, D. J., and Yellon, D. M.,** Inability of desferrioxamine to limit tissue injury in the ischaemic and reperfused rabbit heart, *J. Cardiovasc. Pharmacol.,* 13, 608, 1989.

35. **Babbs, C. F.,** Role of iron ions in the genesis of reperfusion injury following successful cardiopulmonary resuscitation: preliminary data and a biochemical hypothesis, *Ann. Emerg. Med.,* 14, 777, 1985.

36. **Myers, C. L., Weiss, S. J., Kirsh, M. M., and Shlafer, M.,** Involvement of hydrogen peroxide and hydroxyl radical in the 'oxygen paradox': reduction of creatine kinase release by catalase, allopurinol or deferoxamine, but not by superoxide dismutase, *J. Mol. Cell. Cardiol.,* 17, 675, 1985.

37. **Badylak, S. F., Simmons, A., Turek, J., and Babbs, C. F.,** Protection from reperfusion injury in the isolated rat heart by postischaemic deferoxamine and oxypurinol administration, *Cardiovasc. Res.,* 21, 500, 1987.

518

38. **Bernier, M., Hearse, D. J., and Manning, A. S.,** Reperfusion-induced arrhythmias and oxygen-derived free radicals. Studies with "anti-free radical" interventions and a free radical-generating system in the isolated perfused rat heart, *Circ. Res.,* 58, 331, 1986.

39. **Bolli, R., Patel, B. S., Zhu, W.-X., et al.,** The iron chelator desferrioxamine attenuates postischemic ventricular dysfunction, *Am. J. Physiol.,* 253, H1372, 1987.

40. **Farber, N. E., Vercellotti, G. M., Jacob, H. S., Pieper, G. M., and Gross, G. J.,** Evidence for a role of iron-catalyzed oxidants in functional and metabolic stunning in the canine heart, *Circ. Res.,* 63, 351, 1988.

41. **Bernard, M., Menasche, P., Pietri, S., Grousset, C., Piwnica, A., and Cozzone, P. J.,** Cardioplegic arrest superimposed on evolving myocardial ischemia: improved recovery after inhibition of hydroxyl radical generation by peroxidase or deferoxamine. A ^{31}P nuclear resonance study, *Circulation,* 78(Suppl. 5), III164, 1988.

42. **Menasché, P., Grousset, C., Mouas, C., and Piwnica, A.,** A promising approach for improving the recovery of heart transplants: prevention of free radical injury through iron chelation by deferoxamine, *J. Thorac. Cardiovasc. Surg.,* 100, 13, 1990.

43. **Green, C. J., Healing, G., Simpkin, S., Fuller, B. J., and Lunec, J.,** Reduced susceptibility to lipid peroxidation in cold ischemic rabbit kidneys after addition of desferrioxamine, mannitol, or uric acid to the flush solution, *Cryobiology,* 23, 358, 1986.

44. **Omar, R., Nomikos, I., Piccorelli, G., Savino, J., and Agarwal, N.,** Prevention of post-ischaemic lipid peroxidation and liver cell injury by iron chelation, *Gut,* 30, 510, 1989.

45. **Van der Kraaij, A. M. M., Mostert, L. J., van Eijk, H. G., and Koster, J. F.,** Iron-clad increases the susceptibility of rat hearts to oxygen reperfusion damage: protection by the antioxidant (+)-cyanidanol-3 and deferoxamine, *Circulation,* 78, 442, 1988.

Index

INDEX